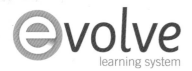
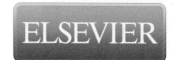
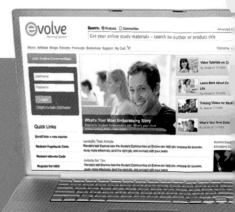

LAVIN'S

Radiography for Veterinary Technicians

Radiography for Veterinary Technicians

Fifth Edition

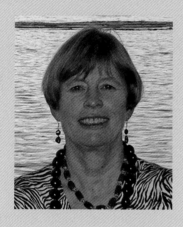

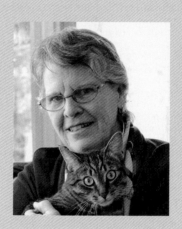

Marg Brown, RVT, BEd Ad Ed

Penn Foster College
Scranton, Pennsylvania
Formerly of Seneca College of Applied Arts and Technology
King City, Ontario
Active Member
Ontario Association
of Veterinary Technicians and Association
of Veterinary Technician Educators

Lois C. Brown, MRT(R), ACR, MSc

Member Canadian Association of Physicists
President
Xray Imaging Consultants Ltd.
Tottenham, Ontario

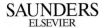

SAUNDERS
ELSEVIER

3251 Riverport Lane
St. Louis, Missouri 63043

LAVIN'S RADIOGRAPHY FOR VETERINARY TECHNICIANS, FIFTH EDITION   ISBN: 978-1-4557-2280-8

Notices

Knowledge and best practice in this field are constantly changing. As new research and experience broaden our understanding, changes in research methods, professional practices, or medical treatment may become necessary.

Practitioners and researchers must always rely on their own experience and knowledge in evaluating and using any information, methods, compounds, or experiments described herein. In using such information or methods they should be mindful of their own safety and the safety of others, including parties for whom they have a professional responsibility.

With respect to any drug or pharmaceutical products identified, readers are advised to check the most current information provided (i) on procedures featured or (ii) by the manufacturer of each product to be administered, to verify the recommended dose or formula, the method and duration of administration, and contraindications. It is the responsibility of practitioners, relying on their own experience and knowledge of their patients, to make diagnoses, to determine dosages and the best treatment for each individual patient, and to take all appropriate safety precautions.

To the fullest extent of the law, neither the Publisher nor the authors, contributors, or editors, assume any liability for any injury and/or damage to persons or property as a matter of products liability, negligence or otherwise, or from any use or operation of any methods, products, instructions, or ideas contained in the material herein.

Library of Congress Cataloging-in-Publication Data or Control Number
Brown, Marg, author.
  Lavin's radiography for veterinary technicians / Marg Brown, Lois C. Brown.—Fifth edition.
    p. ; cm.
  Radiography for veterinary technicians
  Revised edition of: Radiography in veterinary technology / Lisa M. Lavin. 4th ed. c2007.
  Includes bibliographical references and index.
  ISBN 978-1-4557-2280-8 (hardback : alk. paper)
  1. Veterinary radiography. 2. Animal health technicians. I. Brown, Lois C., author. II. Lavin, Lisa M. Radiography in veterinary technology. Revision of (work): III. Title. IV. Title: Radiography for veterinary technicians.
  [DNLM: 1. Radiography—veterinary. 2. Technology, Radiologic—veterinary. SF 757.8]
  SF757.8.L38 2014
  636.089607′572–dc23
                                                                                    2013004017

Vice President and Publisher: Linda Duncan
Content Strategy Director: Penny Rudolph
Content Manager: Shelly Stringer
Publishing Services Manager: Gayle May
Project Manager: Srikumar Narayanan
Designer: Amy Buxton

Printed in China

Last digit is the print number: 9 8 7 6 5 4 3 2

Working together to grow
libraries in developing countries

www.elsevier.com | www.bookaid.org | www.sabre.org

ELSEVIER   BOOK AID International   Sabre Foundation

Contributors

Shannon T. Brownrigg, RVT
Veterinary Technician/Veterinary Assistant Programs
Algonquin College
Ottawa, Ontario, Canada
Equine and Large Animal Radiography

Susan MacNeal, RVT, CVDT, BSc
Veterinary Technician Program
Georgian College
Orillia, Ontario, Canada
Dental Imaging
Dental Radiography

Stephanie Holowka, MRT(R), MRT (MR)
Lead Technologist MEG and 3-D Imaging
Department of Diagnostic Imaging
The Hospital for Sick Children
Toronto, Ontario, Canada
Computerized Tomography
Magnetic Resonance Imaging

Robert Hylands, DVM
Westbridge Veterinary Hospital
Mississauga, Ontario, Canada
Ultrasound

We are excited to present the latest totally modified edition of Lavin's Radiography for Veterinary Technicians. As with the previous text, it continues to focus on teaching the science of imaging used in veterinary and veterinary technology programs. The purpose of the book is to instill a working knowledge of radiologic science as it applies to producing a diagnostic quality image, to prepare radiography students in veterinary technology programs for the certification exam, to assist in the training of veterinary students and to provide a base from which practicing radiographers can make informed decisions about technical factors and diagnostic image quality in the workplace. This text is a mainstay for teaching radiographic anatomy and positioning of all species. It will be a valuable reference for technicians when they have finished their training as well as for veterinarians. The new edition of the Lavin text will provide a thorough, yet practical level of imaging and positioning coverage to equip individuals with the knowledge they need to produce high-quality images on the first attempt.

New Features

The textbook has been totally revamped with all new color photographs and consistent style of color line drawings along with tables and boxes. Each chapter begins with a list of key terms and learning objectives. Points to Ponder, Check it Out, Figure it Out, and Technician Notes have been added as a helpful study tool for students. Key, and other terms, have been defined in the comprehensive glossary that appears at the end of the text. Online enhancement further complements each chapter.

An exciting new feature includes dental radiography. Equipment types (film and digital) and radiation safety is covered in Part One. Positioning and reading the radiograph are covered in Part Two. This will be a particularly useful section for both general veterinary technicians and those who specialize in dentistry.

A major goal of this edition has been to ensure that each chapter is comprehensive so that important information is found in the text without the need to reference other sources. Part One puts theory into practice while each of the chapters in Part Two have been expanded to include not only essential positioning information, but also anatomic references to support the technician in understanding normal anatomic features so that the veterinarian receives accurate images for diagnosis.

Organization

This text is divided into two major parts:

Part One: Diagnostic Imaging

It is particularly pleasant to present to you the results of many research excursions into the ever evolving world of veterinary imaging. This edition presents the field of imaging in a completely new and current light.

With the advent of digital imaging and the Internet, the veterinary profession has embraced technology with enthusiasm. Even as this book was being written advances in technology were taking place and we were, at times, hard pressed to keep up.

Employment opportunities for veterinary technicians and technologists are also expanding into the fields of imaging that were unavailable in previous years. Knowledge of the many disciplines of x-ray imaging is vital to the veterinary technician of today.

There are 17 separate yet interrelated disciplines in the field of medical imaging. It will not be long before the world of veterinary imaging follows this example. The discipline of imaging is driven by the larger field of medical imaging and, from that, new protocols are developed for research into veterinary practice.

New Features

Part One presents the technical side of imaging as clearly and succinctly as possible with little emphasis on theory and greater emphasis on the practical application of the rules and laws which guide our daily lives.

Chapters 1 to 4 present the inner workings of the radiography unit from the source of electricity to the production of x-rays and how we use them. Images of rotating anodes and the principles of transformers, resistance, conductance, and rectification have been presented with actual case studies of possible problems and potential solutions.

Chapters 5 to 9 present a new look at the other side of imaging – the receptor. Film and intensifying screens are explained in a completely new way with the many variables and explanations of this part of imaging explained in detail. Films and screens are still with us in many facilities and the veterinary technician must be prepared to deal with any problems and artifacts that they present as they age.

Chapter 9 looks at the science of computerized radiography and digital imaging. Exciting and fascinating to be sure but 'Caveat Emptor' is the watch word and precedes this chapter.

Chapters 10 to 12 explore the worlds of related imaging technologies that are quickly being added to the diagnostic checklist in the veterinary hospital. Dental imaging, computerized tomography, and fluoroscopy have been on the medical side for many years and now are invaluable to veterinarians.

Chapters 13 to 15 introduce the non–x-ray imaging modalities. Ultrasound, magnetic resonance imaging, and nuclear medicine employ variations of radiation and are common procedures for difficult diagnoses and with the advent of protocols and diagnostic units specifically designed for veterinary use. They are ideal modalities to confirm difficult pathologies, trauma, or rate of healing.

Chapter 16 presents the laws of radiation protection. The protection of the radiation worker and the nonradiation worker is vital. It is also important to supply the correct protection and to be able to assess whether the protection supplied is adequate and intact.

Part Two: Radiographic Positioning and Related Anatomy

This part is divided into the various positioning of small animals, namely small animal abdomen, thorax, forelimb, pelvis and hind limbs, spine and skull. In addition comprehensive chapters on small animal dental radiography, special procedures, large animal radiography, and avian and exotic radiography are included.

The major goal of this section is to ensure that information required for accurate positioning is included so that other texts do not need to be referenced, especially for the related anatomy that I expect our students to be familiar with. Routine, as well as optional views are included. The major emphasis has been on non-manual restraint techniques that improve safety and radiation protection for the radiographer. In practice, radiation safety is often compromised, as veterinary medicine is practically the only health science field in which the radiographer seems to feel the need to restrain the patient while the exposure is being made.

The descriptions in each chapter have been totally expanded. Each chapter includes an outline, learning objectives, key terms, where to measure, the location of the central ray, the borders to include, a step-by-step approach to positioning, further comments and tips to ensure that the perfect image is obtained, as well as a further description of the anatomy related to that part. Technician notes scattered throughout the chapters help stress important points.

The positioning views are accompanied by high quality color photographs, graphic color drawings that visibly indicate the anatomic features and radiographs. Anatomy is an important feature to ensure that proper images will be presented to the veterinarian and aid students in learning anatomy through the integrative application of radiography and anatomy.

The addition of the dental chapter, as well as the expansion of the special procedures, large animal, and avian and exotic sections that contain the previously described features, will definitely make this a one-source reference for radiography in these areas.

As with Part One, this component is essentially linked to the Evolve website. Identification of radiographic and anatomic images, questions, crossword puzzles, word games, and other learning tools for each chapter are on the site. Comprehensive PowerPoints are linked to each chapter. The images as presented in the book are included, as well as a full complement of support for teaching and learning.

Radiography is an exciting field in which the radiographer plays an important part in ensuring that accurate diagnosis is made. With the tools and information presented here, each image should be perfect.

Welcome to the completely revised 5th edition. We hope that you enjoy learning from it as much as we enjoyed writing it.

Acknowledgments

Many people and animals played an important role in this book, and on the evolve website. I have acknowledged some of the clinics and the individuals but there were many more who labored in the background supplying images and general information. Writing, illustrating, and editing a book like this is a monumental undertaking and it would not be possible without the kind encouragement of the veterinary community.

One group that stands out is the entire staff at Westbridge Veterinary Hospital. They were generous with their time and patience as we scanned films and had them pose for pictures; Cathy Buller, DVM, tested the chapters in her teaching modules.

I would also like to thank Arvind Singh H.N.D Mech (UK) at Raymax Medical Corp in Brampton, Ontario; Rikki Tikki Tavi (AKC) CDX, RE, OA, NAJ; (ASCA) CD. R.S.-N, J.S.-N; CPE #CTL1-R, Mascot and Champion (6 points), an Australian Shepherd from Ulster Park, New York. And a great many thanks to Deven Greves for bringing Rikki to the pages of this book as our mascot. His personality continues to shine on in the online sections of the book and his quadruped friends certainly make difficult topics a pleasure to understand.

Finally, my thanks to the animals who patiently posed for images and donated their radiographs to a worthy cause. Special thanks to my own cats, Microchip, Mr Chivers and, particularly, I Curious Tiberius who scanned every page and meowed his approval throughout the proofreading.

Our mascot did a wonderful job of guiding the exercises and creating a learning environment throughout the book. Thanks to Rikki Tikki Tavi and his owner and trainer Sally Gaston.

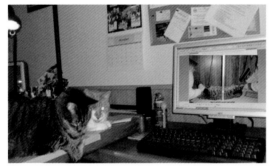

Microchip and Chivers editing

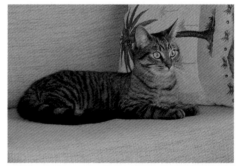

I Curious Tiberius on break

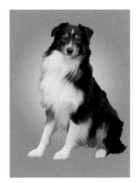

Rikki Tikki Tavi

Lois C. Brown

There are many people that I would like to acknowledge and thank in the production of this book. I appreciate all of your contributions and input, and hope I have not forgotten anyone.

I wish to recognize my former colleagues of the Veterinary Technology program at Seneca College in King City Ontario. You are a great team and have always been a wonderful support system. Since I have moved on, the support still continues, as does the willingness to help. Many thanks to Ace, Sam, and Spud for agreeing to be the models used for most of the positioning pictures in this portion. Of course thanks to their owners for allowing us to take copious photographs. I would like to thank my former and current students as well. Never have I worked a day in my life thanks to you and your enthusiasm, questions, and willingness to learn. You were a constant source of motivation and joy. I learned and continue to learn from all of you. Thank you for helping with this text.

Thanks also to Jennifer King, RVT, of Algonquin College, who helped edit the chapters and gave me great suggestions. To the contributors of the chapters as recognized above, especially Sue MacNeal, RVT, CVDT, BSc, as well as Shannon Brownrigg, RVT, Sue Carstairs, DVM, Evelyn Kelly, RN, MRT(R), ACR, BSc, and to MA. G.K. Smith, DVM and Mandy Wallace, DVM, a big thank you.

I wish to express my appreciation to those who contributed to our photo gallery. These include Katrina White, RVT, for taking many of the positioning photographs, Joshua Schlote, BS, LVT, Carolyn Bennett, AHT, Tara Wochesen, RVT, Seth Wallack, DVM, DACVR, and Vetel Diagnostics. Thanks to the Ontario Veterinary Group hospitals particularly Tara Sefton, RVT, Manager of OVG and Jennifer Baird, plus all of your other colleagues who contributed; Dana Greves, RVT and Jenn White, RVT and to Rick Axelson, DVM. A special thanks to all of you for your photographs and assistance. To those of you who helped edit the chapters and gave suggestions but wished to remain anonymous, a heartfelt thanks.

Of course huge credit is extended to the editing team at Elsevier, especially Teri Merchant and Shelly Stringer. Teri, your patience, sense of humor, encouragement and ever helpful ideas made the project a pleasure. You will be missed. Shelly, you are a real pleasure to work with and I look forward to further projects in the future. Thanks also to our Project Manager, Srikumar Narayanan. The lithography department of Elsevier, Deven Greves, and especially Jeanne Robertson (http://www.robertsonillustration.com), your images are awesome. Your contributions will greatly enhance the learning.

Lois, your perspective and enthusiasm were enlightening and I look forward to our new friendship.

Marg Brown

Abbreviation "e" indicates figures available in the online content.

Figure 2-2: From Ianucci JM and Howeton LJ: *Dental Radiography: Principles and Practice*, ed 4, St Louis, 2012, Elsevier.

Figures 2-3, 2-4, 2-5, 2-6, 3-2, 3-10, 4-8, 4-11, 4-24, 4-25, 4-26, 4-30, 4-31, 4-33, 4-35, 5-19, 9-5, 9-6, 12-2, Table 9-3: From Bushong SC: *Radiologic Science for Technologists*, ed 10, St Louis, 2013, Elsevier.

Chapter 4 chapter opener: Courtesy of U.S. National Aeronautics and Space Administration (NASA).

Figures 4-9, 4-10, 4-17, 4-19: Courtesy of Raymax Medical Corporation, Brampton, Ontario.

Figures 4-27, 4-34A, 5-7, 5-11, 7-2, 7-3, 7-4, 7-12, 7-15, 7-16, 7-17, 7-18, 9-7: From Fauber T: *Radiographic Imaging and Exposure*, ed 4, St Louis, 2013, Mosby.

Figure 4-28: Courtesy Philips Medical Systems. In Bushong SC: *Radiologic Science for Technologists*, ed 10, St Louis, 2013, Elsevier.

Figure 4-32: Courtesy GE Healthcare. In Bushong SC: *Radiologic Science for Technologists*, ed 10, St Louis, 2013, Elsevier.

Chapter 5 chapter opener: Courtesy of Animage-LLC, Fidex Imaging, Pleasanton, California.

Figure 5-20: From Wikipedia. http://en.wikipedia.org/wiki/Phosphorescence.

Figure 5-29: Courtesy of James Duhaime, St Clair Veterinary Facilities, Toronto.

Figure 5-30: From Fauber T: *Radiographic Imaging and Exposure*, ed 3, St Louis, 2008, Mosby.

Figure 5-33: Courtesy Carestream Health. In Bushong SC: *Radiologic Science for Technologists*, ed 10, St Louis, 2013, Elsevier.

Table 5-1: With assistance from Leo Reina, X-ray Cassette-Repair Company, dba Reina Imaging, Crystal Lake, Illinois.

Chapter 7 chapter opener: Courtesy of Westbridge Veterinary Hospital, Mississauga, Ontario.

Figure 9-2: Courtesy Fujifilm Medical Systems, USA, Inc., Stamford, Connecticut. In Fauber T: *Radiographic Imaging and Exposure*, ed 4, St Louis, Mosby, 2013.

Chapter 12 chapter opener: Fidex Veterinary CT, FL, DR Scanner, Courtesy Animage, LLC.

Unless otherwise noted, images are courtesy of the following: chapters 1 through 16: Lois Brown; artwork by Deven Greves; chapters 17 through 23, and 25 through 27: photographs and radiographs were taken at Seneca College of Applied Arts and Technology, King City, Ontario; chapter 24: Susan MacNeal, Georgian College, Orillia, Ontario; drawings for chapters 17 through 27: Jeanne Robertson.

Figures e13-1, e13-2, e13-3, e13-4, e13-5, e13-7, 13-1, 13-3, 13-4, 13-5, 13-6, 13-7, 13-9, 13-10, 13-13, 13-14, 13-16, 13-18, 13-19: Courtesy of R. F. Hylands DVM.

Figure 13-3: Ultrasound courtesy of R. F. Hylands, line drawing courtesy of B. Blevins.

Figure 14-3: Courtesy Magmedix, Inc., Ritchberg, Massachusetts.

Figures 17-1, 20-1, 26-1B: Modified from McBride DF: *Learning Veterinary Terminology*, ed 2, St Louis, 2002, Mosby. In Colville T and Bassert J: *Clinical Anatomy and Physiology for Veterinary Technicians*, St Louis, 2008, Elsevier.

Figures e8-2, 17-3, 20-5A, 21-13C, 23-12B, 25-14: From Lavin L: *Radiography in Veterinary Technology*, ed 4, St Louis, 2007, Saunders, Elsevier.

Figures 18-3A, 18-16, 18-17B-E, 19-29A, 22-2C, 22-7C, 26-1C, E, 26-11, 26-16C, 26-60B, C, 27-34B, 27-35C, 27-39A, 27-41A, Chapter 26 opener: Courtesy Vetel Diagnostics, San Luis Obispo, California, and Seth Wallack DVM, DACVR, AAVR Director and CEO of Veterinary Imaging Centre of San Diego.

Figures 18-3B, 18-16, 18-17, 20-17D, 21-8C, 21-18B, 25-18, 25-19A: Courtesy Rosedale Animal Hospital.

Figures 18-12, 18-13, 21-16A, 26-1F: From Dyce, SA: *Textbook of Veterinary Anatomy*, ed 4, St Louis, Saunders.

Figures 18-5A, 18-6B, 18-10A-D, 18-11A-D, e18-1A, 19-3, 19-5, 19-10, 19-14, 19-18A-D, 20-22C, 20-23C, 22-4C, 22-5C, 22-6C, 22-8C, 22-13C, 22-17C, 22-25: Courtesy Joshua Schlote, BS, LVT, Northeast Community College.

Figures 19-3, 19-4, 19-22, 22-2, 22-11, 22-12, 22-15, 22-16: From Evans H and de Lahunta A: *Guide to the Dissection of the Dog*, ed 7, St Louis, 2010, Saunders.

Figures 19-19, 19-21, 19-24, e27-1, e27-9, 27-14A, 27-15B: Colville T and Bassert J: *Clinical Anatomy and Physiology for Veterinary Technicians*, St Louis, 2008, Elsevier.

Figure 19-24: From Patton KT and Thibodeau GA: *Anatomy and Physiology*, ed 7, St Louis, 2010, Mosby.

Table 19-2: Modified from Morgan JP: *Techniques of Veterinary Radiography*. Ames, Iowa, 1993, Iowa State University Press, and Thrall DE: *Textbook of Veterinary Diagnostic Radiology*, ed 5, St Louis, 2007, Elsevier.

Figures Chapter 19 opener, 20-3B, 20-4C, 20-8C, 20-10C, 20-11C, 20-12D, 20-13C, 20-14C, 20-15D, 20-17C, 20-20C, 21-4C, 21-5C, 21-8C, 21-9C, 21-11C, 21-12D, 21-14C, 21-15C, 21-16D, 21-18C, 21-19C, 21-20B: Courtesy Dana Greves and Jenn White of Mississauga-Oakville Veterinary Emergency Hospital and Referral Group, Oakville, Ontario.

Contents

Diagnostic Imaging

CHAPTER

1

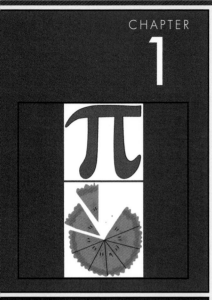

Basic Concepts

The important thing in science is not so much to obtain new facts as to discover new ways of thinking about them.

—William Lawrence Bragg, Nobel Prize in Physics 1915

OUTLINE

LEARNING OBJECTIVES

When you have finished this chapter, you will be able to:

1. Describe the arithmetic and the factors commonly used with an x-ray generator.
2. Understand proportionality and the relationships of numbers.
3. Discuss the units of measurement: mass, length, and time.
4. Recognize the scientific prefixes commonly used in imaging.

Arithmetic

When a technician enters the x-ray room to set up the technical factors on the x-ray generator necessary to produce an optimized image, basic knowledge such as fractions, addition, subtraction and multiplication will be involved.

A quick review of these factors will refresh our essential skills in this area.

Fractions

APPLICATION: *Setting technical factors*
Numerator—the top of the fraction; ⅜, ¾.
Denominator—the bottom of the fraction; ⅜, ¹³⁄₁₄.

Addition and Subtraction

The denominator denotes the number of divisions of the whole. For example, ¼ indicates that the pie is divided into 4 sections, and you will receive 1 piece.

To add two fractions with "like" denominators, add or subtract the numerators and keep the same denominator.

$$1/10 + 2/10 = 3/10$$

Back to the pie … If I divide the pie into 10 pieces and you get 1 piece and your friend gets 2 pieces, there will be 10 − 1 − 2 = 7 pieces or ⁷⁄₁₀ of the pie remaining.

To add two fractions with unlike denominators, find a number that is divisible by both denominators; then convert the two fractions to the same denominator:

$$1/5 + 1/4 = 4/20 + 5/20 = 9/20$$
$$1/2 + 1/3 = 3/6 + 2/6 = 5/6$$

Whole Numbers

APPLICATION: *Setting technical factors on the x-ray generator*

As equipment becomes more sophisticated, fractions are replaced by whole numbers. Throughout the book we will use the algebraic notation for multiplication: A • B.

5×10 will appear as $5 \cdot 10$. When two letters are used, the dot (•) is eliminated, as in AB.

Proportionality (Variation) of Numbers

Proportionality is defined as the relationship between two numbers.

APPLICATION: *Choosing the settings on the x-ray machine, calculating distance, measuring chemistry, calculating radiation doses.*

There are two types of proportionality, direct and indirect.

Direct Proportionality

Direct proportionality means that the first quantity is a multiple of the second quantity. For example, say I have a basket of 25 apples to use in a pie … If I add an apple each time my friend removes an apple, we can say that the number of

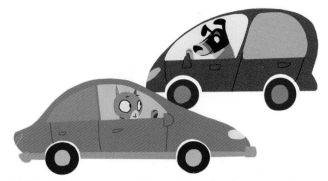

FIGURE 1-1 Driving to and from work is indirectly proportional to the speed of travel. As the speedometer registers higher, the travel time is shorter.

apples added equals or is "directly proportional to" the number of apples removed.

Any factor can be applied to a direct proportion; 1 apple to 1 apple or 2 apples to 4 apples.

Indirect Proportionality

Indirect proportionality means that as one quantity gets larger, the other quantity gets smaller. Thus their product remains the same but each value is different. You are very aware of this every day on your way to work. The time taken for the journey to work is inversely proportional to the speed of travel. As your speedometer registers higher your travel time is shorter. The distance to work is the constant, thus fulfilling all the rules of proportionality (Figure 1-1).

We will visit this very important concept many times when we examine the effects of radiation and radiation doses.

Units of Measurement

APPLICATION: *Setting techniques, measuring patients, raising or lowering the x-ray tube.*

The primary fundamental units of measurement are mass, length, and time.

Mass

Standard unit for mass is the pound (lb) [kilogram (kg)] (Figure 1-2). We do not use mass very much in radiography so we will leave this one alone just now since the other two are very important.

Length

Standard unit for length is the meter (m) (Figure 1-3). Some of the applications for this unit are the measurement of the thickness of the patient; of the distance from the x-ray tube to the patient; and of the distance from the x-ray tube to each wall when we determine the protection we require for the walls of the x-ray room.

Time

Standard unit for time is the second (s) (Figure 1-4). Applications for this unit are time of exposure; time of

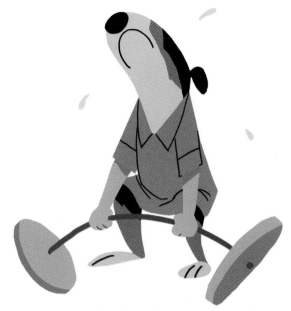

FIGURE 1-2 Mass of an object denotes its weight in either pounds or kilograms. (10 lb weight = 4.5 kg)

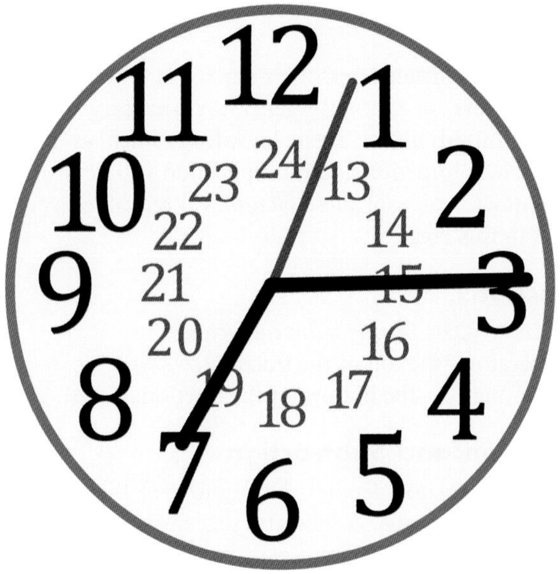

FIGURE 1-4 Standard unit of time. In health care the 24-hour clock is the preferred nomenclature.

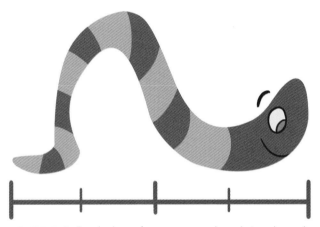

FIGURE 1-3 Standard unit of measurement is the inch. In radiography we measure patients in centimeters.

TABLE 1-1	Common Prefixes	
FACTORS	**PREFIX (SYMBOL)**	**APPLICATION**
10^6	Mega- (M)	Megavolt
10^3	Kilo- (k)	Kilometer, kilovolt
10^{-1}	Deci- (d)	Decimal
10^{-2}	Centi- (c)	Centimeter
10^{-3}	Milli- (m)	Millimeter

injection of contrast media; and time for processing the image.

Prefixes

The metric system uses various prefixes to denote increase and decrease of the original value. Common prefixes used in radiography are shown in Table 1-1. The S.I. Units (International System of Units) of measurement specific to the field of radiation and radiation dose will be described in depth in Chapter 16.

SUMMARY

In this chapter we have reviewed basic mathematical concepts and learned that these simple formulae will be applied in order to control and optimize the radiographic image. The units of measurement that are used to measure our patients and then set the controls on the generator have also been identified. It is important that the units of measurement are correctly identified and notated when they are related to the imaging process.

The Atom and Radioactivity

Nothing exists except atoms and empty space; everything else is opinion.

—Democritus, Ancient Greek Philosopher, 460–370 BCE

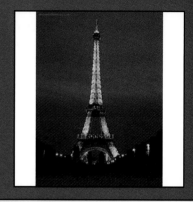

OUTLINE

LEARNING OBJECTIVES

When you have finished this chapter, you will be able to:

1. List the elements most important in radiography.
2. Summarize the history of atomic theory.
3. Understand atomic structure, electrons, protons, and neutrons.
4. Recognize the concepts of ionization, radioactivity, and isotopes.

APPLICATIONS

The application of the information in this chapter is relevant to the following areas:

1. The production of x-rays.
2. Imaging in nuclear medicine.
3. The foundation for contrast media.
4. The components of films, screens, and x-ray tubes.

CHAPTER 2

KEY TERMS

Atomic mass

Atomic number

Atoms

Compound

Electron binding energy

Electron rings (shells)

Electrons

Elements

Fundamental particles

Gluons

Ionization

Isotope

Neutrons

Nucleons

Protons

Quarks

Radioactive decay

Radioactivity

The Elements

It's really not rocket science! Why, actually it is!

Many years ago, or "once upon a time," the ancient Greeks philosophized that there were four substances: earth, air, water, and fire. They further proposed that each of these substances could be altered by the four essences: wet, dry, hot, and cold. Then they decided that every particle of matter could be subdivided many times until all that was left was a unit called an atom, meaning indivisible [*a* (not) + *temon* (divisible)]. The Greeks then represented each type of atom by a symbol (Figure 2-1).

The basis of the table of the elements used today was ingeniously devised by a Russian scholar named Dmitri Mendeleev. He demonstrated that if all the basic elements were arranged in order of increasing mass, a periodic repetition of similar chemical properties occurred. In his day only 65 elements had been identified, and he arranged them in a table that contained eight groups. There were a number of holes in his table but the organization was ingenious. The periodic table that is recognized today contains 114 elements; 92 are naturally occurring and 22 have been artificially produced (Figure 2-2).

In order to understand the basics of radiation we must review the atom and its components and then learn where some important elements, made up of these atoms, are positioned on the periodic table of the elements.

Atomic Theory

While Mendeleev was putting all the elements into the correct slots on his chart, other physicists were attempting to understand how these elements were shaped and then how they interacted with one another. In radiography we use only a few of the elements listed; however, a knowledge of the overall history of the discovery of the elements is important.

Dalton, a British physicist, thought that each atom had a "hook" and "eye" so that they could physically "hook" onto each other. In the 1890s, J.J. Thompson realized that there was some connection with the electrons; thus, he devised a "plum pudding" sort of atom with the electrons acting as a negative charge and the rest of the pudding a formless mass of electrical energy (Figure 2-3).

Finally in 1913, Niels Bohr devised the atomic theory that stands to this day. The atom is a miniature solar system in which the "sun," or nucleus, has a positive charge containing protons and neutrons. The negatively charged electrons are miniature "planets" rotating in specific orbits around the nucleus and held in place by the balanced electrical charges.

The atom is mainly empty space, very similar to our solar system. If the nucleus of the uranium atom were the size of a basketball, the path of the electrons would involve travel of more than 8 miles (12.8 km) away from the nucleus!

Atomic Structure

From what we now know, the structure of the atom involves three very important particles: the proton, the neutron, and the electron (Figure 2-4).

Although the atom has been determined to be quite divisible, with a nod to the ancient Greeks we still use their term. Physicists have now discovered that the nucleus of the atom consists of nucleons, which are protons and neutrons composed of quarks held together by gluons. Digging this deep into atomic theory goes beyond what we require to produce x-rays, so let us examine the fundamental particles of the atom.

Because atomic particles are very small, their mass (size/weight) is expressed as atomic mass units (amu). These numbers are expressed as whole numbers for convenience. One atomic mass unit (amu) is equal to 1/12 of a carbon-12 atom.

The Electron

Each atom contains at least one electron (Figure 2-5). This particle is usually pictured in orbit around a nucleus. What holds it in place is its negative charge. The mass or size of an electron is very small (9.1×10^{-31}). Because precision is not necessary for our studies, we will assume that the atomic mass unit (amu) of an electron is zero.

The electron orbits are arranged in very specific rings or shells containing a limited number of electrons. The maximum number of electrons in each ring is determined by the following formula:

$$2n^2$$

where *n* = the shell number.

For example:

Shell 1 contains $2 \cdot 1^2 = 2 \cdot 1 = 2$ electrons; this represents a helium atom (H)

Shell 4 contains $2 \cdot 4^2 = 2 \cdot 16 = 32$; electrons; this represents a germanium atom (Ge)

The rings (or shells) of the electrons are identified by letters of the alphabet, starting with the letter K, so the fourth shell is N.

Electrons may be added to, or subtracted from, their orbits around the nucleus. Because they encircle the nucleus

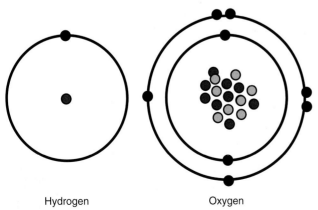

FIGURE 2-1 The symbols for hydrogen (H) (*left*) and oxygen (O) (*right*).

Hydrogen   Oxygen

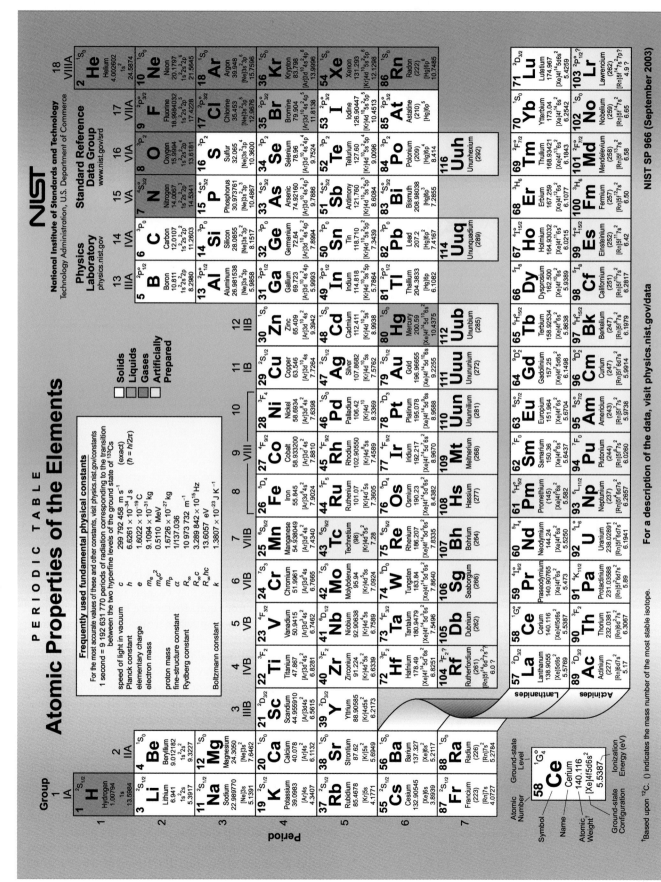

FIGURE 2-2 A periodic table of the elements.

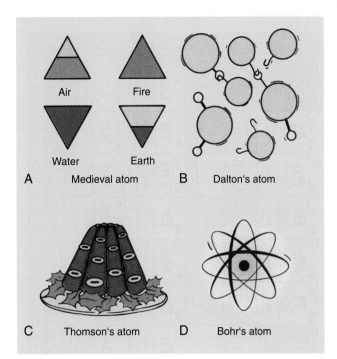

FIGURE 2-3 The stages of the atom through the ages. **A,** The medieval atom. **B,** Dalton's hooks and eyes. **C,** Thomson's plum pudding. **D,** Bohr's atom.

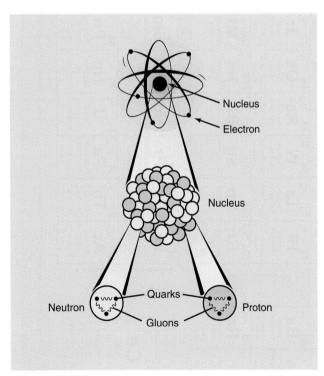

FIGURE 2-4 The current understanding of the structure of the atom, which contains a nucleus of positively charged protons and neutral neutrons surrounded by negatively charged electrons.

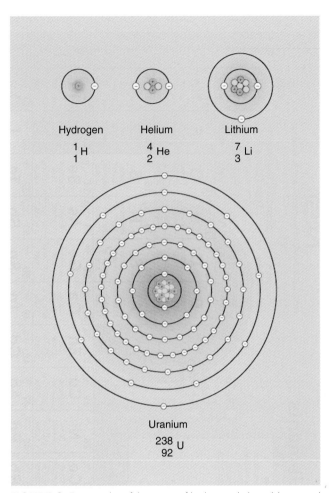

FIGURE 2-5 Examples of the atoms of hydrogen, helium, lithium, and uranium. The protons and neutrons are contained in the nucleus; the electrons orbit in specific rings outside the nucleus.

and some of the electrons are at a relatively great distance from the nucleus, the rings may be quite unstable, giving up and acquiring electrons quite frequently. It is these exchanges that become very important when we discuss the production of x-rays.

The energy that maintains the electrons in their shells is the electron binding energy. The closer the electron is to the nucleus, the higher is its binding energy. The binding energy in each shell depends on the number of electrons and the position of the atom on the periodic table.

The Proton

The proton is a positively charged particle within the nucleus of the atom. Typically, the positive charge of the proton equals the negative charge of the electron. Because the neutron (the third member of the trio) has no charge, the atom has no electrical charge or is electrically neutral.

The number of protons within the nucleus determines the atomic number of the atom. It is represented by the letter **Z.** This number becomes very important when we discuss radioactivity.

The Neutron

The neutron is the third member of the trio and the determinant number for the atomic weight of the atom. The mass of the neutron and the proton together is about 1836 times greater than that of the electron. The total number of protons and neutrons together in an atom is called the mass number and is represented by the letter **A**.

Atomic Weight

Once the elements were identified and Mendeleev and other scientists found their places in the Table of the Elements, it became interesting to note that as the elements progressed along the periodic table, their characteristics formed a unique pattern.

As the atomic number (Z) became higher, the "weight" of the atom became greater and the ability to affect other elements became stronger. For example, barium, with an atomic weight of 56, was considerably heavier than carbon, with an atomic weight of just 6. When these observations combined with experiments with the newly discovered x-rays, it was found that the heavier elements effectively masked the effect of the x-rays. When lead (Z = 82) was introduced between the radiation source and the object being examined, the radiation effect was blocked by the lead.

It is important to note that lead does not completely block x-radiation. It filters the radiation so that the majority of the beam is blocked. Radiation still penetrates lead, and we will explore this issue in chapter 16 on Radiation Protection.

Atomic Nomenclature

The atom has now become fairly complex. We have ascertained that it contains a nucleus made up of neutrons and protons. The neutrons have no charge and the protons have a positive charge similar to the negative charge on electrons. This makes up a stable atom.

The atom can become unstable if we remove electrons or if the number of neutrons changes to form an isotope.

Atomic Representation

Elements are represented in an organized scheme (Figure 2-6) that incorporates the chemical symbol with the atomic mass, the atomic number, the number of atoms per molecule, and the valence state of the atom. Right now we are concerned only with the letters to the left of the X, those indicating atomic number and atomic mass.

Combinations of Atoms

Atoms combine regularly to form molecules, which in turn combine to form compounds. From our earliest experience we know that 4 atoms of hydrogen and 2 atoms of oxygen become 2 molecules of water, as follows:

$$2H_2 + O_2 = 2H_2O$$

Common table salt is a combination of sodium and chlorine (Na + Cl).

Finding naturally occurring elements is relatively rare. Mining gold and silver is quite complicated, whereas pure oxygen and pure hydrogen are also not available naturally. In fact, about 95% of the earth and its atmosphere consist of about 12 to14 naturally occurring elements.

Ninety-eight percent of living animals consist of oxygen, hydrogen, carbon, and nitrogen. Of these, oxygen and hydrogen in the form of water make up 80% of the mammalian body.

The Orderly Organization of Matter

The atoms represent the smallest particle of an element. The molecules are the smallest particle of a compound. The molecules then combine to form tissue, and it is this tissue that we examine when we use an imaging system.

Isotopes

An atom that has the same atomic number but a different atomic mass number is an isotope. An isotope contains the same number of protons but varying numbers of neutrons. Most elements have more than one stable isotope. This feature becomes important in imaging, when we discuss contrast media, nuclear medicine, and oncology.

Radioactivity

Before we leave the explanation of atoms and molecules, it is important that we discuss radioactivity. Some atoms exist in an abnormal state of excitement. Because all matter tries to reach stability, particles and energy will be emitted from the nucleus of an abnormally excited atom, and the matter will transform itself into another atom. This process is called radioactive disintegration or radioactive decay. This process is particularly important in nuclear medicine and is discussed further in the section on nuclear medicine.

Ionization

The natural state of an atom is electrically neutral. However, the farther away from the nucleus the electrons revolve, the lower the electron binding energy, until at various times electrons are removed completely from the atom. Because

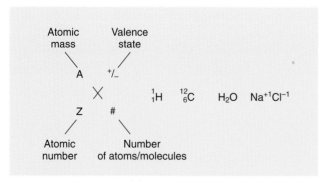

FIGURE 2-6 Protocol for representing atoms in a molecule.

this removal causes an imbalance in the electrical charge (a negative electron has been removed so the atom now becomes positively charged), the atom is said to be ionized. In the production of x-radiation, this is a very important step, because the electrons are "boiled" off the cathode by the heat of the filament circuit.

SUMMARY

In this chapter we have discussed the components of the atom and interactions between these components. Isotopes and radionuclides have been introduced as well as combinations of atoms and molecules.

Electrostatics and Energy, Magnetism and Electricity

KEY TERMS

Ampere
Contact
Continuum
Current
Cycles
Electrification
Electromagnetic
  spectrum
Electromagnetism
Electromotive force
Electrostatics
Energy
Free electrons
Frequency
Friction
Homeostasis
Induction
Magnetism
Matter
Ohm
Particles
Period
Potential difference
Resistance
Sine waves
Wavelength
Waves

LEARNING OBJECTIVES

When you have finished this chapter, you will be able to:
1. Discuss the concept of matter and energy.
2. Define and describe electromagnetic energy.
3. Define and describe particle-wave theory.
4. Define and describe sine waves, wavelength, and frequency.
5. Discuss and describe properties of x-rays.
6. Recognize the laws of electrostatics.
7. Describe contact, friction, and induction.
8. Differentiate between conductors and insulators.
9. Describe electric current.
10. Discuss resistance, potential difference, and voltage.

APPLICATIONS

The application of the information in this chapter is relevant to the following areas:
1. The production of x-rays.
2. Choosing the best x-ray unit for your clinic.
3. Activating the x-ray unit.
4. Setting technical factors.
5. Processing films.
6. Silver recovery.
7. Electrical concepts in digital imaging.

The world in which we live can be categorized to the point at which all things are either matter or energy. Matter is defined as the substance that comprises all physical objects. Energy is defined as the ability to do work.

Electrostatics and Energy

Electricity is really just organized lightning.
—George Carlin, American comedian (1937–2008)

Matter

The principle characteristic of matter is mass or weight. Weight involves gravity. The principle characteristic of energy is movement or motion. As we explore the production and effects of radiation throughout this book, it is important to remember that the combination of matter and energy in the universe is a constant. Matter can become energy and energy can become matter, but neither can be created or destroyed. Each can only be changed in form.

Energy

Work is the result of force acting upon an object over a distance. Power incorporates a time factor into the equation. The same amount of work is required to lift a puppy to a specific height whether you take 1 minute or 10 seconds. However it requires more "power" to lift the puppy quickly (short time) than it does to lift it slowly (long time).

There are many types of energy: mechanical, chemical, thermal, nuclear, electromagnetic, and electrical. The last is the type that we will explore in this chapter.

Electrical Energy

A light bulb demonstrates the conversion of electrical energy into light, or radiant energy. A hair dryer converts electrical energy into thermal energy.

Electromagnetic Spectrum

Various forms of energy had to be organized in some way, and physicists decided to do so by first determining the amount of energy in each type of electrical excitation and then placing that type of energy on a continuum or electromagnetic spectrum. In the same way that light as a form of energy is organized in a rainbow (Figure 3-1), electromagnetic radiation is organized on the electromagnetic spectrum with the rainbow as a very tiny portion near the middle (Figure 3-2).

Early researchers did all their experiments with visible light, so they placed light energy in the middle of the spectrum. Soon it was discovered that energy could be invisible. Using the rainbow as a template, the researchers described ultraviolet light and infrared light. *Ultra-* in this case was above or beyond the violet color of the rainbow, whereas *infra-* was under or below the energy of the red color at the

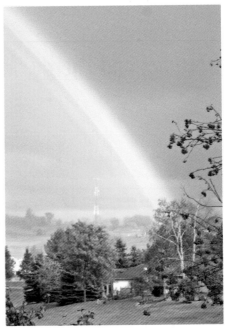

FIGURE 3-1 A rainbow shows all the colors in the visible light portion of the electromagnetic spectrum.

opposite side of the rainbow. It was also discovered that the human eye can see very little of the entire spectrum. The major portion of the spectrum we see only as the effect that the energy has on the universe and the matter around us. This is very important in designing and building a radiography room and a darkroom in which to process films.

Once these energies were identified, the further energies of radio waves, television waves, and radar were placed on the spectrum, and further along the spectrum toward the "ultra-" side, we find x-rays, gamma rays, and cosmic rays.

Particle-Wave Theory

Identifying and quantifying these energies was difficult. Starting with the description of energy as a wave (Figure 3-3) is more logical than the description of energy as particles.

Scientists described energy as waves washing onto an ocean beach. The energy is seemingly endless. The waves can be long and low or they can be high and frequent (Figure 3-4). So wave theory was born.

Waves have a measurable height and a measurable frequency. At the sea shore, the time between the crests of the waves crashing onto the beach or the distance between crests can be measured. The distance between the individual crests, or troughs, is called wavelength. The scientific symbol for wavelength is λ, the 11th letter of the Greek alphabet.

Frequency

The rapidity with which the waves hit the shore is called frequency. A period is the time taken to complete one complete wave; one crest or high point and one trough or low point; or one cycle of the wave (Figure 3-5).

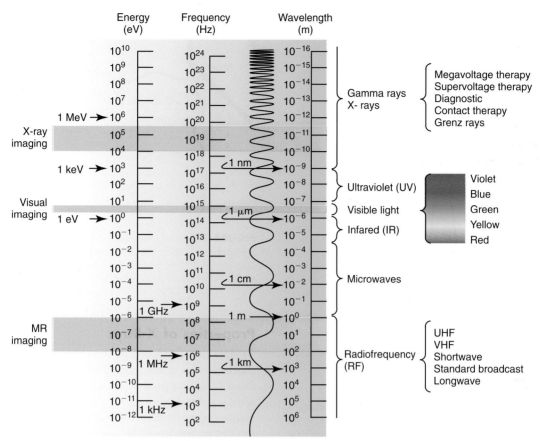

FIGURE 3-2 The entire electromagnetic spectrum is much larger than just the visible light portion. This chart shows the values of energy, frequency, and wavelength for all portions and identifies the three imaging windows.

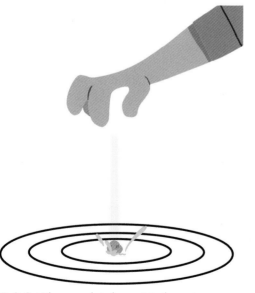

FIGURE 3-3 When a rock is thrown into the water, waves result as the energy is dissipated through the water and the rock comes to rest.

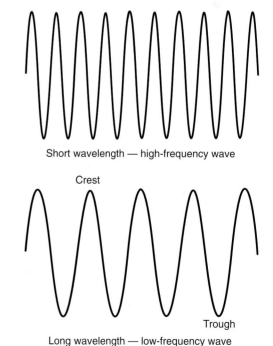

Short wavelength — high-frequency wave

Crest

Trough

Long wavelength — low-frequency wave

FIGURE 3-4 *Top* and *bottom,* Waves in a body of water have measurable heights and measurable frequencies.

Timeline

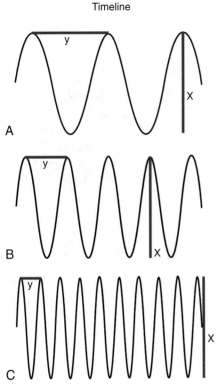

FIGURE 3-5 These three sine waves have different wavelengths. **A,** Long wavelength, **B,** Medium wavelength, **C,** Short wavelength. The shorter the wavelength, the higher the frequency as measured over time. The height of the wave from crest to trough is the amplitude (x), and frequency (y).

A sinusoidal (sine) wave is the tracing of the crests and troughs that the waves describe as they travel through the ocean. The symbol for frequency is the hertz (Hz). Sine waves have a high point and a low point with time being the constant that runs through the middle. This is very important when we set our x-ray unit and choose the time over which the x-rays will be produced.

Sound waves travel invisibly through space, sometimes louder than we appreciate (thunderstorms and very loud music). In practice, electromagnetic waves can travel through a vacuum without losing energy. This property is particularly useful when we activate the semivacuum x-ray tube to produce x-rays.

Energy in Radiography

Some scientists thought of energy in packages or miniparticles. This was particularly true when they were using high-frequency energies such as x-rays or gamma rays (Figure 3-6). In these cases the energies acted more like individual particles than like waves. The photon particle carries a specific energy that depends on frequency. In a photon particle, the energy and the frequency are directly proportional. If the energy is doubled, then the frequency is doubled. When energy is described as particles, it is possible to mathematically quantify this relationship and the amount of energy required to perform work.

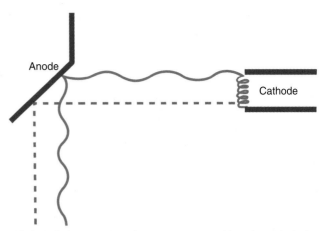

FIGURE 3-6 In an x-ray tube, energy is emitted from the cathode (on the right) as waves by one definition and as particles by another definition. The photons of energy are magnetically drawn to the anode (on the left) when the circuit is activated.

Properties of X-Rays

As Rœntgen developed his experiments and identified the characteristics of the new rays that he was investigating, he listed 12 unique properties. Although he thought that these were just the beginning of a list of properties, his experiments and scientific investigation were so thorough that to this day no one has added to the original list. It is important that we learn the contents of the list because we will encounter these characteristics throughout the balance of the text.

Rœntgen's Properties of Rays

According to Roentgen, x-rays:

1. Are highly penetrating invisible rays that are a form of electromagnetic radiation.
2. Are electrically neutral and therefore not affected by either electric or magnetic fields.
3. Can be produced over a wide variety of energies and wavelengths (polyenergetic and heterogeneous).
4. Release very small amounts of heat upon passing through matter.
5. Travel in straight lines.
6. Travel at the speed of light, 3×10^8 meters per second in a vacuum.
7. Can ionize matter.
8. Cause fluorescence (the emission of light) of certain crystals.
9. Cannot be focused by a lens.
10. Affect photographic film.
11. Produce chemical and biological changes in matter through ionization and excitation.
12. Produce secondary and scattered radiation.

SUMMARY

Thus far we have explored energy in the form of electrical waves and particles. We have also started on our exploration of radioactivity and the identification of x-rays. Now we will proceed to the application of these waves and particles as we work toward understanding the x-ray unit.

Magnetism and Electricity

I have not failed. I've just found 10,000 ways that won't work. To invent, you need a good imagination and a pile of junk.
—Thomas A. Edison, American Inventor, 1847–1931

Electricity Becomes X-Rays

Atoms contain both positive and negative charges. The proton in the nucleus of the atom is positively charged, whereas the electron encircling the atom is negatively charged. The atom always strives to achieve homeostasis, or balance, with the negative charges balancing the positive charges.

The electron is vulnerable to forces outside its orbit, and electrons may be cast off from their orbits to join forces with the orbits of neighboring electrons. If many of these electrons leave the atom, and other electrons do not take their place, the atom will assume a positive charge because there is an excess of positive protons as a result of the missing negative electrons.

Electrons may also be ejected from the atom and float freely in space, not associated with an atom at all. These are called free electrons. All of these actions and reactions take place over very brief periods. The charges that hold the electrons in their orbits are very weak; the bonds are easily broken and reunited. Electricity concerns the movement of the electrons.

Electrostatics

In winter, or in a dry atmosphere, a walk across a rug and then the touch of a friend can become a shocking experience. The charge of free electrons has built up on your body such that when you encounter an object that will accept the charge (a conductor), a metallic object or the arm of a friend, the negative charge dissipates in the form of static electricity, or electrostatic charge (Figure 3-7).

The term electrification describes the process of electron charges being added to or subtracted from an object. The negative charge built up because your feet have literally "scooped up" extra electrons causes an exchange of electrons the moment you are within "shocking" or connecting distance of your friend. This is the way radiation is produced in an x-ray tube but on a far greater scale.

Laws of Electrostatics

The five laws of electrostatics are very important to the field of x-ray exposure. During the discussion of electric charges, electrical energy will be referred to as packets of electron energy and not as waves of energy.

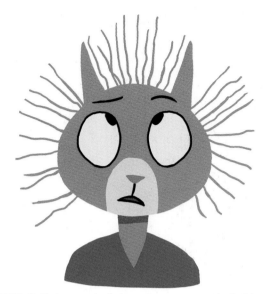

FIGURE 3-7 As a result of electrostatic energy, individual hairs are negatively electrically charged and repel one another until the free electrons are discharged.

Positively charged protons are tightly bound within the nucleus of the atom. Negatively charged electrons are bound by relatively weak bonds and are sometimes free to roam about waiting to join up with an atom that has an incomplete number of electrons. However, it is important to note that the total positive charge of the protons and the total negative charge of the electrons are equal in strength. They just reside in two different places in the atom.

The five laws of electrostatics are as follows:

1. **Like charges repel; unlike charges attract.** This is the principle of an electric circuit and functions as an x-ray tube is prepared to make an exposure. It is also fundamental basis of magnetism.
2. **The inverse square law** (Figure 3-8). This is perhaps the most important concept in the field of imaging. It is applied frequently during the set up of an x-ray unit and in the selection of technical factors. *The intensity of the x-ray beam is inversely proportional to the square of the distance from the source.* This is a very useful concept when a very-low-powered x-ray unit is used. The x-ray tube is moved closer to the subject, intensifying the amount of radiation. One-half the distance intensifies the radiation by four times. Also, when the light is very dim, if the distance is halved, we will receive four times the illumination (Figure 3-9).
3. **Distribution.** The charges reside on the external surfaces of conductors and equally throughout nonconductors.
4. **Concentration.** The greatest concentration of the charges is on the surface where the curvature is sharpest (Figure 3-10). This law may not be all that important to our production of x-rays, but it is very important to a stockman herding cattle into a holding pen or a police officer using a stun gun, such as the one illustrated in the figure. The two contacts at the end of the gun are attached to

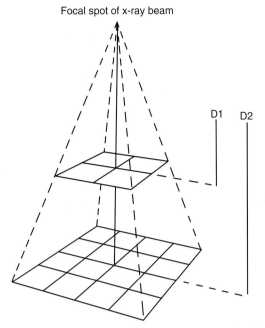

Focal spot of x-ray beam

D1   D2

FIGURE 3-8 D1 is the first distance from the light source (focal spot). D2 represents what happens when the distance is doubled: The light covers four times the area. The intensity of the light on each square at D2, however, is one quarter that of the light on each square at D1.

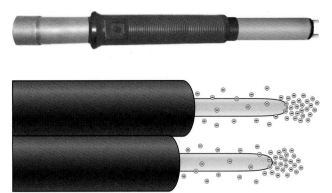

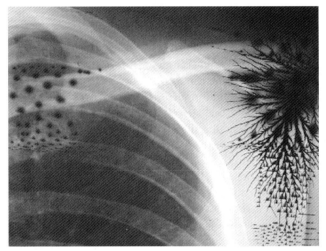

FIGURE 3-10 A cattle prod demonstrates that the concentration of charge will reside on the surface where the curvature is greatest—in this case at the ends of the two contacts.

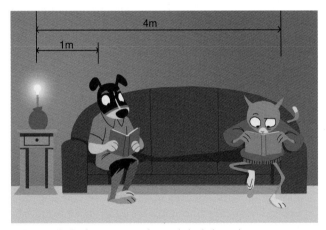

4m
1m

FIGURE 3-9 The person reading with the light at close range can see quite well. When the light is farther away, the intensity of the light is reduced considerably.

two wires, which are ejected from the gun, contacting the victim and releasing a "stunning" amount of voltage.

5. **Movement.** Only negative charges move along solid conductors. The positive charges are tightly bound within the nucleus of the atom

Electrification

An object can be electrified in three different ways: contact, friction, and induction.

Contact

The first method, contact, we have already discussed, in the example of crossing the rug and shocking your friend. Excess

FIGURE 3-11 An example of several types of electrostatic electricity (friction) recorded by a radiograph.

electrons collected on the surface of your body, giving you a negative charge (Law #3). These electrons then concentrated on the point of your finger (Law #4). The discharge occurred when your finger came close enough for the spark to "jump" or discharge onto the body of your friend, who is electrically neutral or possibly slightly positively charged (Law #1).

If we were to take a photograph at the very moment that you touched your friend, or if the room was sufficiently dark, we would see a very brief spark of light as the electrons discharged onto the friend's arm.

Figure 3-11 demonstrates what happens if an x-ray film is put onto the feed tray of a film processor in a very dry atmosphere. Static electricity that has built up on the tray will discharge onto the film. The film is a recording medium so it will record the exact amount of discharge from the encounter. Static electricity is an example of radiant energy.

Friction

Friction (see Figure 3-7) is a type of electricity that occurs when one object is rubbed against another. Electrons travel

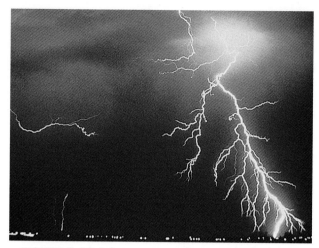

FIGURE 3-12 Lightning is an excellent example of induction.

from one object to the other owing to differences in the availability of the electrons on each object. Cold, dry atmospheres are great producers of static electricity. A buildup of static electricity can be demonstrated when hair is electrified by running a comb through it when it is very dry. The hair builds up an excess of electrons, and because like charges repel, the individual hairs literally stand on end trying to get as far away from one another as possible. Wetting the comb will provide a conductor for the electrons to distribute themselves appropriately, and the hair will then return to its pre-electrified state.

Induction

Induction is the most important concept of electrification because it is the principle used in the operation of electronics and also in the production of x-rays. Induction (Figure 3-12) uses the concept of electrical fields, which we have previously described, acting upon each other without actual contact. In the case of contact and friction, the two opposing forces actually touched each other and a discharge of energy was the result.

Induction uses the force fields of the electrons of one object to cause a reaction in the opposing object without any contact. The very best example of this activity is lightning. The clouds build up a terrific amount of excess electrons as they form into thunderheads. The ground is neutral, and the discharge of the electrons from cloud to ground is instantaneous and very loud. So even though the clouds do not touch the ground, an electric current is generated between cloud and ground.

This energy and the power of the effect of this energy is what we use in transformers, x-ray tubes, and electric motors.

Conductors and Insulators

Certain objects conduct electricity very easily. This is why we use copper wire in our homes and why we do not play with electric toys in the bathtub. Water and copper are very effective conductors of electricity.

Other objects are used as insulators because they do not conduct electricity very easily, if at all. Rubber, plastic, and glass are good insulators. This is why the copper wire in our homes is insulated with a rubber covering.

When an x-ray unit is constructed, the manufacturers make sure that the areas that are touched by the staff in the x-ray room are very well insulated from the power of the electric current on the outside of the control panel.

Electric Current

In the early 1800s a Frenchman named André-Marie Ampère described electric current as packages or a quantity of electrons flowing past a point in time. Because he described many of the principles of electricity the unit of current, the ampere or "amp" bears his name.

Diagnostic imaging uses milliamperes (mA) to regulate the number of electrons used to produce x-ray photons. Every x-ray generator in existence today contains an mA selector on the control panel. This adjustment determines the number of electrons that will flow past a given point. Increasing the mA will produce the effect of darkening the image or increasing the density. Decreasing the mA will decrease the density of the image. In fact an increase of double the mA will cause a directly proportional increase in the density of the image.

Resistance

If every object in the world were a good conductor of electricity it would be a very difficult place in which to live. Therefore, we require some method of reducing the amount of current flow. The opposite of current flow is resistance. A German physicist, George Ohm, researched resistance at the same time as Ampère was investigating electric currents. Because of his contributions in this field, the ohm as a unit of resistance is named after him.

First let us look at one other factor that Ohm identified as very important in his research, potential difference.

Potential Difference

Potential difference causes the electrons to travel from one end of a wire to the other. If we use a garden hose as an analogy, then the hose is connected to a generator (the faucet). When the hose is stored there is very little water throughout the hose itself but a great deal of potential water in the faucet. When the faucet is turned on to allow water to flow, there is a potential difference along the length of the hose. One end has no water and the other has a lot of water with more coming in all the time. The potential difference is the measurement of the full hose compared with the empty hose.

The one item that restricts the flow of water along our hose is the diameter of the hose itself. A small hose causes a lot of resistance to the water as it rushes along. A larger hose gives little resistance (Figure 3-13). From this analogy we can conclude that a very large wire produces little resistance to

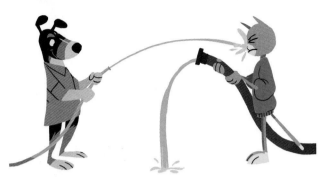

FIGURE 3-13 Principle of resistance. Different-sized fire hoses provide various amounts of resistance depending on their diameters. With the same amount of water flowing through the hose, the smaller diameter hose provides greater resistance than the larger-diameter hose.

the current flowing along it, and a very small wire produces a lot of resistance.

Voltage

At the same time that Ampère and Ohm were doing their research into electricity, another physicist in Italy identified the unit of potential difference. Alessandro Volta recognized electromotive force. It is this force that draws the electrons from an area of excess electrons at one end of a circuit to an area deficient of electrons at the other end of the circuit. The term for potential difference used to denote the strength of the electron flow is the volt, named for Volta.

SUMMARY

We have now been introduced to the essence of the x-ray unit. Electricity must have a circuit in order to be activated. There must be a potential difference between one end of the circuit and the other. There must be electron flow and by default there will be resistance within the circuit.

We now have all the tools in place to put the circuit together and generate enough power to ensure that we will build a useful generator of radiation. We must always be aware of the vast amount of electricity generated when the technical factors are set to produce an exposure to radiographic receptor.

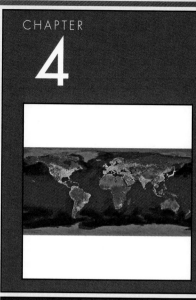

Diagnostic X-Ray Production

If it weren't for electricity we'd all be watching television by candlelight.

—George Gobel, American Comedian 1919–1991

OUTLINE

KEY TERMS

Alternating current
Amperage
Anode heel effect
Anode
Cathode
Circuit breaker
Circuit
Direct current
Exposure switch
Ground
Heat dissipation
Hertz
High frequency
Line voltage
 compensator
Power
Pulses (timer)
Rectifier
Resistance
Rotating anode
Rotor
Stationary anode
Target
Transformer
Voltage
Watt
X-ray tube

LEARNING OBJECTIVES

When you have finished this chapter, you will be able to:

1. Understand power and the use of watts, voltage and resistance.
2. Understand electricity and the components of the electrical circuit.
3. Be familiar with direct and alternating current.
4. Know the difference between transformers and rectifiers.
5. Understand the construction of the x-ray tube.
6. Understand heat dissipation, the activation of the exposure switch.

APPLICATIONS

The application of the information in this chapter is relevant to the following areas:

1. Production of radiation using electricity.
2. The use of electricity in radiography and all the other imaging modalities.
3. The application of switches circuit breakers, transformers, and rectifiers in the production of radiation.
4. The use of transformers to increase and decrease the voltage of the incoming power to the x-ray unit.

Diagnostic X-Ray Production

An electrical circuit cannot exist without potential difference (voltage), resistance (ohm), and amperage (current). Because these units are interrelated, they can be formed into an equation, and if one of the items is missing, there is no circuit (Figure 4-1).

Power

The unit of power is a watt, named after James Watt, a Scottish scientist and engineer. He lived during the same time as Ampère, Volta, and Ohm, and presumably they all worked on electricity separately but were aware of one another's work. Communication was not as convenient then as it is today, so quite often inventors did not realize that someone else, in another part of the world, was coming to the same conclusions that they were developing. Frequently, they would publish a paper and then communicate via letters and patents applications.

One watt is defined as 1 ampere flowing through a circuit at 1 volt per 1 second. When we speak of power, it is a combination of amperes and volts, as follows:

$$\text{Current in Amperes (I)} \times \text{Volts (V)} = \text{Power (W)}$$

or

$$I \cdot V = W$$

Most household appliances use between 500 and 2000 watts. The circuit panel in your home is probably rated at 100 or 200 amperes. These numbers become very important during a new installation of x-ray equipment at a veterinary clinic. Most installed x-ray units in veterinary clinics are equipped to use a maximum of 125,000 volts and a maximum of 300 milliamperes of electricity.

Using $W = I \cdot V$, we can calculate the power rating quite easily, as follows:

$$W = 0.3 \times 125,000 = 37,500$$

$$W = 37,500 \text{ watts or } 37.5 \text{ kilowatts}$$

Most generators in veterinary clinics sold in North America today are rated at a minimum of 30 kilowatts. All circuits in buildings have a safety wattage limitation, and it is important to know this value when a new clinic is being planned or if old equipment is being replaced.

The Electrical Circuit

The power that is generated to activate x-ray units and other electronic devices originates at a power plant. The power is transmitted over vast distances with transformer stations along the way to boost the power that is lost through transmission.

What matters most to the veterinary clinic is the transformer mounted very near the veterinary clinic and supplying power to the entire clinic. Quite often the local transformer station is within a few miles of the veterinary clinic, and an auxiliary transformer is mounted on a hydroelectric pole or within a transformer on the ground just outside the clinic.

The X-Ray Circuit Is Actually a Circle

Another item that is vital to electricity is the circuit itself. A circuit (Figure 4-2) is essential to produce electricity. There must be a connection in order to turn the system on or off. Every time we close the switch on a lamp, a circuit is completed and the light comes on. If we "break" the circuit, the light goes off. This can happen anywhere along the circuit. For example, if the light bulb "burns out", the fine wire that forms the cathode of the lamp, will literally burn out in the heat of the electron flow; the circuit is interrupted, and the light will not function. The same thing will happen if a mouse eats through the cord. Unfortunately for the mouse, in the brief instant that the cord breaks, the mouse will conduct the electricity and will receive a shock powerful enough to kill it.

On/Off Switch

All x-ray units are supplied with an on/off switch. Two other items are very important in ensuring that the correct amount of power is available for the final x-ray exposure, the wall switch and the line voltage compensator.

Wall Switch

Prior to the on/off switch for the x-ray unit itself is the wall switch (Figure 4-3A). It is very important, and in fact, the

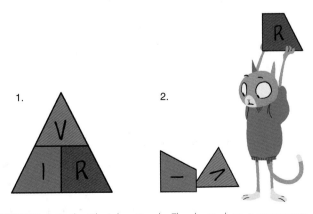

FIGURE 4-1 The Ohm's law triangle. The electrical circuit components are interrelated. If one component is not functioning, there is no current flow. V, voltage; I, current; R, resistance.

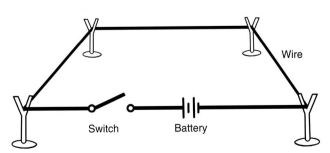

FIGURE 4-2 Example of a simple circuit, consisting of a wire connecting a switch and a battery. Rural electric fencing is an example of a simple circuit.

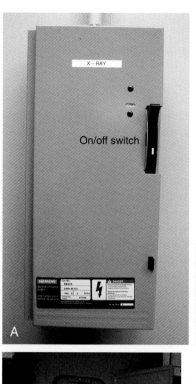

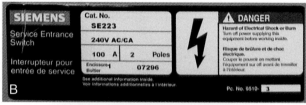

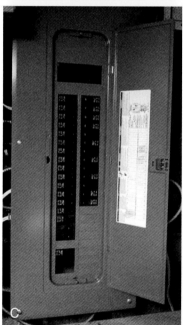

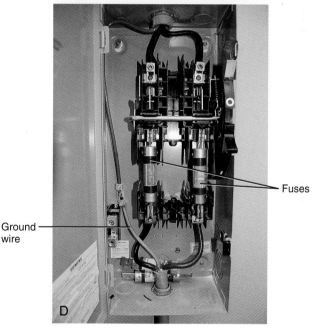

Fuses

Ground
wire

FIGURE 4-3 **A,** The wall switch must be mounted at eye level close to the control panel. **B,** The label on the outside notes the voltage (240 V) and current rating (100 amps) for Canada (AC/CA). 240 volts is the maximum voltage the fuses will handle before they disconnect the circuit. **C,** An example of a circuit breaker panel. Each switch represents a circuit throughout the building so that power can be interrupted in one area and maintained everywhere else. A #2 wire from the electrical panel to the x-ray unit will disconnect the unit from the panel if an overload occurs. **D,** On the inside of the box the two fuses are connected to the two 110-volt lines to provide 220 volts to the radiography unit. The ground wire is green on the inside of the box.

law in most countries that the x-ray unit be installed with a separate wall switch mounted at eye level (about 5 feet) above the floor within reach of the x-ray generator. This is in place so that (if for some reason) there is an equipment malfunction and the xray unit timer does not terminate the exposure function, then the power can be shut off from the disconnect switch on the wall.

Line Voltage Compensator

The line voltage compensator (Figure 4-4) is standard equipment on every unit. On some older units still in use today, a compensator is mounted on the control panel. Newer units compensate automatically. This device is usually connected through the kilovolt (kV) meter and has a method of increasing or decreasing the incoming line voltage. In older units

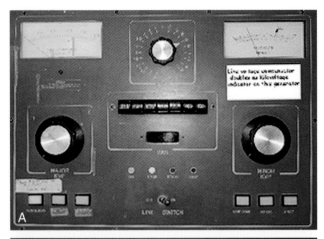

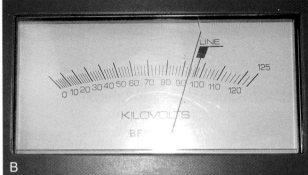

FIGURE 4-4 **A,** Line voltage compensator on a Bennett x-ray unit circa 1985–1990. The indicator on the top right doubles as the kilovoltage indicator as well as the line voltage indicator. The line switch (on/off) is located in the middle of the panel at the bottom. **B,** The switch to read the line voltage is situated on the right side of this x-ray unit. The knob to reset the line voltage is beside it. The indicator needle should be set on the line rather than to the left of the line. The line voltage should be checked at least once per month to ensure that the correct kilovoltage is supplied.

the incoming line voltage was not always as stable as it is today, and also the incoming lines to a facility were limited, so often another piece of equipment was installed using the x-ray equipment power line. At this point there would be a draw on the line and the voltage to the x-ray generator would have to be boosted using the line voltage compensator.

Circuit Breakers: Amperage and Ground

When the power first arrives at the x-ray unit, it immediately encounters the circuit breaker (Figure 4-3C). This is a power supply to the x-ray unit. This circuit breaker is very similar to the panel located in any house. It has replaced the older fuse boxes in most areas. A series of switches are connected to the power lines going out to each room in the facility. Every room, every electric socket, and every switch must be connected to a circuit breaker.

Once the power is brought into the clinic, it arrives at the circuit breaker panel. A circuit breaker will accept current (amperage) up to a certain point—its rating. Once the maximum quantity of power is reached, the circuit breaker disconnects, and power to the electronic device is interrupted until it is manually reset (Figure 4-3C). A fuse works

exactly the same way except that when it reaches its power limit a small piece of metal inside it melts, and the fuse must be replaced with one of equal value.

Amperage

Another factor that is vitally important is the current (amperage) of the circuit. If the current demanded by wthe x-ray generator is in excess of what is available, an overload light is displayed and no exposure is possible until the demand is reduced. The current in a radiography generator is labeled as milliamperage (mA). On very old units, an exposure is possible but the unit will produce only its maximum mA and not the mA requested by the operator.

Most veterinary x-ray generators require a 100-ampere service fused at 80 amperes (see Figure 4-3A). If this is not available, then 80 amperes fused at 60 amperes may be substituted; although this arrangement will limit the power at the higher end of the technique chart, it is workable. When insufficient power is supplied and a secondary step-up transformer is not installed, the #2 wire on the circuit breaker will disconnect the power and thus prevent overheating of the unit. Circuit breakers are very important parts of the x-ray unit and must never be bypassed because of inadequate service from the installer/manufacturer or the power company.

Ground

If the circuit is to remain safe for everyone to use, it needs to be grounded. This means that there is an alternate route for the electricity to flow if the circuit is broken inappropriately. The original electrical circuit is directed to a ground wire attached to an object that will absorb excess electrons and therefore redirect the current flow. The flow of electrons will stop with the broken circuit, but the excess electrons that are still flowing are then redirected to the ground wire. In Figure 4-3D, the ground wire is the green wire on the left side inside the box.

Because the nominal voltage coming into most buildings is 110 volts, it must be doubled to 220 volts in order to connect enough power to supply the x-ray circuit. This is done by connecting two 110-volt power lines coming into the building to the x-ray unit: An equipment manufacturer will request, "Two live lines and one ground."

Direct Current and Alternating Current

In a flashlight, batteries are installed in a tube. They have to be in a certain orientation so that when the switch connects the circuit the unit produces light through the light bulb (Figure 4-5). This is an example of direct current. Direct current requires a source situated very close to the end user. A car battery and a flashlight use direct current. However, if power is to be transmitted over vast distances, then a source that transmits a very low current paired with a very high voltage is less expensive and much more efficient.

Early pioneers working with electric current discovered that it was cheaper and easier to produce an alternating current. Alternating current (Figure 4-6) produces one

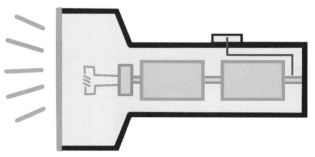

FIGURE 4-5 A flashlight is an example of direct current at work. The batteries carry the voltage. When the switch is closed, the current travels through the batteries and the contact plate to the light bulb, which emits radiant energy in the form of light.

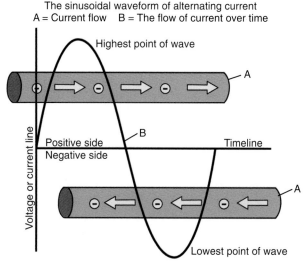

FIGURE 4-6 An example of alternating current. The electrons flow through the coil (**A**), creating one positive portion and one negative portion (**B**) of one cycle.

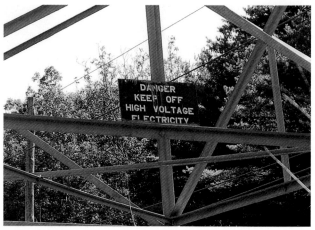

FIGURE 4-7 An example of Hydroelectric Transmission lines alongside a New York Highway. The sign warns potential climbers of High Voltage.

positive pulse and then one matching negative pulse. It was discovered originally that the most efficient way to transmit power was to pair the pulses at 100 cycles per second.

Power in many countries has remained at 100 cycles per second (50 Hz). The North Americans found that 100 cycles per second produced an unacceptable flicker as the current fluctuated, so they increased the frequency to 120 cycles per second (60 Hz). This fluctuation in power requires the use of transformers. Transformers step up (increase) the power at one end of the journey and then step down (decrease) the power at the destination.

For example, if we are to send 1 million watts of power across a grid to provide electricity to a neighborhood, it is much easier and more efficient to send 1 amp at 1,000,000 volts than 1,000,000 amps at 1 volt. Using transformers at each end of the journey alters the voltage as required (Figure 4-7).

The German scientist Heinrich Hertz, who contributed much to the study of electromagnetism, was honored when his name was chosen for the designation describing the cycles per second of the oscillations of alternating current

(one positive and one negative = one oscillation or one cycle). One Hertz equals one positive cycle and one negative cycle and therefore, in North America, we use 60 cycles per second or 60 Hertz.

In Europe and the Caribbean, 50 cycles per second are used, translating to 50 Hertz. So when the factors are set to the shortest time on a single-phase generator in Europe, the time would be set at 1/100 second. In North America, the shortest time on a single-phase x-ray generator is based on 60 cycles per second or a fastest time of 1/120 second.

Transformers

Transformers (Figure 4-8A, B) receive power from the incoming power lines and literally transform the power to the x-ray tube. They do this by using the turns of a wire around a central core (Figure 4-9) or around two magnetic cores with close proximity to each other (Figure 4-10).

In this way they either increase or decrease the voltage in a circuit. The method of electrification in the transformer is induction. For example, 100 turns on the primary and 200 turns on the secondary produce twice the voltage; or 100 turns on the primary and 50 turns on the secondary produce half the voltage.

There are three transformers in the x-ray circuit (Figure 4-11): the autotransformer, the high-tension transformer, and the filament transformer.

The first two transformers increase the incoming voltage. The first is the autotransformer. This is the kilovoltage selector and it allows the technician to select the kilovoltage required to produce a radiograph. The autotransformer has a central core and taps from which the kilovoltage is selected.

The circuit then proceeds to the high-voltage transformer (see Figure 4-11). This unit is the final step-up transformer to boost the voltage to the x-ray tube. For a successful exposure to take place, the voltage must be raised from the original incoming 220 volts to a maximum 125,000 volts. This is a very powerful transformer.

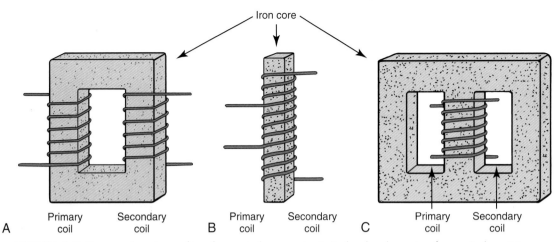

Iron core

A
Primary coil   Secondary coil

B
Primary coil   Secondary coil

C
Primary coil   Secondary coil

FIGURE 4-8 There are three types of transformers in the x-ray circuit. **A**, the closed core transformer, **B**, the autotransformer. This is used mainly to raise and lower kilovoltage. **C**, the shell type transformer. This has largely replaced the older closed core transformer as it is more efficient than the original closed core.

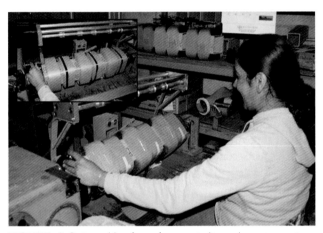

FIGURE 4-9 Assembly of transformer windings, three at one time. Inset shows the copper wire being wound onto a spool. Each layer has a paper cover. There is an A side and a B side for the step-up mains transformer.

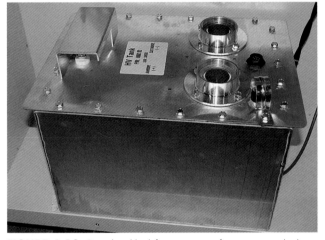

FIGURE 4-10 Completed high-frequency transformer set into the base of the generator cabinet for a small animal radiography unit. The wound coils are contained in the tank that is submerged in oil. The bright red plugs contain the positive and negative high-tension cable receptors.

The final transformer is the filament transformer. This is a smaller step-down transformer which produces the voltage to the filament of the x-ray tube. The x-ray tube works like a very sophisticated light bulb. The small wire that is visible in the bulb of a light is the cathode. It produces light depending upon its power rating, or wattage. The filament (cathode) of the x-ray tube produces electrons in a cloud depending on the factors selected by the technician. The filament must reach a certain temperature in order for the exposure to take place. The filament transformer produces this temperature.

Rectifiers

The one problem with alternating current is that the current is pulsed. In other words, there is one positive pulse and then one negative pulse. This equals one complete cycle. Just as we described the wave forms in Chapter 3, there is a crest and a trough to electrical waveforms. If the current is to remain at 60 cycles (or 60 positives and 60 negatives) there

is a problem when the circuit is connected to an x-ray machine. The x-ray tube can receive only positive pulses because the current can flow only one way through the x-ray tube. Therefore, it receives only one half of the current. Originally, this worked well for the early x-ray units. They worked on the principle of half-wave rectification (Figure 4-12).

The equipment manufacturers invented a method by which the negative portion of the circuit was changed into a positive charge by use of a device called a rectifier circuit (Figure 4-13). Rectifiers redirected the current flow on the negative portion of the cycle to become positive, and the entire 60 cycles per second now traveled through the x-ray tube to produce radiation. This is important because if half of the rectifying circuit is not functioning, only half of the current travels through the tube and only 50% of the expected radiation is produced.

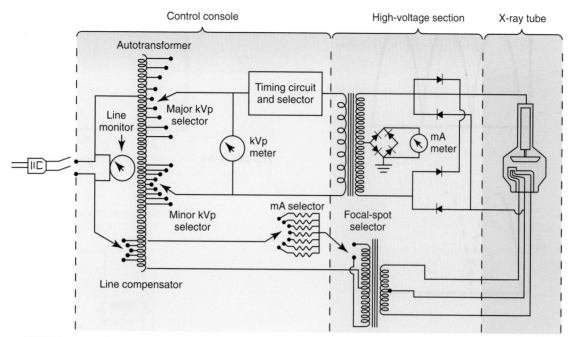

FIGURE 4-11 The complete radiography generator circuit. The three transformers are labeled. Notice that the kV auto-transformer is a single-core transformer. The high-tension transformer is a dual-core step-up transformer, and the filament transformer is a dual-core step-down transformer.

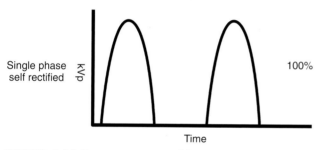

FIGURE 4-12 The negative portion of the wave is suppressed. There is no current flow during the negative phase. This is also called half wave rectification.

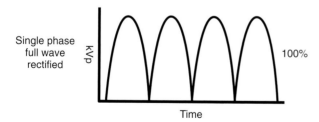

FIGURE 4-13 Single-phase full-wave rectified. The negative pulses have been rectified and the circuit is continuous. There is still a drop in current between each pulse, which limits the output.

One final problem remained when the cycle reached a low point between the pulses. The power output was not consistent. This produced a problem in some units where the circuit did not return to zero following each exposure; therefore, only part of the wave or cycle was used in a subsequent exposure (Figure 4-14).

This problem was resolved by adding to the circuit to ensure that each exposure started at the beginning of a pulse and finished at the end of a pulse. X-ray units built after 1970 have this feature. Units built prior to 1970 may not have this feature. The best insurance on the older units is to block off the lowest time station, usually 1/120 of a second. This would be one complete pulse normally, but if the unit is not set up correctly, it could represent only part of that pulse and therefore only part of the exposure.

Three-Phase Circuits

Another solution to the dips of power in the waveform was to add in two more pulses of power offset from the first pulse and also from each other to make the drop in power much less significant (Figure 4-15). This change produced a small ripple effect in the power but it made the output of the x-ray unit much more effective. The problem that now occurred was that the x-ray unit has became much more sophisticated and requires a great deal more power when it is installed. These units are not used in veterinary medicine except in large veterinary hospitals, where very high amounts of exposure are necessary to image large animal chests and abdomens (see Chapter 6).

High Frequency

Another less expensive and better alternative to the power drop problem is to use high-frequency pulses (Figure 4-16). In this case many phases are overlapped continuously, and the ripple stays very low with continuous output. It costs a little more than the original single-phase units but the

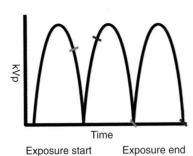

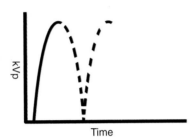

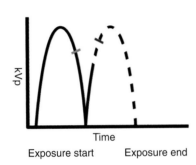

FIGURE 4-14 Example of incorrect exposure due to faulty timer. The timer must reset to zero after each exposure.

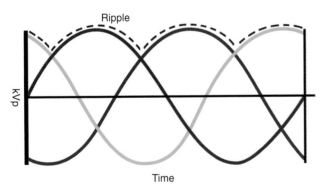

FIGURE 4-15 This is an example of three-phase power. The circuit now has three overlapping circuits and therefore very little loss of power when the cycle reaches zero. The small fluctuation at the top of the waveform is called ripple.

benefit of more x-rays for each exposure allows the technician to reduce the overall exposures, saving wear and tear on the x-ray unit and reducing the overall dose. Radiation dose and dose reduction are addressed in the section on techniques and technique charts (Chapter 6).

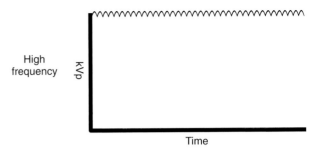

FIGURE 4-16 This is an example of the waveform of high frequency. There is a 3% ripple effect with virtually continuous output.

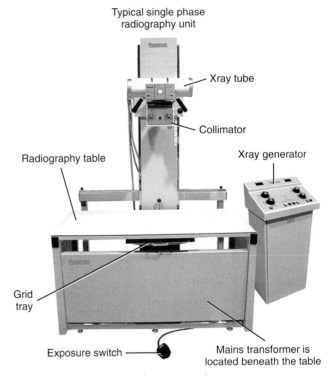

FIGURE 4-17 Typical x-ray unit with separate generator.

The Outside of the X-Ray Unit

We have looked at the inside of the x-ray unit. Let us have a look at the outside of a typical x-ray unit and then relate the dials and controls to what we have learned so far. In Figure 4-17, the generator is separate from the x-ray table and the tube. Note the three items essential to every x-ray unit: the control panel (sometimes called the generator), the x-ray tube, and the high-tension transformer (sometimes called the mains transformer) located beneath the table.

The unit also requires a dedicated power line. The x-ray unit cannot share a power line or source with another piece of equipment that draws a lot of power. The power that is required to activate a standard installed x-ray unit is 100 amperes fused at 80 amperes on a 220-volt single-phase power line. Its minimum power rating is 30 kilowatts.

On some units the generator is mounted above the table (Figure 4-18). This is fine if the staff is reasonably tall but it

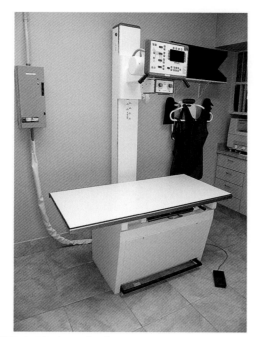

FIGURE 4-18 The Sedecal Veterinary X-ray Unit. The transformer is beneath the table; note that the operator controls are mounted in front of the x-ray tube. With short staff members, this arrangement can present a challenge.

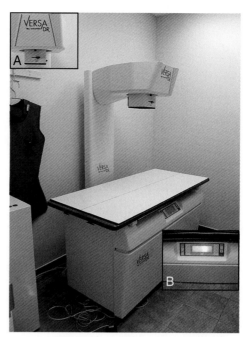

FIGURE 4-20 The Innovet line of high-frequency generators. **A,** Note that the x-ray tube and wires are encased within the tube stand. **B (inset),** Technique selection is located on the front of the table. The x-ray generator and transformer are located beside the table.

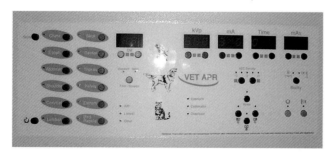

FIGURE 4-19 The operator console of a high-frequency generator with anatomical programming. This unit is the size of a computer keyboard and may be mounted in front of the x-ray tube, as in Figure 4-18.

can be very awkward if the technician is short because the readouts can be difficult to see. On the unit shown in Figure 4-17, the control panel of the generator is mounted near the x-ray tube.

In Figure 4-20 the generator is mounted with the high-tension transformer beside the x-ray table, and the x-ray tube and wiring are encased in the tube stand. (See inset Figure 20B).

Large Animal Portable X-Ray Units

Equine veterinarians must have the facility to travel to their patients and radiograph them on site. To do this, a small version of a full-sized x-ray unit has been developed. These units are not as powerful as the small animal units and they do not have the milliamperage that the larger units have.

However, because equine legs and feet are usually the areas of concern, the units are quite adequate.

In a large animal unit, the generator, transformers, and x-ray tube are all miniaturized and compressed into a very small space (Figure 4-21A-C). The newest unit on the market features a completely wireless system that combines digital radiography and portable large animal radiography (Figures 4-22 and 4-23A, B).

Diagnostic X-Ray Production

The x-ray circuit is now in place to receive incoming power. The step-up transformers will supply power to the cathode side of the x-ray tube. The filament circuit will heat the cathode to reach temperatures in excess of 2200° C (3900° F). The x-ray tube receiving this power is constructed not only to produce the electrons but also to convert those electrons into x-rays.

First we will examine the components of the unit and then discuss how everything works together.

The X-Ray Tube

There are various types of x-ray tubes for different applications. When x-rays are produced, the heat of the interaction of the photons and the anode is extreme. Each tube is sold based primarily on its future application. Small animal veterinary x-ray tubes are not as sophisticated as an x-ray tube installed in large animal facility, where the units are rated at 1000 mA three phase, 12 pulse, and are called upon to produce continuous x-rays for minutes at a time. Each x-ray tube has the same components but the differences are mainly

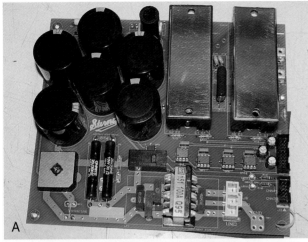

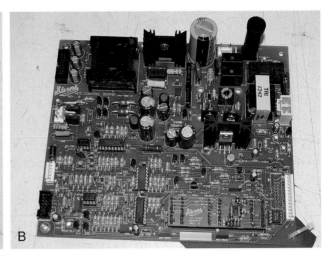

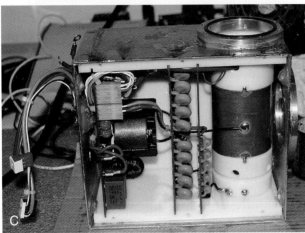

FIGURE 4-21 Components of a large animal x-ray unit. Each component duplicates the small animal unit. They are smaller and do not offer as many options for technique selection.

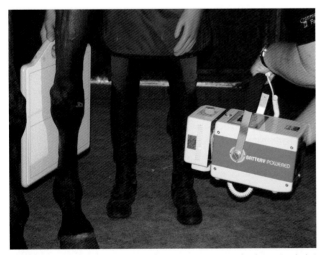

FIGURE 4-22 Wireless digital equine imaging. The laser (*red dot*) ensures the correct distance, and the lack of cords simplifies the imaging process.

to do with the cooling systems. Since the very first commercial x-ray tubes, the ratio of x-rays to heat has been very low; typically 99% heat and 1 % x-rays. This ratio has not changed over the last 100 years, but the method of heat transfer has enhanced the longevity and reliability of x-ray tubes.

The x-ray tube consists of a glass enclosure that houses a specialized anode and cathode (Figure 4-24). The glass enclosure is a special heat-resistant glass. PYREX is one brand of glass manufactured for x-ray tubes. The standard x-ray tube is approximately 30 cm long and approximately 20 cm in diameter. The external housing enlarges the tube to about 50 cm long and 30 cm in diameter.

The Cathode

The cathode of the x-ray tube is typically has two filaments (Figure 4-25). The filaments are very similar to a standard light bulb filament. They are made of thoriated tungsten, which can withstand very high temperatures without melting. The melting point of tungsten is 3410° C (6170° F). The large focal spot is typically 1.4 mm in width and about 1 cm in length. The small focal spot is typically 0.7 mm in width and 0.75 cm in length. Which filament is used is

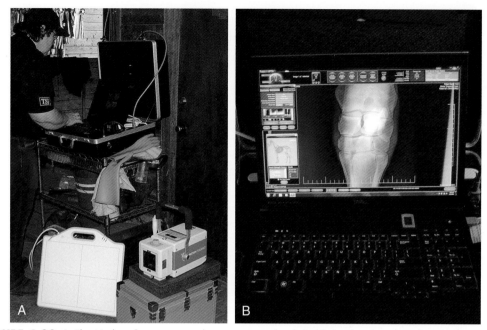

FIGURE 4-23 **A,** The Medison battery-operated x-ray unit paired with the Thales digital wireless plate. **B,** The image is sent wirelessly from the digital plate to the computer.

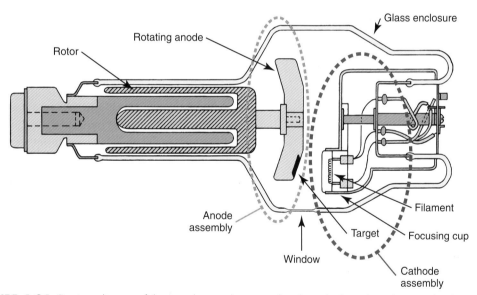

FIGURE 4-24 Cutaway diagram of the typical x-ray tube to visualize the cathode and anode. Note that the cathode is offset from the anode so that the electron beam is directed toward the outer ring of the rotating anode. The angle of the anode will deflect the beam at 90° towards the patient.

determined by the milliamperes on the x-ray generator by the technician.

The filaments are very carefully positioned opposite the anode in a small cup-shaped device called the focusing cup in such a way that they are aimed directly at the anode (Figure 4-26). The focusing cups are slightly negatively charged to focus the electrons that are boiled off the cathode filaments. The beveled edges are both designed to focus on very small areas on the anode. It is here, on the focal spot of

the anode, that x-rays are produced and it is from here that the exceptional amount of heat must be dissipated.

When the circuit is activated, the filament transformer sends electricity to the cathode (see Figure 4-24). The cathode temperature quickly rises and electrons are "boiled off" the cathode filament in a reaction called thermionic emission. The cloud of electrons that is produced is called a space charge, and the whole process is called space charge effect.

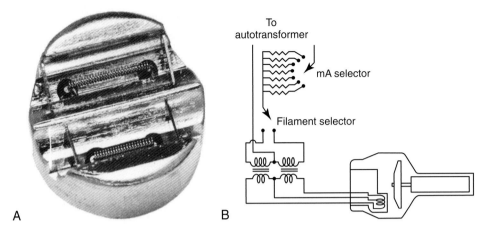

FIGURE 4-25 A, Cathode assembly. Note that the two filaments are much like a standard light bulb filament. **B,** The wiring diagram for the filament selector and the cathode assembly. Note that the cathode is offset so the photon beam is directed toward the beveled edge of the anode.

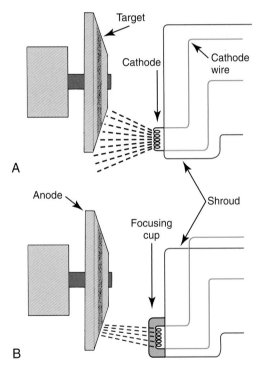

FIGURE 4-26 A, Without a slightly negative charge on the focusing cup, the electron beam spreads beyond the anode. (Similar charges repel one another in a mutually electrostatic repulsion.) **B,** With a focusing cup that is negatively charged, the electron beam is focused toward the target.

The Anode

The Rotating Anode

There are two types of anodes: rotating and stationary. Small animal installed x-ray units use rotating anodes and large animal portable units use stationary anodes. The anode material used for both stationary and rotating is tungsten or a tungsten molybdenum alloy. Tungsten has a high atomic number (74) and is well positioned on the table of the elements to absorb electrons and heat. Higher-grade anodes use a tungsten/rhenium alloy that hardens the anodes and makes them less vulnerable to overheating.

Mounted within the rotating anode is the target of the x-ray tube. Alloying the target area of the anode with tungsten/rhenium makes it more heat resistant and therefore longer-lasting than tungsten alone. The rotating anode is mounted on a stem that in turn is mounted on ball bearings. The entire structure rotates very rapidly once the circuit is closed, and the anode is prepared to receive electrons.

The anode serves several important functions. It mechanically supports the electron target. It serves as a thermal dissipator by directing the heat emitted in the production of x-rays along the stem as well as rotating so that the photons are not always focused on the exact same spot. It is also an electrical conductor. It receives the electrons emitted by the cathode and transmits them back to the high-voltage generator to complete the circuit.

The target of the x-ray tube is mounted on the disc of the anode. The outer edge of the disc is beveled at a very specific angle in order to direct the x-rays down toward the object being radiographed (Figure 4-27).

The Rotor Circuit

The rotor circuit is activated at the same time as the filament transformer starts to heat the cathode. The rotor turns the rotating anode. It will reach speeds of 3200 to 3600 revolutions per minute. The inside of the rotor shaft contains very-high-grade stainless steel bearings that are manufactured to withstand extremely high temperatures as heat is dissipated from the rotating anode.

As the x-ray tube ages, these bearings can distort and develop flat edges when they become very hot and then rest in one position. Because the bearings move rapidly when the rotor is turning the noise can become extreme.

If the bearings seize and the rotor does not rotate, the heat is directed to one tiny spot on the anode, the focal spot. The accumulated heat will crack the overheated anode

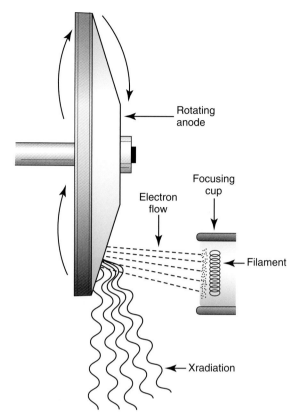

FIGURE 4-27 A rotating anode receiving electrons from the cathode and converting them to x-radiation, which is diverted toward the patient. The structure is a tungsten molybdenum alloy to assist in dissipating heat.

(Figure 4-28A-D). Usually at this point safety interlocks prevent further exposures.

The Stationary Anode

Equine portable units have a stationary anode (Figure 4-29). Because a lot of heat is produced during the exposure, the stationary anode must have an efficient method of dissipating heat as well as absorbing the photons and converting them to x-rays. The stationary anode is composed primarily of copper with a wide stem and a tungsten insert to handle the x-ray conversion and the high amount of heat produced during the exposure.

The end of the stationary anode is angled to direct the beam to the patient. Because the anode is not rotating to dissipate the heat, the technician must be careful to follow the warning and ready lights on the unit so the heat may dissipate between exposures.

The Line Focus Principle

The line focus principle (Figure 4-30) describes how the electrons interact with the anode and change direction so that the x-rays are directed toward the patient being radiographed.

The angle of the bevel on the outer edge of the anode and the resulting change of direction of the radiation is called the line focus principle. If the angle of the anode is less than 15

degrees from the vertical, the resulting x-ray beam will be very narrow and the image will have higher resolution. If the angle is greater than 15 degrees, the beam will be wider, resulting in less heat focused on a very small focal spot and decreasing the "bloom" effect on the focal spot. The typical angle for x-ray tubes in North America is 11 degrees. Depending on the angle of the anode and the choice of large or small focus, the size of the focal spot may become very small and therefore the sharpness of the final image has high resolution.

Off-Focus Radiation and Heat Bloom

When the exposure switch is closed, the electromagnetic function of the circuit takes effect. The cloud of negatively charged electrons is drawn across to the positively charged anode at a great rate. The interactions are in effect during the length of the exposure, and the stream of electrons interacts not only with the actual target but also with the areas of the anode immediately adjacent to the target. Occasionally the electrons "bounce" off the target anode and are then attracted back but at a point beyond the focal spot (Figure 4-31A). For this reason it is very important to ensure that the area of the glass envelope of the tube is supplied with a collar of lead so that any extra focal radiation, or radiation produced outside the actual focal spot, is absorbed by the collar and does not appear on the image as an artifact (Figure 4-31B).

Heat Dissipation

When the target is exposed to radiation over a number of exposures in a short time, the anode can become exceptionally hot, usually 1000° C to 2000° C (1832° F to 3632° F). With repeated exposures the focal spot will dissipate heat into the area immediately surrounding it, and this effect will enlarge the effective focal spot. The descriptive term for this is heat bloom. This is not likely to occur in a veterinary clinic because concurrent exposures rarely happen rapidly during the course of the day. Each x-ray tube is supplied with an anode cooling chart when it is installed. This chart graphically illustrates the cooling period necessary between exposures to prevent overheating of the x-ray tube. Large animal portable units typically have a safety shutoff that prevents overheating. In Figure 4-32, the anode cooling chart indicates that an interval of 5 minutes should be allowed for 60,000 heat units. Heat buildup can be a factor if the unit malfunctions, as evidenced in Figure 4-28.

To calculate heat units, multiply as follows:

Voltage • Current • Time • Constant (which in the case of a single phase unit would be 1.0) = Heat Units

At 80 kV • 200 mA • 0.20 Seconds • 1 3200 heat units, heat dissipation requires less than 1 minute. However, if continuous exposures were made, the heat buildup would be a multiple of that result, and at 23 exposures the heat units would exceed the safety factor.

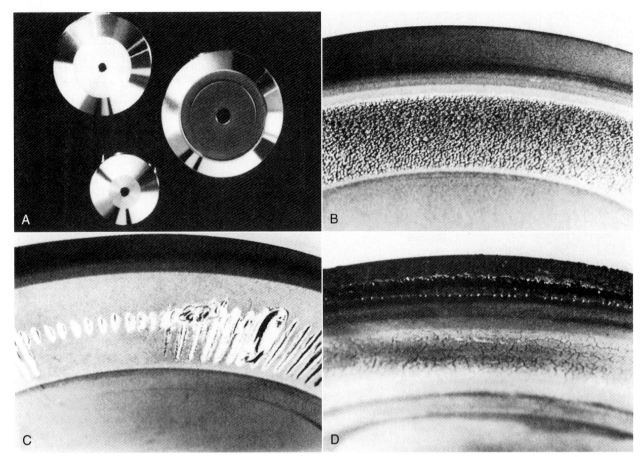

FIGURE 4-28 Effects of an x-ray tube overheating the anode. **A,** Three examples of new anodes; and three examples of anodes after failure. **B,** Slow rotation due to bearing damage; **C,** Repeated overload or overheating of the anode; **D,** Exceeding maximum heat storage capacity.

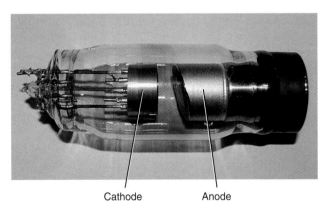

Cathode   Anode

FIGURE 4-29 A stationary anode with a tungsten target.

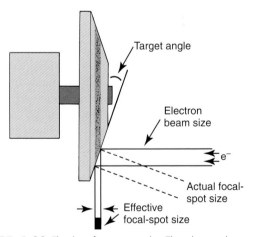

FIGURE 4-30 The line focus principle. The electron beam travels toward the anode. As it hits the target, it is converted to x-radiation. This radiation is directed downwards toward the patient, but because of the angle of the anode, the effective central ray is narrower, making the focal-spot size effectively smaller.

The Tube Rating Chart

An additional chart that is useful to determine the maximum exposure on an x-ray unit is the tube rating chart (Figure 4-33). This chart indicates the x-ray tube limits based on the equation mA • kV • time for the x-ray unit. In Figure 4-33, the maximum exposure at 200 mA is 80 kV and .005 seconds. This would not be a suitable unit for a clinic whose patients

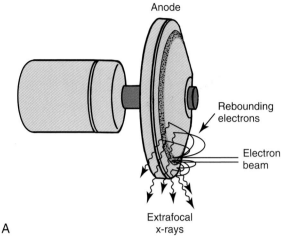

Anode

Rebounding electrons

Electron beam

Extrafocal x-rays

A

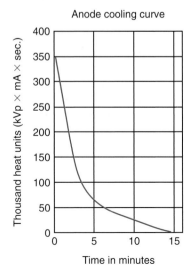

B

FIGURE 4-31 A, The production of off-focus radiation. B, Off-focus radiation has produced an image of the dog's ears beyond the limits of the collimator (*arrows*).

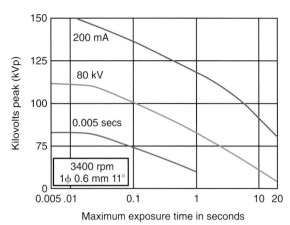

FIGURE 4-33 A tube rating chart for the small focus on a single-phase 150 kV, 200 mA unit.

Anode cooling curve

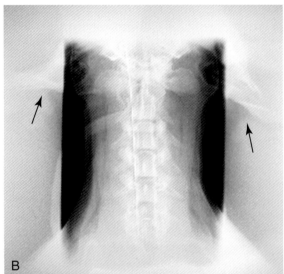

FIGURE 4-32 An anode cooling chart. Dissipation of 3200 heat units between exposures takes less than 1 minute.

included very large dogs, but it may work very well for a cat clinic.

Focal Spot Bloom

Another factor that affects the sharpness of the image is bloom. When the anode is bombarded with radiation it becomes very hot. The heat dissipates through the surrounding metal, but if the exposures continue throughout the day and the tube is not allowed to cool, the outer edges of the focal spot become hot enough to expand the size of the focal spot even though the heating effect of each individual exposure does not exceed the rating chart. A focal spot that started the day at 0.3 mm × 1 cm after several exposures can bloom to 0.45 or 0.5 mm. This will cause the image to lose sharpness, reducing resolution. The cause of the unsharpness is the increased area of the focal spot, as illustrated in Figure 4-34A. The effect is demonstrated in Figure 4-34B.

A focal spot bloom may also occur on a very old x-ray tube. The edges of the focal spot become enlarged and the images start to lose sharpness.

The Anode Heel Effect

Because so few x-rays are produced per exposure, it is important that the x-ray beam is used efficiently. The bevel of the angled anode limits the amount of x-rays being produced on the stem side of the anode; therefore, the intensity of the radiation is greater on the cathode side than on the anode side. This effect, called the anode heel effect, becomes important when a patient is thicker on one end of its anatomy than on the other. The thicker end of the animal should be placed on the cathode side to take advantage of the greater amount of radiation at that end. In Figure 4-35, the head end of the table with the higher amount of radiation would be to the right, and the foot end to the left. With any new or unfamiliar installation, it is important to note the anode and cathode positions of the x-ray tube and to ascertain the correct orientation. If one is not sure, a call to the service engineer should answer the question.

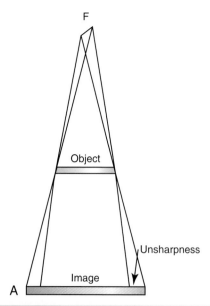

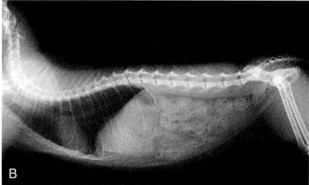

FIGURE 4-34 A, The geometric effect of an enlarged focal spot. B, The image loses resolution and unsharpness predominate.

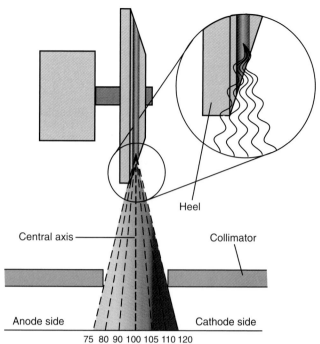

FIGURE 4-35 The anode heel effect. The radiation on the cathode side of the central ray is more powerful than the radiation from the anode side of the central ray.

The Exposure Switch

Finally, the exposure switch is the unit that sets the sequence of events in motion to produce the x-ray exposure.

Most small animal x-ray units have one two-stage exposure switch (Figure 4-36). The first stage activates the rotor and boosts the filament circuit and the transformers. The second stage activates the exposure through the x-ray tube. Technicians should become familiar with the noises that the x-ray unit makes when an exposure is in progress. If the first stage switch is engaged the rotor noise should become evident. If there is no rotor noise the switch should be released and reset. If the rotor does not activate, an exposure should not be attempted because there is risk of damaging the x-ray tube. If the rotor does not activate the anode and cause it to rotate correctly, the entire exposure it will be directed to one very small focal spot on the x-ray tube. This event will eventually melt the anode because the rotating anode tube is not manufactured to accept the full exposure in the same way as a stationary anode tube.

Figure 4-30 shows two examples of anodes that have been overheated and destroyed.

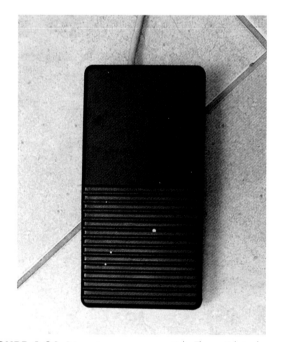

FIGURE 4-36 A two-stage exposure switch. The switch is depressed partway to initiate the rotor circuit and then all the way to initiate the x-ray exposure.

The exposure switch should be tested on a regular basis (annually) to ensure that it disconnects when the foot pedal is released. This "dead man" safety factor is a legal requirement to ensure that the x-ray beam is terminated at the end of an exposure.

If the first stage switch is activated and the sound of boiling liquid (actually oil) is heard, the exposure switch must be released and the attempt to expose the x-ray detector terminated. It is likely that the x-ray tube has "shorted out" and the filament circuit is overheating the cooling oil in the x-ray tube housing. This situation is very unsafe because the tube could explode if the full force of the tube voltage were applied.

Tube heat overload is an indication that the x-ray tube is overheated and will require a few seconds to cool before another exposure is attempted. This occurrence is very common on large animal mobile units. Waiting for the "ready" signal is a very important part of the radiography protocol that prolongs the life of the x-ray tube by not overheating it continually.

Exposure Switch Variations

There are several variations of exposure switches. A single-stage switch may be wired in so that the rotor begins when the generator is turned on. This is not ideal because the rotor should be activated only when the exposure is about to be made. If this is the case, the unit should be turned off between exposures and activated only when the exposure is about to be made.

The single-stage foot switch may also be wired in so that when it is depressed it initiates the rotor. There will be a safety delay until the rotating anode achieves the necessary speed. This installation is not efficient and should be revised as soon as possible because animals being radiographed are not necessarily cooperative and initiating the exposure depends on the timing when there is minimal patient movement.

Another variation is the hand switch. Most human units are activated with a hand switch. The technologist stands behind a screen and instructs the patient. When such a unit is sold to a veterinary facility, the hand switch should be replaced with a foot switch. Occasionally on a unit with an added foot switch, the hand switch is still active. This can be useful if there is a problem with the foot switch; the hand switch can be used during the time the service engineer is on the way.

SUMMARY

The x-ray unit is connected to a power supply that enters the building via a circuit breaker panel. There are three transformers in the circuit as well as a rectifier circuit. These controls enable the technician to select the correct technical factors to produce an image and ensure that the current travels through the x-ray tube in the correct direction. The filament transformer, which is activated prior to the exposure, ensures that the cathode of the x-ray tube is heated correctly in order to produce the free electrons necessary to close the circuit and produce x-rays. The anode attracts these negative electrons, which are drawn across to the target area, producing 99% heat and 1% x-rays. The line focus principle ensures that the x-rays are directed onto the object being radiographed. The anode heel effect uses the more powerful part of the x-ray beam at the cathode end of the x-ray tube.

CHAPTER

5

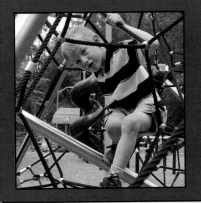

Imaging on Film*

It is change, continuing change, inevitable change, that is the dominant factor in society today. No sensible decision can be made any longer without taking into account not only the world as it is, but the world as it will be.

—Isaac Asimov, Russian/American Author, 1920–1992

OUTLINE

LEARNING OBJECTIVES

When you have finished this chapter, you will be able to:

1. Identify cassettes, screens, and film, and understand how they work together to produce an image.
2. Understand the purpose of screen and film speed and screen colors and how they affect the image.
3. List the characteristics of various commercial cassettes and screens.
4. Understand latent image formation.
5. Know the causes and prevention of artifacts on films.

APPLICATIONS

The application of the information in this chapter is relevant to the following area:

1. Producing x-ray images (radiographs) for evaluation and diagnosis.

*Disclaimer: Throughout this chapter, the author has referenced various commercial companies and their products. These references are not intended to favor or disparage any particular name brand but to point out problems that may arise and of which the customer should be aware during the use of the products. Every product that has survived in the market has merit, but it also may have flaws that are not evident within the first decade of its use.

Section One dealt with the functions of the x-ray unit and how x-rays are produced via an electric circuit through the x-ray tube. This chapter introduces the other side of imaging, the image receptor (Figure 5-1). Every x-ray image is produced using two completely separate systems. The x-ray generator produces the x-rays and the receptor receives the x-rays and produces the actual image.

> **POINTS TO PONDER** It is very important to remember the two separate components of the x-ray system. If one component is changed, say the receptor side, it is not always necessary to change the second component, the generator, transformer, table, and x-ray tube.

When we review various image receptors, we are immediately aware of how much imaging has changed over the years (Figure 5-2). As new concepts evolve and are manufactured, they are tested in the marketplace. This always leads to upgrades as each new x-ray unit is challenged by its supporters and its competitors. Every unit that is successful in the veterinary clinic has some merit. It may be smaller or larger, faster or more efficient to use, but each design changes as the imaging community demands even more convenience and better imaging.

Since Roentgen discovered x-rays just over 100 years ago, the field of imaging has evolved to encompass areas that could not have been imagined in the 1800s (Figure 5-3).

> **POINTS TO PONDER** The age and appearance of the generator make little difference to the final image. As long as the generator is calibrated correctly and the technical factors are correct, a 50-year-old generator will produce the same image as a brand new generator, all other factors being equal.

X-ray film was the common receptor until a few years ago. Now computers have taken over the medical imaging world, and veterinary clinics are rapidly following this trend.

A superior image is achievable only if a basic understanding of technical factors is incorporated into the process. The concept of simplifying the selection of technical factors beyond the control of the operator and to allow the computer to manipulate the image reflects the technical ignorance of the commercial vendor and the operator. A good solid background in radiation production and protection is vital if good imaging practices are to be maintained. We will address these specific issues when we discuss technique charts and digital imaging.

> **POINTS TO PONDER** Just as a camera must be set correctly to record the perfect image, so must the x-ray generator. A local camera store would be seriously remiss if they sold a digital camera with the concept that there is no need for operator training and support, or if the camera store told the proud new owner that there is no need to adjust the settings because every image can be optimized with post-processing. In photography, as in radiation imaging, if the image data is not recorded correctly, it cannot be created with post-processing.

A Brief History of Terminology

The term photography derives from the Greek words *phos* (genitive: *photós*) light, and *gráphein*, to write. From this the term radiographer denotes the technician or technologist who "writes with radiation." The very earliest term for radiographer, "skiagrapher," described a shadow writer, which is also appropriate.

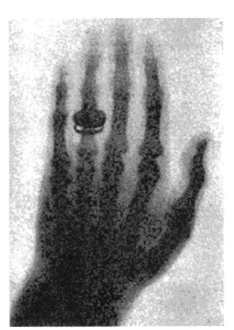

FIGURE 5-2 Imaging then. The first radiograph, the hand of Mrs. Roentgen. It also contains the first artifact; can you identify it?

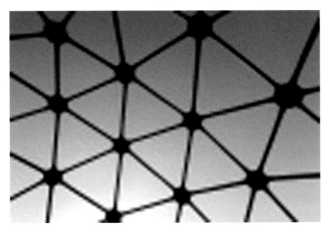

FIGURE 5-1 Imaging on film, any film, is similar to building a geodesic dome.

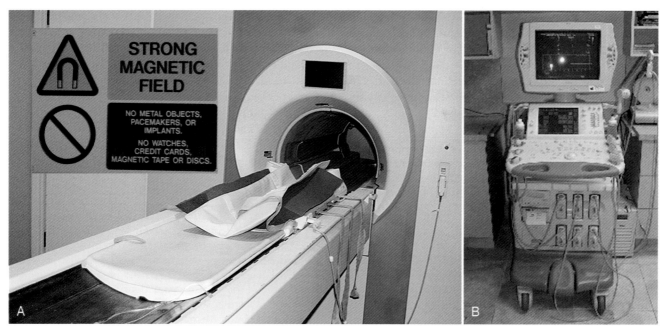

FIGURE 5-3 Imaging now. Magnetic resonance imaging (**A**) have evolved from radiography and (**B**) ultrasound, although neither modality uses x-rays to produce images.

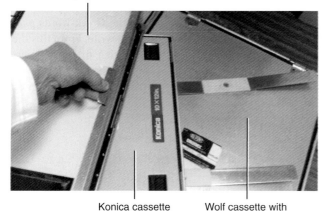

Kodak always yellow on back

Konica cassette
Double deck

Wolf cassette with
DuPont Hi Plus screens

FIGURE 5-4 Three different manufacturer's cassettes. Sometimes intensifying screens from a different manufacturer are mounted inside the cassette. Note that the cassette front shows where the film identifier is located; the cassette back identifies the type of intensifying screen enclosed.

FIGURE 5-5 Cassette fronts and cassette backs.

Film-Based Imaging

There are three receptor components to every film-based imaging system: the cassette (the film holder) (Figure 5-4), the intensifying screens (permanently installed within the cassette), and the film. Because each item is an integral part of the imaging system, the description of one item is incomplete without mentioning the other two. Each one is laterally important, so we will start from the outside and work in.

X-Ray Cassettes

The x-ray cassette is a film holder that has been designed to contain one pair of intensifying screens, attached to the front and back sides of the cassette, and one sheet of film of the appropriate size, which is placed between the screens.

The cassette front (Figure 5-5) is the side nearer the patient. The cassette back (Figure 5-4) is the side farthest from the object of interest. The cassette back usually contains the intensifying screen information. When the cassettes are opened they are placed on the counter with the face (or front side) down.

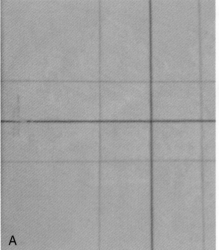
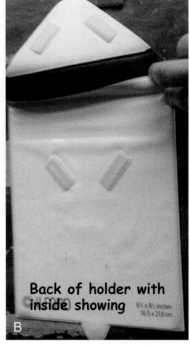
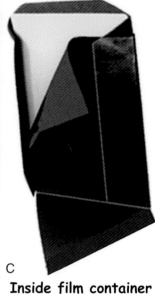

Front of holder   **Back of holder with inside showing**   **Inside film container flap folded down and screen installed**

FIGURE 5-6 A to C, Film holders were originally made of cardboard and later plastic. They usually had a paper liner and can still be used for small body parts (wings and rodent's feet).

Early cardboard and later plastic holders were used to encase the thinner and more flexible film since, unlike photography, the radiation penetrated the film holder (Figure 5-6). These holders were vulnerable to repetitive handling, and it soon became evident that a more substantial product was necessary. With the introduction of intensifying screens, the entire package needed to be protected by a holder that was sturdy and unbendable because the emulsion of the intensifying screen could be damaged if it was folded or bent.

The metal/Bakelite x-ray cassette was introduced in the 1930s. These film holders were substantial, addressing the problem of protection for the film. Transporting cassettes to and from the processing area required wheeled transport because multiple cassettes were very heavy. Manufacturers finally developed a cassette that met all the necessary criteria. An x-ray film cassette:

- must be sturdy so that it doesn't crack under the heavy weight of a patient or several cassettes in a pile.
- must not break apart in very cold conditions (equine radiography).
- must withstand considerable abuse during the course of many years of service.
- must be inflexible; must not warp if the patient's weight is unevenly distributed on the front.
- must have secure latches that do not come undone inappropriately, exposing the film to light.
- must have a radiolucent front that will not produce artifacts on the film.
- must have a balanced weight from back to front so that the cassette does not warp with age.

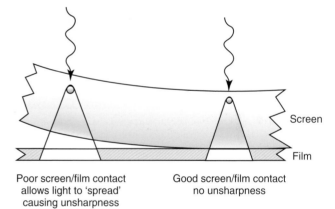

Poor screen/film contact allows light to 'spread' causing unsharpness   Good screen/film contact no unsharpness

FIGURE 5-7 The principle of poor film/screen contact.

- should contain a leaded foil back to absorb scattered radiation emitted from the patient.
- should contain some method of ensuring that the x-ray film is in good contact across the entire intensifying screen on both sides of the cassette (usually either foam or felt). Film/screen contact is essential to high resolution (Figure 5-7).
- must have material on the outside that is washable and impervious to most cleaning solutions, blood, and other effluents.

Film/Screen Contact

The intensifying screens must be held in the cassette in close overall proximity to the film. Any air gaps between the screen

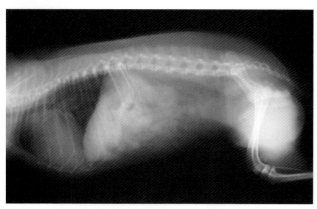

FIGURE 5-8 An image produced with poor film/screen contact. The structures are visible but appear fuzzy.

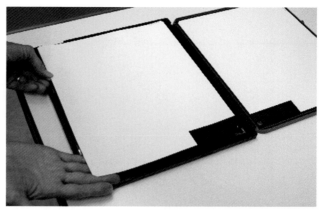

FIGURE 5-10 The front screen with the metallic backing is lifted and pulled forward, replicating the action of the magnetic rubber on the back screen. The front screen may be lifted to eliminate dirt and dust that may be trapped between the screen and the front of the cassette.

Magnetized rubber back
Metal foil fixed to back of screen

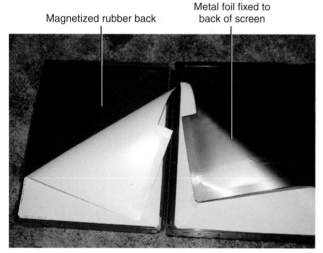

FIGURE 5-9 Agfa cassettes have a magnetized rubber back to "pull" the front screen forward to enhance film/screen contact. This design met with limited success.

and the film will result in a fuzzy image (Figure 5-8). Early cassettes had metal bars that locked under the edges of the cassettes (see Figure 5-4). These bars assisted with good film/screen contact, but many operators' fingers were pinched between the bars and the edges of these cassettes. This method was abandoned in favor of sliding bars that clipped closed (but also clipped open on the larger cassettes at inappropriate times).

Agfa cassettes (Figure 5-9) were made of a lightweight plastic that made the cassettes lighter to carry, but the overall design detracted from good film/screen contact. An Agfa cassette is equipped with a magnetized rubber insert on the back of the cassette and a metallic film beneath the screen on the front of the cassette. The front screen is loosely held in place so that it can be drawn to the magnetized back (Figure 5-10). The engineering was critical and expensive. The magnet, over time, lost its holding strength and contributed to loss of film/screen contact. These cassettes are clearly marked (they are bright orange and black) and should be

checked with a screen contact test tool regularly or if a problem is suspected (Figure 5-11).

Most companies use foam rubber, which is glued to the back of the cassette, holds the screen evenly and permanently with the correct amount of pressure against the front screen, and maintains the film in between in good film/screen contact.

> **POINTS TO PONDER** All cassettes are vulnerable to problems and should be reviewed every 6 months. The films should be removed in the darkroom (or the cassette should be left unloaded after use). The cassette should be examined under room light to ensure that the foam rubber has maintained its integrity and that the hinges and latches are in good working order. The screens should then be cleaned with gauze dampened with distilled water to remove any dust or fingerprints. The cassettes should be stood upright on the table top for a minimum of 10 minutes until the screens are completely dry.
> A record should be kept that notes any problems observed during the inspection.

Kodak cassettes (Figure 5-12) were rugged and sturdy with rubber edges and hinges, which worked well when they were new; as they aged or were subjected to extreme temperatures, however, the rubber hardened and cracked on the hinge side, and the cassette broke apart. Kodak also slightly bent the back of the cassette to improve film/screen contact. This worked well; however, it put extra strain on the hinge side which also compromised the rubber.

> **POINTS TO PONDER** Kodak cassettes can be turned around and used back to front if a particularly large anatomical area is being radiographed. We will discuss this effect further in the section on grids (see Chapter 8).

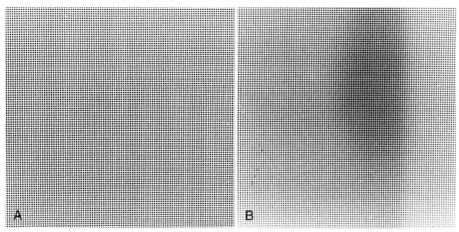

FIGURE 5-11 A, Confirming film/screen contact using a wire mesh test tool. B, The fuzzy area on the image demonstrates poor film/screen contact. A speck of dirt lies at the center of the reduced screen contact.

FIGURE 5-12 Split back on Kodak cassettes. Note that there is an intentional bend in the back of the cassette, designed to ensure good film/screen contact.

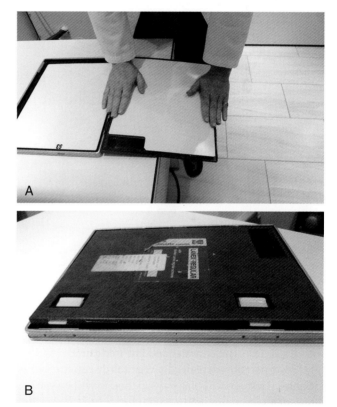

FIGURE 5-13 Correcting the decreased bend in a DuPont cassette. A, Place the back of the cassette lengthwise on the edge of a counter. Carefully press down firmly but gently on the overhanging side of the cassette. B, Test the cassette closure after each attempt to ensure that the tension is intact and that it has not been overbent.

DuPont also bent the back of the cassette slightly to enhance the film/screen contact. Over time, the bend decreased as the cassette was opened and closed hundreds or even thousands of times. This is easily corrected by placing the cassette over the edge of a table and lightly, carefully pressing gently but firmly on both ends of the back of the cassette (Figure 5-13). The other major problem with the DuPont cassette was the very tiny "handle" (Figure 5-14) that was added to assist the operator in opening the cassette. This worked well if the cassette back popped up when the cassette was opened but if the bend was eliminated and the cassette was opened without the back rising slightly it became very difficult to open the cassette once it was unlocked. Carefully rebending the cassette solves this problem.

Any kind of foreign material (Figure 5-15) will block the light of the screens from reaching the film. This is a particular problem with older Fuji cassettes. Fuji cassettes (with bright green backs) worked very well and were also used as replacement cassettes when the cassettes of other manufacturers broke down. Problems arise as the Fuji cassettes age; the rubberized foam, which provided excellent film/screen contact, breaks down (it is particularly vulnerable to commercial screen cleaners). The tiny bits of black foam cover the screens, which the technicians try to remove by cleaning, which then compromises the foam even more, causing myriad areas of radiolucency ("white dots") on the x-ray images. The only solution is to replace the cassette. The

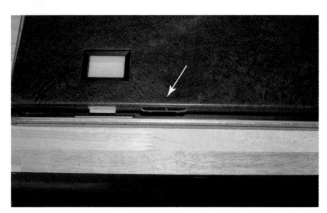

FIGURE 5-14 Back of a DuPont cassette with close-up of the tiny handle (*arrow*).

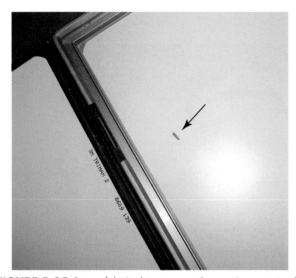

FIGURE 5-15 Piece of dirt (in this case a moth; *arrow*) on an intensifying screen will mask the light from the screen, causing a minus density artifact in the image beneath the foam.

screens are probably in good condition and can be installed into a replacement cassette once the black foam is removed with the use of distilled water and lint-free gauze.

3M Corporation developed a very sturdy cassette with a locking/latching system that was superior. It has become the cassette of choice for replacement of old, broken cassettes from other manufacturers.

> **POINTS TO PONDER** If the cassette breaks or is compromised, the intensifying screens are not necessarily damaged. They can be moved into another cassette that is still usable or into a new cassette shell.
> Changing screens is addressed in the section on intensifying screens.

Cassettes must be handled with care to ensure that the front remains undamaged and radiolucent. Any foreign material introduced into the cassette shell may show up superimposed on the image. Patient effluent, barium, or

contrast material can leak between the front of the cassette and the back of the screen. If seepage occurs, the screen and backing must be removed and cleaned thoroughly. Distilled water and gauze are the best cleaning agents because the screen emulsion may absorb other cleaning agents and thus be rendered useless.

Mud, dust, hay, and straw have been found between the screen and the front of the cassette in veterinary radiography practice. If an artifact is demonstrated in the same place on every image and the cause is not visible when the cassette is opened, then it is most likely that the culprit is between the foam backing of the screen and the front of the cassette. Agfa cassettes have a loose screen mounted on the front side of the cassette and are particularly vulnerable to this problem. The screen should be carefully raised, and the entire screen pulled towards the hinge. The cassette can then be examined with the use of a flashlight to reveal foreign material (Figure 5-10).

Intensifying Screens

Very soon after Roentgen discovered x-rays, he noticed that a paper covered with barium platinocyanide reacted quickly to the x-rays, converting them to light. Because he already knew that film is more sensitive to light than to x-rays, the logical conclusion was to convert the x-rays to light after they had penetrated the patient and to record the resulting image on glass plates coated with an emulsion that would maintain the image.

Barium platinocyanide was the first material used as an intensifying screen. Other physicists carried on his research, and in February 1896, the first commercial intensifying screen was developed. Thomas Edison, the founder of General Electric, applied for the first US patent; however, intensifying screens became widely used throughout the world within months of Roentgen's discovery of his rays.

Manufacture

The intensifying screen is composed of a base with an emulsion painted onto it. Often there is an adhesive layer that glues the emulsion to the base. Originally, the base was composed of cardstock, which was easily destroyed. Currently the base is a plastic/polymer, which is virtually indestructible. The emulsion adheres to the base with an adhesive layer. Removing the screens from one cassette to install into another cassette can be difficult, as some screen emulsions peel off the base and flake away as the screen is removed (Figure 5-16).

Characteristics

When the x-ray photons penetrate the front of the x-ray cassette and arrive at the intensifying screen, they are immediately converted to light by the phosphor in the emulsion of the screen. The intensity and color of the light depend on the components of the phosphor. This is one of the most important areas of imaging with film/screens. The speed (or rate) at which the x-rays are converted to light by the individual phosphors is called the intrinsic conversion efficiency

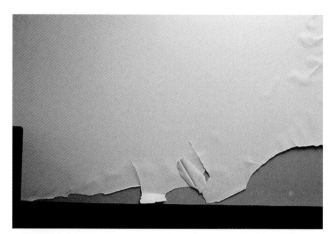

FIGURE 5-16 The screen emulsion may peel away from the base and flake.

FIGURE 5-17 Example of density 1.0 film.

of the phosphor. Each screen is rated by how fast or how slow the conversion occurs. It is this number that determines the speed of the screen (screen speed) or how fast that particular screen converts radiation to light.

Calcium tungstate emulsion (the older technology) has a 30% to 40% conversion efficiency.

The rare earth emulsion (the newer technology) has a 50% to 60% conversion efficiency. This means that less exposure time is required to produce an image on the film using rare earth intensifying screens than using film and calcium tungstate screens.

In order to make a comparison among the screens produced by each manufacturer, the concept of screen speed classifications was introduced. A standard film and rigidly controlled processing was used to test the system speeds. The speed of the system was measured by the amount of radiation required to produce a certain specific density on a film. The density chosen was 1.0 (Figure 5-17). This density is exactly in the center of the visible density range and is the density that is imaged in the middle of the ilium or in the

center of the cranium in a lateral skull on a correctly exposed radiograph.

Film has infinite resolution, so if the film alone, contained in the appropriate light-tight filmholder, is correctly exposed and processed under perfect conditions, a near perfect high-resolution image will be produced.

Problems arise because of the time of the exposure necessary to acquire that image. Original exposures in the early 1900s were measured in minutes rather than parts of seconds. Patients are not always cooperative, hearts beat, lungs move ribs, and abdominal contents roil and gurgle their way through the system, so a faster, more efficient method needed to be invented. An added benefit to using intensifying screens was the enhancement of contrast. When film alone is used on body parts greater than 12 centimeters, the amount of radiation required to expose the film causes scattered and secondary radiation to reduce the contrast dramatically to the point at which the anatomy is compromised, making diagnosis from the film nearly impossible.

The measurement of the rate at which the intensifying screen converts the x-ray photons to a produce a specific density on a film compared with the exposure necessary to produce that density without the use of intensifying screens is called the intensification factor. One example of a reduction in exposure time would be the technical factors required for a VD radiograph of a large (32 cm) dog's abdomen. All other factors being equal, the time required with no intensifying screens would be approximately 4 minutes (240 sec). The time required using 400-speed intensifying screens would be 1/10 sec (0.10).

$$IF = \frac{\text{Exposure without screens}}{\text{Exposure with screens}} = \frac{240}{.10} = 2400$$

The intensification factor is usually associated with a reduction in patient entrance dose, but the example here using time will suffice.

Until the 1970s calcium tungstate ($CaWO_4$) was the phosphor of choice for producing intensifying screens. In the 1970s a scientist at 3M in Minnesota was experimenting with phosphors during her research to collect light from distant stars. Several phosphors were identified as being very efficient at capturing photons. These phosphors all belonged to the group of elements known as the rare earths, so-called because of the difficulties encountered when extracting them from the earth. This discovery was shared throughout 3M, and the first rare earth radiographic intensifying screen was developed. In the early days, system speeds of up to 1200 were produced by 3M, but owing to a number of factors, the company settled on a 400-speed system. The first rare earth intensifying screens were marketed in the late 1970s by 3M. Kodak and DuPont followed soon after in the early 1980s.

Rare earth phosphors produce three to four times the amount of visible light per absorbed photon than the calcium tungstate phosphors. This means that the technical factors and thus the amount of radiation necessary to produce the same image density (optical density 1.0) may be considerably reduced with the rare earth phosphors.

Blue Systems	Green Systems
Screens Emit Violet Blue light	Emit Green or Blue-Green light
Require Blue receiving film	Require Green receiving film
Demonstrate various speeds of conversion efficiency	Usually demonstrate single speed of conversion efficiency

FIGURE 5-18 Blue systems versus green systems.

The older calcium tungstate screens are still available but are not recommended for use in any medical or veterinary facility.

The Blue/Green Question

Until 1981 all radiography film was manufactured to react to blue light from the blue-emitting intensifying screens (Figure 5-18). In 1981 Kodak introduced the rare earth Lanex intensifying screens, which emitted green light (Figure 5-18B). This event threw the imaging world into mass chaos. Now the competitive film companies, who were just perfecting the blue systems, had to "play catch-up" and manufacture two completely different emulsions, one intensifying screen emulsion and also a companion film emulsion. Also, Kodak introduced the 24 cm × 30 cm x-ray cassette, which replaced the standard 10 inch ×12 inch (25 cm × 30 cm) cassette. The added metric cassette was a marketing ploy that confuses people to this day.

The green screen technology was definitely a superior imaging system, and the research dollars spent to improve this system have definitely given it an advantage over the blue systems. As of the writing of this edition, blue systems are being phased out and eventually will not be supported as the production of blue-receiving film slows down and eventually ceases.

> **POINTS TO PONDER** It is vitally important to know which color system is in place at the veterinary facility (Figure 5-19). Ordering or accepting a delivery of incorrect film and trying to optimize imaging is a very common problem in the radiography room.

More about Color

A rainbow is the result of light travelling through the atmosphere. Each of the colors of the rainbow is refracted at a slightly different angle. This results in a perfect spectrum of color. Every time light is refracted, whether through a prism of glass, a sudden shower, or a perfect diamond, the colors remain in the same orientation and order. This arrangement is known as the visible light spectrum (Figure 5-19). Infrared is at the far "outside" of the curve with blue and ultraviolet on the "inside" of the curve. Violet morphs to blue then to green, yellow, orange, and red. This order is very important when we investigate x-ray film and intensifying screens. It is

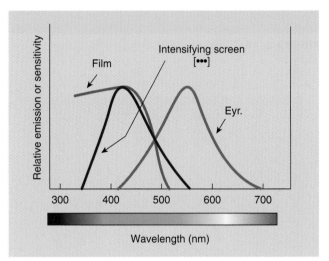

FIGURE 5-19 The importance of spectral matching. The film must be able to "see" the light emitted from the intensifying screen. In this case blue light is emitted and blue film overlaps the emission and therefore reacts to the light. The film would not see green light as it is too far removed, to the right of the spectrum, to be activated. It does however "see" a small amount of the blue light since there is a blue component in the green light.

vitally important when we set up a darkroom and use a safelight (see Chapter 8).

> **POINTS TO PONDER** If the film reacts to only the blue-green side of the spectrum, it will not react to the deepest red part of the spectrum. If it reacts to green, it will react to an orange yellow color because there is a yellow component in the color green. (Blue + yellow = green.)

> **CHECK IT OUT** The easiest way to identify the color of the screen in your facility is to remove the film from each cassette in the darkroom and store it in a light-tight container. Place the **open** cassette on the x-ray table under the x-ray tube, and set the factors on the generator, usually 100 mA, 1/4 (0.25) sec, and 70 kV. It is important to set a long enough time for you to be able to identify the color of the screen while the exposure is being made. Make sure the room is darkened and that the collimator light is off. Now make an exposure and watch for the screen to fluoresce.

The early intensifying screens were made of calcium tungstate ($CaWO_4$), which emits a very pretty blue-violet light. When the rare earth phosphors were developed, the striking difference apart from their rapid conversion efficiency was the color of their phosphor emission, a bright green-yellow. This changed the entire world of imaging. The x-ray film that had been developed to respond to blue light did not "see" the extended portion of the spectrum, the yellow-green portion. Therefore, a new film had to be developed that responded to blue light but also to yellow-green.

POINTS TO PONDER Many facilities today still have a problem confusing the film that is ordered.

Green-sensitive film must be used with green-emitting screens. Blue-sensitive film must be used with blue-emitting screens. Green-sensitive film "sees" the blue light portion of the green screens, but blue film does not react to the green portion of the green-emitting screens. If the incorrect film is used, the technical factors will have to be increased because the imaging is not optimized. This increases patient and staff radiation dose considerably and results in a less than optimal film.

If blue film is inserted between green screens, the images will be dull gray, lacking contrast that does not improve even if the technique is raised or lowered.

POINTS TO PONDER DuPont Quanta V screens were the answer to Kodak's Lanex Regular screens. They were never as successful and were eventually abandoned. The replacement technology led to the introduction of DuPont UV (Ultraviolet) screens, which moved the sensitivity to the left of the spectrum into the ultraviolet range. These screens had limited success. They were mostly successful with extremities and thinner body parts. They do show up in the veterinary market occasionally. The film to be used with these screens, if one attempts to use them, is blue-receiving film. They do not respond well to the light of green-emitting screens even though there is a minor blue component in the green light. Ideally the screens should be replaced.

We will visit this topic again when we discuss radiographic film, both blue-receiving film and green-receiving film. The concept is important and frequently confused.

Screen Speed

The conversion efficiency of the phosphor reflects the components of the x-ray screen, and unfortunately, not all screens are created equal.

With green screen technology, there are two screen speeds, fast and slow. (A medium-speed screen is available but not in general use.) The phosphor thickness is a factor in the screen speed but so is the thickness of the emulsion. Slower systems have thinner emulsions. The faster systems with thicker emulsions produce more photons of light per incident ray than the slower systems. This design reduces the radiation dose to the patient but produces poorer spatial resolution.

When a photographer, using film, takes a graduation picture, for instance, he or she visualizes the fine minute details of the dew on the rose and the twinkle in the graduate's eye. The film speed would reflect this detail at 32 or 64 ASA (American Standards Association). When the graduation party begins and the dancers come out in all their finery, the lights dim and a faster film speed is necessary to record the party. A film speed of 200 or 400 would record the faces of the participants but would not demonstrate the fine detail of the dancers. Later, at a beach party, where a bonfire lights the faces of the partygoers, a film speed of 800 or even 1200 will be sufficient to record memories. All of the film manufacturers agreed on this speed table and produced their films accordingly.

Translating this principle to radiography is consistent. The slower the screen speed, the more detail or higher resolution is evident on the image. However, in order to produce the same density on the film every time, more radiation must be used to produce an image from a slow screen than from a faster screen, just as a longer time must be taken to photograph with a 32 ASA film than with an 800 ASA film.

Over time, many applications were developed using a variety of screen speeds, and mixing and matching screens became quite common. This interchanging of screens was known as asymmetrical systems, and 3M was the company best known for this technology.

POINTS TO PONDER The cassette/screen manufacturers usually labeled the cassettes on the back to notify the user which screens were installed. 3M cassettes are often labeled 2/6 or 6/12; this labeling denotes an asymmetrical system.

In order to compare screen speed, the manufacturers agreed on a numbering system that we still use today. They used the DuPont Hi Speed Screen as a baseline and called it 100-speed class. It must be remembered that each manufacturer had its own concept of the speed of it particular phosphor "recipe," so the speeds were not all exactly the same; this is why we use the term "speed class."

For example, Kodak Lanex screens are a true 400-speed whereas DuPont Quanta 111 screens in the 400-speed class are actually closer to 350-speed. More radiation must be used with the Quanta 111 screens than with the Kodak Lanex screens to produce the same density on a film.

Table 5-1 lists the common manufacturers with the names and speeds of their systems.

Luminescence

Intensifying screens react to the incoming radiation by a process called luminescence. The photons of the x-ray beam are converted to light when they reach the emulsion of the screen.

TABLE 5-1	Table of Screen Manufacturers and Their Speed Classifications			
MANUFACTURER	**SCREEN NAME**	**SPEED CLASS**	**COLOUR OF PHOSPHOR**	**RARE EARTH?**
Agfa	Ortho Fine	100	Green	Yes
	Ortho Medium	200	Green	Yes
	Ortho 400*	400	Green	Yes—no longer available
	Ortho	400	Green	Yes
DuPont	Par	50	Blue	These screens were produced from 1960 to 1980 and are now obsolete. The speed of the screens has diminished to the point that they should no longer be used ever.
	Hi Speed	100	Blue	
	Hi Plus +	200	Blue	
	Lightning Plus	150	Blue	
	Quanta 11	300	Blue	Yes —no longer in use
	Quanta 111	400	Blue	Yes
	Quanta V	400	Green	Yes
	Quanta UV	400	Ultra Violet	Yes
Fuji	G4	200	Green	Yes
	G8	300	Green	Yes
	G12	400	Green	Yes
	HR	400	Green	Yes
Kodak	Xomat	200	Blue	No
	Fine	100	Blue	No
	Lanex Fine	100	Green	Yes
	Lanex Med	200	Green	Yes
	Lanex Regular	400	Green	Yes
	Lanex Fast	600	Green	Yes
Konica	KMC	200	Blue	Yes with type HB film
	KMC	400	Blue	Yes with type A film
	KF	100	Green	Yes
	KM	300	Green	Yes
	KR	400	Green	Yes
	KS	600	Green	Yes
3M Corp	2 or 3	100	Green	Yes
	6	200	Green	Yes
	12	400	Green	Yes

*Old Agfa screens often donated to a veterinary clinic demonstrated phosphorescence and would fog the film in the cassette as it waited to be used. Agfa's Ortho 400s had the most frequent problems.
3M corporation developed the technology to use the rare earth phosphors for intensifying screens and therefore had many more varieties and combinations than are listed here.

There are two types of luminescence: fluorescence and phosphorescence. Fluorescence is an instantaneous reaction that lasts exactly as long as the phosphor is stimulated. Phosphorescence (Figure 5-20) occurs when the phosphor continues to emit light after the stimulation has ceased. This is not desirable in medical imaging and is termed screen lag or afterglow.

Screen Aging Response

As intensifying screens age over time, the response of the phosphor reduces in brightness and speed, so that a screen that responded to the incoming radiation 100% when new will respond only 50% by age after 15 or 20 years.

The response of the screen both in brightness and over time is called screen speed. Technical problems arise as the products age, particularly with the technique chart. If older screens from various manufacturers are used in one clinic, the screens may react very differently and the images produced can vary widely in density and contrast. This is often the reason why a particular cassette is discarded, because "it doesn't work properly." Actually, it may be reacting to the x-ray beam correctly according to its manufacture, original screen speed, and age. It is very important to know which screens are in use at the veterinary facility and whether they are matched for screen speed and age.

POINTS TO PONDER Intensifying screens age very differently, and this feature greatly affects the imaging from cassette to cassette if a variety of different manufacturer's screens have been accumulated (Figure 5-21). The difference in the density from one image to the next could be as great as 800% with the use of identical technical factors if different screens are employed and/or if screens of varying ages are used.

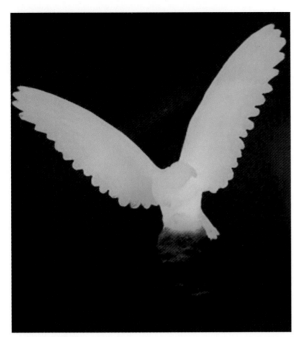

FIGURE 5-20 Phosphorescence: an example of a glow-in-the-dark eagle. The paint is often used on watch dials and glow-in-the-dark toys.

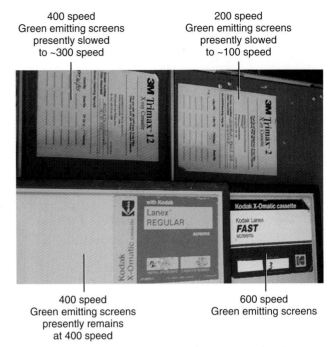

400 speed
Green emitting screens
presently slowed
to ~300 speed

200 speed
Green emitting screens
presently slowed
to ~100 speed

400 speed
Green emitting screens
presently remains
at 400 speed

600 speed
Green emitting screens

FIGURE 5-21 Various cassettes and screen speeds. The Lanex screens retain their original speed throughout their lifetime. Most other screens deteriorate in speed.

> **CHECK IT OUT** To identify the uniformity of the intensifying screens in your facility, first ensure that the generator is correctly calibrated and has good reproducibility. Next, place one cassette containing film on the tabletop and center it beneath the central ray. Open the collimators to the size of the cassette. Set the generator to 50 kV, 100 mA, 1/30 sec (3.3 mAs). (This is a typical technique for a 400-speed system. If your system speed is different according to the chart in Table 5-1, then adjust the mAs accordingly.)
>
> Process your film and record the density. Adjust the technique if necessary until the image is density 1.0 (Figure 5-17). Now, using the same technique, test all of the cassettes. (If you had to adjust the technique, then retest the original cassette.) Check the speed of the intensifying screens and compare them using the same illuminator with the room lights turned off. Slower screens produce a lighter image; faster screens produce a darker image. Ideally, all images should be the same density.

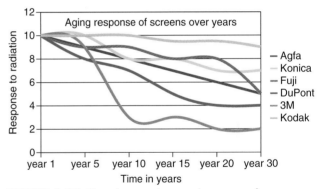

FIGURE 5-22 Chart depicting the typical responses of screens over 30 years. This is not the result of a controlled experiment but rather an observation over 50 years of imaging consultation.

Figure 5-22 roughly illustrates the reduction in speeds of intensifying screens as they age. This is not the result of a scientific experiment but rather illustrates years of observation and technical consultation in many different clinics and medical facilities under various circumstances.

If there is a mixture of various manufacturers' screens in the facility, there is most likely a wide variation in the speeds of the intensifying screens. In this case, adherence to a standard technique chart is impossible, as is the production of consistent, optimized radiographs.

Intensifying screens are frequently replaced in cassettes but the change is not necessarily noted on the outside of the cassette. A cassette label may note that it contains Quanta 111 Screens installed in 1982; the actual screens may be Fuji HR or Kodak Lanex Regular installed very recently.

> **POINTS TO PONDER** If there is a problem with imaging, the first place to investigate is always the film/screen combination. It is common for the incorrect film to be ordered or even supplied by the film dealer. Checking the film/screen combination is the easiest place to start the investigative protocol.

Screens are always labeled in very fine print on the edge, usually along the long side (Figure 5-23). The imprinting is very tiny and sometimes hard to read, but it is essential that the operator is aware of the phosphor emission color and the screen designation.

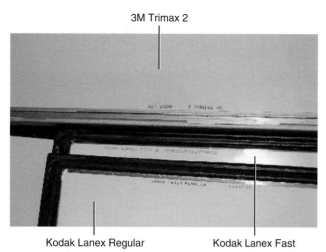

3M Trimax 2

Kodak Lanex Regular   Kodak Lanex Fast

FIGURE 5-23 Screen Stencils: 3M and Kodak. The numbers identify when the screen was manufactured and the batch number.

Screen Artifacts

Screen manufacturers occasionally produce a product that works well in the dry, clean atmosphere of a human hospital but develops major problems when it is sold to a clinic in a dusty or humid environment or does not age well beyond the first year of its use.

DuPont Quanta 111 and Quanta UV screens are examples of this problem. In the late 1980s the company changed the formula for the production of the Quanta 111 screens. The new formula worked well in the dry atmosphere of a medical facility but it had a tendency to absorb moisture, which caused swelling of the emulsion of the intensifying screens (Figure 5-24). The swelling appears as tiny raised points usually along the edges of the screen at first and then gradually working their way toward the center of the screen. It may appear as bubbles as well, and the emulsion may peel off in severe cases.

The lattice network of the undeveloped image is very tenuous, and the tiny points of the swollen emulsion shatter the newly formed network. This appears as tiny points of "unexposed" or clear film on the final image. These minus-density "points or dots" seriously compromise the image.

The screen cannot be repaired or dried out because the swelling is irreversible.

The best example of the effect of humidity in my experience was in the office of a large animal veterinarian who placed an autoclave in the darkroom with the Quanta 111 screens and cassettes. Steamy autoclaves should always be placed well away from both films and screens.

Chemistry Spills

Loading and unloading of the cassette in a veterinary facility are always completed in a darkroom. This may be a room specifically set up to process films or it may be the radiography room, which has been adapted to double as a darkroom. Darkrooms can be very small, cramped, and inefficient. It is very important that, in any darkroom, the cassette is opened and the film is removed without any possibility that

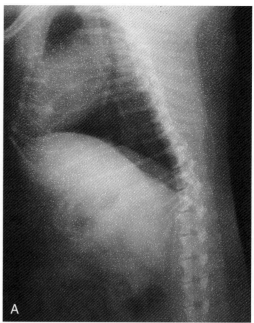

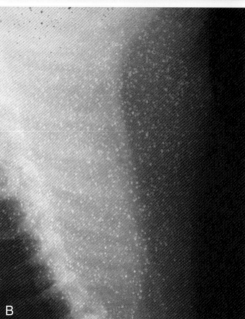

FIGURE 5-24 A and B, Example of Quanta 111 screen artifact. The pinpoint swellings of the screen emulsion desensitize the lattice network in the film and produce a null exposure artifact.

chemistry will be splashed on the intensifying screens (Figure 5-25). The protocol in a very small darkroom should be as follows: the exposed film is removed from the cassette; the cassette is closed; the film is placed in the developer or automatic processor; the replacement film is removed from the box and inserted into the cassette.

Smudges on screens mask the light from the screen and prevent its full intensity from reaching the film. If the smudge overlays anatomy, the smudge can replicate pathology such as a renal or bladder calculus. If a pathologic finding is demonstrated in exactly the same place on several radiographs, a screen artifact should be suspected.

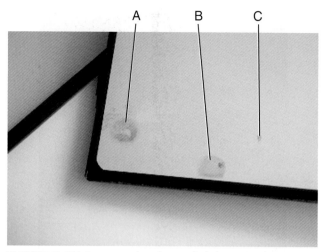

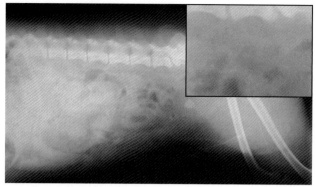

FIGURE 5-27 Screen emulsion becomes worn over many years. The thinning emulsion is not as effective at converting x-rays. The lighter areas on the film replicate the wear areas of the screen. The insert demonstrates an enlarged part of the indistinct image due to screen wear.

FIGURE 5-25 Screen smudges from spilled chemistry. A can be fixer or developer or both; B can be near the outside edge or in the middle; a small drip (C) may look like pathology on a radiograph.

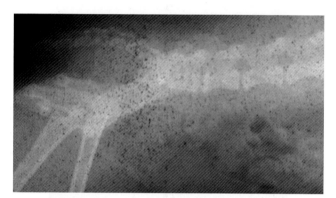

FIGURE 5-26 Screen cleaners can build up residues, which eventually cause artifacts on the film as they mask the light from the screens.

Screen Cleaners

A number of commercial screen cleaners have been introduced over the years. There are also a several home remedies for cleaning screens. A commercial screen cleaner can stain a screen if the particular brand does not match the brand of the screen. Screen cleaners can also leave a residue that builds up over the years and causes artifacts on the image (Figure 5-26). If screen cleaners are mandatory for whatever reason, they should be used once per year followed by a distilled water rinse to remove the residue.

Home remedies such as alcohol and other cleaning agents should never be used on screens because they can dissolve the protective layer and damage the emulsion.

The best screen cleaner that is readily available is distilled water, which is used as follows:

1. Open the cassette and remove the film in the darkroom.
2. Lay the open cassette on the x-ray table.
3. Dampen a 4″ × 4″ (10 cm × 10 cm) gauze wipe with distilled water. The gauze should be damp, not wet.
4. Wipe the screen lightly in one direction then wipe again at 90°. The screen should be very slightly damp with no

visible water marks. Any surface dirt or dust is removed by this technique.
5. Stand the cassette upright on the table and leave it to dry for at least 15 minutes. The cassettes should be stood upright in order that dust in the room does not settle and adhere to the screens.

> **POINTS TO PONDER** Commercial screen cleaning agents are often specific to the manufacturer and can stain screens that are manufactured by other companies.
> Screen cleaners often build up a residue, which eventually becomes visible on the images. Distilled water and lint-free gauze are the best combination to use to clean screens.

> **POINTS TO PONDER** It is very important that a screen is completely dry prior to reinserting the film. Film emulsion is manufactured to absorb moisture rapidly, and any remaining moisture on the screen would be absorbed into the film emulsion and would adhere to the screen, ruining the film as well as the screen.

Stains and scratches that have penetrated the emulsion of the screen are not removed by the technique just described. If the emulsion from the screen is missing, there is no way to repair the screen.

Older screens exhibit wear artifacts (Figure 5-27). Over many years of use, the emulsion of the screens thins and then disappears completely as thousands of films are inserted into and removed from the cassette.

In both cases, the screen should be replaced with one of similar speed.

Radiography Film

Several companies manufacture film, and several more cut and sell the film. The one standard among all these companies is the film size (Table 5-2).

TABLE 5-2	Table Outlining Film and Cassette Sizes; Metric versus Inch*	
FILM SIZE IN INCHES	**FILM SIZE IN CENTIMETERS**	**TYPICAL IMAGING USE**
6 × 8	18 × 24	Available in limited quantities
8 × 10	20 × 25	Equine and extremity
10 × 12 (25 cm × 30 cm)	24 × 30	Equine and feline, also skull and extremity
11 × 14	28 × 35	General radiography
	30 × 35	General radiography
14 × 17	35 × 43	General radiography

*Some of the inch sizes do not have an equal-sized metric partner, as is the case with the cm sizes.

Film is sold in very specific sizes to match the sizes of the cassettes. It is important to know what size cassette is in use in the facility and then to order the appropriate size film.

Kodak's introduction of the 24 cm × 30 cm film and cassette made the industry even more complicated. Film price is based on the square inch of the product. A box of 25 cm × 30 cm film (traditionally 10 inches by 12 inches) is more expensive than the 24 cm by 30 cm film introduced by Kodak and now sold universally. 25 cm × 30 cm film will fit into a 24 cm × 30 cm cassette only if it is cut down to size in the darkroom; 1 cm must be removed from the long side. This is a lengthy procedure and unnecessary if the correct size is originally ordered. Also, it is expensive to order the incorrect film in terms of both time and money.

World's First Human Portrait

The earliest x-ray images were produced in a darkened room using an emulsion painted onto a glass plate. This system was very much like the early days of photography, when glass plates and draped cameras recorded family portraits.

In 1839, Robert Cornelius, a Dutch chemist who immigrated to Philadelphia, took a daguerreotype portrait of himself outside his family's store and made history: He made the world's first human photograph!

It soon became obvious that clearer, more usable film bases were necessary to enable photographers to record historic events.

The earliest image receivers were glass plates. These plates had a light-sensitive emulsion but were very awkward and heavy. The glass tended to shatter easily, injuring the operators and destroying the image.

Prior to World War 1 (1914–1918), there was a shortage of good quality optical glass. The glass plate manufacturers investigated film bases that would be flexible and unbreakable.

Cellulose nitrate was introduced as a film base in 1914. A major problem with this material was its flammability; after several tragic hospital fires in which patients and staff died because of the noxious emissions from the breakdown of x-ray products, a nonflammable base, cellulose triacetate, was introduced in the 1920s. One problem with cellulose

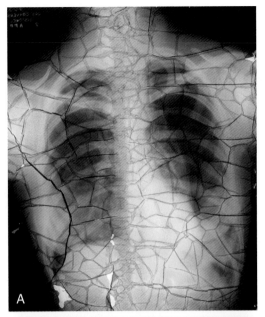

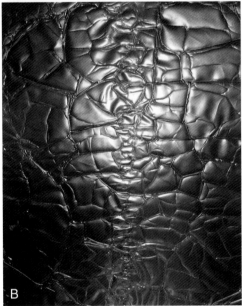

FIGURE 5-28 A, Cellulose acetate base; human chest radiograph. B, The film base has slowly shrunk over a period of 40 years, buckling and bubbling the fragile emulsion layer.

triacetate that did not show up until years later was its tendency to shrink when it was stored for long periods of time (Figure 5-28).

The old emulsions on the original film bases took a very long time to react to light or x-rays, and some exposures took as long as 10 minutes. Processing the images was a lengthy procedure. So along with the new film bases, more and more efficient emulsions were investigated.

The cellulose triacetate base was used into the 1960s, when DuPont introduced the film base that is in use today. Along the way the company also invented Nylon, Dacron, Kevlar, and many other related substances, but their major achievement in imaging was the invention of Mylar. Mylar has been used in medical imaging for about 50 years. Prior

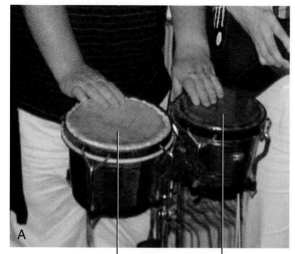

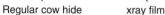

Regular cow hide   xray film

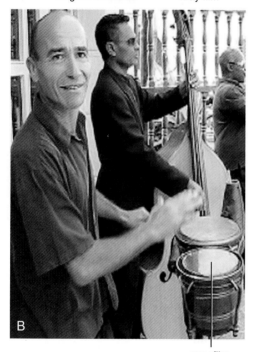

xray film

FIGURE 5-29 A and B, One use for recycled radiography film!

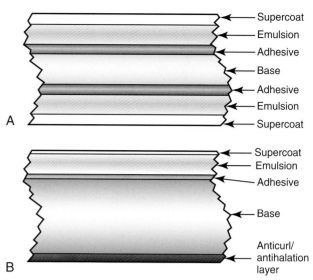

FIGURE 5-30 Cross-section of (A) double-emulsion film and (B) single-emulsion film.

Composition of Radiography Film

The x-ray film base is translucent and flexible. Light-sensitive film emulsion coats either one (single-emulsion film) or two sides (double-emulsion film) of the base (Figure 5-30). Between the base and the emulsion is an adhesive layer that is so thin it is basically incorporated into the emulsion layer. The supercoat is a hard protective gelatin layer on top of the emulsion that protects the image from the rigors of processing. This is only somewhat effective, so film should always be handled with respect because the emulsion on a preexposed film and the image on a post-exposed film is very tenuous and easily compromised.

Double-emulsion film contains a dye layer that prevents crossover effect from the light of one intensifying screen affecting the opposite emulsion (Figure 5-31).

Single-emulsion film requires an anticurl/antihalation layer on the nonemulsion side. Halation is the effect of the light being reflected off the back of the film base and affecting the image by causing a shadow effect (Figure 5-32). The antihalation layer is removed during film processing. Single-emulsion film is easily identified even in the darkroom under safelight conditions. The side with the emulsion is dull, and the side with the anticurl/antihalation layer is very shiny.

Double-emulsion film is used in general radiography. Single-emulsion film is used in special applications, such as high-resolution imaging and in laser imaging printing for computed tomography and magnetic resonance imaging.

Film Base

The base material that holds the emulsion of the film must be strong yet flexible. It must bend without stretching, and it must be stable throughout changes in temperature and humidity. It must be rigid enough to hang on an illuminator and yet flexible enough to travel through an x-ray processor. Most of all, it must be consistently and uniformly optically translucent. It must permit the transmission of light without adding any artifacts to the final x-ray image.

to the introduction of Mylar, if the film became caught in a processor, it would tear apart and be destroyed. With the introduction of a film base that was nontearing and inflammable, the x-ray film became virtually indestructible.

POINTS TO PONDER Recycled radiography film has been used in many applications once its life in the medical world is complete, including in gardening, to prevent drainage from raised beds; as windows in third-world countries, and as heads of bongo drums (Figure 5-29)! When the time comes to dispose of used film, the radiographer should always make sure that the recycler is actually destroying the film by shredding or should remove any patient identifiers from each film.

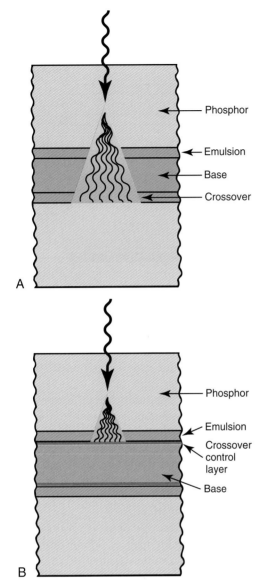

FIGURE 5-31 A and B, Dye layer (orange layer) that prevents crossover from one emulsion to the other.

The film base must also be thin enough that when the image is produced, there is no crossover effect (reflection) from one side of the image to the other (see Figure 5-32).

In the 1960s it was discovered that the addition of a slight blue tint to the film base enabled the radiologist reading the images to work for longer periods without experiencing eyestrain and headaches from the glare of the illuminators transmitted through the lightly exposed or unexposed portions of the film (see Chapter 7).

Film Emulsion

An emulsion (Figure 5-33) is a material that is coated onto the film base by means of an adhesive material to bind it to the film base. Film emulsion starts with very-high-quality gelatin. Yes, that is the same gelatin that is used in cooking and JELL-O. The gelatin used in this application is very high quality and completely translucent. The photosensitive

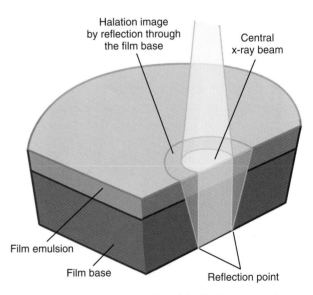

FIGURE 5-32 The halation effect. If the film has two emulsions and no antihalation layer, there will be a crossover effect.

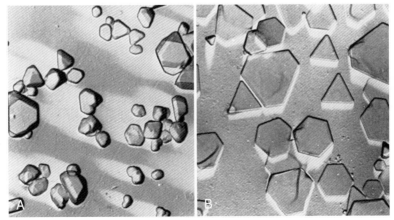

FIGURE 5-33 Magnified portion of the film emulsion. (**A**) Represents old technology silver halide crystals; (**B**) new technology using tabular grain silver halide crystals.

products within the emulsion are mainly silver bromide (about 95%–98%), silver iodide, and silver chloride. There is very little silver chloride in film emulsion today. Collectively, the term silver halide is used to describe the components of the emulsion.

The gelatin base must allow the processing chemicals to infiltrate the emulsion and react with the silver halide crystals to produce the image. It must be uniform; its thickness is usually .0002–.0004 inch (5–10 μm), depending on the manufacturer, and it must be flexible enough to permit bending without stretching as the film winds its way through an automatic processor.

The Supercoat

The outside of the film is protected by a tough coating of hard protective gelatin, the supercoat, that has been treated to prevent tearing, scratching, and abrasions to the film as it is loaded into the cassettes and then processed either manually or automatically. The film can be damaged by rough handling as it is removed from the film box and placed into the cassette (Figure 5-34).

It is important to note that once the film is wet, the gelatin absorbs moisture and the supercoat becomes vulnerable to scratches and abrasions (see Chapter 8).

Latent Image Formation

POINTS TO PONDER This theory is called the Gurney-Mott theory after the two scientists who first postulated how the image is formed within the emulsion. It has never been proven and therefore is still a theory of image formation.

The film emulsion with the silver halide particles suspended in a gelatinous layer also contains sensitivity specks (centers), small physical imperfections within the network of the silver halide. It is these small areas that become magnets for the silver particles to adhere to one another and form an image.

POINTS TO PONDER It is important to note that if the silver halide were perfect, without any imperfections (sensitivity specks), the image would not form and the film would exit the processor with no discernible image. When film is first manufactured, it must remain in the warehouse for a time in order for the sensitivity specks to settle within the emulsion. This process is called aging or seasoning.

According to theory, the latent image is formed within the emulsion of the x-ray film when the x-rays and light activate the silver particles in the film emulsion. The silver particles are attracted to the sensitivity specks by electromagnetism. It is believed that there must be at least three silver atoms to each sensitivity speck in order for the image to form. The term latent image refers to the image that is formed but is invisible until it is processed either manually or in an automatic processor. This new arrangement of silver halide particles is called the lattice network. It is a tenuous arrangement and may be easily destroyed.

Its structure is much like the jungle gym in a park (Figure 5-35). The joints of the bars are the sensitivity specks. High-detail film contains more sensitivity specks than general radiography film and therefore produces a more detailed image. The silver compounds now wait until they are processed in order to produce a manifest image.

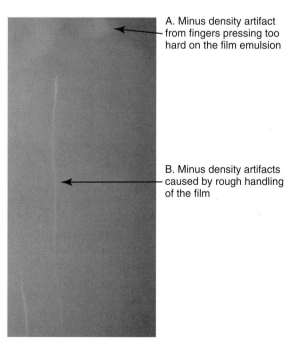

A. Minus density artifact from fingers pressing too hard on the film emulsion

B. Minus density artifacts caused by rough handling of the film

FIGURE 5-34 Abrasions on image resulting from film mishandling by roughly removed from the film storage box.

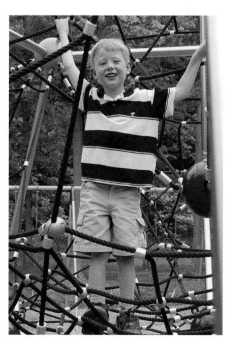

FIGURE 5-35 A lattice network. It is similar to the lattice network that forms when an image is produced on a film. The balls and joints are the sensitivity specks drawing the silver ions together to form the network or lattice.

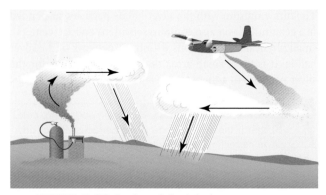

FIGURE 5-36 Seeding of clouds by human intervention.

The lattice network forms very much like the seeding of clouds to cause rain. The water droplets require impurities in the clouds to form rain, and these impurities can be added naturally by the wind raising dust clouds or mechanically by an airplane dropping dust onto the cloud (Figure 5-36). In this case the impurities—sensitivity specks—are built into the film emulsion, and the catalyst to start the process of latent image formation is the introduction of photons of light and x-rays. The actual physical process is still somewhat a mystery, but it is known that the image forms around the sensitivity specks electromagnetically and that at least three freed silver atoms must be deposited for a clump of black metallic silver to be formed by chemical development later in the processor.

The latent image is fragile. Just like the Tinkertoy maze of long ago, the network is very easy to break. Dropping a cassette from a height will destroy the network and cause an artifact of streaks radiating from the point of impact. Time will also cause the latent image to start to fade, although it does take a fairly long time (in excess of 24 hours) to fade completely. The lattice network will form a denser (darker) image the more it is exposed to radiation, light, and heat. A continuous heavy pressure on the unexposed film will prevent the lattice network from forming or break down what has already formed, leaving a clear area outlining the area of the pressure. This is why the film and cassettes should always be stored in an upright position in the darkroom and never flat on the counter.

Base + Fog

When the film is originally manufactured it will process completely clear except for the base + fog that is inherent in the film manufacture. After the film seasons, or matures, to the point that it can be sold and put into practice, it will develop a low fog level. In other words, if a brand new film out of a new box is processed, it will have a very low density, usually an optical density of (O.D.) 0.10 to 0.15. This is the evidence that the sensitivity specks are active and will convert any radiation into metallic silver during processing. Whenever film density is discussed, the base color and the fog level are always included as part of the image (e.g., density 1.0 plus base/fog).

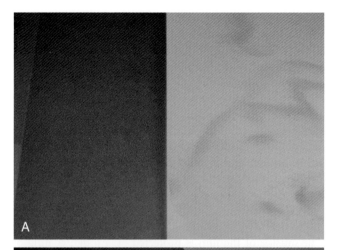

FIGURE 5-37 There are two film/screen systems on the market today. Green is the color of preference, but some facilities still use blue. Four brands of film are illustrated here, two blue and two green. **A,** Blue light receiving film is physically green. **B,** Green light receiving film is physically violet.

The base/fog level is usually minimal in unexposed film. However, if the film is exposed to unsuitable storage conditions and then exposed to radiation, the base/fog will be dark enough to compromise the contrast of the radiograph, because the clear areas will no longer be visible, having been replaced instead by a fog density of 0.20 to 0.29.

Film Response to Light

Film Colors

Modern film responds to the light emitted from the intensifying screens. This light may be either blue or green. This is an area that causes the most confusion in any veterinary facility. It is also one of the most important concepts in the practice of film/screen imaging.

Blue-emitting screens require blue-receiving film. Confusion arises when the blue dye used in the base "mixes" with the yellow color of the emulsion. The film becomes physically green in color (Figure 5-37A).

In order to prevent confusion with the physical appearance of the film and also to add an antihalation dye to the green-receiving film, the manufacturers all agreed to a violet dye for the green film (Figure 5-37B).

Rather than preventing confusion, this step added to it, and to this day, green-receiving film is physically violet and blue-receiving film is physically green.

Film Speed

Because the manufacturers already had an emulsion in place they decided to see whether they could increase the speed with which the film reacted to the x-ray photons. This was somewhat successful but mostly the speed decreased.

DuPont took advantage of the speed reduction and marketed a very successful combination of half-speed film and full-speed screens (Cronex 10T [now Agfa 10T] and Quanta 111 Screens). This combination is still in veterinary facilities today, although the image quality has degraded considerably with the age of the screens. Konica and Fuji followed suit with Konica HB and Fuji RX-U.

3M had been using various film/screen combinations prior to that and had reasonable success. What is important for our purposes is that there may still be some half-speed film stored away somewhere that may arrive at your facility.

The other film that may be available today in certain geographic locations is extremity film and/or single-emulsion film. It is important to note that single-emulsion film has emulsion on one side and an antihalation layer on the other side.

Single-emulsion film reacts to radiation and light from the screens only on the side with the emulsion, and it is far slower than double-emulsion film. Single-emulsion film is used in certain specific applications in which exceptional detail is required. It may be used in some equine practices when tiny spurs, spicules, or hairline fractures are suspected. It can also be used in wildlife practices to diagnose fractures on the wings of birds or within reptiles. Single-emulsion film requires considerably higher doses of radiation to produce an image, so it is definitely not recommended for routine veterinary examinations. Typically it is only available in 8 in × 10 in, 24 cm × 30 cm, and 10 in × 12 in sizes.

Other films, such as duplicating film and laser films, are not in wide practice in veterinary medicine. It is always good practice to examine every box of film that has been delivered from the supplier to ensure that the correct film has been shipped. The type of film and the code number are clearly marked on the front and/or side of the film box.

Film Speed and White Box Film

Film speed is the most difficult factor to control in the production of the film itself. Mixing emulsions is a little like following a recipe from a list of dissimilar ingredients. A little of many different components, depending on the manufacturer, are mixed in with a lot of gelatin.

If the mix is slightly "off" either way, the film may react a little too quickly (fast) or a little too slowly (slow). Each manufacturer has a specific benchmark for the reaction time of the film, and each batch of film is tested against this

FIGURE 5-38 Two examples of "white box" packaged film. The film in these packages was manufactured in Belgium (Agfa Film) and finished in the United States. Other film may be manufactured in the United States (Kodak film).

benchmark. If the speed of the film is within ±10% of the perfect speed, it is accepted and boxed with the manufacturer's label.

At this point the film is in huge rolls, about two feet (0.61 m) in diameter and about 80 to 100 feet (24.4–30.5 m) long.

If the speed of the entire roll of film is beyond the 10% parameter up to a point of non-acceptance as defined by each manufacturer (usually ±25%), it is sold off as white box film (Figure 5-38). The film is then cut to various sizes and boxed in white boxes with a film dealer's label. It is important to remember this process when images never seem to be quite right; some are too dark and others are too light for the same size animal under the exact same processing conditions. Because the white box packagers deal only with originally rejected film, they may easily mix films of different speeds in one box. A box of 100 sheets may have film that failed the quality control standards because it was too "slow" mixed in with film that failed because it was too "fast". The easiest solution is to purchase film with the original manufacturer's label on the box. The few dollars saved by buying white box film is not necessarily a cost saving when a diagnosis is missed because of poor image quality.

Typically, the original manufacturer is identifiable on the white box by where the product was manufactured. Because it is law that the country of manufacture be noted on every product, the label will state "Manufactured in USA (Kodak film)" or "Manufactured in Belgium (AGFA film)." This information only serves for general interest and definitely does not reflect on the product of either manufacturer.

Resolution

In radiography, recorded detail is measured and expressed as resolution. Resolution in radiography is the ability of the viewer to distinguish separate line pairs. A line pair is described as one black line and one white line in an image.

Line pairs are expressed as lp/mm. The test tool that is used is a resolution test pattern (Figure 5-39). Very-high-resolution images are 30 to 35 lp/mm (for extremity and mammography images in medical imaging). Standard full-speed x-ray film with appropriate 400-speed screens is typically 8 to 9 lp/mm. Advertised line pairs in digital imaging is typically 4 to 5 lp/mm.

The question of resolution is important throughout all areas of imaging. It is what defines a system. The system in this case being the cassette, intensifying screens, film, and all the other factors that are included in the process. It becomes even more important when digital imaging is considered. The comparison between digital imaging and film/screen imaging is always, primarily, about resolution.

X-ray film alone has virtually infinite resolution. When a veterinarian looks at an image and attempts to diagnose a hairline fracture, he/she is looking at the combination of the technical factors used to produce the image, the cassette front, the film, the intensifying screens, any tabletop artifacts, the grid, processing artifacts, the patient's anatomy, and, finally, the illuminator. Each of these factors can degrade the image and yield a far less than perfect result.

We will deal with the tabletop, the grid, and the illuminators in other discussions of equipment and accessories (see Chapter 6), technical factors (see Chapter 7), and processing and processing artifacts (see Chapter 8).

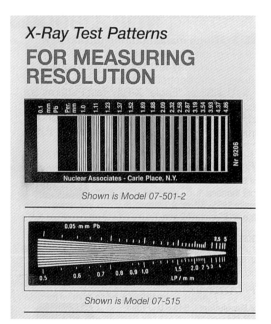

FIGURE 5-39 Two typical test tools for measuring resolution defining line pairs/mm (*top*) and one white line—one black line (*bottom*).

Storage: Cassettes, Screens, and Films

Storage of the products we have just studied is very important. The film and chemicals must be stored on a rotating basis so that the first product in is the first product out. This is also known as FIFO storage.

Film

Film boxes must always be stored on edge and not flat on a counter (Figure 5-40A). Film is sensitive to pressure both before and after it has been exposed to radiation. Dropping a cassette with exposed film can destroy the lattice network and ruin the image. Heavy pressure on the film can also destroy the film's capability to form a lattice network, resulting in no image in the area of the pressure.

Film must be protected from light leaks and from radiation (Figure 5-40B). It is important to note the expiration

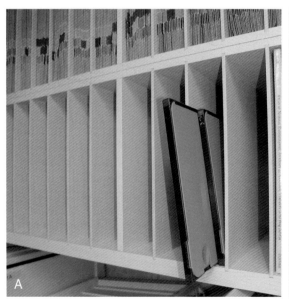
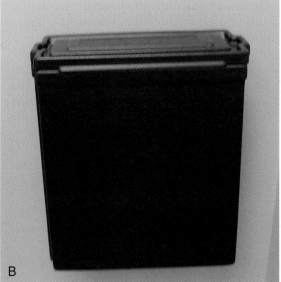

FIGURE 5-40 **A,** Cassettes should be stored upright on a counter or in a cabinet protected from radiation. **B,** Open boxes of film should be stored in a light-tight film bin.

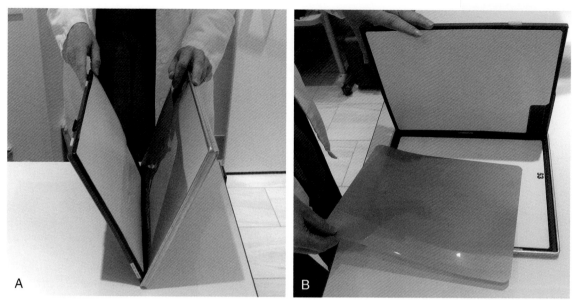

FIGURE 5-41 Proper way to remove film from a cassette. **A,** Stand the cassette on edge and let the film fall away from the screen. **B,** Now lay the cassette on its front and gently remove the film from the cassette.

date on the boxes. If the facility has several different sizes of cassettes and film, some of the film may age beyond its expiration date.

When a film is manufactured and finally presented to the market, it has aged and is ready to be used. The emulsion on the film is an unstable entity ready to react within parts of a second to any stimulus. Heat and aging will all darken the film without any exposure to radiation. It is important to store film at room temperature and not allow it to overheat or expose it to chemical fumes. Film that has aged beyond its expiration date starts to darken as the fog level rises. At first this darkening does not interfere with the image. However, as the fog level rises, the darkening increases dramatically and the resulting image loses contrast because the clear areas of the film will no longer be visible. (We discuss film fog again in Chapter 6).

Cassettes and Screens

Cassettes should be stored upright in a cupboard without possibility of exposure to radiation. They should not be stored on the floor, where they could be knocked over or subjected to spills and liquids. They should not be stored in a pile on a counter because the pressure of one cassette on top of another will affect the film. Also, pulling a cassette out from under a pile of cassettes exerts extra wear and poses the risk of damage to the cassettes. The cassettes should be loaded with film and ready to be used. It is important to ensure that the correct film is used in each cassette.

Screens should be protected when the film is being removed from the cassette (Figure 5-41). Sliding the film in the cassette will cause wear artifacts on the screen. If the film is not readily removable, the cassette should be held on edge to allow the film to separate from the screen naturally.

Cassettes should be loaded with film and kept closed in the darkroom in order to protect the integrity of the screens. Humidity and dust adversely affect the screen and compromise the image.

SUMMARY

The tools that the radiographer requires to produce an image have been discussed in this chapter. Various x-ray cassettes and screen types have been presented along with some of the problems inherent in selecting the correct combination necessary to produce an optimized image. Screen/film combinations along with the blue versus green problems have been reviewed.

Latent image formation, base/fog, and general film fog have been discussed. Finally, the importance of correctly storing and handling these products has been outlined. An optimized system is possible only if the correct products are matched, purchased, and used correctly.

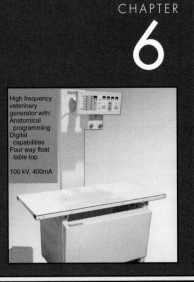

High frequency
veterinary
generator with:
Anatomical
 programming
Digital
 capabilities
Four way float
 table top

100 kV, 400mA

CHAPTER

6

Producing the Image

Pleasure in the job puts perfection in the work.
—Aristotle, Greek critic, philosopher, physicist, and zoologist, 384–322 BC

KEY TERMS

Contrast
Density
Expiration date
Fog
Grid tray
Inverse square law
Log book
Measurement
Positioning
Radiographic contrast
Scattered radiation
Secondary radiation
Subject contrast
Tabletop
Technique chart

OUTLINE

LEARNING OBJECTIVES

When you have finished this chapter, you will be able to:
1. Recognize exposures on film.
2. Define film fog.
3. Define density and contrast.
4. Know the difference between subject contrast and radiographic contrast.
5. Know how to establish a technique chart.
6. Understand the causes and prevention of artifacts on films.

APPLICATIONS

The application of the information in this chapter is relevant to the following areas:
1. Producing x-ray images (radiographs) for evaluation and diagnosis.

The production of an optimized radiograph is an art and a science. The main objective of all imaging systems is to demonstrate the differences in tissue density. Air, water, fat, tendons, muscle, and bone all have different tissue densities, and it is this differentiation, this contrast, that must be optimized.

The x-ray generator is the same basic unit now as it was 60 years ago. On a correctly calibrated radiography unit, 70 kilovolts is still 70 kilovolts; 200 milliamperes is just that; all the rest is cosmetics. If the generator has the variables necessary to produce good radiography, there is no need to replace it because a new imaging system is introduced or because it is old and not as attractive as the newer models.

As long as the unit is correctly calibrated, and parts and service are available to keep it that way, there is no need to upgrade to a different unit. A technique chart can be developed to work with any x-ray unit from a large animal portable unit to a highly sophisticated medical model. It is the development of the technique charts that we explore in this chapter. In order to do this, the technique chart section of this chapter is arranged so that the reader may search for the type of chart that matches the model of generator in use at a specific facility. The actual factors may have to be adjusted slightly from the charts presented here due to differences in the incoming line.

The Radiography Unit in Use

Every complete x-ray unit is composed of an x-ray tube, a generator, and a high-tension transformer. Each of the component parts is individual. In a small animal facility, the other necessary component is the radiography table. Some radiography units have add-ons for convenience, such as a cassette holder or a recessed control at the table side, but these are not necessary. The only two components that must be matched every time are the generator and the high-tension transformer. Quite frequently a tabletop becomes scratched, broken, or marred in some way. Most tabletops can be removed and replaced with a new medical-grade, radiolucent tabletop. The new tabletop should be attached to the table with hook-and-loop tape in order to facilitate removal if a kitten escapes and goes exploring beneath the x-ray table or just for cleaning purposes.

A great number of options are available for selection of an x-ray table. The important factors are stability, height, and the ability to install a grid tray. The most important factor is radiolucency. The x-ray photons must be transmitted through the tabletop without superimposing an image of the grain of the tabletop onto the radiograph. If an artifact consistently appears in the same place on every image produced with the cassette in the grid tray and the cassettes are ruled out as a cause, then the next place to look is either the grid (Figure 6-1) or the tabletop.

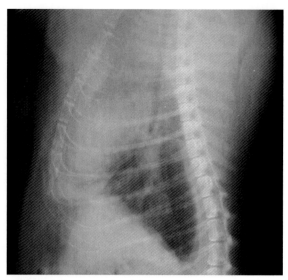

FIGURE 6-1 Illustration of grid deterioration. The image of the grid is superimposed on the chest radiograph. (The nasty, streaky straight lines are a clue to the grid problem.)

CHECK IT OUT Place a 14 in × 17 in (35 cm × 43 cm) cassette in the grid tray, and expose the film using 100 mA, 1/30 sec, and 55 kV. Process the film and examine the resulting radiograph. The image should be a density 1.0 + base /fog, or medium gray. If the image is too dark, repeat the exposure using half the mAs value. If there is a problem with the grid or the tabletop, it will be demonstrated on the film. This method will also work for digital imaging; just expose the plate and examine the image for an artifact.

Film Fog

When the film is originally manufactured, it will process completely clear except for the slight blue tint that is part of the base. After the film "seasons" or matures to the point that it can be sold and put into practice, it will develop a low fog level. In other words, if a brand new film out of a new box is processed, there will be a very low density on the film, usually an optical density (O.D.) 0.10 to 0.15. This is the evidence that the sensitivity specks are active and will convert any radiation produced image into metallic silver during processing. Whenever film density is discussed, the base color and the fog level are always included as part of the image (e.g., density 1.0 plus base/fog).

The base/fog level is usually minimal in unexposed film. However, if the film is exposed to unsuitable storage conditions and then exposed to radiation, the base fog will be dark enough to compromise the contrast of the radiograph, because the clear areas will no longer be visible, replaced instead by a fog density (Figure 6-2A&B).

Film fog is one of the most common problems in any facility. Film can be fogged by light, heat, and radiation in various ways. The recognition of film fog seems

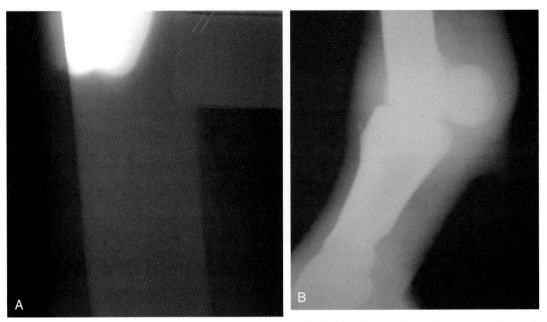

FIGURE 6-2 Film fog. **A,** The fog has obliterated the image, and only the technician's fingers have protected a small portion of the film that remained unexposed. **B,** The fog in this image was more subtle and just eliminated the resolution on the image. It was caused by a wrong color safelight (See chapter 8).

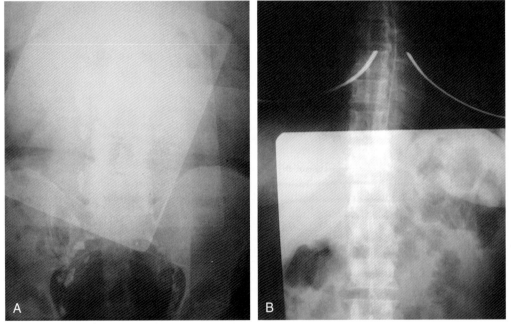

FIGURE 6-3 Examples of film fog on radiographs. **A,** One film lying on top of another in a cassette. **B,** One cassette masking another. These images are from a human facility, evidence that fog can happen anywhere.

to be a difficult concept. When the lattice network has formed within the emulsion, it is eight to ten times more sensitive to radiation exposure than it was originally (Figure 6-3A&B).

The cassettes that have been exposed during an examination should be removed from the radiography room and placed well out of direct or scattered radiation.

Recognition of film fog is often a problem. The image has an overall gray appearance that does not change if the technical factors on the x-ray unit are raised or lowered. Often when the images have been fine and they suddenly become indistinct and overall gray, the first suspicion should be film fog. We also address this problem in Chapter 8 which discusses processing the image and optimizing the darkroom.

One unusual case of fog occurred when a veterinary clinic changed locations. The move went well and the images were satisfactory until a change in the seasons. The sun now set at a lower angle and in doing so penetrated the window of the radiography room. The film bin, which was now located in the direct path of the sunbeams, had a slightly faulty closing mechanism. This was not a problem until the intensity of the sun as it set lower in the sky and further south fogged the top edge of each film as it lay on top of the box waiting to be placed into the cassette.

Exposing an already exposed cassette can cause fog. Another rare occurrence is the phosphorescence of the intensifying screen. Some of the Agfa 400 intensifying screens continued to phosphoresce after they were exposed to radiation. Most of these screens have now been taken out of service, but there are a few around, and they do cause problems as the new, unexposed film is exposed to radiation in the cassette while it sits on the shelf waiting to be used.

Excessive heat in the darkroom or film storage compromises the film because it activates the lattice network. The atoms within the film emulsion start to "develop" the film even if there is no actual light or radiation exposure.

CHECK IT OUT Remove a sheet of film from the box and place it on the counter in a well-lit room. Place a piece of cardboard to cover half of the film. Leave the combination in place for about an hour. When you lift the cardboard, the half beneath the cardboard will be lighter than the half that was exposed to light for the past hour. The lattice network starts to form on its own without being exposed to radiation as long as it is exposed to light. The longer it is exposed in this way, the darker the film will become. It does not become completely black because of the dye in the emulsion.

The film will also start to develop within the box over time as the lattice network slowly begins to form around the sensitivity specks. Latent film fog is a problem with old expired film boxes. Always check the expiration date on the film box and make sure it is used or recycled within 6 months of the "Best Before" date (Figure 6-4).

The Technical Factors

In order to produce an image in the radiograph, the contrast that separates the tissue densities must be optimized. The four factors of exposure (kilovoltage [kV], milliampere-seconds [mAs], distance) must be manipulated in such a way that the tissue absorption of radiation is exactly correct to demonstrate anatomy and pathology and to minimize any external artifact that may obscure the desired result.

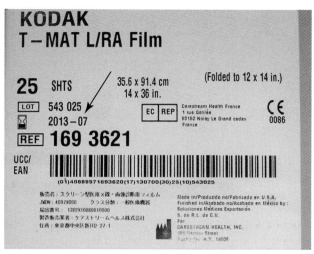

FIGURE 6-4 This expiration date (*arrow*) was current when this image was taken.

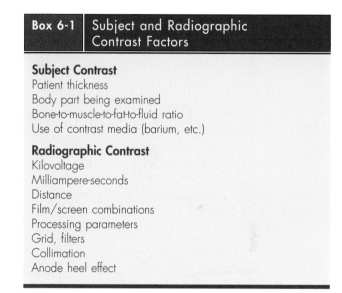

Radiographic Contrast versus Subject Contrast

What constitutes the variables that provide contrast in an image? There are two main areas where contrast may be manipulated. The patient thickness and conformation will determine subject contrast, whereas the mechanical variables available to enhance contrast are collectively called radiographic contrast (Box 6-1).

Distance, Kilovoltage, Milliamperage, Time

The factors that are set on the x-ray unit are four-fold. All of these factors are interdependent and a change in one factor dramatically affects the other three.

Distance and the Inverse Square Law

We referred to the inverse square law (Figure 6-5) in Chapter 3. The lesson learned here is that the distance between the x-ray tube and the image receptor (film or digital plate) is critical. The inverse square law states that the intensity of the radiation at a location is inversely proportional to the square of its distance from the source of the radiation.

This is true in our daily life (refer to Figure 3-10) as well as in the veterinary hospital. If the original distance is 1 and we halve it to 0.5, the intensity of the radiation is four times higher. This can be a very useful tool if the x-ray unit has low power and the body part that we need to examine is very large.

In most small animal hospitals the distance between the x-ray tube and the receptor is preset and marked on the x-ray tube column. Forty inches (100 cm) is the normal preset distance. Occasionally this is altered because of the limitation of the ceiling height or the height of the tabletop. This alteration must be taken into account when the technique chart is established.

The film is exposed in one of two ways in a small animal clinic. The cassette is placed either on the tabletop or into a grid tray beneath the tabletop. The grid tray usually sits approximately 3 inches below the tabletop, and the technique chart must be adjusted not only for the tube-tray distance (source image distance, or SID) but also because of the grid, which is addressed in Chapter 7. Frequently, the operator is encouraged to change the height of the x-ray tube, lowering it when the cassette is placed in the grid tray and raising it when the film is on the tabletop. This change is not necessary if the technique chart is adjusted slightly to compensate for the extra 3-inch (7.6-cm) distance, because it must already be adjusted to account for the grid. We discuss the grid factor in Chapter 7.

> **POINTS TO PONDER** Quite frequently the small amount that the tube is raised and lowered is confused in the facility and often the tube is mistakenly lowered for the tabletop exposures and raised for the grid tray exposures. It is far preferable to compensate for the extra distance by adjusting the technique chart, for both the grid and the distance, leaving the x-ray tube stationary.

Kilovoltage, Milliamperage, and Time

> **POINTS TO PONDER** The controlling factors kV and mAs are often referred to as the factors controlling the quality of the radiation (kV) and the quantity of the radiation (mAs). When the kV is increased, the beam is said to be "hardened." When the mAs is increased, the density of the image is directly affected.

The three remaining factors to be set on the x-ray unit are completely interconnected. Each factor has a specific importance to the outcome of the image, and each factor will affect the other factors as well. Kilovoltage mainly affects contrast in the image. It also affects density because too high a kilovoltage will blacken the film and so eliminate any contrast. The mAs value primarily affects density; however, this value, too, will eliminate contrast if set far too high or far too low.

The best analogy for understanding the interaction of the technical factors is represented in the illustration of the game of pool (Figure 6-6). A certain number of balls are racked or

Focal spot of x-ray beam

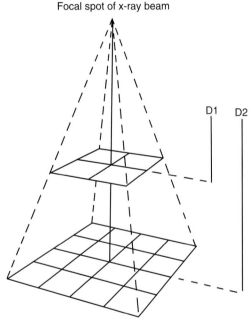

D1   D2

FIGURE 6-5 The inverse square law. When the distance is increased from D1 to D2 (doubling the distance), the amount of radiation on each square is decreased to a quarter of the amount at D1; it is spread over four times the area.

kV - Power behind the cue stick   Whenever a ball hits the side of the table it loses energy in the impact

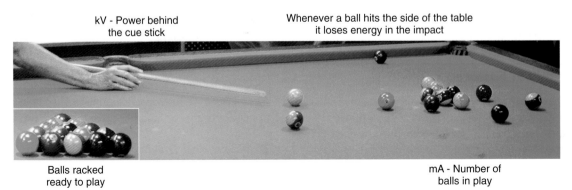

Balls racked ready to play   mA - Number of balls in play

FIGURE 6-6 The game of pool. An analogy of the technical factors of radiation exposure.

positioned on a felt-covered table. A cue ball is aimed at the prepositioned balls, and the cue stick is used to hit the cue ball and scatter the racked balls to put them into play. The scattered balls move according to how much energy is transferred down the cue stick and at what angle that energy is transferred. In radiography, the x-ray photons projected out of the x-ray tube are the balls on the table.

The *kilovoltage (kV)* is the power behind the cue stick. It is how hard the balls are hit. If the balls are hit very hard, they bounce off the edges of the table and as they do so they transfer a little energy to the tableside and move off to interact with other balls or the other side of the table until they come to rest. Each interaction, whether it be with table edges or with other balls, subtracts energy from the initial load until the ball finally comes to rest.

In the world of radiation, energy is transferred when the photons bounce off one another or the atoms within the patient. This energy becomes scattered radiation, or secondary radiation, and it is visualized on the image as nonuseful radiation or is absorbed by another interaction within the animal. The nonuseful radiation contributes to either the radiation dose to the patient or technician, or appears as film fog. When the technique chart is developed, the kilovoltage must be set as low as possible in order to penetrate the body part and keep the scattered radiation to a minimum.

The kilovoltage is responsible for penetration of the x-ray beam. In our analogy, it is the power behind the cue stick. In Figure 6-7, it is obvious how the energy of the x-ray beam affects contrast. If the energy is set so high that it penetrates every tissue, there will be no contrast. Similarly, if it is set so low that it penetrates nothing and never arrives at the film, there will be no contrast on the image.

Figure 6-7 illustrates that kilovoltage greatly affects contrast. The nomenclature on contrast is straightforward. Figure 6-7A has short-scale contrast (black and white). It does not take long to read the image from black to white. Figure 6-7B, which has long-scale contrast (black, gray, gray, white), represents more steps between black and white.

The difficulty arises when the operator states that he/she would like to see more contrast. This means that fewer shades of gray will lead to a higher level of contrast on the image. This can be interpreted incorrectly and cause confusion. More contrast means fewer shades of gray. Less contrast means more shades of gray.

> **POINTS TO PONDER** Contrast is the key word on any radiographic image. If the veterinarian requests more contrast, it is always wise to clarify whether he/she wants to see more shades of gray (long scale) or a shorter-scale, high-contrast, black/white image. Sometimes that is not clear.

Optimizing Kilovoltage

The range of kilovoltages on a general radiography unit is usually between 40 and 125 kV. When the technique chart is developed for the facility, it must be fine-tuned to consider all of the variables inherent in the production of the final image. The main objective in optimizing the technique chart is to use the lowest kV value that will penetrate the region of interest within the body and enhance the tissue contrast surrounding it. Each body part or component can be penetrated by an optimum kilovoltage (Figure 6-8).

Table 6-1 is meant to be a guide for an average-sized animal. For larger animals or for pocket pets and smaller animals, the kilovoltage is adjusted on the final chart. Because kilovoltage is the energy with which the x-ray beam passes through the body, a change in kilovoltage is not in direct proportion with the increase or decrease in tissue. This difference is due to a variation in tissue absorption (tissue fluence).

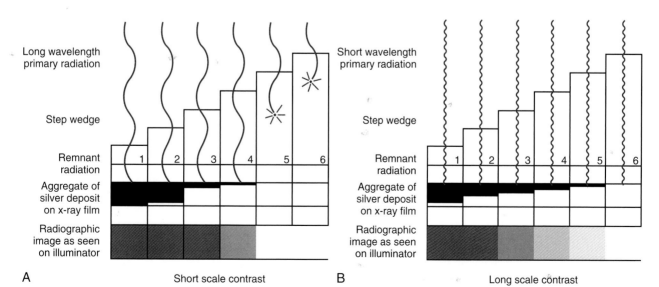

FIGURE 6-7 An aluminium wedge with a series of graduated steps is used in this model. How contrast affects the image: **A,** Low kilovoltage = short-scale contrast. **B,** High kilovoltage = long-scale contrast; with very high kilovoltage, the entire wedge is penetrated and there is no contrast.

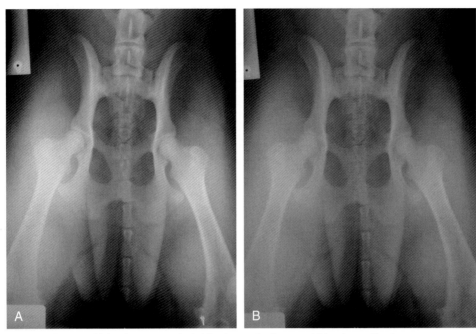

FIGURE 6-8 Optimized kilovoltage versus high kilovoltage. **A,** Optimized kilovoltage. The bony structures are visible and trabecular patterns are well visualized. **B,** High kilovoltage. The bony structures are overpenetrated and now blend in with the muscle tissue. Trabecular patterns are no longer visualized.

TABLE 6-1	Table of Optimum Kilovoltage per Average-sized Body Part for Film and Digital Imaging		
BODY PART	**OPTIMUM kV FOR FILM IMAGING**	**OPTIMUM kV FOR DIGITAL IMAGING**	**NOTES**
Extremities	40-55	55-65	
Cervical spine/ skull	60-75	65-75	
Thorax/abdomen/pelvis	60-80	80-90	For larger animals, the kV may be increased to 95 maximum

The optimum kV is the kilovoltage that penetrates the anatomy so that it is identifiable on the radiographic image. For example, on an abdominal plate, if the anatomy is visible, the spine is evident, and the intervertebral spaces are clearly defined, then the anatomy has been penetrated. Now, to optimize the image, the mAs must be altered. However, if the image is far too light or so dark that the anatomy is obscured, the 15% rule should be employed.

The 15% Rule

The 15% rule is used only to optimize kilovoltage because the body part has not been imaged satisfactorily. It should not be used to increase or decrease density on an image.

To increase penetration: multiply the original kV by 1.15 (kV +15%); for example, 80 • 1.15 = 92kV

To decrease penetration: multiply the original kV by 0.85 (kV −15%); for example, 80 • 0.85 = 68 kV

The application of this rule will increase or decrease the penetration of the region of interest.

This rule will be effective for the kilovoltages between 55 kV and 95 kV, which is the normal range of use in radiography. If the technique chart is optimized and the patient is positioned and measured correctly, the technician will never have to use this formula.

Milliamperage

To return to the pool table analogy, the milliamperage (mA) represents the number of balls on the table. If there are a lot of balls on the table, there will be a high number of interactions and a greater potential to have a dark film (Figure 6-9). If there are very few balls on the table, a light film will result. The mAs value is responsible for density. It is directly proportional; doubling the mAs doubles the density on the film. There is no higher math to calculate when one is determining how to optimize an image using mAs.

On older units the number of choices for mAs was always limited. There may be only two mA stations and 20 time stations or, if a large animal portable is being used for small animal radiography, there will be individual time stations and four or five linked kV/mA stations. This can be frustrating when one is developing a technique chart.

> **POINTS TO PONDER** A major point to consider when purchasing a new generator is the number of time stations and mA stations available. A generator with the highest number of both, or a high-frequency generator with anatomic programming, is ideal.

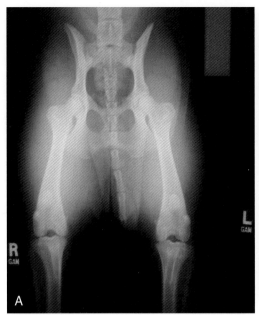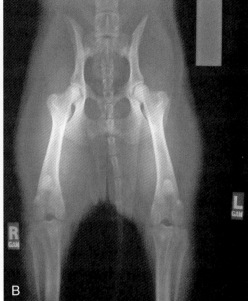

FIGURE 6-9 Optimized mA versus low mA. **A,** The density provides a black background with the bony structures well visualized. **B,** The inadequate mAs value provides a flat image with loss of visualization in the bony structures. Note that the contrast is maintained.

A limited number of stations is workable, but the limitation will be the choices per centimeter of tissue as the chart is prepared. These units will not necessarily produce an optimized image but will take advantage of the forgiveness of the film/screen combination.

Adjusting the Factors

The three factors that may be adjusted on the generator are kV, mA, and time. The limits outlined in Table 6-1 are the standard for an average patient. Figures 6-7 through 6-9 show the result of stepping dramatically outside those limits. This is basically true for digital imaging as well because the computer must adjust for variations in technique beyond what is reasonable. The advantage is that this adjustment can be accomplished without further radiation to the patient. However, when post-processing becomes the norm, information is lost in the translation. We discuss this issue in Chapter 9.

The images in Figure 6-9 represent changes in kV while adjusting the mA to maintain density 1.0 + base/fog in the ilium of the pelvis. They demonstrate that an increase in kilovoltage causes a substantial change in contrast as the x-ray beam becomes "harder" or more penetrating.

The images in Figure 6-10 represent changes in mA while the kV is adjusted to maintain density 1.0 + base/fog in the ileum of the pelvis. They show that a decrease in mAs causes a substantial change in density but does not affect the contrast.

Developing Technique Charts

The Three "Commandments"

Three rules must be followed before one attempts to develop a technique chart for any medical, veterinary, or research facility.

Rule #1

The x-ray unit must be calibrated by a qualified x-ray service engineer. Tests must be carried out on every station that will be within normal range of use to ensure that what is being set exactly conforms to the output of the x-ray unit. There is no point in setting up a chart only to find that 70 kV on one mA station is actually 76 kV and on a second mA station it is 68 kV.

This rule cannot be emphasized enough. There are countless examples of major frustration within the x-ray room that occur because the service engineer did not bother to calibrate the mA stations correctly or the unit has "drifted" over the 20 years since it was last calibrated. Every x-ray unit should be calibrated a minimum of once every 2 years. As the unit ages, it should be calibrated yearly.

> **POINTS TO PONDER** The difference between mA stations must be linear. Because the output of the mA station is directly proportional, 200 mA must produce double the radiation of 100 mA. If the service engineer does not calibrate the unit correctly or does not match the unit to the incoming electricity, it will be impossible to set up and follow a technique chart. Also, each kV station must be matched so that the output of 70 kV at 100 mA is double the output of 70 kV at 50 mA, and so on. This can be determined on the engineer's test tools and should be checked by the veterinary technician before the service person leaves the facility.

Rule #2

The technique chart is set up to reflect the thickness of the body part that is being radiographed. It is not intuitive! That is to say, the animal must be placed in position on the x-ray table prior to being measured. Figure 6-10 demonstrates a possible difference in measurement of 7 cm between when

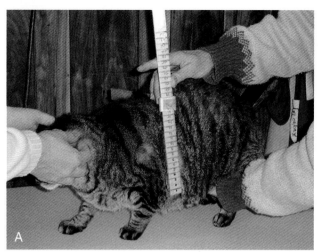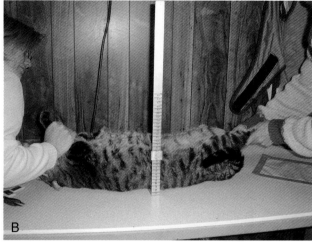

FIGURE 6-10 Microchip being incorrectly measured (16 cm) (**A**) and then correctly measured (8 cm) (**B**). The staff will don leaded aprons, thyroid collars, and gloves to complete the radiograph.

Microchip was not measured correctly and when he was held in position and measured accurately. This represents a huge difference in technical factors.

> **POINTS TO PONDER** Measuring correctly cannot be stressed enough. The x-ray unit is not intuitive. It will produce the radiation that is requested for the measurement that is preset. The difference in measurement at one clinic for one dog measured separately by seven people was 17 cm! (Incidentally, every person obtained a different measurement, depending on how the dog accepted the person with the calipers.) Training the staff to measure uniformly with the animal in position resulted in consistently optimized radiography.

Rule #3

The measurement must be made at the area of particular interest. The central x-ray must enter the body part that was measured. If the area of interest on a greyhound or a whippet is the bladder (8 cm) and the dog is measured at the level of the kidneys (17 cm), the image will be far too dark.

If the area of interest is on a dog with a very high chest-to-abdomen measurement ratio, then the widest part and the narrowest part should be measured and the technique set at the midrange (e.g., for a chest measurement 20 cm and pelvis measurement 10 cm, technique should be set for 15 cm). The central ray would then enter the midrange of the abdomen (see Chapter 18). Anode heel effect can be used in this instance (see Chapter 4).

> **POINTS TO PONDER** The x-ray generator will only deliver the amount of radiation that is requested by the operator and it will not take operator error into account when the exposure is made. Measuring the patients correctly is fundamental to the use of a technique chart. The amount of tissue that is to be penetrated is finite. It is not a guessing game and has no relation whatsoever to the weight or species of the animal.

Producing a Working Technique Chart

> **POINTS TO PONDER** The technique chart is a tool, and it provides **suggested** techniques on the basis of anatomy and positioning. The factors that are presented are completely dependent on the accuracy of the technical staff. The radiography unit does not discriminate between species, a prime rib roast, or your great aunt Tilly. It only produces an image based on accurate and precise measurements.

As we begin the discussion on setting the technical factors on the generator, it is vital that we review the objective of any radiograph produced by any imaging system. The objective is to enhance the differences in tissue density of our subject.

A basic knowledge of veterinary anatomy is essential to setting up a technique chart. Historically, veterinary technique charts were based on human technique charts. A lot of the early x-ray units were purchased from hospitals and clinics that were upgrading their single-phase generators. There are still many human systems installed in veterinary clinics.

The animal chest anatomy is quite different from the human chest anatomy. The human heart is much narrower and takes up far less space in the chest cavity. This is mainly because of our upright stance and greater overall heart-to-lung ratio, which produces maximum contrast on a radiograph. The typical human chest is always imaged upright at 6 feet (180 cm) or more. Because of these differences, the human technique charts do not transfer well to veterinary charts, which normally use a consistent distance of 40 inches (100 cm) with a prone or supine animal.

In technical terms, the tissue density of the animal chest is very similar to the animal's abdominal density; the heart occupies a great proportion of the chest, and there is a fairly even mix of muscle tissue, air cavities, and bone. The techniques for chest and abdomen can be virtually the same.

Manipulating Technical Factors

At the start of this chapter we discussed the codependency of each of the factors: kV, mA, time, and distance. The following example helps illustrate how to manipulate a factor for a particular result:

You have produced a good image but the veterinarian now requests that you increase the contrast to image an obscure bladder stone. All other factors taken into consideration, the optimum kV for the abdomen was 80 kV. 70 kV will penetrate the bladder, but what do you do with the mAs, since the density on the first film was fine?

When increasing kV, multiply by 15% (80 • 1.15 = 92) and divide the original mAs by 2.

When decreasing kV, multiply by 15% (80 • 0.85) and multiply the original mAs by 2.

Technical Rules

Rule #1

When you are having difficulty with your images and you request a calibration by a service engineer, *always* make sure that a staff member at the clinic meets with him/her in the x-ray room and verifies the numbers on the meters. 70 kV must be 70 kV (±1 or 2 kV either way is not a problem; ±5-10 kV is a problem). The kVs *must* be verified on each mA station individually.

The output of 100 mA *must* be 50% of the output of 200 mA. The output of 300 mA *must* be three times that of 100 mA. Unfortunately, many service engineers are not as conscientious as they should be; hence this is the first technical rule.

Rule #2

Review the three "commandments" of calibration, positioning, and measuring. A technique chart cannot be optimized unless these rules are followed.

Rule #3

If the region of interest is not demonstrated and the technique chart is usually accurate, reposition and remeasure.

Rule #4

When you have an image that is unsatisfactory, always adjust the mAs first, assuming that you have penetrated the region of interest, but not before you have reviewed rule #3.

Rule # 5

If the film is very light and it is usually satisfactory, check the temperature of the chemicals, either in the tank or in the developer of the processor (see Chapter 8).

Rule #6

If the image is dull gray and does not improve with a change in technique, assume that the film has been fogged and look for light leaks in the darkroom or an opened or broken cassette (see Chapter 8).

The Technique Chart

In this chapter the technique chart for film radiography is discussed. The chart for computerized radiography and digital imaging is discussed in Chapter 9.

There are several ways to set up a technique chart and there are many, many charts in many animal hospitals from hand scribbles on the wall to very sophisticated charts that are laminated and colorful.

Every imaging department is slightly different and all of the factors discussed in previous chapters must be taken into consideration. Just because a technique chart works in one clinic does not mean that it will produce optimized images in a neighboring facility. Most equipment suppliers will supply a technique chart with a new radiographic unit. Some of these charts have been set up by sales people with a business degree and no concept of all the factors that are components of the image. Therefore some charts are suitable and some are not. Typically, if the images are good for a 10 cm abdomen measured and positioned correctly, then the chart should be extrapolated and should produce optimized images for any size animal for that particular unit and the film screen combination that accompanies it.

Anatomic Considerations

Skull and Cervical Spine

Both the skull and cervical spine represent bone and tissue with high contrast tissue densities. They do not require high kilovoltage.

Chest, Thorax, Abdomen, Lumbar Spine, Pelvis

The chest, thorax, abdomen, lumbar spine, and pelvis are similar in the differences in tissue density—a mix of air, fat, tissue, muscle, and bone. These body parts will be difficult to image if very high kilovoltage is used because the potential for photons producing secondary/scattered radiation increases as the thickness of the animal increases. It is important to keep the kilovoltage as low as possible and to increase the mAs proportionally as the tissue thickness increases.

Extremities

The tissue-to-bone ratio in extremities is high and the body parts are thin. A low kilovoltage is indicated.

Pocket pets and birds should be radiographed with similar technical factors to the extremities of cats and dogs unless a special film/screen combination is used.

Tabletop versus Grid Tray

One other issue that has not been discussed is use of the tabletop versus the grid tray. That will come in Chapter 7. Here, it is a factor in the chart. Any body part that measures less than 12 cm will be radiographed on the tabletop. Any body part that measures 12 cm or greater will be imaged with the cassette either beneath the tabletop in the grid tray

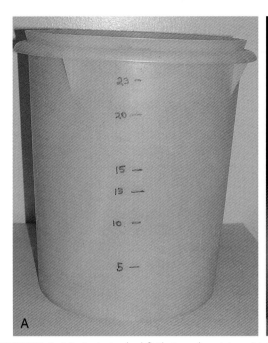
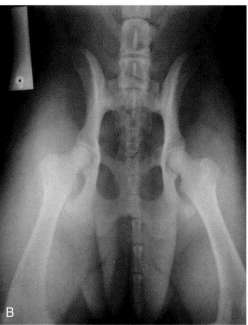

FIGURE 6-11 **A,** A standard flat-bottomed container. Note the standard measurements on the side. These duplicate extremity, skull, and abdomen equivalents since the water level can be altered easily. **B,** A correctly exposed pelvis and hips on a large dog; note the density immediately superior to the acetabulum. This is a standard density, 1.0 + base/fog.

(with a grid installed beneath the tabletop) or using a grid taped to the cassette. The use of the grid and precautions are covered in Chapter 7.

Finally, a "standard patient" is a flat-bottomed plastic bucket to which we will add water in varying depths (Figure 6-11). Measure the water by using a ruler or tape measure inserted into the container. The standard container produces an image that is uniform and is not complicated by positioning or inaccurate measurement.

Standard measurements are as follows:

Extremity: 4 cm 48 kV@ 4 mAs

Skull, etc.: 6 cm 48 kV@ 4 mAs; 12 cm 68 kV @ 5 mAs in grid tray

Thorax etc.: 8 cm 50 kV@ 3 mAs; 12 cm 74 kV @ 9 mAs in grid tray

Check to establish the speed of your system (films/screens, processing temperature). The techniques previously listed are for a 400-speed system processed correctly on a recently, and correctly, calibrated generator. The film should appear medium gray.

If the images turn out very light using these techniques, you may have a 200-speed system or the temperature in your processor may be incorrect. Start over and recheck the speed of the system, the calibration of the unit, and the processing parameters.

POINTS TO PONDER If the image is unsatisfactory, there is always a reason. Ninety percent of my consulting calls are problems with processing and not obeying the three technique chart "commandments."

Completing the Chart

Provided that the densities on the test images were satisfactory, each of the techniques may be extrapolated. Fill in the blanks on your chart. Increase 2 mAs for every 3-cm increase in density, and increase 2 kV for every 2-cm increase.

Take careful measurements, and record the results in your clinic log book. Always make sure that the patient is measured correctly and that the techniques are logged correctly. The only way to optimize the chart is to monitor it carefully, correctly, and consistently.

Small Animal Technique Charts

The charts shown in Figure 6-12 A&B are in use in many clinics in North America. They are set up to be used on the specific units identified in the legends. These units must be correctly calibrated; the patients must be correctly measured and correctly positioned, with obedience to the rules outlined previously.

The use of a large animal portable unit in a small animal radiography clinic can produce acceptable images; however, the lack of technique selection and the limited mA values (usually maximum 30 or 50) can be frustrating.

Nonstandard Radiography Units (Alternate Charts)

If the radiography unit is limited in the number of mA stations or time stations, then adjustments have to be made within the chart to compensate for the lack of variables. Figure 6-13 demonstrates typical charts that will work well for the older Summit Innovet units, which have two mA stations and limited time stations.

GRID NOW (vertical label between table-top and grid sections)

Chest / Thoracic spine / Shoulder	Table top					
CM	6	7	8	9	10	11
mAs	3		4		5	
kVp	52		54		56	

Use whatever mA station will give you the correct mAs																	
CM →	12	13	14	15	16	17	18	19	20	21	22	23	24	25	26	27	28
mAs	12		15			18		22			24			26		28	
kVp	62	64		66		68		70		72		74		76		78	

Abdomen / Lumbar spine / Pelvis	Table top					
CM 4	6	7	8	9	10	11
mAs	5		6		7	
kVp	50		52	54	56	

CM	12	13	14	15	16	17	18	19	20	21	22	23	24	25	26	27	28
mAs	12		15		18		22		24		26			28		32	
kVp	64	66		68		70		72		74		76		78		80	82

Skull / Cervical spine	Table top					
CM	3	4	5	6	7	
mAs	4		4		6	
kVp	50		52		54	

													Abdomen lumbar/pelvis continued				
CM →	8	9	10	11	12									29	30	31	32
mAs	8		10		12									34	36	38	40
kVp	56		58	60	62									84	86	88	90

Limbs and stifles	Table top					
CM	1	2	3	4	5	6
mAs	4		5		6	
kVp	48	50		50		

All limbs are table top																	
CM	7	8	9	10	11	12											
mAs	7		8		9												
kVp	50		50		52												

**It is essential that the animal is measured in the position that it is to be x-rayed.
**Central Ray enters at the point of measurement
A ** Read chart from left to right** ©

Small Animal Technique Chart 400 speed - High Frequency Unit

GRID THIS SIDE (vertical label between table-top and grid sections)

Chest / Thoracic spine / Shoulder	Table top					
CM	6	7	8	9	10	11
mAs	.5		1		2	
kVp	50		52		54	

Use whatever mA will give the correct mAs																	
CM →	12	13	14	15	16	17	18	19	20	21	22	23	24	25	26	27	28
mAs	6		8			10		12			14			16		18	
kVp	62	64		66		68		70		72		74		76		78	

Abdomen / Lumbar spine / Pelvis	Table top					
CM 4	6	7	8	9	10	11
mAs	.5		1.0		2	
kVp	54		56	58	62	

CM	12	13	14	15	16	17	18	19	20	21	22	23	24	25	26	27	28
mAs	6		8		10		12		14		16			18		20	
kVp	62	64		66		68		70		72		74		76		78	80

Skull / Cervical spine	Table top					
CM	3	4	5	6	7	
mAs	2		3		4	
kVp	50		52		54	

													Abdomen lumbar/pelvis continued				
CM	8	9	10	11	12									29	30	31	32
mAs	8		10		12									25	27	29	31
kVp	56		58	60	62									84	86	88	90

Limbs and stifles	All limbs are table top					
CM	1	2	3	4	5	6
mAs	2		3		4	
kVp	46	48		50		

All limbs are table top																	
CM	7	8	9	10	11	12											
mAs	4		5		6												
kVp	48		50		52												

**It is essential that the animal is measured in the position that it is to be x-rayed.
**Central Ray enters at the point of measurement
B ** Read chart from left to right** ©

FIGURE 6-12 A, The single-phase chart. The completed radiography chart for a small animal clinic using a single-phase unit, 400-speed system, and correct processing. B, High-frequency chart to be used with correct processing, correct measurement, and a 400-speed film/screen system on a correctly calibrated unit.

Chest	mA							Please refer to the notes which accompany this chart prior to using													
Thoracic spine	CM	6	7	8	9	10	11		12	13	14	15	16	17	18	19	20	21	22	23	24
	Sec	.1		.15		.15		→→	.15		.20			.25		.30			.35		
Shoulder	kVp	60		60		60		G R	70	70		70		70		70		80		80	
Abdomen	mA							I	mA												
Lumbar spine	CM 4	6	7	8	9	10	11	D	12	13	14	15	16	17	18	19	20	21	22	23	24
	Sec	.1		.2		.25		→	.15		.20		.25		.30		.35		.40		
Pelvis	kVp	60		60	60	60			70	70		70		70		70		70		80	
Skull	mA							N	mA												
	CM	3	4	5	6	7		O	8	9	10	11	12								
Cervical spine	Sec	.1		.1		.1		W	.15		.20		.20								
	kV	60		60		60		→	70		70	70	70								
Limbs and stifles	mA								All limbs are table top mA												
	CM	1	2	3	4	5	6		7	8	9	10	11	12							
	Sec	.05		.05		.05			.08		.08		.08								
	kV	60	60		60				60		60		60								

**It is essential that the animal is measured in the position that it is to be x-rayed.
**Central Ray enters at the point of measurement
A ** Read chart from left to right** ©

Chest	Table top 100 mA								300 mA																
Thoracic spine	CM	6	7	8	9	10	11		12	13	14	15	16	17	18	19	20	21	22	23	24	25	26	27	28
	mAs	2.5		3.3		6.7		→→	7.5		10			15		15			25			25		30	
Shoulder	kVp	48		50		52		G R	68	70		72		74		78 80 kv's inc due to mAs				80		82		84	
Abdomen	Table top 100 mA							I	300 mA																
Lumbar spine	CM 4	6	7	8	9	10	11	D	12	13	14	15	16	17	18	19	20	21	22	23	24	25	26	27	28
	mAs	2.5		3.3		6.7		→	7.5		10		15		15		15	25	25			30			
Pelvis	kVp	48		50		52			68	70		72		74		78	76	74		80		82		84	86
									KV's changed due to mAs																
Skull	Table top 100 mA							N	300 mA													Abdomen lumbar/pelvis continued			
	CM	3	4	5	6	7		O	8	9	10	11	12									29	30	31	32
Cervical spine	mAs	3.3		5		6.7		W	7.5		10		15									30	33	36	40
	kV	50		48		50		→	60		62	64	66									88	90	92	94
Limbs and stifles	All limbs are table top 100 mA								All limbs are table top 100 mA																
	CM	1	2	3	4	5	6		7	8	9	10	11	12											
	mAs	1.7		3.3		5			7.5		10		15												
	kV	46	48		50				48		50		52												

**It is essential that the animal is measured in the position that it is to be x-rayed.
**Central Ray enters at the point of measurement
B ** Read chart from left to right** ©

FIGURE 6-13 A, The large animal portable chart (used for small animal radiography). Note that the time stations and kV stations are limited; therefore, the images will not always be optimized but they will be diagnostic. B, Specially adapted Summit Innovet chart. Notice that the kVs are adjusted for chest and abdomen because the time stations are limited.

Body part	Size/view	kV	mAs	Grid (if used)
Navicular	**AP**	**74**	**2.5-2.8**	**4.0-5.0**
Coffin	A.P.	74	.8	
Coffin Jt/foot	Lat	74	.5	3.2
Coffin Jt./foot	Obl.	74	.5	3.2
Fetlocks and	**A.P.**	**74**	**.5**	**2.5-4.0**
splint bone	lat	74	.6	
	Obl	74	.5	
	Flexed lat	74	.5	
Knees	**A.P/Lat/Obl**	**74**	**.5**	
	Flexed lat	74	.5	
	Skyline	74	.5	
Hock	**A.P.**	**74**	**.8**	
	Lat/Obl.	74	.6	
	Flexed lat	74	.6	
	S1 talus	74	.5	
Stifle	**Lat Jt.**	**76**	**1.2**	**4.0-5.0**
	Lat patella	76	1.0	
	A.P.	80	3.2-5.0	8.0-10
Elbow	**Lat**	**74**	**.8**	
	A.P.	74	1.0-1.2	
Shoulder		**80**	**6.2-8.0**	
Thoracic sp./	**T 1-3**	**76**	**.5-.8**	
withers	T 4-6	80	.8-1.8	
Cerv. sp.	**Foal C1-C2**	**76**	**.6**	
	Foal C3-C4	76	.8	
	Foal C4- C6	78	.8	
Skull	**Incisors/Wolf**			
	teeth	**74**	**.5**	
	Malaise	74	.8	
	A.P.	76	1.0-1.6	
	Jowl	74	1.2	

**All these techniques are set up for 30" distance
All views are full size horse unless otherwise noted

FIGURE 6-14 Typical large animal portable (equine) technique chart.

All of the charts have been developed for a 400-speed film/screen system and a correctly calibrated radiography unit. The images were developed either manually or automatically using correct time temperature development.

Equine Radiography

Equine radiography is typically carried out on location using a large animal portable radiography unit that is specially adapted to be transported from location to location. The technique chart shown in Figure 6-14 will work well with standard units, and a digital chart is included in the digital imaging chapter.

The unit must be calibrated correctly, and the wearing of leaded aprons, thyroid collars, and gloves are essential for any personnel in the vicinity while the examination is in progress.

Also, each unit is equipped with a measuring device that must be used to ensure that a consistent distance is used for each view.

The cassettes must be protected both before and after the exposure is made, and a method of separating exposed cassettes and unexposed cassettes must be used consistently so that there is never a question as to whether a cassette has been used or is available for an exposure.

The technique chart illustrated in Figure 6-14 is a typical chart for a typical large animal unit. The system speed is 400-speed class, and the films were processed in an automatic processor.

The Radiography Log Book

Legally, the clinic must keep a record of every patient radiographed. The log book (Figure 6-15) must include the

Date	Film #	Client	Breed	Area of body	Measure-ment Cm	kV	mA mAs	Time	Comment

FIGURE 6-15 A radiography sample log book page.

patient's name, identifiers, the views taken, the measurements, and the technical factors. Leaving a space for a comment is often useful.

The log book must be completed every time a patient is radiographed. The technical factors and measurements are critical to maintaining a working technique chart. If a problem arises and the technique chart is completed correctly, it is much easier to diagnose.

The technical factors must be entered as the images are completed. Guessing techniques based on past images is not an option.

SUMMARY

The technical factors that were introduced and discussed in Chapters 3-5 have now been put to use. It is vitally important to approach the technique chart with a scientific mind. The settings on the unit indicate the correct settings in order to produce an optimized image. If a service consultant is on site, the first place he/she will look is the log book.

Each facility is unique, but the universal truth is that 70 kV is 70 kV, and the generator and the technical factors set on the generator must be accurate and reproducible.

Optimizing the Image

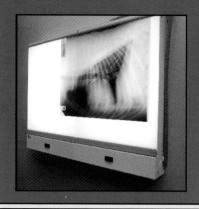

Fix your eyes on perfection and you make almost everything speed towards it.

—William Ellery Channing, American writer, 1780–1842

OUTLINE

KEY TERMS

Blur
Central ray
Collimation shutters/leaves
Collimator
Collimator indicator
Compensating filters
Distortion
Filtration
Grid
Grid deterioration
Grid ratio
Grid tray
Illuminator
Illuminator mask
Inherent filtration
Line pairs/inch (Grids)
Line pairs/mm (Resolution)
Motion
Off-focus radiation

LEARNING OBJECTIVES

When you have finished this chapter, you will be able to:
1. Define motion, distortion, magnification, and blur.
2. Understand the purpose of filters.
3. Define collimation.
4. Understand the purpose of illuminators.
5. Know how to use grids.

APPLICATIONS

The application of the information in this chapter is relevant to the following areas:
1. Optimizing the images (radiographs) to aid in diagnoses.

We have discussed the science of image production in the previous chapters. Now we will cover all the procedures that coalesce to produce the art of radiography: the optimized image.

In this chapter we refer to the central ray (Figure 7-1). This is the x-ray beam that is produced off the central point of the focal spot of the anode and directed at 90 degrees to the image receptor.

It is essential to ensure that the most cooperation possible is obtained from the patient. If an animal is so ill or terrified that it tremors continuously, obtaining an optimized radiograph will be very difficult unless the animal can be reassured or sedated to the point at which it will be cooperative. Many veterinary facilities are limited to 1/120 of a second on their radiography units, and at times this is not fast enough to arrest involuntary motion such as tremor.

Other factors, such as magnification, distortion, and blur, can be minimized by understanding the principles behind these factors. The use of collimation and grids reduces the scattered radiation.

Filtration eliminates a certain amount of secondary radiation. The use of a correctly set-up illuminator is a very easy fix to enhance the review of the image.

Motion, Distortion, and Magnification

Motion

Motion is an enemy of resolution. Unsharpness resulting from patient motion may be voluntary or involuntary. Reducing involuntary motion or waiting a few extra seconds until the patient settles is very important to good radiography. Diagnosis is impossible if the patient appears to be

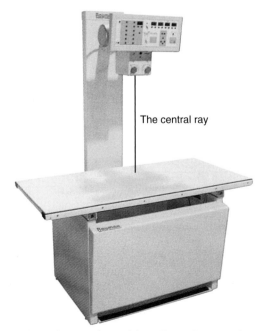

The central ray

FIGURE 7-1 The central ray of the radiography unit is the point at which the x-ray beam enters the patient.

leaving the table as the exposure is made. This is also true if a wagging tail is moving across the image. The use of sandbags and rolled towels can support body parts that are unstable and out of the region of interest. Sandbags can be obtained commercially or, if someone in the facility can sew, they can be made quite easily. Be aware that sandbags are not radiolucent and should never be placed where they will obscure the region of interest.

> **CHECK IT OUT**   A sandbag can be made out of heavy vinyl. A piece 15 in (38 cm) long and 15 in (38 cm) wide will make a sandbag 15 by 5.5 inches (38 × 13 cm). The vinyl should be folded over twice on each seam, and the seams should be oversewn so that the sand does not leak out over time. Colorful slipcovers can be sewn and secured at the top with hook-and-loop (Velcro) strips. This would make a standard size sandbag. Larger or smaller sizes are also useful. If no one at the facility can sew, sandbags and foam blocks for positioning can be purchased from commercial suppliers.

Blur

Blur is another factor in patient motion and may be useful when imaging a particular body part that is obscured by overlying anatomic structures. Blur is the principle of computerized tomography; we investigate this principle in depth in Chapter 11. In general radiography, imaging the bodies of the thoracic spine is made easier by allowing the patient to breathe normally and setting a long (1 to 2 sec) exposure time. Because the ribs move during this exposure time, they are blurred and indistinct, whereas the thoracic spine, which moves very little and is in line with the central ray, stays in focus. The milliampere (mA) value will have to be adjusted so that the milliampere-seconds (mAs) value remains the same but the time of exposure is increased.

> **POINT TO PONDER**   The mAs must be constant no matter what factors are used to produce the image. 100 · 0.10 = 10 mAs; 25 · 0.40 = 10 mAs. In order to use a 1-second exposure, the mA should be set at the lowest possible setting, and the kV should be decreased, if necessary, through the use of the 15% rule.

Distortion

Distortion (Figure 7-2) is the foreshortening or elongation of a body part due to angulation of the body part, the x-ray receptor, or the tube. Distortion can be useful when one body part obscures the area of interest. For example, on an upper lateral chest view, if the upper shoulder obscures pathology of the lower humerus, the x-ray tube may be angled obliquely so that the upper shoulder is projected away

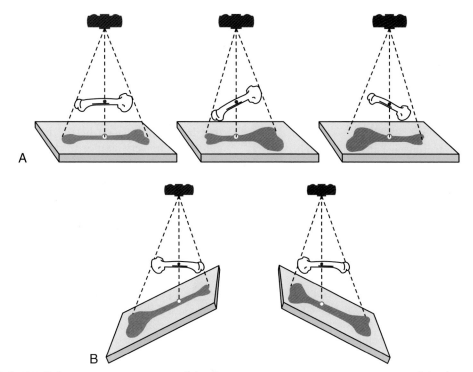

A

B

FIGURE 7-2 Distortion. **A,** Part not parallel to the image receptor. **B,** Image receptor not parallel to the part.

from the lower humerus. The patient may also be rotated slightly to demonstrate pathology. Useful distortion is practiced regularly in dental radiography, as we shall investigate in Chapters 10 and 24.

For the most part, distortion is not useful if it results in elongation or foreshortening of the region of interest. Shape distortion can occur from inaccurate positioning of the central ray. If the region of interest is the chest and the central ray is directed to the abdomen, the anterior ribs will be projected superiorly and the shape of the chest will be distorted. It is very important that the region of interest is centered beneath the central ray of the x-ray tube.

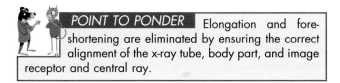

POINT TO PONDER Elongation and foreshortening are eliminated by ensuring the correct alignment of the x-ray tube, body part, and image receptor and central ray.

Magnification

Magnification (Figure 7-3) of a body part is reduced if the body part is placed as close as possible to the image receptor. The source-image distance (SID) on most veterinary radiography units is 40 inches (100 cm). If the object is closer to the x-ray tube than it is to the image receptor, the object will be magnified. In everyday practice the actual measurement of an object in question is not an issue. However, if one is interested in the size of an object, such as a bladder stone or

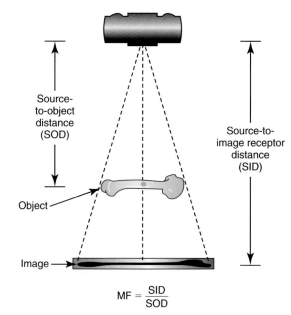

Source-to-object distance (SOD)

Source-to-image receptor distance (SID)

Object

Image

$$MF = \frac{SID}{SOD}$$

FIGURE 7-3 Example of magnification of an image structure. MF, magnification factor.

kidney stone, then the source-object distance (SOD) would have to be calculated by determining the distance of the object from the image receptor by measuring on the lateral view and subtracting the distance of the object from the image receptor. This method will determine the magnification factor by applying the formula MF = SID/SOD.

Filters and Filtration

Once radiation became useful in general radiography, the problem of scattered radiation and secondary radiation had to be addressed. As body parts being examined become larger, the technical factors increase, and the problem becomes even more evident.

When radiation enters the patient, it does so as a heterogenous beam. In other words, when 70 kV is set at the generator, that is only the effective kilovoltage. There are five ways of measuring kilovoltage on a meter, because diagnostic radiation produces a beam with many energies. For practical purposes, the 70-kV beam contains radiation representing 70 kilovolts. It also contains other photons of varying amounts of energy that are absorbed within the patient and others that scatter from the patient as secondary or scattered radiation. Because this radiation is not useful, it must be filtered out either before it enters the patient or after it exits the patient as scattered radiation from within the patient.

The best method to filter out the soft or lower-energy radiation before it reaches the patient is through aluminum filtration.

Inherent Filtration

The radiography unit is equipped with added filtration when it is installed. Before the x-ray beam exits the port of the x-ray tube, it is attenuated by the glass envelope of the tube, by the oil surrounding the tube, and by the mirror inside the collimator (the beam restrictor located just below the x-ray tube); this is the inherent filtration.

Added Filtration

The beam is then further attenuated by the added filtration that has been installed by the manufacturer. The federal guidelines are very clear as to the amount of filtration that must be installed in each radiography unit. This added filtration may be adjusted according to the typical procedure in the radiography room. The Canadian and US federal guidelines specify a minimum of 2.5 mm of aluminum for x-ray units operating above 70 kV.

Measuring the Half-Value Layer

An indirect method of measuring the amount of filtration is with a radiation dosimeter and sheets of aluminum. The principle is to measure the amount of aluminum filtration that reduces the original intensity of the x-ray beam by 50%.

The original intensity of the primary beam is measured using a dosimeter. Plates of high-grade aluminum are added into the primary beam until the original dose is reduced by half. This amount of filtration is the half-value layer (HVL) (Figure 7-4).

Special Filters

Other filters may be added to the primary beam to enhance the imaging process. These are known as compensating filters. A wedge filter (Figure 7-5) may be added to the collimator with the thicker part over the thinner area of the abdomen if the region of interest is the upper abdomen of a dog with a large discrepancy between the measurement of the pelvis and the inferior aspect of the ribs. The technique set is for the inferior rib measurement, and the x-ray tube is positioned over the region of interest, at the level of the spleen and kidneys.

Many other filters are available both to even out the discrepancy between areas of the body and to absorb scattered and secondary radiation.

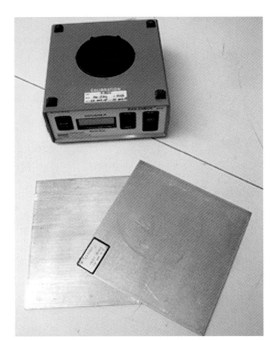

FIGURE 7-4 The setup to measure the half-value layer (HVL). A radiation dosimeter measures the amount of radiation exiting the tube. The pieces of aluminum filtration are added until the original dose is reduced by 50%.

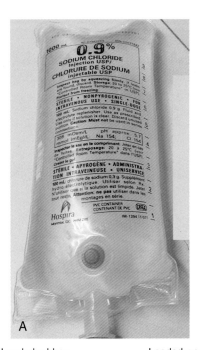

A

Leaded rubber
cassette divider

Leaded wood
cassette divider

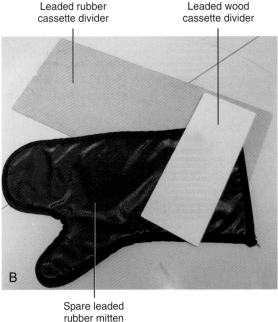

B

Spare leaded
rubber mitten

FIGURE 7-6 A, Simple intravenous saline bags absorb scattered radiation if the region of interest is on the outer aspect of the anatomy. B, Special lead blockers also work well as long as they are not pushed under the patient, because if they were, they would block primary radiation. Leaded rubber gloves and cut-up pieces of lead apron also serve this purpose.

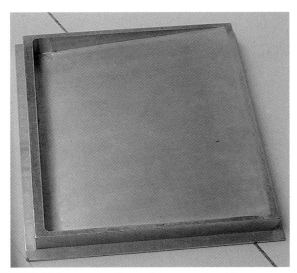

FIGURE 7-5 A wedge filter will even out the difference in tissue measurement. It is attached to the collimator with the thickest end at the thinner part of the patient. The technique set is the measurement of the thicker body part.

Filtration to eliminate scattered radiation is as simple as laying a mask of leaded rubber on the tabletop along the lumbar spine for a lateral exposure. The leaded rubber absorbs the scattered radiation and prevents it from reaching the image receptor. Other effective filters are large intravenous saline bags and plastic bags filled with flour or rice. The advantage of the saline bags and flour bags is that they are radiolucent and do not produce an artifact on the image (Figure 7-6).

Collimators

The unit immediately beneath the x-ray tube is the collimator. There are many, many varieties of collimator (Figure 7-7). They have one standard function and that is to produce a light beam that is coincident with the x-ray beam and covers the region of interest. It is very important that the light beam is centered and within 0.50 inch (1 cm) of the area of the x-ray beam.

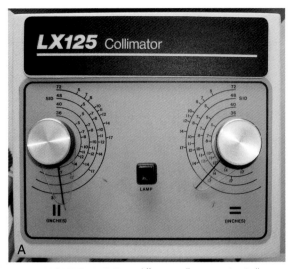
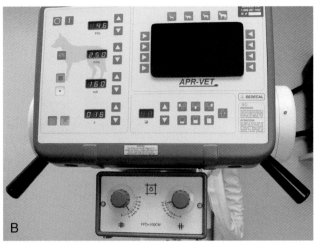

FIGURE 7-7 Two different collimators. **A,** Collimator for Raymax LX125 (Raymax Medical, Brampton, Ontario, CA). Note the indicators for height and film size on the front. **B,** The collimator for SEDECAL APR VET (SEDECAL USA, Inc., Arlington Heights, Illinois) is mounted directly below the generator control panel.

Collimation Indication

There is a graph on the front of many collimators. In front of the graph are the two knobs that elongate or close the internal shutters. The graph indicates the various cassette sizes and the position at which the knob should be turned to open the shutters to the desired cassette size at the selected distance.

The collimator indicator is not available on all collimators, particularly the older models. If it is there, it should be accurate. A good protocol to follow is to collimate to the film size prior to placing the animal on the table.

> **CHECK IT OUT**   Place a cassette on the table-top and activate the collimator light. Note the size of the cassette, and turn the knobs to match the cassette size. Are they coincident? Or are they slightly wider and longer than the cassette size? If the latter situation is the case, then the collimator was probably set for the cassette in the grid tray.

An added advantage to most collimators is their ability to focus the x-ray beam by reducing scattered radiation.

> **POINTS TO PONDER**   As the collimation increases, the beam size becomes smaller and the amount of scattered radiation is reduced. As the collimation decreases, the area radiographed becomes larger, the field size increases, and the potential for scattered radiation is higher.

Collimation and Contrast

As the radiation area decreases, the amount of radiation scattered from the region of interest decreases. If the scattered radiation reaches the film, it is not useful radiation. Its only effect is to increase the base density and reduce the contrast between the base density and the imaged structures.

TABLE 7-1	Effect of Changing Factors*	
	INCREASED FACTOR	
Field Size	Collimation	
Patient dose	Increase	Decrease
Scatter radiation	Increase	Decrease
Contrast	Decrease	Increase
Density	Increase	Decrease

*Increasing the collimation narrows the field of view. Increasing the field size is the same as opening the collimator shutters.

If collimation restricts the beam size dramatically, the technical factors may have to be increased slightly to accommodate the restriction of some of the useful radiation (Table 7-1). To change the density, only the mAs should be increased, not the kV.

Collimator Testing

If the collimation shutters or leaves do not close correctly, the resulting radiograph may not be exposed over the necessary area of the film. The quickest method to test a collimator is to use a 10 × 12 in (25 × 30 cm) cassette, as follows.

1. In the darkroom, remove the film from the cassette and place it in the storage box.
2. Place the open cassette on the table beneath the collimator light, and turn on the collimator light. Center the front screen to the center of the light. Close the shutters so that approx 2 inches (5 cm) of the outside edges of the screen remain unlit.
3. Straighten out four large paper clips or use four lengths of wire. Place these items at the edges of the lighted area of the screen.
4. Set the generator at 50 kV, 100 mA, and at least 0.50 second. You need the radiation to light the screen long

enough to assess the coincidence of the radiation to the wires on all four sides.

5. Put on a leaded apron, thyroid collar, and gloves, and position yourself so that you are able to see the cassette clearly the collimator light must be off prior to exposure. Make an exposure, and view the position of the lighted screen in relation to the wires.

This test may also be carried out using a cassette with film installed. Center the film on the tabletop as instructed. Center the wires as instructed. Use 50 kV, 100 mA, and 1/30 sec. Using a 400-speed system, process the film normally, and review the position of the wires in relation to the position of the radiation field.

The standards for collimator coincidence state that the distance from the light field to the x-ray field must be within 1% of the distance to the image receptor. At 100 cm, a 1-cm offset is allowable.[1-3] Service on a collimator in the clinic setting is somewhat complex, because the shutters are constructed to function as a unit and must not obstruct the field of view. It is important, therefore, to protect the collimator, particularly an older collimator, from damage by animals kicking out as they are positioned for ventrodorsal views.

> **POINTS TO PONDER** Older collimators were not equipped with the metals to absorb scatter that the newer collimators have as part of their manufacture. When the collimator is being tested, place a loaded cassette next to the test cassette, and process both films. If there is scattered radiation on the test film, it is likely that the collimator is not absorbing scattered radiation as it should. This will be evidenced by a decreasing density on the film from the near side to the far side of the film as it was positioned next to the test cassette. The older Videx models of collimators were notorious for this problem.

Collimator Problems or Scatter from the Patient?

The collimator is the last filtration system of the x-ray beam before it reaches the patient. In some cases, when the beam is collimated, there is a shadow of the patient's anatomy on the image beyond the edges of the collimator.

This may be caused by scatter from the patient itself. If the "splash" of radiation is larger when the patient being radiographed is large and is not visible when the patient is quite small, the problem is most likely scatter from the patient. Placing a lead strip along the side of the patient prevents this scatter from affecting the image.

If parts of the patient's anatomy are clearly visible, such as a leg or the spinous processes in an otherwise collimated spine, then the fault is most likely *extrafocal radiation* (see Chapter 4) *or off focus radiation* (Figure 7-8). This is radiation that is created by the photon stream outside the actual focal spot. It may be due to a defect in the design and manufacture of the collimator or to high technical factors.

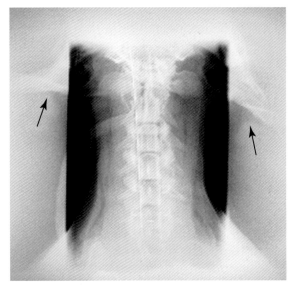

FIGURE 7-8 Evidence of extrafocal radiation (*arrows*).

Scattered Radiation

The radiation produced in this manner has much lower energy than the usable photon stream. Scattered radiation does not have the capability of producing an organized image beyond the limits of the collimator. The presence of scattered radiation is the main reason that anyone within the room at the time of exposure should be appropriately gowned and gloved (see Chapter 16).

Changing the Collimator Light Bulb

Whenever service of any kind is required on the radiography unit, turn off the generator at the wall. *Never* open the generator panel or any part of the radiography unit without a qualified service person in attendance, *except* to change the collimator light bulb.

When the radiography unit is new, it should be supplied with a spare collimator light bulb. The replacement bulb should be kept in a very specific place, and its location should be noted on the x-ray generator. Whenever the light bulb is changed, a new one should be ordered right away. Collimator lights are usually supplied by x-ray service companies or they can be ordered online (just type in the alphanumeric code of the bulb followed by the words "light bulb" in your search engine). Always make sure that the voltage of the bulb you are ordering is the same as the one you are replacing. The wattage should also be the same, but the voltage is more important.

If you are not sure which bulb to order, check the back of the collimator (Figure 7-9). There is usually a label specifying voltage and wattage. If there is no label, then carefully follow these instructions:

1. Make sure the generator is turned off at the wall switch.
2. Search for a coverplate on the collimator. It is usually on the back or on the side.
3. Remove the coverplate. Typically the light bulb is evident. On some collimators, the shutters must be closed to

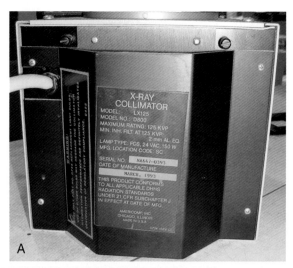

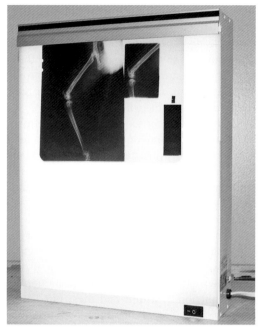

FIGURE 7-9 **A,** Cover plate on the back of a collimator. **B,** Note the lamp type instructions. This collimator label also includes the amount of filtration inherent in the components of the collimator.

FIGURE 7-10 A typical stand-alone illuminator. This illuminator may stand on a table, may be mounted on a wall, or may be inserted into the wall between the upright joists.

expose the bulb. Other collimators have a small black box that must be removed. Carefully note the position of the box before you remove it.

4. Once the light bulb is exposed, remove it, noting whether it required turning or just a gentle tug to do so. This is very important. Some light bulbs are mounted between what appears to be two steel plates. If you look very closely you will see a slight opening for the end of the new bulb. Some light bulbs have a bayonet mount and require turning as well as pulling to remove them.

5. Check to ensure that the bulb you are replacing is identical to the new bulb. The code numbers or letters may differ but the wattage and voltage must be the same.

6. The new light bulb will probably be a halogen bulb, so it is important not to touch it with bare hands or fingers. The bulb usually comes wrapped in a plastic cover from which the bottom may be cut away, revealing the insertion end of the bulb. Using the cover, gently and firmly insert the bulb in the exact spot from which you removed the old bulb. Then remove the plastic cover.

7. Once the bulb is firmly in place, turn on the main power, and test that the bulb is working.

8. Turn off the power again, and reaffix the collimator coverplate.

Illuminators

Illuminators (Figure 7-10) are used to transmit light evenly through a specially produced glass in order to identify and interpret radiographic images. It is vital that the illuminators are checked regularly for optimum brightness. The American Society for Testing and Materials (ASTM) provides an accurate description of the purpose and optimum brightness

of an illuminator. This is regarding industrial radiography but the standards are appropriate for General Radiography:

"The luminance of the transmitted light shall not be less than 30 candelas per square meter for film densities equal to or less than 2.5 optical density and not less than 10 candelas per square meter for film densities greater than 2.5 optical density. If the illuminator has a diffusing screen, the light shall be sufficiently divergent so that both eyes of the observer receive rays from all parts of the screen. The maximum illuminator luminance, and divergence and diffusion of light shall be tested to meet the requirements prescribed."[4]

The illuminator in the veterinary facility is the means by which the veterinarian and often the client view and discuss the results of the radiographic examination. It is very important that the conditions under which the radiographs are interpreted are of the highest possible quality.

The illuminator glass should be cleaned regularly whenever the countertops and shelves are dusted. A cleaning solution such as a standard glass cleaner may be used on the diffusion glass. The switch must be a safety switch and must be checked to ensure that it is not worn or faulty.

At least once per year, the glass panel should be removed, and the illuminator box dusted and cleaned. The bulbs should be checked for brightness and consistency. If one bulb is faulty, all of the bulbs should be replaced at the same time.

Illuminator Specifications

The inside of the illuminator must be painted a bright white in order to reflect as much light as possible toward the diffusion glass. Illuminators are available with wooden or stainless steel boxes but these are not suitable because they absorb photons of light and diminish the amount of light available to view the images.

The color of the light bulbs must be "daylight" or very light blue–tinted bulbs to match the color spectrum of the radiographic film. Commercially available bulbs may be purchased at a hardware store. It is important to note that bulbs are also available with a green, yellow, or pink tone, which are not suitable for viewing radiographs.

CHECK IT OUT A combination of correct color and brightness enhances the contrast of the radiographs. As a quick test to reveal whether the color of the illuminator bulbs in the facility is correct, review a radiograph hung on the clinic illuminator. Now go to a window on a cloudy, bright day and review the same radiograph (this is the same color as the daylight light bulb). If the image looks the same, then the light bulbs are most likely daylight. Most fluorescent bulbs are labeled at one end with the manufacturer and the color.

An illuminator that is not working correctly or does not transmit the light effectively can seriously compromise the reading of a radiograph.

Illuminator Position

An illuminator may be mounted on the wall or positioned within the wall so that the front is flush with the wall. The films are hung from holders at the top of the illuminator, and these should be checked regularly to ensure that they do not catch and hold the film so firmly that it cannot be hung and removed without incident.

The illuminator should be positioned in the room so that the overhead light may be switched off. This way there will be no backlighting to reduce the brightness of the light transmitted from the illuminator.

Illuminator masks (Figure 7-11) should be available to cover any part of the illuminator panel not covered by the film, so that all available light reaching the eye of the clinician is directed through the radiograph.

CHECK IT OUT To construct radiographic masks, remove a sheet of film from the film box in the darkroom. Close the box and return it to the holder. Turn on the light in the darkroom, to expose the film. Process the film normally. The film will be completely black and will act as a mask for radiographs hung on an illuminator. Ensure that you have enough masks to cover any size area that is not covered by the normal-sized films.

For dental films, produce the mask and cut out a hole the size of the dental film in the middle of the mask. Cut out as many holes as necessary. Return the cutouts to the film and tape them in place. Place the tape along the bottom of the hole so that the cutout can drop down when the hole is in use by the dental radiograph and be returned to position when it is not in use.

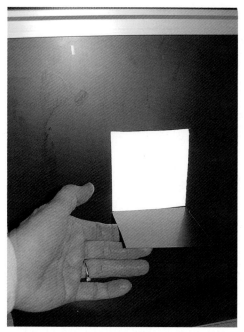

FIGURE 7-11 Illuminator mask. Keep the piece that is cut out and use it to mask that hole. Then you can make the mask cutout fit other sizes of film. Make the cut out close to the middle of the illuminator to ensure you have the brightest light.

Grids and Grid Trays

In the very early days, Drs. Potter and Bucky invented a device in which vertical strips of metal interspaced with a radiolucent material (newspaper was used at one time) were enclosed by metal straps and mounted into an oscillating tray that was connected to the exposure switch on the radiography unit. The tray contained the x-ray cassette with the film enclosed. The strips were positioned vertically to the axis of the table. This was the birth of the grid that we use today. They named the entire unit the Potter-Bucky diaphragm. The colloquial term "Bucky tray" has lingered in the profession, but the device has long since been replaced by a stationary grid in the veterinary profession and we now use the term grid tray.

The original Bucky tray had to be set (or cocked) prior to each exposure; when the exposure was made, the lock released and the tray moved across the face of the cassette. This somewhat complicated contraption worked on the principle of the windshield wiper moving across the car windshield during a rainstorm. Your eyes do not focus on the windshield wiper but rather through the window to the road outside. Drs. Potter and Bucky speculated that if the grid moved rapidly enough the strips would not be visible and any scattered radiation that was not projected vertically through the strips would be absorbed by them, thus eliminating scatter and improving contrast. The device worked well originally, and Dr. Bucky in particular made a name for himself that persists to this day.

A couple of problems arose when this technology transferred to the veterinary market. The Potter-Bucky oscillating device made a fairly loud noise as it was released. Once the

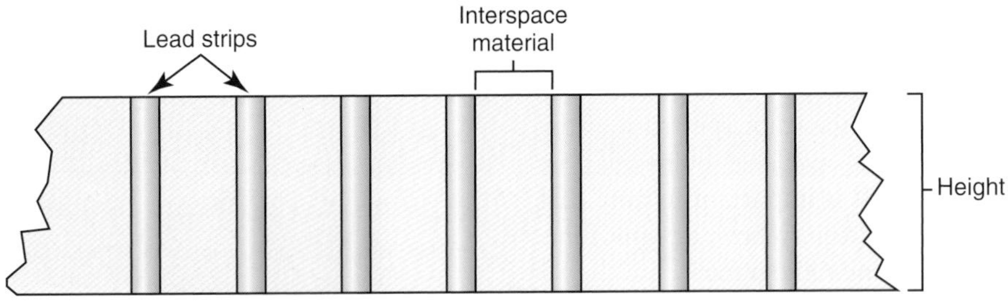

Lead strips

Interspace material

Height

Grid ratio: $\dfrac{\text{Height}}{\text{Width of interspace}}$

FIGURE 7-12 Grid ratio is the ratio of the height of the lead strips to the distance (interspace) between them.

spring was converted to a motor, the whirring noise of the motor was bothersome to some animals. The other problem was the timing of the original units. The exposure time had to be 1/10 of a second or longer for the strips to move rapidly enough to blur out the image. Most veterinary exposures must be far less than 1/10 of a second, so grid lines are a problem.

Over many years, the grid itself was refined and improved. The metal strips were replaced by more sophisticated materials, and the interspace material was upgraded with the invention of polyesters. The grid was so effective that various models are manufactured for specific applications. Grid nomenclature is very important, and knowledge of the type and ratio of the grid in any veterinary clinic is vital.

Grid Nomenclature

Every grid manufactured throughout the world is imprinted or labeled with the grid ratio, the lines per inch, and the manufacturer.

> **CHECK IT OUT** Remove the top of the x-ray table carefully. Most tabletops are screwed to the frame either on top of the table or beneath the table. Most medical-grade tabletops are screwed to the frame beneath the table. Remove the screws carefully. The tabletop can always be reattached with strips of adhesive-backed hook-and-loop (Velcro) tape.
>
> (If the tabletop does not come off easily and it is necessary to change the grid, contact a service person to remove the grid from beneath the tabletop.)
>
> The grid is seated above the grid tray. The grid lines should run parallel to the length of the table. There should be a line etched or drawn on the grid indicating the direction of the lines. A label or etching on the front or top of the grid indicates the grid ratio and the line pairs per inch.

Grid Ratios, Line Pairs/Inch

A ratio is expressed as a number with a relationship to a second number; the ratio of 25 apples to 5 apples is 5:1. It is always expressed with a colon (:) in between the two numbers.

As grids were used in various procedures, the manufacturers made ever more sophisticated grids. The best way to identify them was by expressing a ratio of lines of the

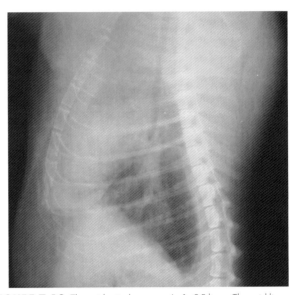

FIGURE 7-13 The grid ratio here was 6:1, 85 lines. The grid lines are obvious on the radiograph, and the grid has started to deteriorate, placing a pattern on every image and obscuring a correct reading of pathology.

material used to "clean up" the scatter (Figure 7-12). So grids became 5:1, 6:1, 8:1, 10:1, 12:1, 16:1. It was soon discovered that grids with the lower ratios did not "work" as well as the grids with higher ratios. Also, the grids with very high ratios—16:1—and higher were useful only for very specific applications and not for general radiography. The higher-ratio grids eliminated the scattered radiation but they also eliminated some of the useful beam, thereby increasing patient radiation dose. (If some of the useful beam is eliminated then technical factors would have to be increased thereby increasing patient dose.)

The problem with expressing the grid ratio alone is that it does not specify the number of line pairs (lp) per inch. A grid may have an 8:1 line ratio, but if the lines are spread too far apart they will show up on a radiograph (Figure 7-13). Because the ratio numbers identify the height of lines or strips in comparison with the space between them, the number of lines or strips is important.

In the veterinary field, grids of 8:1 and 10:1 103 lp/inch work the best. The scatter control is good without the need to increase the radiation dose by too much to overcome the clean-up of the grid.

Grid Deterioration

Older grids deteriorate over time and will overlay an image of their degradation on every film that is exposed in the grid tray (Figure 7-14). The image on a film with grid deterioration usually demonstrates streaking lines travelling in the direction of the grid lines. The interspace material can degrade and disappear, leaving minus-density artifacts on the image.

There is no way to repair a grid, and any grid more than 25 years old should probably be replaced.

Parallel versus Focused Grids

The original grids were manufactured with parallel lines running in the vertical direction of the table (Figure 7-15). A problem arose when larger cassette sizes became available

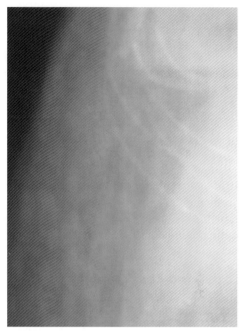

FIGURE 7-14 Grid deterioration up close. The mottled pattern is the absence of the interspace material. Newsprint was frequently used as interspace material. Over time it would disintegrate.

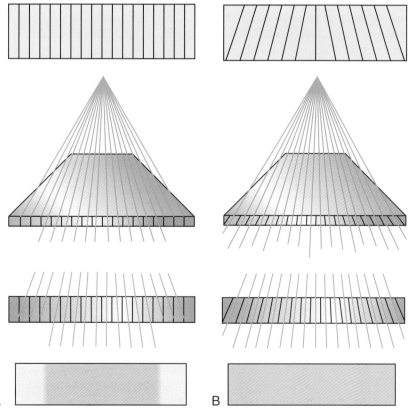

FIGURE 7-15 A, A parallel grid absorbs the radiation at the edges of the image. B, The focused grid allows the rays to pass through to the outer edges of the image.

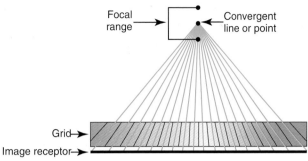

FIGURE 7-16 A focused grid. The lead lines are angled coincident with the divergent primary rays. The focal length is now preset, and the focal range is slightly above and slightly below the convergent point. Typically, a 40-inch focal length grid has a focal range of 34 to 44 inches.

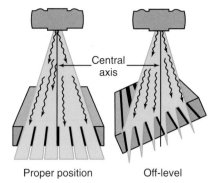

FIGURE 7-17 A focused grid raised on one side of the table. One side of the grid acts as a parallel grid; the other side absorbs the primary and secondary radiation.

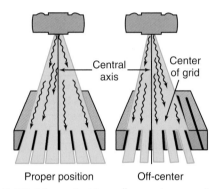

FIGURE 7-18 A focused grid set off-center does not allow the radiation to penetrate the grid correctly, causing off-center cutoff.

and the collimators opened to a 14-inch lateral width. The edges of the image became clear, and the grid cut off the useful radiation reaching the edges of the film.

Grid Focus and Focal Length

Grid manufacturing techniques became more sophisticated, and the newer grids were manufactured with the lines tilted slightly to match the divergent x-rays of the primary beam (Figure 7-16). These focused grids allowed more primary radiation to reach the film than the older parallel grids, but they also introduced another variable that had to be addressed. The divergent rays of the x-ray beam exit at a prescribed distance from the grid (40 in or 100 cm). The problem occurred if the primary beam was moved to 6 feet (180 cm). The angled strips would absorb the radiation incorrectly. Another problem occurred with equine radiography when the x-ray unit was held too close to the grid. So the manufacturers produced grids specific to certain focal lengths. The common grid for a veterinary clinic is a 34 to 44 in (86 to 112 cm) focal length.

Grid Installation

The grid is installed beneath the tabletop above the cassette. A grid tray is usually in place under the table. The cassette is placed in the grid tray, and the folded metal edges of the grid tray will support the grid. An older installed grid may be screwed in place, glued in place, or just set on the guides in the hope that the table will not be moved to dislodge the grid. Grids have even been held in place by paper clips and chewing gum!

When the grid is to be replaced, the size of the grid tray is important. The grid should overhang the edges of the cassette slightly to effectively absorb the scattered radiation and not be visible on the image. For example, an 18 in (46 cm) × 18 in (46 cm) grid will cover a 14 in × 17 in (35 cm × 43 cm) cassette.

Strips of adhesive-backed hook-and-loop (Velcro) tape work well to attach the grid to the grid tray. It may be necessary to cut the strips to a width of 0.5 in (1.27 cm) lengthwise

so there is no chance that they will catch on the cassette as it is drawn in and out of the tray.

Grid Artifacts

Positioning the grid is also critical because it must be exactly in the center of the table or, in equine radiography, the central ray must be centered exactly on the center line of the grid. The grid must also be installed flat on the grid tray, exactly parallel to the port of the x-ray tube. If it is tilted slightly from one side to the other, it will allow the radiation on one side to pass through but will cut off the radiation prematurely on the raised side (Figures 7-17 through 7-19).

The Effect of a Grid on Technical Factors

The grid absorbs some of the primary beam as it impacts directly on the lead strips. The grid conversion factor (GCF) is the formula that determines the increase in technical factors to compensate for this absorption. As the grid ratio increases, the radiographic density decreases, and vice versa.

The mAs value changes according to Table 7-2. However, this table should not be necessary if the technique chart is set up correctly at the original installation.

The formula is as follows:

$$\text{Grid Conversion Factor} = \frac{\text{mAs with the grid}}{\text{mAs without the grid}}$$

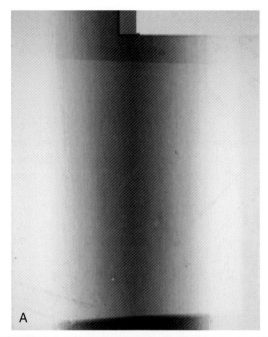

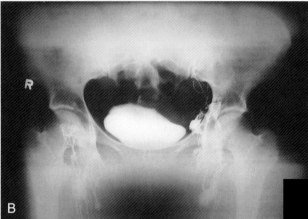

FIGURE 7-19 A, A focused grid installed upside-down. The divergent rays are absorbed, and only the central rays affect the film. **B,** The grid has been installed upside-down and also rotated 90 degrees. The grid lines should run parallel to the tabletop.

Two Imaging Tricks When No Grid Is Available

A grid should always be included in the radiography inventory. However, some sites do not have a grid installed. The following two suggested methods function as a

TABLE 7-2	Grid Conversion Factors*
GRID RATIOGRID	**CONVERSION FACTOR NUMBER**
5 to 1	2
6 to 1	3
8 to 1 & 10 to 1	4
12 to 1	5
16 to 1	6

*Grid conversion factor: multiply the mAs by the grid conversion factor number for each grid ratio

very-low-ratio grid and may help clean up some scattered radiation, but they should never be regarded as a replacement for a grid.

Air Gap Technique

One way to reproduce the effect of a 5:1 grid is to move the patient approximately 8 in (25 cm) away from the cassette. The easiest way to do this is to have the patient stand on the table 8 in (25 cm) from the cassette. Angle the x-ray tube at 90 degrees to the tabletop. The 8-inch air gap will absorb some of the scattered radiation from the patient and replicate the effect of a low-ratio grid.

Remember that moving the patient away from the film will also result in magnification, which could affect resolution.

Reverse Kodak Cassette

The cassette manufactured for Kodak is a distinctive bright yellow on the back. If the cassette is turned over so that the patient is lying on the back of the cassette on the tabletop, the yellow back will replicate the absorption of a 5:1 grid.

SUMMARY

This chapter contains the basics of optimizing radiographic images. Motion, blur, distortion, and magnification have been discussed. The installation of a grid is a necessary factor in the reduction of scattered radiation affecting the image. All of the options discussed in this chapter are essential to produce the best images possible, no matter what radiography unit and technique chart are used.

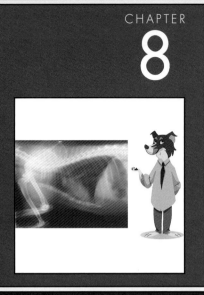

Processing the Image

It is an old maxim of mine that when you have eliminated the impossible, whatever remains, however improbable, must be the truth.*

—Sherlock Holmes, Character of Arthur Conan Doyle (1859–1930)

OUTLINE

LEARNING OBJECTIVES

When you have finished this chapter, you will be able to:
1. Understand darkroom specifications.
2. Understand the purpose of developer and fixer.
3. Explain the process of washing and drying.
4. List some causes of artifacts.
5. Understand processor construction and processor quality control.

APPLICATIONS

The application of the information in this chapter is relevant to the following areas:
1. Optimizing images (radiographs) to aid in diagnoses.

*Sherlock Holmes could have been referring to film artifacts!

The final phase of the production of the image is processing. Ninety-eight percent of all artifacts on an image occur during this process. In this chapter, manual and automatic processing methods are discussed, as well as the architecture and layout of a suitable darkroom in which to carry out the procedures. Suggestions for new facilities are also included.

A Word about Chemicals

In these days of conversion to digital radiography, the chemical suppliers have been hard hit as human hospitals and clinics convert their systems and cancel their chemical contracts. Because these contracts were their main source of income, these companies have switched to selling other products to support that business and the production of chemicals has reduced considerably. Also, the components of the developer and fixer have been altered to remove any product that does not directly involve actually processing the films. Along with the antisludge and antifrothing components, some manufacturers have removed most of the odor masks. The smell of the chemicals has emerged to a point at which it is objectionable to stay in the darkroom for any length of time. The suggestion to address this problem is to search out a brand of chemical that has not removed the odor mask. They are quite easy to find. The fixer is the worst culprit, and sampling various brands of fixer is quite straightforward as long as the chemicals from two different companies are not mixed together.

A further solution to the odor problem is to increase the ventilation in the darkroom. An added fan and keeping the darkroom door open when it is not in use is also helpful. A light-tight air vent window is available. This mesh window, which is installed in the darkroom door at eye level, allows air but not light to pass through. It is available from any supplier of photography equipment as well as from radiography accessories suppliers.

Automatic processing also helps reduce the odor to a degree because the chemical containers remain covered during processing.

Darkroom Layout

In a new clinic, it is useful to make the radiography room light-tight and to place the processor in one corner of the room. The patient can be removed during the processing of the film or can stay on the table as long as the room is lit with two safelights so that the patient may be monitored under the safelight conditions.

The darkroom as an individual room must be large enough that an adult can enter, open a 14 in × 17 in cassette on a counter, and place it either on a hanger or in the processor without risk of spilling chemicals on himself/herself or the cassette (Figure 8-1). A minimum darkroom size of 5 feet (1.5 m) by 7 feet (2.13 m) is sufficient to position the processor or wet tanks. One extra foot (30 cm) in both directions would be an ideal minimum.

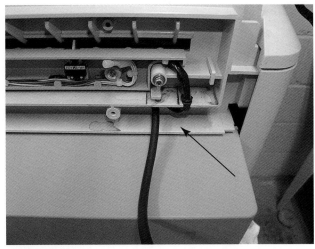

FIGURE 8-1 Chemicals spilled on the processor between the feed tray and the developer. This chemical could easily seep down onto the processing boards, causing a malfunction and an expensive repair.

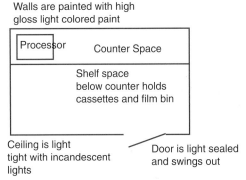

FIGURE 8-2 A typical darkroom layout. The wet side is on the left and the dry side on the right. Ventilation is achieved through a door vent and a ceiling exhaust fan that is light-tight.

The darkroom door should be hung to swing out from the darkroom. In a minimum-sized darkroom this is not an option. The technician has to walk into the darkroom and close the door. He/she has to fit inside without any possibility of bumping into the processor or wet tanks. Once the processor is in position and the tanks are filled, it is very easy to jostle the processor and cause overflow of chemicals from one tank to another or, worse still, the developer to be splashed onto the control boards, destroying them completely and causing the processor to malfunction (Figure 8-2).

The space should have a counter top large enough to open a 14 in × 17 in (35 cm × 43 cm) cassette. The processing area should be removed from the dry film area so that there is no chance of chemicals being transferred to the cassettes and screens.

The temperature in the darkroom should be maintained at 68° F (20° C). The humidity should be maintained at 40% to 60%. The door to the darkroom should be left open when it is not in use. This practice will maintain the temperature and humidity and will also ensure good airflow. If the

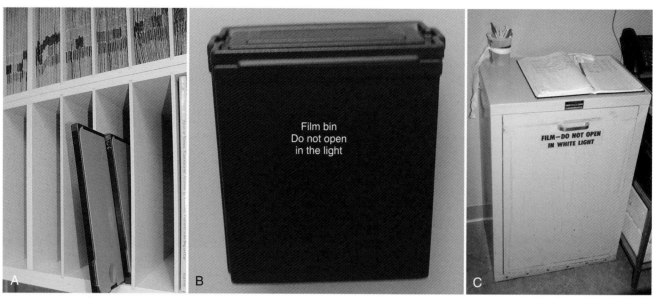

FIGURE 8-3 **A,** Cassettes are stored upright above the processor. The films are stored above the cassettes. **B,** A plastic film bin for use in the darkroom. **C,** A steel film bin for use in the radiography room.

darkroom is sealed too tightly, it may be difficult to close the door. A light-tight airflow pass-through is available.

The cassettes and film boxes must be stored upright and well away from the chemical storage (Figure 8-3A). Ideally a film bin should be mounted on the wall in order to store the film out of the light and accidental exposure (Figure 8-3B). A metal film bin must be used if the processor and film are located in the radiography room (Figure 8-3C). Scattered radiation will penetrate a plastic film bin unless the bin is located a minimum of 10 feet from the source of the scatter.

The walls should be painted a light reflective color in order to take advantage of as much light as possible from the safelight. The countertop should be positioned between 29 inches (74 cm) and 33 inches (84 cm) above the floor.

Ideally the replenishment tanks are positioned beneath the tabletop processor. If this is not possible, they should be accessible both for cleaning and for "topping up" chemicals.

Film should be used on a first in/first out basis so that the boxes are rotated systematically and the film does not become stale dated. Chemicals should be stored in their original containers until they are used. Extra chemicals should not be stored in the darkroom but rather in an appropriate storage place in the facility.

The darkroom should be cleaned regularly as part of the quality assurance program in the clinic. Dust and dirt accumulate on the processing tray and will affect the film emulsion as it is being processed. The darkroom is not a cloakroom, and coats and linens should be stored elsewhere.

It is better use of the space to place the processor in the radiography room rather than in a very small, cramped darkroom and run the risk of chemicals splashing onto the cassettes and screens.

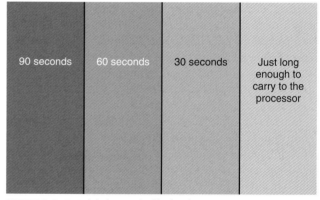

FIGURE 8-4 Safelight test. The film has been pre-exposed and placed beneath a cassette in the darkroom. The exposure time has allowed the film to fog. The darkroom should be resealed, and the test should be repeated.

Darkroom Integrity

The door of the darkroom must be light-tight. The darkroom must be completely dark. **This is nonnegotiable.** If the door is closed and after 5 to 8 minutes of moving about in the pitch-black dark the technician sees no visible light leaks, the integrity of the darkroom is confirmed. The human eye requires about 5 to 8 minutes to adjust to the darkness after being exposed to a lighted room.

Light is very pervasive, and it is vital that all light is eliminated. Even if the human eye does not readily see the light the film will "see" it instantly and record it as fog.

Safelight Test

The unexposed film does not react to light as readily as an exposed film. A film that has been exposed to radiation is eight to ten times more reactive to any type of fog than an unexposed film. A safelight test (Figure 8-4) is always performed with an exposed film; it is exposed film that is vulnerable when it is being placed on the processor feed tray. The safelight test is performed as follows:

1. Expose a film in a cassette using 50 kilovolts (kV), 3 milliampere-seconds (mAs) on the tabletop.
2. Take the cassette to the darkroom and place it on the counter.
3. Turn the safelight on, secure the darkroom, and open the cassette.
4. Remove the film from the cassette, and place ¾ of the film beneath the cassette, leaving ¼ exposed to the safelight. Count to 30 seconds.
5. Slide the next ¼ of the film out from under the cassette, and count to 30 again. Now ½ of the film has been exposed to the safelight.
6. Repeat this once again so that ¾ of the film has been exposed to the safelight.
7. Immediately remove the rest of the film from under the cassette, and process it.

The last ¼ of the film was exposed to the safelight for just the length of time it took to take the film to the processor. If there is a problem with the safelight, the areas exposed to the safelight will be darkened in proportion to the length of time that they were exposed to the light plus the amount of the original exposure. The total length of exposure time is 1.5 minutes.

FIGURE IT OUT The darkroom integrity was intact, yet the films were being fogged. I requested that a record be initiated on which the staff recorded the usual size of patient, and so on, and also the time of day and the weather conditions when the technicians entered the darkroom to process film. The clinic was located in a converted house, and the darkroom, at the front of the house, had a large window that was tightly covered by a dark vinyl/faux leather material. The clinic was manually processing films.

According to the record, the films were being fogged between 1 and 4 PM on sunny days. Other times of the day there was no problem, and on cloudy or rainy days there was no problem. The clinic faced south, it was summertime, and the sun at that time of the year was shining directly at the front of the clinic. The intensity of the sun penetrated the thick vinyl and coincidentally reflected off a mirror on the back of the door opposite the window. The vinyl, it turned out, was a very, very dark green, which matched the color spectrum of the film and at that time of day under those conditions fogged the film.

Safelight Specifications

The color spectrum that the film responds to is at the ultraviolet/blue-green side of the spectrum. The most common film in use today is green light–receiving film. Blue light–receiving film is being phased out, and so when a facility purchases or replaces a safelight, the light emitted from the safelight should be dark red (Figure 8-5) with no orange or yellow.

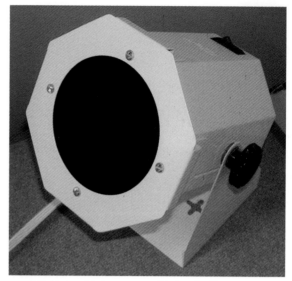

FIGURE 8-5 A red light–emitting safelight. The filter is very important and must match the spectral sensitivity of the film.

Old safelights prior to 1981 were Wratten series 2B red-brown. Once green-receiving films were marketed, the safelight color had to change because the red-brown tint has a yellow component and the color green is made up of blue and yellow. The safelight should be mounted on the wall a minimum of 4 feet (1.22 m) above the working surface where cassettes are loaded and unloaded.

Film Identifiers

The traditional veterinary identification (ID) labels and labeling tape are slowly being phased out because they are not as efficient now that a lead replacement material is being used. The electric or battery-operated photoidentifier is preferable, and the information is much clearer on the images than those produced by the older method. Individual lead lettering is certainly sharper still but very time consuming because each patient's information must be set up individually.

An electric or battery-operated photoidentifier works in conjunction with the cassettes. The following steps must be taken before the labeler (Figure 8-6) is used:

1. Choose a corner of every cassette and put a black label over each screen in the appropriate corner. These blockers will prevent the radiation from affecting the film in that area. (Use the same label position on every cassette in the facility)
2. The cassettes should then be labeled on the outside over the blocked-off portion so that patient anatomy and identifying markers are not positioned over the blocker.
3. ID labels must be printed, including the patient's name, date, ID number, the name of the veterinary facility, and the address of the facility. This is required legal information in most countries and must be visible on each film.
4. Once the film is exposed, take it to the darkroom and remove it from the cassette. Place the film in the photomarker and stamp it with the patient's identifiers.

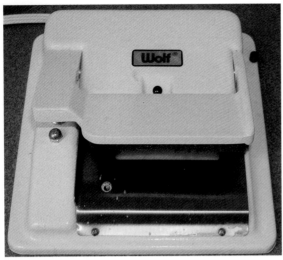

FIGURE 8-6 An ID labeler ready to be used.

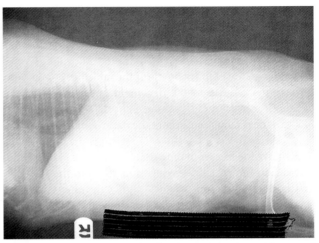

FIGURE 8-7 Film processed with exhausted developer. The overall image lacks correct density and contrast; it has a washed-out appearance.

5. With this method, each film is identified prior to processing. This is by far the most efficient method of identifying individual films.

Secondary film identifiers, such as right and left markers, positioning markers—VD, DV, upright—time of day, and so on, must all be positioned within the radiation area and must be clearly identifiable.

Radiography Log Books

A radiography log book must be maintained by the facility. This will ensure that the examination, the technical factors and the patient identifiers, date, name, owner's name, patient measurement, examination, acquisition number, and technical factors are recorded for inspection, for reexamination, and by any radiation inspector surveying the clinic. Each of the factors must be entered each time as an aid to quality control within the clinic.

Processing the Film

Film processing in the radiography department is very similar to any photographic process. The film must be immersed in developer, which will convert the latent image to a visible image. The film is then transferred to the fixer, in which the unexposed emulsion is removed from the film base, leaving the developed image intact. Washing the film removes all the waste chemical components from the film base and the retained emulsion. Finally, drying the film completes the process.

This process occurs either manually with the use of wet tanks and hangers or through an automatic processor.

Developing the Image (Figure 8-7)

The purpose of the developer is to cause the latent image to become a manifest image. This change is achieved by immersing the film in a chemical solution. The chemicals have two main components and then several other auxiliary components. This is the first step in the process.

> **POINTS TO PONDER** The components of the developer and fixer have changed dramatically over the years. The chemical manufacturers have developed products that mix together and meet most municipal hazardous waste standards. In most communities, therefore, the chemicals are safe to dispose of in small effluent quantities down the drain with the other waste products from the facility.
>
> Each facility should review the chemical waste guidelines with its municipality and must always have the component sheets from the chemical manufacturer on hand in the clinic. The hazardous waste sheets for most chemicals are available online and are always available from the manufacturer.

Developer Components

The two main components in the developer are phenidone and hydroquinone. Their main function is to reduce the silver halide in the film emulsion to metallic silver by donating additional electrons to the sensitivity specks in the latent image centers. The other and equally important function is to amplify the amount of metallic silver on the film by increasing the number of silver atoms in each latent image center. Unexposed silver halide in the film emulsion does not react to the chemicals because it has not been ionized and therefore will not accept electrons from the developing solutions. Table 8-1 lists the developer components and their functions.

Time Temperature Developing

If the developer solution is overheated or if the film is left in the solution for an extended time, the unexposed crystals start to react to the solution and a "developer fog" occurs. This is why timing the exposure of

TABLE 8-1	Developer Components and Their Functions		
AGENT	**CHEMICAL**	**FUNCTION**	**KEY TO REMEMBERING**
Developing Agent	Phenidone	Fast-Produces the gray densities, stable, and long lived	**Ph**enidone—**ph**ast—mainly grays
Developing Agent	Hydroquinone	Slow—produces blacks; increases contrast on the image; sensitive to temperature, oxygen, and aging	**Longer** name—**longer** time—mainly blacks The sensitive one, reacts to time, temperature and air and will be the first to become exhausted
Activator	Sodium carbonate	Stabilizes the pH; maintains acidity	**Bi**carbonate of soda stabilizes the acidity in your stomach if you have eaten rich food
Restrainer	Potassium bromide	Decreases the reduction of the unexposed silver halide	This is the stopper—**POTAS**Sium (read it backwards)
Preservative	Sodium sulfite	Decreases sensitivity to oxidation	
Hardener		"Glues" the emulsion to the base to reduce scratches in the processor	
Solvent	Water	Makes up about 98%–99% of the solution	

TABLE 8-2	Fixer Components and their Functions		
AGENT	**CHEMICAL**	**FUNCTION**	**KEY TO REMEMBERING**
Fixing agent	Ammonium thiosulfate	Clears away unexposed silver halide	This causes the rotten egg smell—
Acidifier	Acetic acid	Stops development	Vinegar
Preservative	Sodium sulfite	Prevents a reaction between fixing agent and acidifier	Same as developer
Hardener	Chrome alum, potassium aluminum sulfate, or aluminum chloride	Hardens the emulsion	Similar to what is in your deodorant! As a drying agent
Solvent	Water	Makes up about 98%–99% of the solution	

the films to the chemicals and the temperature of the chemicals is very important, particularly in manual (nonautomatic) processing.

The manufacturers of chemicals produced a solution that is optimized for manual processing at 68°F (20°C). It is not a coincidence that this is also the average temperature in a veterinary clinic. The chemicals do not have to be heated or cooled prior to use.

The technique chart should be optimized so that the film is processed at 4 minutes in the manual developer at 68°F (20°C). If the image appears too quickly or too slowly, the technique should be adjusted, not the temperature of the chemicals.

The hydroquinone works slowly to build up the blacks and therefore enhance the contrast of the image. If the solution is either too hot or too cold, the hydroquinone does not function correctly and the image is compromised.

Fixer

The main purpose of the fixer (Table 8-2) is to remove the unexposed silver halide from the film base and ensure that the image that has been developed remains intact and permanent. The fixer also stops the development of any unexposed crystals of silver halide (by removing them from the film base), and it further hardens the image to the base. If the film is not fixed correctly, it exits the processor with a milky or even pink appearance (Figure 8-8).

POINTS TO PONDER The developer is highly alkaline, and the fixer is highly acidic. Both of these chemistries must be treated with great respect. An eyewash station must be positioned close to the processing area and must be checked by the quality assurance officer in the clinic regularly. When the chemicals are being handled, it is essential that the personnel are equipped with protective safety goggles. These are available and inexpensive to purchase at any hardware or department store. A drop of fixer concentrate can melt the lens of the eye in seconds.

Washing

The film travels through the fixer and into the wash tank. It must be thoroughly washed to preserve its archival quality. Staining or fading results if the film is not washed with flowing water.

The wash should ensure that clean water flows through the processor as the films are being washed. This takes place by a process called diffusion. The wash water contains less thiosulfate than the fixer and so the chemicals in the fixer are diffused into the wash water. The water must move about the film so that a concentration of fixer does not build up next to the film. This is achieved by the action of the rollers and fresh water running through the tank. If the wash water is not turned on, the film will be stained. This staining is

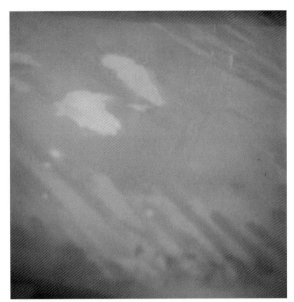

FIGURE 8-8 Film processed with exhausted fixer. The film has a milky appearance and may even appear to be pink from the dye used in the green-receiving film.

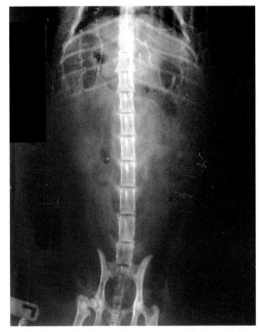

FIGURE 8-9 This film has a few processing faults; sulfiding is very evident on this image as the result of inadequate washing.

evident on a film that is reviewed several weeks after it has been dried and stored. Sulfiding and staining are the result of poor washing (Figure 8-9).

Drying

The dryer temperature should be set on the processor to ensure that the films are not tacky or sticky. If the dryer temperature is optimized and the films are still slightly

TABLE 8-3	Development/Fixer Washing Guidelines*	
PROCESS	**TIME**	**TEMPERATURE**
Developer	4 minutes with agitation	68°F (20°C)
Fixing	8 minutes with agitation	68°F (20°C)
Washing	12 minutes with agitation	68°F (20°C)

*Applies to manual processing only.

damp, adjusting the replenishment rates may be a solution. Approximately 85% to 95% of the moisture should be removed from the films as they travel through the dryer. If they are too hot when they emerge, the film base may become fragile and crack.

Manual Processing

There are still some low-volume sites that process film manually. The chemicals used in manual processing are the same as for automatic processing, except that the temperature and time are very different (Table 8-3).

Cleanliness is essential in this procedure because it is very easy to splash chemicals onto the cassettes and screens. In the manual processing area, the cassettes are never left open. The exposed film is removed, and a fresh film is inserted into the cassette immediately. The exposed film is then readied for processing.

Chemical fumes can be irritating, and the chemicals itself are dangerous to ingest or splash into one's eyes. Safety glasses should be worn by anyone processing film or replenishing chemicals. A 14 in ×17 in (35 cm × 43 cm) film is lifted almost parallel with the eyes when the hangers are moved from tank to tank. It is very important that the technician is careful not to splash chemicals during this procedure.

Procedure

The tanks are always checked for correct temperature (68°F [20°C]) and the chemicals are agitated immediately prior to processing of the films. This is the only time to agitate the chemicals. Agitating the chemicals prior to radiography is premature, and the chemicals will have settled by the time the film is introduced into the tanks. The stir rods are very specific to the chemicals. One stir rod is all that is necessary. It must be made of stainless steel. Any other substance would absorb the chemicals over time and contribute to contamination of the developer. The end of the stir rod is a flat plate with holes punched through it. The technician stirs the chemicals using a vertical motion. The up-and-down activity reduces the tendency for the chemicals to overflow the tanks, but it also brings the stratified liquids up from the bottom of the tank to mix thoroughly. Ten to 15 vertical motions are all that is necessary to completely mix the chemicals.

Film Hangers

The film is removed from the cassette and identified (if a photo id labeler is used). It is then hung on a film hanger. The film hangers have flexible clips at the top and stationary clips at the bottom. The film is hung on the stationary clips first and then on the flexible (spring-equipped) clips at the top. Some hangers have channels into which the film is slid. These are rare, however, and are also difficult to keep clean.

Develop

The film is introduced into the chemicals slowly and steadily. The hanger is held by the top (handle), and once the film is completely immersed, it is agitated in an up-and-down motion several times to ensure that any air bubbles that have entered with the film are removed. The timer is set for *4 minutes*. At 2 minutes the film is agitated up and down once again. This moves the chemicals directly next to the film away and places fresher chemicals against the film. At 4 minutes, the film is agitated once up and down and then moved to the intermediary wash tank. It is agitated once or twice to arrest the development and remove some of the developer; then it is placed in the fixer tank.

Fix

The film is placed into the fixer tank with the same method. It is introduced slowly and steadily and then agitated up and down. The timer is set for *8 minutes*. At 2 minutes the light may be turned on, and the film may be checked. If there is still unexposed emulsion on the film, the fixer is no longer fresh and should be changed once the films are processed. At 4 minutes, the film should have cleared completely and may be viewed momentarily by the staff on an illuminator. Once the film is reviewed, it must be put back into the fixer to complete the fixing process.

It is essential that the fixing process is complete to ensure the archival quality of the image.

Wash

The film is removed from the fixer and lowered into the wash tank. It is preferable for the wash tank to have flowing water. Ideally, the water should enter from the bottom of the tank and exit from the top through a stand-pipe placed in the drain.

The entire film, including the hangers, must be immersed in each solution. The fixer cleans the developer out of the clips of the hangers, and the wash removes the fixer from the hangers and leaves them clean for the next film.

As the clean water flows over the film, it is washed by a diffusion process. The wash water contains less thiosulfate than the fixer, so the chemicals in the fixer are diffused into the wash water. The water must move around the film so that a concentration of fixer does not build up next to the film. Hanging the films in static clean water will work only if the films are agitated frequently during the wash time.

The wash time is *12 minutes* with flowing water. Once again, it is important to wash the films to ensure archival quality. If the used fixer is not removed, the films will turn yellow/brown within weeks (see Figure 8-9).

Running a hose over the films for 2 to 3 minutes in a bathtub is not sufficient to wash the films thoroughly. This problem is evident on in a film reviewed several weeks after it has been dried and stored. Sulfiding and staining are the result of poor washing.

Dry

The film must be dried either by hanging the films in a dryer cabinet or by allowing them to dry naturally in the air of the clinic. Eighty-five percent to ninety percent of the moisture in the film emulsion is removed during drying. If too much moisture is removed, the emulsion will crack, compromising the quality of the image.

The film is now ready to be reviewed and stored permanently.

The hangers may be hung on a hanger rack, and the films may be air dried. If the processing is completed correctly, there are no artifacts on the films. The drying process takes several hours because even though the films feel dry to the touch, the emulsion takes longer to dry completely. If the films are placed in the envelopes too soon, they will stick together and will be impossible to separate.

The Automatic Processor

The first automatic processors were very clumsy, awkward, and very heavy. The racks of rollers required to move the film, through the chemicals were exceptionally heavy, to the point at which a crane or electric pulley was used to lift the racks for cleaning. There are still some very primitive processors in clinics today, but for the most part, they are very expensive to maintain owing to lack of parts. They are now being replaced by lighter and simpler processors.

The automatic processor (Figure 8-10) facilitates the routine of producing a manifest image on the film. It must do so quickly, efficiently, and without imprinting an artifact or scratching the emulsion during the process.

The rollers that transport the film must be close enough together to move the film but far enough apart that they transport the film without imprinting a pressure artifact or otherwise scratching the emulsion. The rollers must be made of the right material so that they are hard enough to

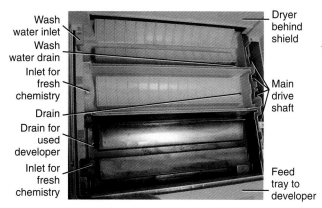

Wash water inlet
Wash water drain
Inlet for fresh chemistry
Drain
Drain for used developer
Inlet for fresh chemistry

Dryer behind shield
Main drive shaft
Feed tray to developer

FIGURE 8-10 The inside of a Konica SRX 101A Processor.

transport the film without absorbing chemicals and imprinting the stale chemicals onto films processed later in the day; they must be soft enough that they do not damage the fragile wet emulsion.

The processor must also be built so that it transports the film evenly and continuously with no hesitation through the developer, fixer, and wash and then into the dryer. It must be able to renew the chemicals so that they are always fresh and are not contaminated by previous film emulsions. It must maintain temperature and speed so that each part of each film remains in solution just long enough to develop the correct amount and then carry on to the next process.

The processor must be built small enough to fit into a small workspace. This means that the film may have to bend around the rollers so that it travels in an undulating pattern, which may be highly exaggerated in a large hospital processor or slightly undulating in a small tabletop processor.

POINT TO PONDER Every time a roller comes into contact with the film, it has the potential to damage the emulsion and imprint an artifact on the film. The more rollers there are, the easier it is for them to damage films. Cleanliness and quality control of the processor are vital, especially if the processor has many rollers. In most veterinary facilities, tabletop processors work well. When one is purchased, a processor with as few rollers as possible should be purchased.

The Feed Tray

The feed tray is situated at the entrance of the processor. The film is placed either horizontally or vertically on this tray, and from there it is accepted into the processor by means of the motor drive. The feed tray is situated very close to the surface of the developer. When a film enters the feed tray it is within 1 to 2 inches (2.5 to 5 cm) of the developer. It is essential that the film is placed squarely on the tray. Once it enters the processor it *must not, under any circumstances,* be drawn back onto the tray. There are a few reasons for this, as follows:

- Typically, the replenishment switches are situated just at the edge of the entrance to the processor. If the film is drawn back, it will deposit developer onto these switches.

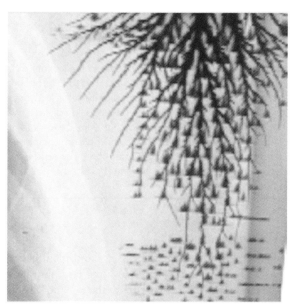

FIGURE 8-11 Static from a feed tray. Note the flat lines produced when the film was placed onto the feed tray.

When the developer dries it is very sticky. If even one of the replenishment switches sticks open, it will pump the replenishment chemicals continuously through the processor until the tanks are empty. Then, if this problem is not noticed in time, the pump will burn out because there are no chemicals flowing through it (Figure 8-14).

- If the film has entered the developer rack and it is pulled backwards, it may lift the rack off the gears and not only damage the gears but also compromise the position of the rack for the next film.
- If the film has entered the developer and is drawn backwards onto the tray, the developer solution is then smeared on the tray. There it will adversely affect the next film that is placed on the feed tray.

The feed tray may be stainless steel or plastic. Either way, if the air in the darkroom is dry, static may build up on the tray and discharge when a film is placed on it. The feed tray should be wiped with a fabric softener cloth at the beginning of the day to prevent static buildup (Figure 8-11).

Processor Systems

The film has now entered the processor and is affected by several systems. Each system is vital to the production of the final image. Table 8-4 outlines the systems. We will examine each in turn.

Transport System

There are several varieties of film processor on the market. The unit that is used to demonstrate the internal workings in this book is a Konica model.

Processors may have many or few rollers. The fewer the better, and this model has very few. The film is guided by the roller angles and the guide shoes (Figure 8-12). This particular method of travel is termed "undulating" because the film is guided in a wavelike path.

TABLE 8-4	Automatic Processor Systems
SYSTEM	**FUNCTION**
Transport system	Chain or gear mechanism moves the rollers in order to transport the film through the processor.
Replenishment	Two pumps are set to replenish the chemicals (developer and fixer) so that it maintains consistent pH and solution concentration throughout the day.
Recirculation	Mixes the fresh chemicals with the working solutions so that the films are processed evenly.
Thermostats	Two—maintain a consistent temperature in the working solution and in the dryer.
Silver recovery	Not part of the processor but an essential unit placed in the outgoing fixer line.

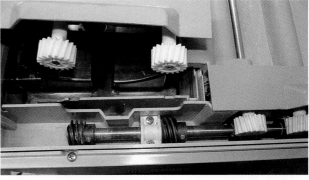

FIGURE 8-13 The rollers of the racks. These rollers are made of a specialized material that does not absorb chemicals over time and will not swell or shrink during their lifetime.

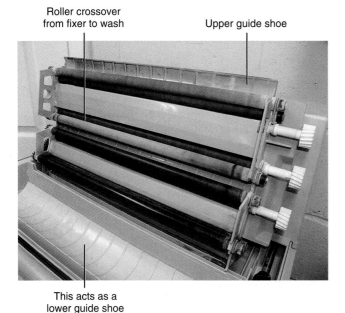

Roller crossover from fixer to wash

Upper guide shoe

This acts as a lower guide shoe

FIGURE 8-12 The transport system. The main drive is below, and this picture shows one rack in place and the other raised to show the gears, which will mesh with the drive shaft when it is put in place.

All rollers in a processor must move at the same speed. They are positioned so that they move the film through the various stages of processing evenly and without hesitation. Larger processors use a system of offset rollers and a vertical transport system. The film enters the processor and is transported by means of the entrance roller assembly into the developer tank. At the bottom and top of each turn, there is a large roller (called a sun roller) that turns the film 180 degrees and sends it back up the assembly to meet a guide shoe at the top, which then turns it back down through the fixer. A unit of this size is most efficient when it is processing 150 films per hour. A typical veterinary clinic, even a busy clinic, does not handle that volume of films, and so a tabletop processor is quite adequate.

The most efficient and easiest processor to maintain is one with very few rollers and an efficient reliable transport system. The Konica SRX model (see Figure 8-10) is an example of this processor type. There are few rollers, and each one is easy to see and assess if there is a problem. The roller assembly is fairly easy to take apart and service, because each rack assembly is easily lifted out of the processor and washed. Daily maintenance is quite simple. The main drive motor on a tabletop processor is connected to a simple geared shaft that fits to the gears on the roller assembly (Figure 8-13). This arrangement ensures that all rollers turn at exactly the same speed.

A broken or worn gear may cause an inconsistency in the rotation of the gears. This problem is easily identified by lifting the lid of the processor and watching for a hesitation or "bumping" of the rack assembly.

Replenishment System

The chemicals in the working tanks become exhausted as the chemicals interact with the silver halides in the emulsion of the film. The developer also interacts with air reducing its effectiveness (Figure 8-7).

The fixer becomes exhausted for several reasons. It is weakened from the introduction of silver halides that it removes from the film base. It also is weakened by the introduction of developer contained in the film emulsion and carried over from the developer.

The film is processed by the fresh chemicals in the individual tanks. It is important that fresh chemicals are introduced as the old, used chemicals are removed. The dimensions of the film and the method by which they are fed into the feed tray determine the amount of replenishment. The switches for replenishment are situated at the back end of the feed tray, immediately next to the developer.

There are two replenishment pumps. One for the developer is set to deliver approximately 60 mL of chemicals for every 14 inches (35 cm) of film. The second pump for the fixer is set to deliver approximately 110 mL of chemicals for every 14 inches (35 cm) of film.

The reason for the discrepancy in the amounts is due to the fact that the film entering the developer is dry and is

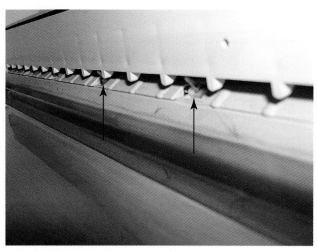

FIGURE 8-14 On this processor, four small fingers (arrows point to two of them) are pressed down when the film slides through the feed tray into the developer. The replenishment pumps stay activated while these fingers are depressed.

FIGURE 8-15 A treelike shadow overlays the entire film. This occurred because the developer replenisher was introduced into the developing tank and not into a recirculation tank. The fresh developer affects the film and activates the developing process, but the older chemicals take longer to accomplish development. The solution to this problem was to install a diversion for the new chemicals so that they mixed with the old chemicals before they reached the film.

affecting only the developer. The film then carries contaminant (developer) into the fixer and also removes fixer when it leaves. So the fixer requires more replenishment in order to keep it fresh and replenish what is removed.

A second form of replenishment is called "flood replenishing." This means that the chemicals are replenished at timed intervals independent of the amount of film used. This arrangement works well if a low amount of film is being processed through a large processor. Because the volume of chemicals is great and the film volume is low, it is much more difficult to maintain stability and concentration of the chemicals. This system is not available on many tabletop processors but it is available on most free-standing processors.

Recirculation System

When the fresh chemicals are delivered to the working tank, they must be introduced gradually and in a separate portion of the tank from where the film is travelling. The fresh chemicals are much more active and will react faster with the emulsion on the film. This can cause a plus-density artifact on the film—in other words, a pattern of the spray of the new chemicals across the film.

In some tabletop processors, the working chemicals in the processing tanks are directed into an auxiliary tank within the processor. It is here that the fresh chemicals are introduced to the working chemicals, and together they enter the working tank. Some processors have a baffle system so that the chemicals are introduced and immediately directed away from the film being processed. Figure 8-15 is an example of the artifact produced when the baffle is accidentally removed during cleaning.

Thermostats (Heating and Cooling System)

There are two main thermostats in the processor. One maintains the temperature of the chemicals, and the other the

temperature of the dryer. Heating coils may be placed in the bottom of the developer and fixer tanks, or the heaters may be placed in the recirculation system. It is essential to maintain a constant temperature in the developer and fixer tanks because the activity of the processing solutions depends directly on the temperature.

The dryer temperature is important to ensure that the films exiting the dryer are dry and not sticky to the touch. They must not be overheated as the emulsion may crack and split.

The typical temperature of the solutions in the developer and fixer is 97°F (36°C). Typical dryer temperature is 131°F (55°C).

Silver Recovery

It is the function of the fixer to remove the unexposed silver halides from the film base. This removal results in a high concentration of silver halides floating in the fixer. A silver recovery unit (Figure 8-16) removes the silver from the effluent of the processor as it exits the fixer tank.

> **POINTS TO PONDER** A good method to test whether the silver recovery unit needs to be replaced is to place a copper penny in its outflow. The copper penny is electrolytic and attracts the silver ions, which plate onto the copper. If the penny turns silver, it is time to replace the cartridge.

Metallic Replacement

The silver recovery unit typically used in veterinary clinics consists of a glass jar containing steel wool. The effluent from the fixer tank enters the jar on one side and is directed through the steel wool. The silver in the fixer solution replaces the iron in the steel wool by giving up electrons to the silver halides, and the metallic silver fuses to the iron.

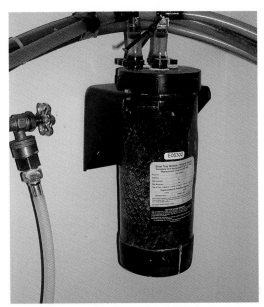

FIGURE 8-16 A silver recovery unit is attached to the outflow of the fixer tank.

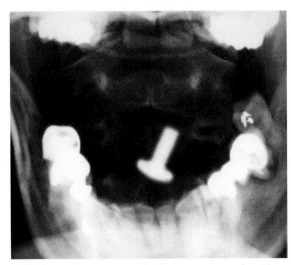

FIGURE 8-17 This is an example of an equipment artifact. The small screw fell out of the collimator shutter onto the collimator window. It was not noticed until the image was processed. Because of the distance to the patient, it is also magnified.

Electrolysis

A second method of silver recovery is an electrolytic process that is used mainly for large volume units. A very low current flows through a unit equipped with metal plates. The negatively charged silver ions bind to the plates. This method is the easiest way to collect the metallic silver; however, if the current is flowing and there is no silver, the fixer may start to break down, and because the main component of fixer is sulfur, a terrible odor may be the result.

Film Storage

The finished processed image is now available for viewing and storage. Films should be stored in individual envelopes specific to each patient. They should be stored upright in slotted shelves. Films contain a fair amount of silver and are very heavy to sort through if they are stored in a pile. Because the envelopes rarely contain only one size film, the piles become unwieldy if they are not stored correctly. They should be stored in a temperature-controlled area (68° F [20° C]). If the humidity is too high, the emulsion absorbs the moisture and the films stick together. They are virtually impossible to separate unless they are soaked in water. However, if there was insufficient hardener in the processing chemicals, soaking the films in water will only serve to lift the emulsion off the base. Ideal humidity in the storage room is 40% to 60%.

Processing Artifacts

Ninety-eight percent of all film artifacts are produced in the processor or by manual processing. We will review the majority of common problems and hope you will be entertained by a few very unusual artifacts.

Artifacts may be categorized into three groups: equipment artifacts, processing artifacts, and handling artifacts.

Equipment Artifacts

Examples of most equipment artifacts are illustrated throughout the text. The chapters in which these artifacts appear are noted beside the artifact type. The radiographic equipment can imprint many artifacts on the image. The most common artifacts are from those listed here.

Equipment Malfunction

The following equipment malfunctions create artifacts (see Chapter 7):
- Collimator parts on the window (Figure 8-17)
- Collimator incorrectly positioned (see Chapter 7)
- Collimator positioning marks incorrect (see Chapter 7)

Tabletop

The following tabletop problems create artifacts (see Chapter 6):
- Incorrect material used (plywood)

Bent or Broken Table Top Grid

The following grid problems create artifacts (see Chapter 7):
- Incorrect ratio for the examinations performed
- Incorrect focal length for the table tube distance
- Old deteriorated grid
- Old deteriorated interspacing material
- Incorrect positioning
- Upside-down placement

Intensifying Screens

The problems with the intensifying screens create artifacts (see Chapter 5):
- Damaged screen
- Poor film/screen contact

Old or Worn Screen Cassette

The following problems with the cassette create artifacts (see Chapter 5):

* Front old or damaged
* Dirt between the front and the screen
* Contrast media between the front and the screen
* Warping of the cassette
* Faulty latches

Foreign Body

Foreign bodies in the following locations create artifacts (see Chapter 5):

* Within the cassette
* Within the collimator
* Between the table and the grid

Processor Artifacts

Processing is the single greatest cause of artifacts on the films. As already stated, 98% of all film artifacts are due to problems with processing. The emulsion is softened and the rollers must touch the film as they transport it from tank to tank. The distance between the rollers is very narrow, and if a roller should swell it will place a plus- or minus-density mark on the film. Artifacts are categorized within the sections as visible by reflected light (looking at the film as a page out of a book) or by transmitted light (reviewing a film hung on an illuminator). Most artifacts are visible by transmitted light.

The illustrations here (Figure 8-18) are extreme examples but they are valid and should be recognized.

Transport Artifacts (Transmitted Light)

Plus density—these marks are darker than the surrounding emulsion.

Minus density—these marks are lighter than the surrounding emulsion but still maintain emulsion (Figure 8-19A).

Scratch marks—the emulsion has been removed from the base either prior to processing or within the processor.

Pick-off—the emulsion is picked off (removed from) the film base and redeposited on another area of the film. This leaves a tiny hole in the emulsion. This problem is not as evident on double-emulsion film as on single-emulsion film (Figure 8-19B).

Hesitation marks—the rollers are moving unevenly, and the film hesitates slightly. These marks can be mild (plus- or minus-density lines) or severe (the emulsion is removed from the base).

Chatter—two or more gears need to be replaced the plus- or minus-density marks are not deposited in a specific pattern.

Pi lines—these plus-density marks are specific to the circumference of the roller that caused the artifact. (Hence the term *pi*, the mathematical constant related to a circle's circumference) (see Figure 8-19).

Guide shoe marks—fine lines on either the leading edge or the trailing edge of the film. They are caused by the "snapping" of the film against the film guides as it travels out

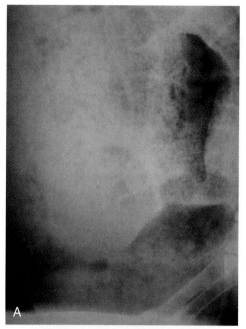

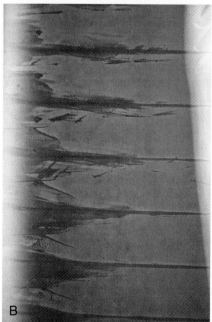

FIGURE 8-18 **A,** A radiograph of a goat abdomen. This image has many artifacts: technique, handling, and processing. **B,** The upper developer rollers were washed and not dried, imprinting their dampness onto this image. Processor maintenance is an art.

of one tank and into another. The marks are very faint and can be matched against the guide shoe indentations in the processor.

Chemicals Artifacts

Dichroic fog—the film appears to have an oily pattern of color in reflected light. This is caused by leaking or dripping of fixer back into the developer.

Under-replenishment—a flat and poor-contrast film; often films are damp when they exit the processor.

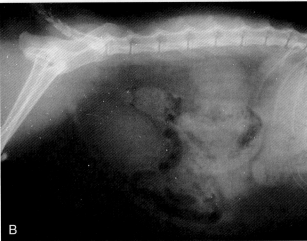

FIGURE 8-19 A, Pi-lines are caused by a swelling of the processor roller. They may be either plus- or minus-density lines. The roller is easily identified from the measurement of the circumference of the roller; hence the name "pi." **B**, Pickoff occurs when the processor rollers are not clean. The emulsion is picked off by the dirt on the rollers and usually deposited somewhere else on the film.

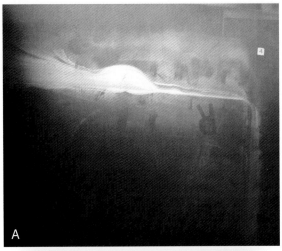

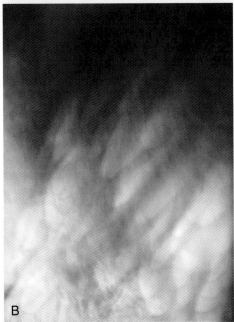

FIGURE 8-20 A, Silver has plated out onto the film as the fixer lines were crimped and replenishment had ceased. **B**, An example of incorrect mixing of developer in a manual tank.

Temperature too cool—images are dull and lack contrast; the hydroquinone is too cool to function correctly.

Temperature too warm—images are dark and dull, lack contrast; developer will exhaust quickly and turn dark brown.

Fixer not replenishing correctly—silver plating on the images (Figure 8-20A).

Fixer overconcentrated—fixer precipitates on the rollers, causing scratches, and in the gears.

Fixer exhausted—films are milky white or pinkish, and feel grainy and rough.

Fixer tank empty—films are either green (blue-receiving film) or mauve/pink (green-receiving film); there is an image but it blackens quickly.

Incorrect mixing—the film has a blur pattern of minus and plus densities (Figure 8-20B).

Wash water tank empty—films are milky and look streaky in reflected light.

Wash water tank not circulating—films appear dirty and streaky, archival quality is compromised, and films turn yellow within 2 or 3 weeks.

Handling Artifacts

Causes of artifacts on film may turn into a Sherlock Holmes–type adventure into the mysterious. This is where good record-keeping and good darkroom practices pay off in good rewards. Some of the causes of handling artifacts are as follows:

- Foreign objects in the cassette
- Dust on feed tray
- Double exposure
- Film fog—from heat, age, and so on

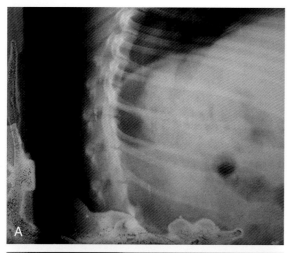

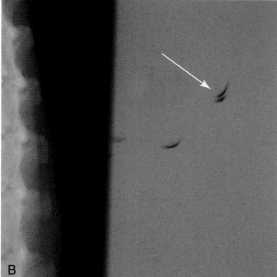

FIGURE 8-21 A, Barium behind the screen imprints its shape on the image. **B,** Fingerprint creases are caused by flexing the film roughly; they may be plus or minus density.

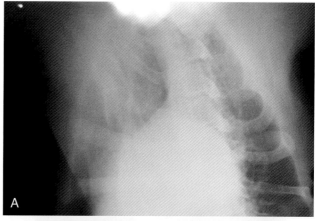

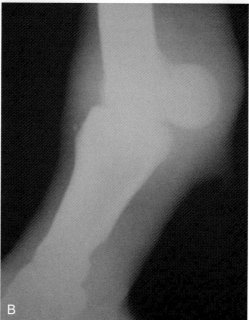

FIGURE 8-22 A, Film fog on an image from a small animal clinic. The fingers holding the film have protected it from light leak in the darkroom. The balance of the image has a fog overlay. **B,** Film fog on an image from a large animal darkroom. This was the result of an incorrect safelight filter.

- Scattered radiation fog
- Secondary radiation fog
- Extrafocal radiation
- Static—smudge, spot, or tree static
- Sweaty fingerprints (Figure 8-21)—creases to film, the image 8-21 does not demonstrate sweaty fingerprints. It does demonstrate creases to film and they are both handling artifacts, but the film creases got left off the list and they are very common.
- Darkroom conditions (Figure 8-22):
  - Safelight filter
  - Safelight wattage
  - Safelight color
  - Safelight distance from films

- Chemical odor
- Darkroom integrity

SUMMARY

This chapter has discussed processing the image and all of the problems associated with chemicals, films, screens, and cassettes. It is important to also refer to the Evolve website, where you will find more examples of artifacts that have occurred in other facilities, both human and veterinary. The entire chapter is well represented by the chapter quotation.

Computerized Radiography: Digital Imaging

The digital camera is a great invention because it allows us to reminisce. Instantly.

—Demetri Martin, American Comedian, b. 1973

KEY TERMS

Charge-coupled device
Imaging plate
Photodiode
Photomultiplier tube
Photostimulable luminescence
Photostimulable phosphor
Storage phosphor screen
Storage plate
Thin-film transistor

LEARNING OBJECTIVES

When you have finished this chapter, you will be able to:

1. Know the difference between computerized radiography and digital imaging.
2. Understand the fundamentals of computerized radiography.
3. List the basics of direct digital imaging.
4. Understand the purpose of the charge-coupled device camera.
5. Understand digital technique charts.
6. Know the difference between windowing and leveling, and between contrast and density.
7. Know the rules to follow when purchasing a digital system.
8. Understand the software variables.
9. Understand picture archiving and communications systems.
10. Know how to look for artifacts in the images.

APPLICATIONS

The application of the information in this chapter is relevant to the following areas:

1. Producing digitized x-ray images (radiographs) for evaluation and diagnosis.

Caveat Emptor: Let the Buyer Beware

The Latin phrase *caveat emptor,* which means "Let the buyer beware," has always been appropriate but never so much as in this time of conversions to digital imaging. This chapter informs you how the systems function and the reasoning behind the development of many of the systems in place today. This discussion will, hopefully, encourage each potential purchaser of computerized and/or digital radiography systems to research the product thoroughly and to view many images produced on the system of his or her choice before purchasing the system.

Following are the ten commandments of digital imaging purchase. We have compiled these commandments over several years of consultation with vendors and purchasers. Hindsight is always 20/20. Caveat emptor!

1. *First reviews:* Researching digital imaging is a fascinating look into possibilities. Just as with everything else, it is vital that you as the researcher remain fully grounded in reality. The vendors are all very pleasant and agreeable. They, too, have to buy groceries and send their children to school. They have a vested interest in your clinic. It is vitally important not to allow emotions to cloud your objectivity. At the end of the day, one of the vendors will win the contract and the others will not. That is your decision, based on the best interests of your clinic and your staff.

2. *Narrow the possibilities:* Research first on the Internet. Find out what is available and where all the vendors are located. Remember, this is much like Internet dating. If you decide to purchase a digital system, you will be committed to your vendor and your happiness with your images will very much depend on the system and the expertise that that company has to offer. You will also depend very much on the commitment of the individual service person that the company provides. You will deal with him or her on a daily basis initially.

3. *Visit the sites that have systems installed:* It is worth the drive, or the flight, to see the potential system in which you are interested. Visit competitors' sites and ask the purchaser why this system was chosen over all the others. Ask to see images … a lot of images. Request extremity and bony anatomy views. Abdomen images are always impressive unless the system is very bad. Check out contrast on chest images, and play with the windowing and leveling. Decide whether a hairline fracture would be visible. It is a rare digital system that demonstrates a hairline fracture in bony anatomy.

4. *Check out the service, cost, and location:* An assurance from the vendor that "We will look after you" is not enough. Does the vendor have a service department or company near where you are situated? Are they even in the same country? If the head office is in a different country or across the continent, is there a local qualified service engineer who can service not only the digital system but also the x-ray generator? If the system breaks down (and they all do), what is the guaranteed "down time"? How will they service the unit? Will they supply a replacement product while yours is being serviced? Is there any warranty on the part that is being serviced or on the replacement part? Ask to speak with a client who has had his or her unit serviced. Discuss holidays and weekends. Is the service department available "24/7"?

5. *Warranties:* Discuss the warranties in depth. No system is infallible. Most are very reliable, but if the system breaks down or the image is unsatisfactory from the start, only a company with a good service record can help restore it. The price of a digital system is too high for it to be used as a backup computer because the images are pixilated from the first day and there is no one to service it. Also, again, is there a warranty on any part that has to be returned to the manufacturer for service? This issue is vital and worth repeating.

6. *Licenses and upgrades to the software:* Licenses and upgrades are the areas in which a number of digital system vendors add on to the cost of the original system. Also, what is the cost of licensing two, three, or four computers within the same clinic? Extra work stations should be billed only for the price of the computer. This is not a separate system; it is piggybacked to the main system. Separate computers are merely slaves to the main system. There is no reason that the clinic should be invoiced for an auxiliary system when slave computers feed from the same software. Upgrades should be automatically added during the period of the warranty. Once the warranty is finished, an agreement may be reached as to the price of future software upgrades.

7. *Service contracts:* The vendor has sold you the digital equipment. The only way that the vendor can make more money is through service contracts. A service contract with any x-ray company is designed to cover the most expensive piece of equipment that needs to be replaced during the time of the contract. Typically, service contracts do not cover glassware (the x-ray tube). Any service contract that covers the digital imaging plate is going to be prohibitive costwise and probably unnecessary. Read and discuss any service contract very thoroughly. Make very sure you are aware of what is, and is not, covered.

8. *Lease to own or time payment plans:* The technology is moving forward quickly, and imaging is improving because the competition in this field is fierce. It is not the veterinary market that drives the technology but, rather, the medical market. The veterinary market benefits from the research. However, it is also important that the digital unit pay for itself in a timely manner. By the time a 5-year loan taken out on a piece of equipment 5 years ago has been paid off, the veterinary clinic is left with a paid-for dinosaur in technology. Speak to your potential vendor about trade-ins or upgrades to your unit.

9. *Remember that the digital unit is the image receptor:* A correctly calibrated radiography unit of any age is quite capable of delivering the radiation necessary to produce digital images. The clinic does not need to upgrade

the radiography unit if it is correctly calibrated and serviceable. The digital system is replacing only the detector portion of the radiography system.

10. *The golden rule of business:* Make sure that the unit you purchase is a good business decision for the clinic or hospital. Does it make good business sense to purchase a unit, and can the number of radiographs produced each month pay for the monthly payment on the equipment? It is unwise to expect the other areas of the hospital to contribute to the purchase of a digital radiography unit.

> **POINTS TO PONDER** An associate veterinarian purchased a clinic with a three-year-old Digital Imaging System. The amount owing was $68,000. When it malfunctioned she was given the choice to repair the digital plate for $50,000 or replace the plate for $68,000. If she chose to repair the plate it was no longer under warranty because it was a used plate. For further information on what can go wrong (and right) refer to the Evolve website.

Introduction to Computerized and Digital Radiography

Traditionally, the imaging process involved several steps: positioning the patient, measuring the patient, setting the technical factors, making the exposure, processing the film, and then reading and archiving the images.

Computers started to change these traditional steps quite slowly at first. The changes came first in fluoroscopy and the related modalities nuclear medicine and ultrasound. These modalities were already using a closed system for viewing the images. It was possible to print out the images, usually on special single-emulsion film, so that they could be archived, but if there were a way to store the images in the system it would be much more efficient and economical. The original storage devices were enormous and worked very much like the juke box that was familiar in those days. The files were

stored on discs or tape and retrieved by an arm moving to a tape and placing it in the correct position to be played.

As technology progressed and the data became much larger with use, everything needed to be scaled down. Now we have the images and data in the hospitals and clinics today. The images can be stored on a personal computer with exchangeable hard drives. The backup images are often stored in data banks anywhere in the world. Because of technology, we now realize that the future of imaging is limitless.

Computerized Radiography

The first step in the journey toward digital imaging was computerized radiography (CR). There are many similarities between CR and traditional imaging (Table 9-1). They both use a cassette that must be processed in a separate unit (Figure 9-1). The cassettes protect the screens from light and abuse. They both require postprocessing to archive the images. The only step that CR eliminates from the traditional protocol is reloading the film into the cassette. This is taken care of by the CR reader, which not only reads but also clears the image and prepares the screen for the next image. The CR cassette is available in all the same sizes as those for film/screen imaging.

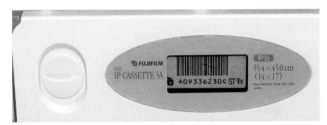

FIGURE 9-1 The computerized radiography cassette is similar to a traditional radiography cassette except that (1) it opens only at the top to allow the screen to be drawn out to be read and (2) the cassette identifier is imprinted in a window at the back of the cassette. This identifier links the patient acquisition numbers to the cassette.

TABLE 9-1	A Comparison of Protocols	
TRADITIONAL FILM/SCREEN IMAGING	**COMPUTERIZED RADIOGRAPHY (CR)**	**DIRECT DIGITAL IMAGING (DDI)**
Load cassette	Prepare the cassette	—
Prepare photoidentifier	Enter patient's data	Enter patient's data
Position patient	Position patient	Position patient
Measure patient	Measure patient	Measure patient
Set technique/make exposure	Set technique/make exposure	Set technique/make exposure
Process film	Process image	—
Reload cassette	—	—
Hang the film	Post the image	—
Read the film	Read the image	Read the image
—	Postprocess the image	Postprocess the image
Archive the film	Archive the image	Archive the image

In the patient timeline, only one step is removed from the traditional process with CR. Four steps are removed with DDI. An additional step is available with CR and DDI.

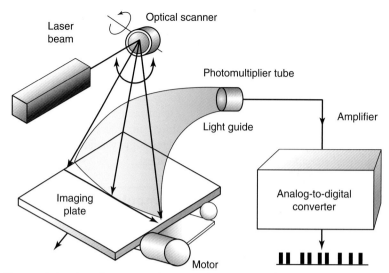

FIGURE 9-2 The neon-helium laser beam scans the exposed CR imaging plate to release the stored energy as visible light. The photomultiplier tube "sees" the light, amplifies it, and converts it to an electrical signal. The electrical signal is picked up by the analog-to-digital converter, which converts the analog data to digital data. It is these digital data that appear on the hospital or clinic's monitor.

A single screen in the CR cassette acquires and stores the image, ready for processing, thereby eliminating the need for film. The function is the same as in film/screen imaging, except that the screen retains the image instead of transferring it to film.

The similarities end when we compare how the images are acquired, processed, and then viewed.

The Imaging Plate

Inside the CR cassette is a single intensifying screen that traps the image by means of a photostimulable phosphor. In this form the screen is referred to as an imaging plate (IP). This is a distinct advantage to CR. The cassettes can be easily substituted for film/screen imaging, and any imaging equipment can be used. Tabletop exposures are possible so radiation doses for extremities may be kept low.

The front of the imaging plate is coated with a photostimulable phosphor (PSP), usually barium fluorohalide. This phosphor reacts instantly to the x-ray beam and also to light. When the electrons within the PSP are stimulated by the x-ray beam, they become metastable. Approximately 50% of the electrons return immediately to their stable state, giving off a prompt emission of light. The other 50% remain unstable and give up their unstable state over time. This feature is important because it is this 50% that holds the patient's image on the IP until it is stimulated by an infrared (laser) light (Figure 9-2). The laser, which is 50 to 100 nanometers wide, passes over the plate as it is drawn out of the cassette after it has been placed in a reader. The laser causes the remaining unstable electrons to return to their original state with the emission of a shorter wavelength light in the blue area of the spectrum. At this point, the latent image becomes visible.

If the IP is not placed in the reader, the image will fade within 6 to 8 hours as the electrons return to their original state.

TABLE 9-2	Sources of Noise within the Computed Radiography (CR) System
SOURCES OF NOISE IN THE CR IMAGE	**RESULT FROM**
Mechanical defects	Slow scan driver Fast scan driver
Optical defects	Laser intensity control Scatter of stimulating laser Light quanta emitted by the screen Light quanta collected by the optics
Computer defects	Electronic noise Inadequate sampling Inadequate quantization

Once the image has been read, the IP is flashed with an intense white light. This light returns all the unstable electrons to their ground state, preparing the IP to be used again immediately. The IPs work best if they are used immediately after processing.

The plates should always be flashed every morning because they may retain a previous image or they may be "fogged" by background radiation. Fogging of the PSP is possible from direct radiation or scattered radiation, heat stimulation of the IP, or light leaks within the cassette.

The spatial resolution on the image depends entirely on the cross-sectional diameter of the laser. The laser beam tends to spread as it leaves the source, so it is collimated by a lens system that keeps it to a 100-µm diameter.

Sources of Image Noise

Noise is greatest in CR at the lower levels as a result of background fog and scattered radiation. Table 9-2 lists sources of noise in the CR system.

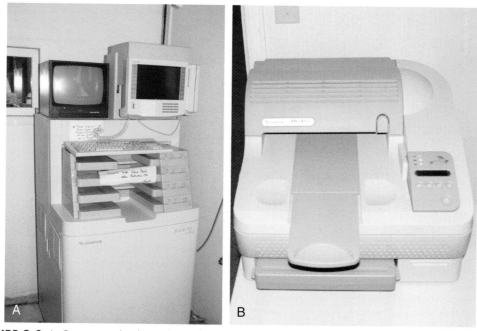

FIGURE 9-3 **A,** Computerized radiography reader. Note the trays for various sizes of cassette. The configuration of the trays is the choice of the veterinarian. **B,** The laser film printer, which produces hard copy images for the clients.

Image Dose

The principal source of noise on the image is scattered radiation. The dose curve in CR radiography is directly linked to technique. This means that as the IP is stimulated, the response of the plate is immediate. The output of the CR image is constant throughout the diagnostic imaging range of techniques. This may easily lead to overexposure, because technique charts are supplied by vendors who are ignorant of the ALARA (as low as reasonably achievable) principle. It is very important that a technique chart is maintained that sets the technique and therefore the dose to an ALARA level. Typically, traditional technique charts at a 400-speed system are acceptable for CR.

Advantages

The elimination of the wet processor and the processing chemicals is a distinct advantage. The wide latitude regarding technical factors and the short wait for the image display are two further advantages. The cassettes are replaceable at a reasonable cost. There is also an environmental advantage to any type of digitized imaging, in that the chemicals associated with traditional film processing are eliminated.

Disadvantages

There are disadvantages to CR as well. The imaging plates are consumables and therefore need to be serviced and replaced when they become worn or when "ghosting" of previous images cannot be erased. The plates are prone to the effects of scattered radiation and should be flashed before each use if radiography in the clinic or hospital is limited. Noise at low levels of radiation is bothersome, but newer technology promises to reduce this factor.

Another disadvantage is the intermediate step of having to process the image in a laser reader (Figure 9-3). This step delays the viewing process and also requires one more piece of (expensive) equipment that must be maintained and serviced.

Digital Radiography

Direct digital radiography evolved from the computerized radiography model. The scientists reasoned that if all that was standing in the way of directly reading the image from a monitor was the photostimulable phosphor, then they should develop a system that is stimulated directly within the mechanics of the plate itself and then read directly, immediately, from the screen.

Now, with this system in place, the acquisition of images eliminates several steps in the film/screen imaging process. CR eliminated just the "reloading the cassette" step in the film screen process. Digital radiography eliminates the entire "processing and hanging" steps as well as the cassette preparation step (see Table 9-1).

Digital radiography was developed from research into a highly light-sensitive device designed for military use in the 1970s. The device was attached to a computer and was mainly used in astronomy and digital photography. The unit, named a charge-coupled device (CCD) (Figure 9-4), had several advantages. It was light sensitive and had a wide dynamic range.

Sensitivity of the CCD is its ability to detect very low levels of visible light and this feature made it valuable in radiography using its sensitivity to detect low patient radiation dose. *Dynamic range* is the ability of the detectors to respond to a wide range of light intensity. This replicated the dynamic

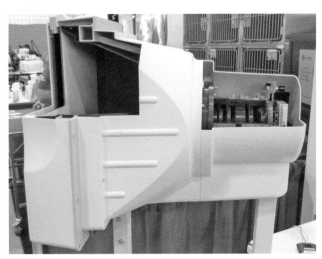

FIGURE 9-4 A charge-coupled device (CCD) camera cut away to show the grid, the automatic exposure control, and the cesium iodide screen. The scintillation light from the cesium iodide phosphor is efficiently transmitted through fiberoptic bundles to the CCD array, the camera chip, and the computer boards at the back. The result is high x-ray capture and good resolution, up to 5 line pairs per millimeter (lp/mm).

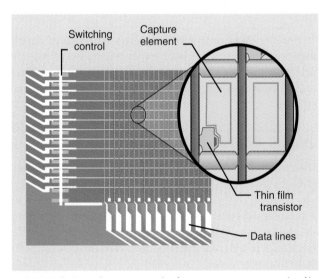

FIGURE 9-5 A photomicrograph of an active matrix array–thin film transistor digital radiography image receptor with a single pixel highlighted.

range of the 400-speed film/screen system. There was one advantage of the CCD over the film screen response: The response of the CCD was completely linear and therefore could detect far more stimulus than the phosphor in the film screens, allowing for a much greater range of sensitivity.

Mechanics of Digital Imaging

The detector of a digital system is a scintillation phosphor that is spread across a supportive plate. This plate rests on a thin-film transistor (TFT). The plate transfers the radiation signal to the digital receptor (DR). The DR is fabricated into individual pixels (picture elements) (Figure 9-5), which convert the radiation into electronic components and transfer the data to the software via the datalines extruding from each pixel.

The end goal of any imaging system is to achieve a highly diagnostic radiograph that enhances all the differences in tissue density while achieving the lowest radiation dose possible. This goal was difficult to reach in the early days of digital radiography, because the system of detectors was very slow and the computer had to be prepared to receive the image. Some sophisticated systems now achieve approximately 400 film/screen system speed.

The limitation of this type of digital imaging is the pixel size, which limits the resolution.

> **POINTS TO PONDER**   *A great dilemma:*
> The technique charts supplied by various otherwise reputable vendors are worrying in the extreme. Setting a technique of 85 kilovolts (kV), 300 milliamperes (mA), and 1/120 sec for either a kitten's paw or a cat's 10-cm abdomen illustrates the ignorance of the vendors and the problems that are encountered by the staff when they trust such charts.
>
> This is an ethical dilemma. From these charts every image must be postprocessed, adding time to the original examination. When postprocessing is a factor in every image, there are losses in data. Adjusting windowing and leveling for every image compromises the information on the image. Also, some of the images are beyond unreadable. The high kV has penetrated every tissue evenly, eliminating any chance of enhancing contrast. The scattered radiation produced by a 110-kV exposure for a 16-cm abdomen is enough to add to the radiation dose on the technician's dosimeter.
>
> The ethical problem lies in the fact that the system is installed. There is no "do-over," and the images are unreadable. Does the veterinarian order images that he or she knows cannot be read because the digital unit must be paid for? Does he or she have the image post-processed as best as possible and then revert to the old system of diagnosing clinically because the images are so poor? What about the technicians who have worked at the clinic for 10 to 20 years and are now seeing dose readings on their radiation dosimeters for the very first time because of excess amounts of radiation?

The Thin-Film Transistor and Pixel Capture

The acquisition of the image is variable as technology moves forward. Acquisition is important to the manufacturers because it is here that the image is acquired and transferred to the computer. The vendor is always anxious to have the sharpest resolution and the highest-contrast image. It is often the software that allows this to happen.

The percentage of the pixel that is actually affected by the capture element is 80%; the other 20% contains the TFT and the data lines. This means that the 20% of the pixel element does not contribute to the actual image but must be filled in by the computer. As the pixel size is reduced, the spatial resolution improves, but the patient dose must be increased to compensate for a reduction in fill factor and to maintain signal strength.

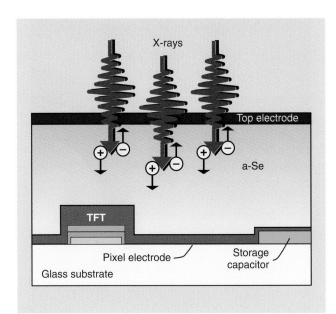

FIGURE 9-6 The use of amorphous selenium as an image receptor capture element eliminates the need for a scintillation phosphor. This plate is approx 200 μm thick and is sandwiched between charged electrodes.

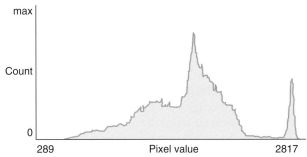

FIGURE 9-7 A histogram showing number of each of the gray values from left to right (the horizontal axis). The total number (count) of each pixel value is added up vertically.

TABLE 9-3	Approximate Spatial Resolution for Various Medical Imaging Systems	
IMAGING SYSTEM		**SPATIAL RESOLUTION (LINE PAIRS/MM)**
Magnetic resonance imaging		1.5
Computed tomography		1.5
Digital radiography		4
Computed radiography		5
Film screen radiography		8-9

Direct Digital Radiography

A solution to the problem just described came with research into digital mammography on the human side. Mammographic film/screen imaging was enhanced by a slow high-resolution system. The dose for each individual exposure was great but the spatial resolution was optimized.

An amorphous selenium (a-Se) plate was developed (Figure 9-6). The incoming radiation interacts directly with this plate. There is no intervening scintillation phosphor. The a-Se plate is sandwiched between two charged electrodes. X-rays that reach the a-Se plate are collected by a storage capacitor and remain there until the signal is read by the switching action of the TFTs. All of this happens very quickly and results in an image within seconds of the radiographic exposure.

Spatial Resolution and Contrast Resolution

Every image is a combination of spatial resolution (the image in space) and contrast resolution. Spatial resolution is expressed in line pairs per millimeter. It is the ability to visualize a high-contrast black line that is separated by an interspace of equal width (see Chapter 5). Contrast resolution is expressed as the values of black and white. The highest contrast available is an image that is completely black and white with no intervening shades of gray. The descriptor for contrast resolution is *dynamic range*.

The end result of digital imaging should logically create a high-resolution image. However, it is important to note that the limitations of pixel size and monitor output always result in an image that does not have the spatial resolution of film/screen technology (Table 9-3).

Digital Image Processing

The digital data are collected and sent to the digital processor (the computer) as an electronic signal. These data are evaluated and manipulated by the software before they are displayed. The software uses the data to construct a histogram. This is a graphic display of the image. Think of it as alphabetizing every pixel, plotting them on a graph from lightest to darkest and taking into account the number of all pixels that represent the same dark/light value. Images of extremities are high on the light values and on the dark values with very low levels in between. An image of the abdomen peaks in the gray areas and is low on both very light and very dark.

Often digital cameras provide a histogram of the image displayed (Figure 9-7). A *histogram* is a graphic description of the each pixel value in the image. This histogram is then evaluated to enhance the contrast and brightness of the image on the basis of a known algorithm. The software contains a series of lookup tables (LUTs) that provide a baseline for each examination. For example, if the image is a chest radiograph, the image is enhanced as a high-contrast image and the contrast in the active image is enhanced.

Each digital imaging system depends on a certain variety of algorithms to produce an image. Algorithms are formulas built into a program in order to solve a problem. They are much like the recipe for baking a cake, except that they are more complicated and detailed; they would include the instructions for opening the bag of flour and breaking the egg.

Algorithms are selected on the basis of previous programs and computer codes to enhance the histogram. The service engineer would be the only person to have access to the program at this level, and he or she cannot change anything within the basic programming of the software. The service engineer may apply filters to adjust the histogram but not to change the algorithm.

Dynamic Range

The question remains, Why do the digital images look so much better than film images? Digital images take advantage of the ability of the digital process to create a greater number of shades of gray in the image. It remains a fact that no digital image can resolve an object smaller than the pixel size of the image receptor.

Film/screen imaging has a limited dynamic range. The dynamic range of film/screen technology is three orders of magnitude because the density of the image is read from 0 to 3. This represents a dynamic range of 1000, but the viewer can visualize only 30 shades of gray because of the limitations of the human eye.

The dynamic range of the digital imaging systems is defined by the bit capacity of each pixel. Typical DR systems have a 14-bit dynamic range ($2^{14} = 16,384$ shades of gray). Digital mammography systems and some later digital systems have a 16-bit capacity and therefore image 2^{16} or 65,536 shades of gray. Still, the human eye is not equipped to visualize and appreciate all these features. We are still limited to 30 shades of gray. The advantage of the digital systems is that with edge enhancement and the ability to manipulate the image (which is not available in a film/screen system), the radiograph may be enhanced by postprocessing so that the contrast or brightness is amplified.

Contrast and Brightness (Windowing and Leveling)

The amplification of contrast and brightness enhancement is the most important feature of digital imaging. Window level (see Points to Ponder box) establishes the midpoint of the densities visible on the digital image. Window width controls the range of gray-scale images to adjust the contrast on a digital image.

> **POINTS TO PONDER**   *Windowing* (Figure 9-8) refers to the contrast range of densities, whereas *leveling* (Figure 9-9) refers to density or brightness. It is the use of windowing and leveling that alters the image on the monitor.

Postprocessing and the Service Engineer

If an incorrect exposure is used and the image is compromised because of very low contrast, the operator may alter the contrast and brightness by postprocessing. This is definitely not a substitute for correctly exposing the image using a correct technique chart. It is time-consuming, and some information may be inadvertently lost when the image is manipulated. It is also an example of lack of regard for the ALARA principle, which recommends the lowest radiographic technique in order to reduce dose to both the patient and the operator.

If the correct technical factors are used and the images are still consistently problematic, the system engineer can open

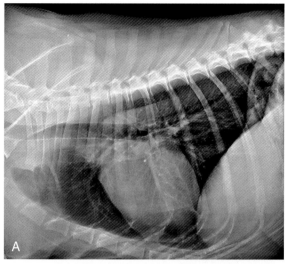

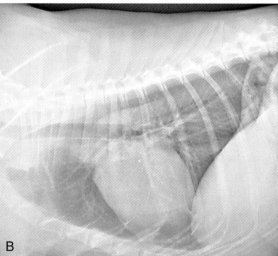

FIGURE 9-8 Examples of postprocessing an image with the use of windowing. As the window is reduced, the contrast flattens out so that the differences in tissue density become less obvious. **A** The image lacks contrast in the areas of the lungs and heart. **B:** windowing the image provides better contrast and demonstrates the vascular areas of the lung tissue.

his or her part of the program and apply filters to enhance the overall images. This is not true for every system. If the software chosen by the vendor is faulty and does not manipulate the data correctly, the image cannot be enhanced even by the experts. These are the programs that will not last in the marketplace as word is spread regarding certain software.

Digital Image Artifacts

Digital imaging artifacts may be produced by the imaging plate, the grid, and mechanical system, or by the software. It is important to identify the cause of the artifact and then to contact the system engineer to correct it. There are few artifacts in digital imaging, mainly because of the way the systems are installed. Typically, artifacts are caused by human error and can be resolved. If there is a definite problem with either the hardware or the software, it must be addressed right away. The system engineer can usually resolve most

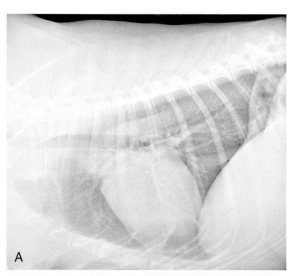

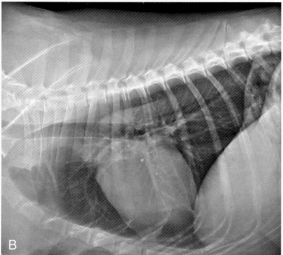

FIGURE 9-9 A change in leveling. As the level increases the overall density of the image becomes greater although the contrast remains the same. **A** This image has good contrast but is overall too light. **B:** Levelling the image maintains the contrast and enhances the anatomy.

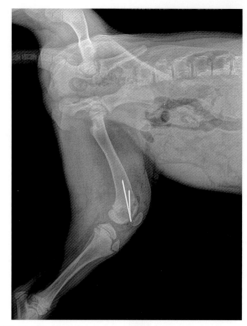

FIGURE 9-10 Digital imaging enables the viewer to surround the image with a black background which eliminates glare from the monitor.

problems online. Hardware problems may be more difficult to resolve.

Picture Archiving and Communications Systems (PACS)

Once the image is produced it must be archived. It is very important to research the archiving of the images carefully. The archive is stored on a computer. Computers fail. Therefore all systems must have redundancy. In other words, the data must be stored in more than one place. The intricacies of data storage are far beyond the scope of this text and are indeed another chapter or even a book.

The simplest means of data storage is the use of interchangeable external hard drives. Most clinics use three hard drives if they plan to store all the images on site. Two hard drives store the day's images, and then the third is traded in at the end of the day and hard drive #1 will be taken home by a designated person. The following day's images are now stored on drives #2 and #3, and then #2 is taken home at the

end of the day. This is complicated, but the system is inexpensive and secures the images locally.

A second means of data storage is off site. Several companies offer offsite computer data storage. They may be located locally, on the same continent, or on the other side of the world. They are efficient and store masses of data from many different modalities. A word of caution: If the company chosen is local do not assume that your data will be stored locally. Many companies act as intermediaries and store the actual images on the other side of the planet. It is wise to know where your data are stored and who controls the storage facility. This is especially true if local politics or turbulent weather cause damage or destruction to storage facilities.

Digital Imaging Monitors

The conditions under which the images are viewed must be controlled in order to take advantage of the optimized image. The room must be darkened so that the ambient light does not affect the contrast on the monitor screen. Most imaging programs are equipped with automatic collimators that blacken the area surrounding the image on the monitor (Figure 9-10). This feature reduces glare and is not as tiring to the viewer.

SUMMARY

Digital imaging either by means of CR or direct DR is a definite leap forward in radiographic imaging. The future is limitless as research continues to provide imaging applications that use technology to best advantage both to limit radiation exposure and to provide high-quality images. The storage of data is an area of research that is ever expanding, and the sophisticated methods of storage become even smaller and more convenient.

CHAPTER

10

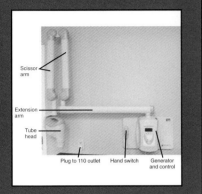

Scissor arm

Extension arm

Tube head

Plug to 110 outlet　Hand switch　Generator and control

KEY TERMS

Chairside darkroom

Computerized radiography

Conversion factor

Direct digital imaging

Extension arm

Extension cone

Lead composite

Processing chemicals

Scissor arm

Stationary anode

Dental Imaging

Lois Brown, RTR (Cdn/USA), ACR, MSc and Susan MacNeal, RVT, CVDT, BSc

Trying to define yourself is like trying to bite your own teeth.
—Alan Watts, British philosopher, 1915–1973

OUTLINE

LEARNING OBJECTIVES

When you have finished this chapter, you will be able to:

1. Describe the dental x-ray unit.
2. Discuss the unique qualities of the dental unit.
3. Explain the use of dental x-ray film.
4. Recognize the unique packaging of dental x-ray film.
5. Name the standard sizes of dental x-ray film.
6. Explain the methods of dental film processing.
7. Recognize computerized, digital, and film dental radiography.
8. Discuss the merits of each system.

APPLICATIONS

The application of the information in this chapter is relevant to the following areas:

1. Radiography of the dental architecture; radiography of extraordinary anatomy using a dental unit.

Dental radiography has become a significant imaging modality in the veterinary clinic. Imaging a patient's teeth and dental architecture has become recognized as an essential diagnostic tool. Dentistry in veterinary medicine has become an important preventive for heart disease and many geriatric pathologies. The dental radiography unit is quickly becoming an invaluable piece of equipment not only for radiography of teeth but also for high-definition imaging of other small body parts.

The Dental Unit

The dental unit is a specialized radiographic unit that has been developed for human use over many years. Most people are familiar with having their teeth 'x-rayed' during a dental checkup.

The veterinary dental unit is a modification of the human unit. The only difference is a veterinary dental overlay on some units and a variation in technical factors. The human dental unit can be converted to a veterinary dental unit merely by placing it in the veterinary hospital. No modifications are necessary.

The generator consists of a small box mounted on a wall (Figure 10-1). Typically, the kilovoltage is preset at 70 kV and the milliamperage at 7 or 8 mA. The operator determines the time according to the size of the structure being radiographed. An extension arm of variable length, usually 20, 60, or 80 centimeters, extends from the box on the wall and swings 180° degrees (Figure 10-2). A standard 110-volt power outlet is required. At the end of this arm is a scissor arm, which is extendable, usually to a distance of approx 48 in (122 cm). At the end of the scissor arm is the x-ray tube. The x-ray tube holder, or hanger, is unique in that it rotates around the stem of the scissor arm. It is also able to rotate about the axis of the hanger approximately 270 degrees.

The Dental X-ray Tube

The dental x-ray tube (Figure 10-3) is a very small stationary anode tube. It is housed in a specialized casing that includes

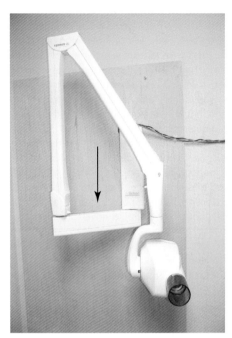

FIGURE 10-2 Main extension arm of the dental x-ray unit moves about the generator in a 180-degree arc (*arrow*). It is normally available in three lengths. This is dependent on the configuration of the dental suite. The x-ray tube is suspended from the end of the scissor arm.

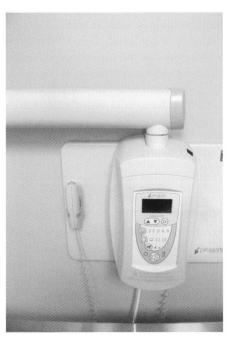

FIGURE 10-1 A veterinary dental control.

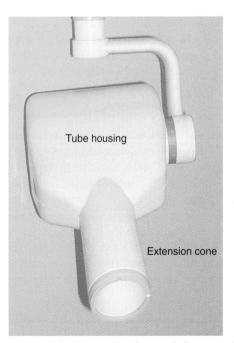

Tube housing

Extension cone

FIGURE 10-3 The dental x-ray tube. The actual tube is a small stationary anode tube. The tube housing is suspended from the scissor arm by a tube hanger that allows for 360 degrees of rotation.

a composite leaded cone projecting out from the housing. The housing encasing the tube is also lead composite material. The extension cone on the newer units is lined with lead composite material. The extension cones on older human units are not always lead-lined and should be checked when they are installed.

> **CHECK IT OUT** The older human units were not legally required to have shielded cones until approximately 1980. If a human unit is purchased for a clinic, it is wise to test the shielding of the cone. Place a cassette or image receptor beneath the cone, which is suspended 4 in (10 cm) above the receptor. Set the technique on the dental unit to 0.05 seconds, or 6 pulses. Process the image. The cone should limit the exposed area to the diameter of the cone, usually 4 to 6 cm. If the exposed area is considerably larger than the cone opening, then the cone is not shielded and must be replaced. Be sure that the exposure is not set too high, which will cause scatter radiation or "splash" and affect the results of the test. The density of the exposed area is medium gray and the image should have should have fairly sharp edges.

The extension cones are supplied in various lengths. This arrangement was originally intended to accommodate various sizes of film. Currently, a standard cone length of 5 to 8 inches is sufficient to accommodate any size dental film. There is no collimator light, so it is important to view the projection of the cone from several different angles to ensure that the cone is positioned correctly. The end of the cone should be positioned at 4 in (10 cm) away from the patient's anatomy. This standard distance assists in maintaining a correct standard technique, because distance is a major factor in establishing a technique chart (see Chapter 6).

When an exposure is made using this unit, there is no rotor noise because the anode is stationary. The x-ray beam is directed toward the animal through the cone, and any extrafocal radiation and scattered radiation are absorbed by the lead composite material.

The Dental X-ray Generator

The original dental generators were very inefficient and used a self-rectifying x-ray circuit (see Chapter 4). Newer technology has made smaller and better circuitry available (Figure 10-4). The dental units produced in the last 10 years, since dentistry became a factor in the veterinary clinic, are very efficient high-frequency units. This efficiency enabled the manufacturers to offer a unit that produced a maximum amount of radiation in a much shorter time. The newer units also became less expensive as these generators were produced using just two circuit boards and more efficient technology.

Dental X-ray Imaging

Three types of image receptors are now used in dental imaging. Film is available, but in small packages rather than

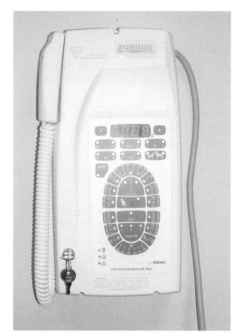

FIGURE 10-4 This generator offers settings for dog, cat, exotics, and paws.

TABLE 10-1	Dental X-Ray Film Sizes	
FILM SIZE	**FILM DIMENSIONS**	**USE**
1	$^{19}\!/_{16}$ in • $^{15}\!/_{16}$ in 40 mm • 24 mm	Not commonly used in veterinary medicine
2	$1^{5}\!/_{8}$ in • $1^{1}\!/_{4}$ in 40.5 mm • 30.5 mm	Commonly used for individual teeth
4	3 in • $2^{1}\!/_{4}$ in 57 mm • 76 mm	Shows tooth alignment or dental architecture

cassettes. Direct digital imaging is available as well as computerized imaging using small phosphor plates, which can be bent to accommodate the patient's dental architecture.

The animal is always anesthetized for dental radiography and cleaning of the teeth. The endotracheal tube inserted for the anesthesia is useful to hold any of the receptors in place. A number of positioning tools are available within the clinic to help with positioning of the patient's head and the image detector. Chapter 24 describes dental radiography positioning.

Film Imaging

Film is commonly distributed in two sizes for dental imaging; size 2 and size 4 (Figure 10-5; Table 10-1). There are several suppliers of dental film and various speed classes of film. It is important when the unit is being set up that one type of film is selected, the exposures are set for that film, and that film should be ordered all the time. Changing the film should be necessary only if there is a consistent supply problem.

If it is necessary to change film brands, a conversion factor should be established and the technical factors must be altered for every exposure. Because time is the only variable, establishing the conversion factor is quite simple; the procedure is as follows:

Fill a glass beaker or flat-bottomed drinking glass with 4 cm of water. Place the original film under the glass, and set the technical factors for a 4-cm mandible. Process the film. The image should be density 1. Density 1 is a silver-gray image. Now place the new film under the beaker, and expose it with the same technical factors. Once that film is processed, compare the densities of the two films using an optimized illuminator (see Chapter 7). If the images look to be the same density, then no conversion factor is necessary. If the newer film is significantly darker than the original film, then the factors must be reduced. Place a second, new film package under the glass, halve the time, and expose and process the film. Once again compare the densities of the films. Continue to adjust the time (milliamperes-seconds [mAs]) until the two films are the same density. Now you have a conversion factor. Reduce all of your exposure times by that factor. For example, if the original time was 0.50 and the new time is 0.25, then the conversion factor is 50%. Reduce all of the exposure times by 50% for the new film. Note: This procedure works only if the techniques were optimized at the start.

Conversely, if the exposure on the new film is very light compared with the old film, then double the time and process the film. If the images are now the same then increase all the factors by 100%.

The film is wrapped in a small paper folder and backed with foil to absorb exiting remnant radiation through the back of the packet (Figure 10-6). The leaded foil in most dental packets has been replaced by a density equivalent foil that is lead free. The film is then encased in a waterproof envelope, usually thin plastic, so that it is not affected by saliva or other liquids in the patient's mouth. Finally, a small indentation is imprinted onto the film package. This allows the technician to identify how the film was placed in the patient's mouth after the film is processed. The back of the envelope has a raised overlap so that the package may be opened easily for processing (see Figure 10-5B).

FIGURE IT OUT The technician had no idea which tooth was identified on the radiograph. It was definitely an incisor, but which one? Her colleague came over to help. "If the film was inserted into the patient's mouth while you held the concave dot and the patient was lying in the DV position, then it must be the right incisor, since the concave side of the dot is always on the side you image" (Figure 10-7). Problem solved.

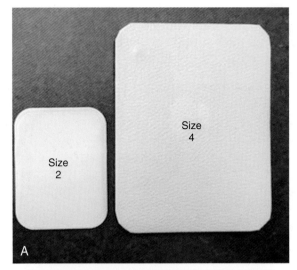

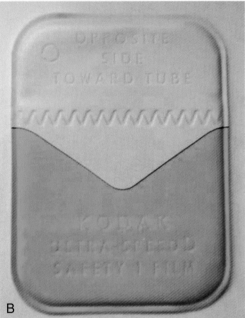

FIGURE 10-5 A, Dental x-ray film. Several sizes are available, but two sizes are commonly used, 2 and 4. B, The back of a dental x-ray film packet. The small handle assists in opening the packet to process the film.

CHECK IT OUT When the dental suite is set up and the film is chosen, the information sheets within the box of film inform the consumer where the film is produced. It is important to check with the supplier, or the manufacturer, about whether lead is enclosed in the packets to absorb scatter or whether a lead equivalent substance is used. If lead is used, the leaded foils should be placed in a separate envelope during processing and disposed of responsibly rather than with the regular garbage.

Dental film is packaged without intensifying screens. Radiographic film has infinite resolution; therefore, a correctly exposed dental radiograph is highly detailed. The film/

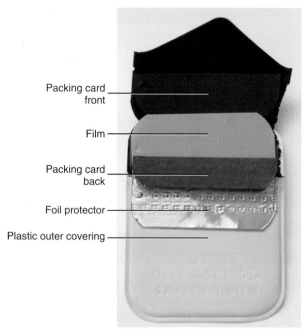

Packing card front

Film

Packing card back

Foil protector

Plastic outer covering

FIGURE 10-6 Inside of dental x-ray film packaging.

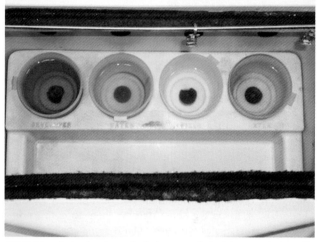

FIGURE 10-8 The chairside darkroom with the lid open. The jars are labeled, *left to right*, developer, wash, fixer, and wash. The intermediate wash between the developer and the fixer acts as a stop bath.

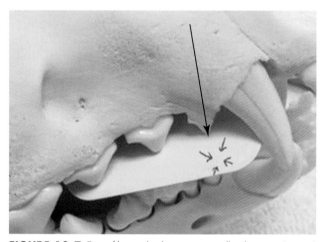

FIGURE 10-7 Every film packet has a very small indentation (*arrows*) to assist in identifying the position of the film when the image was taken.

screen resolution in general radiography is approximately 9 line pairs per millimeter (lp/mm). High-detail extremity film/screen systems in general radiography are 30 lp/mm. Digital imaging is approximately 4 to 5 lp/mm (with other factors affecting the image to enhance it). Dental film has infinite resolution (see Chapter 5).

The fact that intensifying screens are not used in dental radiography increases the technical factors required to produce a diagnostic radiograph. Although the normal kilovoltage required to penetrate a mandible would be approximately 45 to 50 kV in general radiography, the units are preset at 70 or 80 kV in dental radiography.

The time chosen for each of the settings is also considerably higher, and therefore the radiation dose to the patient is higher. The mA is preset at 7 or 8.

Film Processing

The x-ray film may be processed manually or automatically. Dental film processors are available and are used in human dental offices routinely. They are efficient and consistent as long as they are used frequently. If the chemistry is allowed to sit for several days without being used, it will start to evaporate on to the rollers and the developer will oxidize. In short, film processors are a poor choice for veterinary clinics if one considers the digital options available today.

Dental film may also be processed automatically through the clinic radiography processor. There are potential problems with this method because the rollers on some processors are fairly far apart. Therefore, a leader film must be used, as follows; a small radiography film or a larger one cut into four will suffice as a leader.

1. Attach the dental film to the radiography film using autoclave tape, which seems to work well because it is manufactured to hold in hot, damp atmospheres.
2. Overlap the dental film with the small indentation overlapping the leader.
3. Place the tape so that it covers both films but does not protrude over the edge of the leader film.
4. Make sure that it is very firmly sealed to the dental film and the leader film.
5. Place the leader film on the film tray and let it carry the dental film through the processor.

This method is not foolproof and occasionally the films will separate during processing.

A product has now become available that transports dental film through a standard processor. It seems to work well in some processors and not at all in others.

Manual Processing

Dental film is small enough that it can be processed manually with use of a chairside darkroom (Figure 10-8) or a set of jars in the radiography darkroom. The best jars to use are pickle jars because they are short and have wide mouths. The film can be held with dental clips or small forceps.

The safelight and darkroom integrity must be confirmed as intact. The jars are set on a towel on the counter. The developer/fixer that is used for general radiography may be dipped out of the developer/fixer replenishment tanks. The developer should be a very pale yellow.

Dental film usually develops at room temperature in about 30 seconds. Fixing time is longer because the emulsion on dental film is thicker than that on regular film. Fixing time should be at least 1.5 minutes, and washing time is then 3 minutes in running water.

The developer should be used for the dental session and disposed of. If dental examinations are to be done on consecutive days, the developer should be watched closely for signs of contamination. If the developer turns to the color of morning tea, it is contaminated. If the fixer starts to take longer to clear the film than it did at the start of the process, it is exhausted.

FIGURE IT OUT The films were processed perfectly through the processor but the complaint was that they looked milky (Figure 10-9). It looked as if someone spilled milk on them. The answer was that the films were not fixed correctly. The emulsion on dental film is thicker than on regular film, so it requires longer clearing time than is available in the processor. The solution is to slow the speed of the processor, so that all the films take a little longer to process, or to place each film in a fixer jar and refix the films for about 1 minute manually, then washing them and hanging them to dry.

Fast-Acting or Rapid Dental Processing Solutions

Fast-acting and rapid dental processing solutions are available to be used with either the chairside darkroom or in the darkroom itself (Figure 10-10). They are supplied in small amounts, and once they are opened, they should be used quickly. Because they are rapid developers they also become contaminated rapidly owing to the high activity of their components. They are usually only fresh for one dental session.

Developing time is usually 12 to 15 seconds. Fixing time is shortened to about 30 seconds. Washing time is 1 minute.

The economy of these solutions sometimes makes it impractical to use them rather than the standard developers and fixers.

The Chairside Darkroom

If the radiography darkroom is located some distance from the dental operator, processing the films within the x-ray room is possible with use of a chairside darkroom (see Figure 10-8). This unit is equipped with a red translucent panel and four jars held in position in the base of the unit. Prior to the examination, the jars are filled with developer, fixer, and wash. Two jars are used for the wash, and they are filled with water. The jars are always placed in the same order in the unit.

Once the film is exposed to the x-rays, it is taken into the chairside darkroom, which is equipped with light-tight arm holes. The film package is opened, and the small concave dot is identified. The film is hung on a clip at the concave dot (Figure 10-11).

The film is moved through the developer to the wash, then to the fixer and into the wash. The intermediary wash tank serves as a stop bath. The stop bath arrests the activity of the developer and washes off some of the surface developer prior to immersion in the fixer.

Labeling and Storing the Images

Each image must be clearly identified with a permanent marker (extra-fine point) or with a typed label attached to the edge of the film. It is important for future reference to ensure that each tooth is identified correctly and that the film

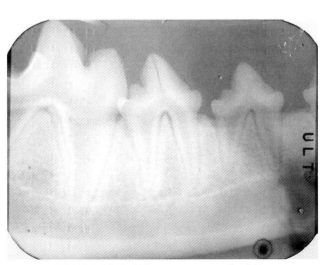

FIGURE 10-9 Milky image on an unfixed film.

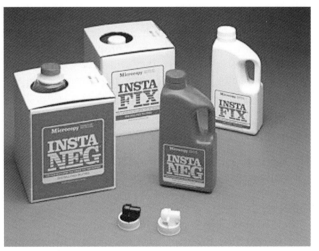

FIGURE 10-10 An example of rapid developer and fixer specifically made for dental processing.

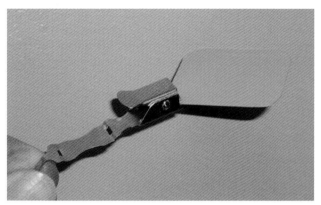

FIGURE 10-11 The film is attached to a clip prior to manual processing.

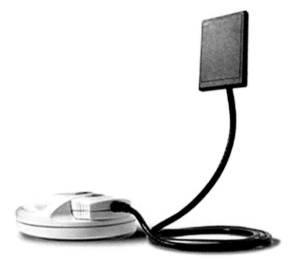

FIGURE 10-13 A direct digital detector. The unit is placed in a plastic sleeve in the patient's mouth. Once the exposure is made, the image appears on the computer monitor within seconds.

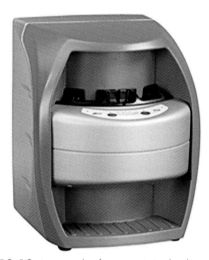

FIGURE 10-12 An example of a computerized radiography processor. The cassettes are similar to standard dental film and are supplied in standard sizes.

is filed appropriately. The films may be filed within a separate envelope in the patient's file or in a completely separate file. A note should be affixed to the patient's chart noting the location of the patient's dental radiographs.

Once the films are completely dry, they can be removed from the hangers and placed in the appropriate file. Provided they are processed correctly, they will have good archival quality and will be available for reference whenever they are required.

Computerized Radiography

The computerized radiography dental unit is similar to a standard computerized unit described in Chapter 9 (Figure 10-12). The dental processing unit is miniaturized and is equipped to process any size dental film. The cassette is a plasticized cover that houses a flexible phosphor plate. The plate is positioned in the patient's mouth, and the image is processed through a reader before appearing on the computer monitor. The image can then be attached to the

patient's file and archived in the picture archiving and communications system (PACS).

The exposures are similar to those for film-based systems because the receptor is a type of intensifying screen.

Direct Digital Imaging

The image receptor for dental direct digital imaging is typically a size 2 detector (Figure 10-13). Size 1 detectors are available but are too small for veterinary use. It is typically attached to a computer via a wire. The computer contains the preloaded program code to convert the image it receives from the detector immediately, without the intervening processing step. The digital detector is supplied with sleeves that prevent liquids from damaging the detector surface.

The exposure in most units is the same as or a little higher than most film-based systems because the digital detectors must be prepared to receive the exposure and then must receive it. All this happens quickly but it is necessary for each exposure. On the newer units, the detectors are prepared to receive the exposure when the computer is set up and the dose then is the same as that in film imaging.

Table 10-2 lists the advantages and disadvantages of the different types of dental receptors.

Dental Exposures

In dental imaging the exposure factors are preset. The only factor that the technician can change is the time, which varies considerably with each unit. Table 10-3 is included here as a guide, but it is consistent. If it is necessary to set up an exposure guide for a converted human unit or if a dental unit has been purchased with no technical guidelines, then this chart may be necessary.

Practicing techniques and positioning is best carried out with a cadaver cat or dog. Cadaver cats seem to work best

TABLE 10-2	A Comparison of Dental Image Receptors' Advantages and Disadvantages	
DENTAL RECEPTOR	**ADVANTAGES**	**DISADVANTAGES**
Film	Inexpensive Easy to use and store Easy to retrieve Switching between sizes is inexpensive within the same receptor type Exceptionally high resolution—far better than either CR or DR	Time consuming—film must be wet-processed Individual storage means that films can be lost Films may be damaged or destroyed accidentally Processing may make it difficult to keep chemistry fresh Must be viewed on an illuminator—difficult to reproduce on a monitor
Computerized radiography (CR)	Different receptor sizes available Receptors are flexible and disposable Images are similar to those of direct digital exposure	Expensive to purchase and maintain; still uses consumables (receptors) Service maintenance for the laser and reader is expensive Possibility of malfunction of the processor at a critical time—service is not necessarily local Intermediate step for processing takes time Plates can be easily damaged because the photostimulable phosphor is very thin; "plate" is removed for processing, so it cannot be repositioned according to its previous position
Direct digital radiography	Less expensive than CR systems because no intermediate equipment must be purchased and maintained Sensor remains in position while radiograph is reviewed so adjustments are simplified if positioning is incorrect No intermediate step—image is displayed within seconds of the exposure Image is high resolution because there is no intermediate limitation A malfunctioning detector may be replaced with a spare from the service provider without interruption of service	Size of the detector is limited to #1 or #2; switching between sizes is very expensive Detector is inflexible so placement is critical The detector may be damaged by rough handling

TABLE 10-3	A Suggested Exposure Chart for Dental Equipment Supplied Without a Technique Chart		
	EXPOSURE (PULSES)		
	MANDIBLE*	**MAXILLA***	**EXTRAORAL MAXILLA***
Cat	8–12	10–14	14–18
Dog (toy)	9–12	10–16	
Dog (small)	12–16	14–18	
Dog (medium)	18–22	20–28	
Dog (large)	22–28	28–36	
Dog (giant)	26–34	32–42	
	EXPOSURE (SECONDS)		
	MANDIBLE†	**MAXILLA†**	**EXTRAORAL MAXILLA†**
Cat	0.13–0.2	0.17–0.23	0.23–0.30
Dog (toy)	0.15–0.22	0.17–0.27	
Dog (small)	0.2–0.26	0.23–0.30	
Dog (medium)	0.30–0.37	0.33–0.47	
Dog (large)	0.37–0.47	0.47–0.6	
Dog (giant)	0.43–0.57	0.53–0.70	

*In pulses for D-speed films. For E-speed films, decrease the exposure to half.
†In seconds for D-speed films. For E-speed films, decrease the exposure to half.

because cats are the hardest to image correctly. Technicians should practice as follows: Use the technique chart as a guide, and position the patient. Take two exposures one at a set time and one at 50% less exposure. Process both films. Now there is a baseline. Adjust all the other techniques on the chart as a multiple of the successful image. The chart is set up so that the top part is listed as technical factors in pulses and the bottom in seconds.

SUMMARY

Dental radiography is a challenging modality. Positioning and correctly imaging each tooth is a challenge. Each patient's dental architecture is slightly different, and therefore the technician or veterinarian must be able to adapt his or her positioning appropriately.

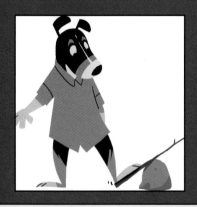

Computerized Tomography

Lois Brown, RTR (Cdn/USA), ACR, MSc and Stephanie Holowka, MRT(R), MRT(MR)

*Part of the inhumanity of the computer is that, once it is competently
programmed and working smoothly, it is completely honest.*
—Isaac Asimov, science fiction writer and biochemistry professor, 1920–1992

OUTLINE

LEARNING OBJECTIVES

When you have finished this chapter, you will be able to:

1. Understand the basic principles of tomography.
2. Discuss the basics of computed tomography.
3. Understand the apparatus of the CT scanner.
4. Correlate tomography with computerized tomography.
5. Have a basic understanding of the application of CT as a diagnostic tool.
6. Describe the concept of three-dimensional reconstruction.

APPLICATIONS

The application of the information in this chapter is relevant to the following areas:

1. The use of computerized tomography in veterinary medicine.

Introduction and History

In the very early days of radiography, researchers were frustrated by the lack of resolution on the images they produced. In the early 1900s, several researchers worked independently in different countries with a common goal, to separate the superimposed shadows that necessarily result when complex structures of differing density are exposed to radiation and the exposure is recorded on a two dimensional image receptor. How could the unwanted shadows be eliminated and the structures of interest be left clear and unobscured?

In June 1921 Andre Bocage filed a patent for an "apparatus for radiography on a moving plate." The first tomography unit had been established. All the other refinements to this original patent have left the original concept of M. Bocage untouched.

Tomography, from the Greek word *tomos* meaning "cut" or "section," has been defined as "a special technique to show, in detail, images of structures lying in a predetermined plane of tissue while blurring or eliminating detail in images or structures in other planes." A further clarification describes the original two-dimensional radiographic image as layers of images piled on top of one another. Pathology or contrast-enhanced anatomy in one layer may be obscured by dense anatomy in an area lying on top of or below the region of interest (Figure 11-1).

If the layers of tissue can be separated and the areas above and below the region of interest are blurred sufficiently, the anatomy in the plane of interest stands out in sharp focus against the blurred background.

The best way to demonstrate the concept is to return to the Jungle Jim playground. The seesaw, or teeter-totter (Figure 11-2), is a good place to start. A child sits on either end of a board. The board is balanced on a central support. The amount the children travel as they ride on the board is determined by the length of the board and also by the angle at the central support. If the children sit still, there is no travel and thus no angle. As the children start to travel through the arc, the angle at the center becomes wider and wider.

Principle of Rotation about a Fixed Point

The region of interest is a fixed point in the anatomy of the patient. The structures above and below that point must be blurred out in order for the region of interest to stand out

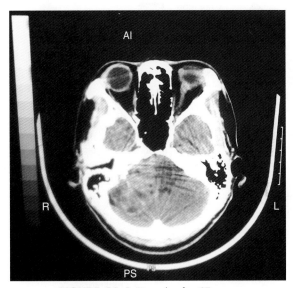

FIGURE 11-1 Example of a CT scan.

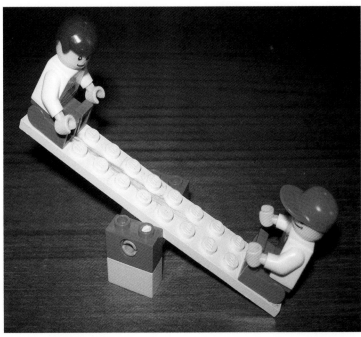

FIGURE 11-2 The concept of the seesaw or the teeter-totter.

in focus (Figure 11-3). If the x-ray tube and the image receptor stay perfectly still, all of the structures will be in focus and the layers of anatomy will be superimposed. If the x-ray tube moves through an arc and the image receptor follows that arc exactly, then the structures at the fixed point will remain in focus and the structures above and below that point will be blurred (Figure 11-4).

In Figure 11-5 the objects at levels A and C are projected onto different areas of the image receptor and are therefore seen as blur. The objects at level B are projected onto exactly the same place on the receptor and are in sharp focus.

The Focal Plane

The focal plane (Figure 11-3) is the section, or layer, at which minimal blurring occurs.

Fulcrum

The fulcrum is the central support in the playground seesaw. It is also described as the central point about which a lever rotates. In tomography, the x-ray tube constitutes one end of the teeter-totter and the image receptor is situated at the other end. The length of the lever does not change, but the

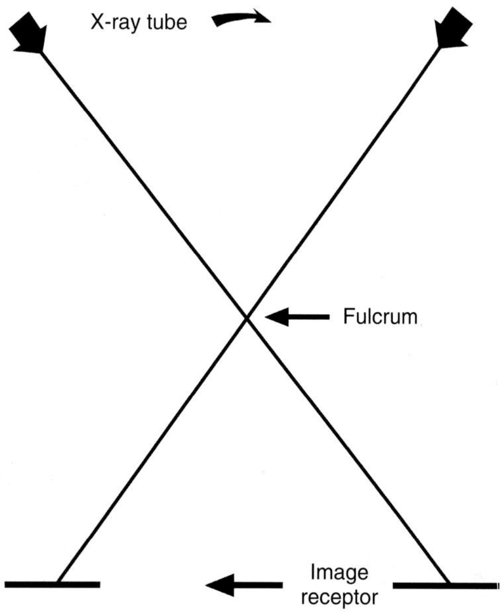

FIGURE 11-3 Rotation about a fixed point.

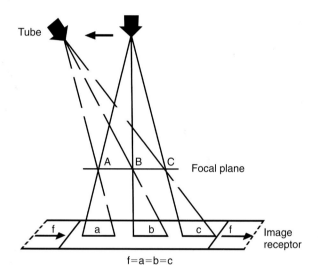

FIGURE 11-4 Blurring of points outside the focal plane. The objects at levels A and C are projected onto different areas of the image receptor and are therefore seen as blur. The objects at level B are projected onto exactly the same place on the receptor and are in sharp focus.

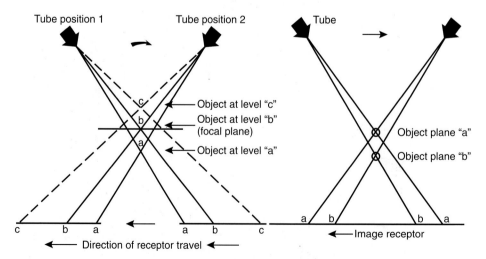

FIGURE 11-5 As the x-ray tube moves coincident with the image receptor, the anatomy on the focal plane is projected onto the same place on the receptor. All other anatomy is blurred. This figure illustrates the fact that during the exposure and consequent tube and receptor movement, there is a "plane" or slice or tissue in focus, and not merely a point within the object.

point about which the lever rotates, the pivot point, can be moved up and down. This then changes the level at which the anatomy is blurred.

> **CHECK IT OUT** Hold a yardstick (meter-stick) vertically in one hand. Grasp it at a midway point, say 18 inches (45 cm). Your hand has now become a fulcrum about which either end of the stick may be rotated evenly. Now move your hand down to the 9-inch (23-cm) mark. The length of the stick has not changed, but the fulcrum has moved significantly and the area of interest is now at the 9-inch (23-cm) mark.

Blur

Blur is the distortion of the resolution of anatomy above and below the region of interest.

Computerized Tomography

The introduction of computers in the mid-1970s transformed standard tomography. The images could now be received and demonstrated on a computer, and the wealth of information far surpassed the routine imaging on film.

CT took the standard analog images on film from conventional tomography and transformed them into digital images with the use of computers.

A *matrix* is a series of boxes or individual shades of information. If a wide matrix is imaged, the result is said to be pixilated (Figure 11-6A). If the boxes of information are very small the image becomes clearer (Figure 11-6B).

When we image structures on a radiograph, we produce a two-dimensional image (length and width of the structure) —a matrix of pixels or picture elements. The computerized tomographic image is a three-dimensional image—a matrix of voxels—that includes the third dimension, depth.

Computerized tomography employs an x-ray machine that acquires images that look like slices in a loaf of bread. As in conventional tomography, the machine uses a moving x-ray tube to create the series of images; however, these machines also require the use of detectors and a computer to do so. Computerized tomography is also known as CT or CT scanning or CAT (meaning computerized axial tomography) scanning. Invented in 1971 (by Sir Godfrey Hounsfield), CT was the first imaging modality that enabled surgeons to noninvasively see the brain. CT has evolved as a technology significantly over its 40-year history, but the basic working principles have remained the same.

Translation to the Computer

An x-ray tube (emitting a fan-shaped beam of x-rays) rotates 360 degrees around a gantry (or opening in the center of the machine) and the patient within it (Figure 11-7). Mounted directly across from the x-ray tube is a series of x-ray detectors that rotate at the same speed around the patient. The x-rays pass through the patient, and the attenuated beam is collected by detectors. The detectors convert the photons to an electrical signal that is fed to an analog-to-digital converter. The digital signal or raw data (also known as scan data) are sent to the computer, which reconstructs the images and presents them in the operator's chosen format. As a CT scanner is taking images, the table also moves in increments

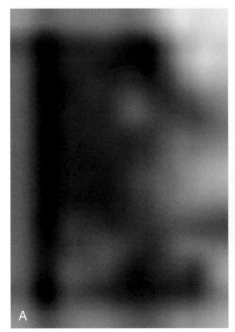 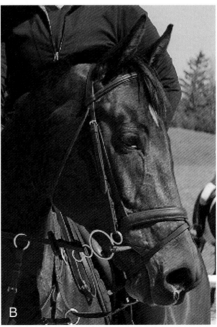

FIGURE 11-6 **A,** The image is pixilated and subject is unrecognizable (37 × 123 pixels/inch). **B,** The matrix is enhanced, the pixels are smaller, and the resolution is superior (750 × 1029 pixels/inch).

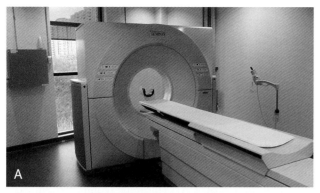

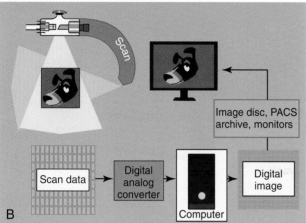

FIGURE 11-7 A, A CT scanner located in a veterinary clinic. Beside the scanner on the right is a power injector, which is used for injecting contrast. **B,** The basic workings of a CT scanner. The x-ray tube rotates around the patient, and this data is sent to the computer. The resultant images look much like slices in a loaf of bread.

set by the operator, and so several images/slices are taken for a complete examination.

> **POINTS TO PONDER**   As the x-ray beam passes through the patient, parts of it are absorbed by the tissues. The amounts that are absorbed by the various tissues are related to the attenuation coefficient of the tissue, that is, how many photons each type of tissue absorbs. In this text, the math is not important; the important part that allows us to view the image is the fact that bone attenuates more x-rays than tissue, and fat and air attenuate about the same amount.

The Hounsfield Genius

It is normal x-ray practice to take at least two views 90 degrees apart of most body parts to display the anatomy free of superimposing structures. In computerized tomography, multiple views or projections are created by the rotation of the x-ray tube and detectors. The detectors are photodetectors that convert the x-ray photons into light and then into electrical currents. Historically, the detectors were vacuum

tubes containing xenon gas; however, modern-day CT scanners use solid state detectors. The data or electrical currents created by the detectors are fed to an analog-to-digital converter and then sent to the computer for reconstruction. The primary method of reconstructing CT images is a process called filtered back-projection. Back-projection is a method of calculating an unknown value from multiples of known values. The multiple views performed by a CT scanner create a number of calculations so great that a computer is required to do it in a timely manner. Take a look at the simplified picture of the process in this picture:

by calculation   x = 1

6	3	7	4
5	2	3	5
5	X	4	5
4	3	7	6

In this simple depiction, one can calculate the value of '*x*' by subtracting it from all of the known values—crosswise and diagonally. The calculated values appear in gray. The computer does a similar process in CT, but in the order of thousands of calculations. A mathematical filter or calculation is applied into the pixel calculations to cancel out any blurring artifact in the final image.

The numbers depicted in the example for back-projection can also be used to demonstrate another aspect of the CT image. When images are reconstructed for CT, they are constructed and displayed as a matrix. A matrix is made up of several pixels or picture elements—the dots in a picture. The resolution of the image is also tied into how many pixels are displayed in a given field of view. In the example of filtered back-projection, the resulting image would have a matrix of 2. The size of a pixel depends on its relationship to the field of view that is displayed.

An image's resolution can be calculated in mm^2 as follows:

Resolution in millimeters = field of view in millimeters/matrix

In most modern-day CT scanners, the standard matrix used is 512×512.

Another factor in the setup of a CT scan image is the slice thickness. The operator chooses the slice thickness according to the anatomy to be displayed. Therefore, each image in CT is a three-dimensional slice of the subject, because the image has length, width, and height (or thickness). Because images in CT are created as slices, the pixels making up the image are actually voxels or volume elements, and the density displayed is averaged into each pixel of each slice. When one looks at a single CT slice, the image has height and width, but one does not look at the picture from the top or bottom. Rather, the thickness of the image is whatever the collimation has been set at the time the slice was acquired. We discuss the slice thickness concept in more detail later.

Each voxel in CT image is also calculated into a density measurement called a Hounsfield unit or CT number. The value is calculated by this equation:

$$\text{Hounsfield unit} = K\frac{\mu p - \mu w}{\mu w}$$

where K is the constant (usually 1000), μp is attenuation coefficient of the pixel, and μw is the attenuation coefficient of water. (An attenuation co-efficient describes the ability of the pixel to absorb radiation. Bone absorbs more radiation and fat and water absorbs less.)

This equation is significant to the CT scan for the following reasons:

1. It converts densities from tiny values of attenuation coefficients to usable units.
2. Every pixel can be therefore interpreted as a particular density that can be utilized in diagnosis or postprocessing.
3. The Hounsfield unit sets up a direct relationship with creating and displaying the images.

Table 11-1 gives the conversions for various attenuation coefficients versus Hounsfield units (HU). From the chart, one can see that the variances between the attenuation coefficients are very tiny, in the order of 10^{-3}. The Hounsfield unit shows demonstrable and consistent differences for each of the tissue densities. This is also key for the visibility of various tissues in the body. On a normal x-ray, bone appears white because it is very dense, and soft tissues appear as shades of gray. It is difficult to see individual soft tissue organs on x-ray because their abilities to absorb x-rays are very similar; also, organs are superimposed on top of one another (Figure 11-8A and B). However, a CT scan is able to show soft tissue organs in cross-sections and in Hounsfield units, such that one can see various organs in Figure 11-8C.

Image Display

Hounsfield units also affect how images are displayed in terms of brightness and contrast. For CT images, the window of an image is the number of shades of gray making up the image (or what would be known as contrast). The level is the midpoint of the range of grays. A brain, for example, may be windowed at 80 HU and leveled at 38 HU. This means that there is white and black making up the image, and 78 shades of gray in between. So how does one come to this number? If 38 is the midpoint, it is half of the number for contrast. So 80 is divided by 2 (or a half), which is 40. Then, to calculate the number of shades of gray visible, you add and subtract 40 from the level of 38: 38 − 40 = −2 and 38 + 40 = 78. This means that all of the shades of gray are visible from Hounsfield units −2 to 78. Bone, which is denser, simply appears as white because its Hounsfield unit is out of the visible range. Air and fat appear as black because again their Hounsfield units are less than what is visible as a gray level.

Let us try this calculation again. As stated before, bone is visible on a brain window only as white, so we use a different window/level (or contrast/brightness) to demonstrate bones.

A typical window width will be 2000. A typical window level will be 250. Half of 2000 is 1000. Now you add and subtract 1000 from 250 to get the visible range of grays.

TABLE 11-1	Conversions for Attenuation Coefficients (AT) vs. Hounsfield Units (HU)	
SUBSTANCE	**μ AT 60 KV (CM −1)**	**HU AT 120 KV**
Air	0.0004	−1000
Fat	0.185	−50 to −150
Water	0.206	0
Blood	0.208	+80
White matter	0.213	34
Gray matter	0.212	38

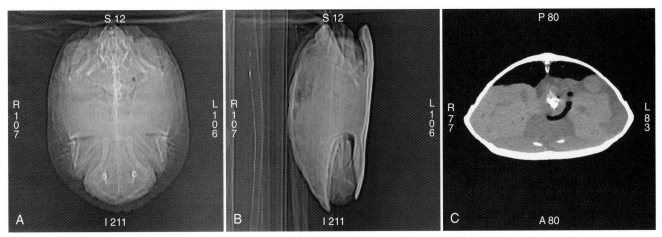

FIGURE 11-8 A and B, Two x-ray images generated on a CT scanner showing how on simple x-rays the turtle is not well demonstrated. This is a classic issue for structures such as the brain and skull in other animals. C, The CT scanner allows one to see the internal organs through the shell. Spleen, lungs, liver, and trachea are all visible on the CT scan.

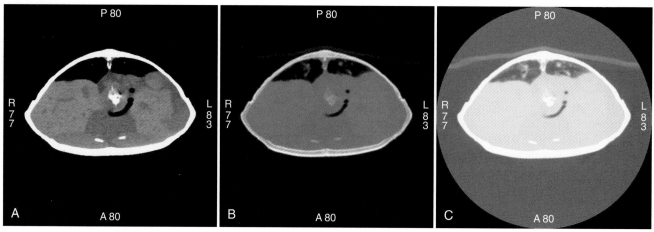

FIGURE 11-9 Same image of the turtle, but different window levels. **A,** The internal organs are best on abdominal windows (W350, L40). **B,** The bone is best on a bone window (W2500, L250). **C,** The lungs are shown on a lung window (W 2000, L–700).

250 being the midpoint means that −750 to 1250 will be visible as shades of gray. Anything below −750 HU will be seen as black, and anything above 1250 will appear as white. This is a considerably wider window level. It is good for showing bone, but the brain is not as visible because there are very few Hounsfield units or shades of gray between white matter and gray matter (Figure 11-9).

Hounsfield units also can be measured with a cursor to help the veterinarian determine the nature of a lesion. For example, when a veterinarian sees a lesion in the lungs, if a cursor reading is −50 HU, then the lesion may be fat. If it is 160 HU, then it is calcium. Blood reads at about 80 HU. Some scanners even have a feature that allows a person to apply a set cursor which will read all of the Hounsfield units for each voxel.

The CT Data

On CT scanners, the operator uses two types of data. The scan data (raw data) collected from the detectors are used to create the images. These data sets tend to be very large, and so storage is usually temporarily on the CT scanner itself. The operator will use the raw data to recreate images as needed, even after the patient is no longer on the table. Once the raw data is removed from the scanner (most scanners perform the removal after a while automatically), new images can no longer be produced. The image data is the data that is sent either to films or to a picture archiving and communications systems (PACS). Modern CT scanners are capable of producing hundreds if not thousands of images.

Just as in digital radiography all images are stored, or archived, in a huge data bank. These banks may be local or they may be anywhere on earth.

For a CT scan operator, there are many ways that a scan or the images from it can be viewed. Some of the considerations that show the thinking behind the various methods are discussed next.

Field of View

In CT scanning, there are two types of field of view (the area seen in the image). There is the *scan field of view* (SFOV), which is the number of detectors that are covered by the x-ray beam. This is important, because if the patient's body part is outside the field of view (or chosen range of detectors), it cannot be reconstructed back. There is also the *display field of view* (DFOV). The DFOV is a key element in the resolution of the CT images. DFOV will be either equal to or smaller than the scan field of view. By decreasing the DFOV, one can increase the ability of the images to resolve structures. Although a maximum SFOV may be set by the manufacturer, the DFOV is a key factor that an operator chooses for his or her CT images (Figure 11-10).

Even after an animal has been scanned and removed from the CT scanner, a technologist can reconstruct the images using the scan or raw data to create images that have a desired DFOV.

Technical Factors Used in CT Scanning and Radiation Dose

Like x-ray units, CT scanners use peak kilovoltage (kVp) and milliamperes per second (mAs) as scanning factors. Typically, the range of kVp tends to be much higher than in regular x-ray—from 80 up to 140 kVp. The mAs value tends also to be much higher, ranging from 10 to 400 mAs. The *scan time* depends on the method of scanning (spiral or conventional) and usually means the time it takes the x-ray tube to rotate 360 degrees around the patient for an exposure. By increasing the mAs, an operator can affect which structures are visualized.

Of course, increasing kVp or mAs also increases the overall radiation dosage given by the CT scanner. One unfortunate aspect of CT scanning is that the higher the technical factors, the prettier the images. CT has much more tolerance for high technical factors than general radiography. In any

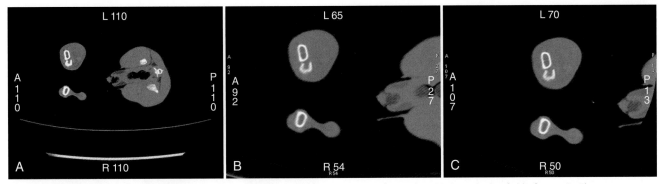

FIGURE 11-10 A rabbit with a tibial fracture. **A,** This image was taken with a 22.0-cm display field of view. **B,** This image was acquired by magnifying the original scan. **C,** This image has the best resolution because the scan data were reconstructed into a 12.0 display field of view.

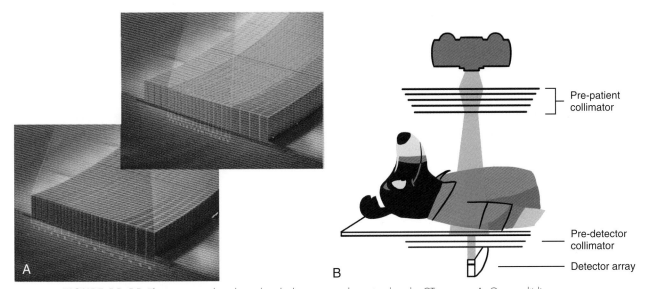

FIGURE 11-11 These images show how slice thicknesses are determined on the CT scanner. **A,** On a multislice scanner ranges of detectors acquire multiple images in a collimation. **B,** The operator selects a slice thickness or detector range. The scanner's pre-patient and pre-detector scanners maintain that slice thickness for the images.

imaging particularly imaging of children, there is a great desire to restrict dosage as much as possible and always adhere to the ALARA (as low as reasonably achievable) principle.

Slice Thickness in CT Scanning

Slice thickness is a technical variable determined by the operator of the CT scanner and is a key factor in the image resolution. The slice thickness is altered by pre-patient and pre-detector collimators. The original CT scanners acquired images in 10-mm-thick slices. If a lesion was less than a couple of millimeters thick, it could be missed by the averaging of the 10-mm slice of anatomy. Modern-day CT scanners with multislice technology are able to acquire images slices thinner than a millimeter (Figure 11-11).

Algorithm or Kernel

An algorithm is a mathematical calculation. It is applied on each of the pixels creating the CT image to enhance certain structures. Some manufacturers give algorithms (or kernels) an actual number. Other manufacturers give these calculations a name. A soft or low-pass algorithm will shift the pixels to enhance structures (like brain) that have very few increments of CT numbers. A high-pass or bone algorithm will alter the images to enhance structures that have sharp edges. The use of an algorithm can be understood when one compares a soft tissue view to a bone view. Even with the proper window/level, a soft algorithm produces a blurry bone image. A bone algorithm on a brain image produces a very grainy, noisy image. In CT scanning, as long as there are raw data (or scan data), a user can postprocess the images multiple times to show various structures.

Multislice CT Scanners

Within the past 11 years, CT scanning has seen a further evolution in the design of the detectors. Most scanners available now have multiple detectors. Instead of a single detector array, the fan beam originating from the x-ray tube is now wider to radiate a larger array of detectors. Modern multislice scanners can have up to 256 detectors in the width of their array. Because of this new technology, larger sections can be obtained in one scan while the images are reconstructed into submillimeter thicknesses. This has allowed most CT scan datasets to be collected as volume scans that can be reconstructed in three-dimensional pictures afterwards.

A key working part in CT scanning is the movement of the table during the CT scanners. Three types of table motion can be chosen. For setting up the scans, a scout view or scanogram may be taken. This looks much like an radiograph and allows the operator to choose the regions included in a scan. For the picture to be taken, the tube and the detectors remain in one location while the table passes through a chosen distance. For the actual CT scanning, the images are acquired in a conventional method or helical/spiral. The operator of the CT scanner has the ability to choose or plan which type of scanning is best for a given image or pathology.

Conventional scanning reverts the original CT scanners. The scanner takes a slice or picture at one location. The table then moves a chosen distance, and another slice is taken. A whole stack of slices can be created in this manner. On the older machines, the x-ray tube was connected by wires and cables to its generator and transformers in a separate box outside the gantry. The tube was therefore limited to moving in one rotation and then back. This motion also took time in CT scanners. Typically, the delay between slices on later model conventional CT scanners was in the order of 3.5 seconds. In the late 1980s, a new phenomenon became available in CT scanning called spiral or helical CT scanning.

The design of the scanner was changed to allow a slipring and brushes (Figure 11-12) to bring power to the CT gantry and x-ray tube. In turn the same slipring/brush assembly gave back information to the CT computers. This arrangement allowed the x-ray tube and detectors to rotate continuously, thus saving a delay between scans. In order for helical scanning to work, the CT scanners also had to compensate for the motion of the scanner by using another calculation called an *interpolation algorithm*. Interpolation is the calculation of an unknown value based on two known values on either side. The scanner is thus able to calculate the slice in a straight plane rather than in how it would appear (like a corkscrew). CT scanner manufacturers have used either a 180-degree or a 90-degree interpolation algorithm to correct helical images. To lessen the CT dose, the helical scanner also allows the technologist to choose a greater table motion than the slice thickness. Pitch is defined as a ratio between the table movement in millimeters and the CT slice thickness. How does this look in calculation?

Pitch = table movement in mm/slice thickness in mm

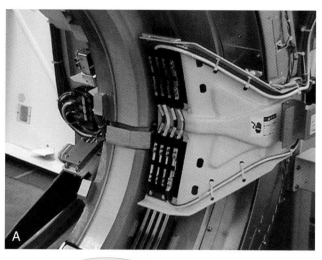

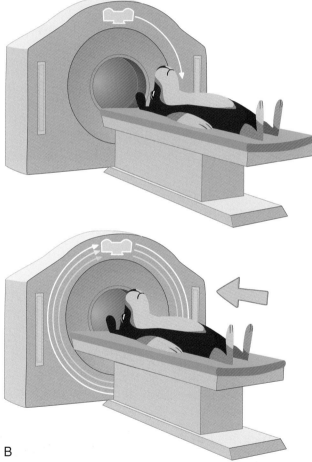

FIGURE 11-12 A, Photograph of slipring and brushes. The brushes are mounted onto the slipring. B, As the x-ray tube and gantry rotate around, the sliprings transfer electrical signals and receive data.

If a table moves 5 mm for a 5-mm slice, then the pitch calculated is 1.

If the CT operator chooses a pitch of 1.5 on a 5-mm slice, the table will move 7.5 mm while scanning 5-mm-thick images. The plus in using pitch is that it drops the radiation dose for the patient while keeping the image resolution. On single-slice CT scanners, the pitch could be increased up to

1.8 with no visible effect on image resolution. Scanner design has changed further with the advent of multiple slice CT scanners. Now the table pitch must also take into account the numbers and width of the detectors chosen.

Prescribing a Scan and Protocols

Just as varied as the region or body area that may need to be scanned are the protocols or scan technical factors used. All CT scanners allow operators to program protocols (labeled for body part or type of scan) and store them in the computer. Technologists may receive a request for a CT scan of the head. They would then enter the name (or select the name from a list created by the radiology information system) and then select the desired protocol. The technologist would complete a scanogram view or scout view (CT version of an x-ray) and from those images prescribe the actual CT scan.

The CT scanner always allows the technologist to make any desired change to a protocol setup as needed. On some protocols, an intravenous (IV) contrast agent may be required. IV contrast agents are iodine-based and enhance veins, arteries, and some entire organs. Angiography can also be performed on CT; by rapidly injecting a contrast agent, an operator can show the arteries and veins in any given part of the body. Abdominal scans typically need a contrast agent so that the organs can be better seen. Contrast agents may also be used to demonstrate infection in extremities. In cases in which a spinal pathology is suspected, a veterinarian may inject a contrast agent into the spinal canal (via a lumbar puncture) to show any disturbances of the spinal cord. This procedure is called a *myelogram*. (Only special contrast agents are used in the spinal canal—more is covered in the contrast chapter.) Fluoroscopy, radiographs, and CT scans may all be part of the imaging of a myelogram.

Indications and Postprocessing for CT Scanning

CT scans used to be the primary modality for imaging the head and spine. Magnetic resonance imaging has supplanted it for this use. CT scanning remains an excellent diagnostic tool for assessing trauma and for body imaging. CT scanning is also good at demonstrating the skeleton. Because of the evolution of the technology, CT scans are performed so that the images can be reconstructed in multiple ways. A single conventional exposure through a multislice scanner can create 32 images of 0.625 mm thickness. Whether the images are collected by a conventional scan or a spiral scan, if they have the same field of view, center, matrix, and algorithm, they function as a volume. This means that several slices can easily be stacked together and reconstructed into any plane or three-dimensional image.

In three-dimensional imaging, there are multiple ways to construct the objects. The simplest reconstruction is to build the image in two dimensions but create it through any plane. The operator can alter the slice thickness on the reconstruction, and the window/level so that he or she can demonstrate what needs to be seen. For a spine, one would always reconstruct sagittal or longitudinal images through it. Typically, several images are constructed along each plane (Figure 11-13).

Three-dimensional images can simply be created by a process called *shaded-surface display*, whereby a three-dimensional object is created by limiting the number of Hounsfield units seen. For bone, one would select 160 HU and upwards. For a skin surface the range might include −200 HU and upwards. These objects can be modified by well-designed software. Another type of three-dimensional imaging is called *volume rendering* (Figure 11-14). This process takes all the range of Hounsfield units and includes them in the picture. The operator can then select what range of voxels are opaque and what are transparent.

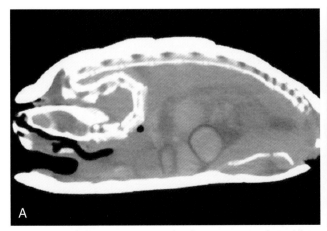
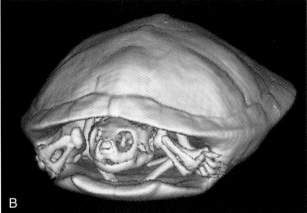

A

B

FIGURE 11-13 A, Sagittal reconstruction of Waddle's spine from axial CT scans. **B,** A three-dimensional picture that is a shaded-surface display image demonstrating voxel values of 160 Hounsfield units and higher. Such three-dimensional images can be virtually angled and cut into to show various perspectives on anatomy.

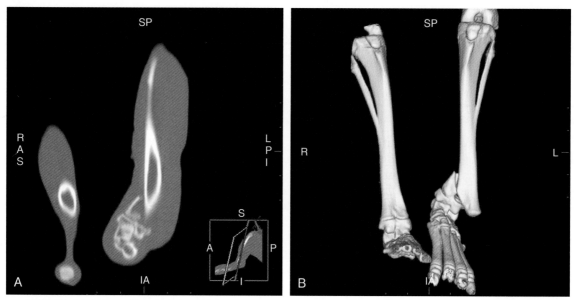

FIGURE 11-14 A, Although the rabbit's fracture is visible in the two-dimensional coronal reconstruction or reformatted image, **B,** the severity is much more apparent on the volume-rendered three-dimensional reconstruction. Tools such as three-dimensional imaging greatly help in the understanding of pathology.

SUMMARY

Computerized tomography is a modality that uses x-radiation to create images in cross-section. It has the ability to demonstrate soft tissue and bone structures. Images can be reconstructed in many formats from CT scanning, including two-dimensional reformat, three-dimensional imaging, and volume rendering. All of these formats can aid the veterinarian in the assessment and diagnosis of the patients.

Fluoroscopy

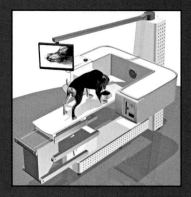

Television is a medium because anything well done is rare.
Television is the triumph of machine over people.

—Fred Allen, American Comedian, 1894–1956

OUTLINE

LEARNING OBJECTIVES

When you have finished this chapter, you will be able to:

1. Discuss the equipment necessary for fluoroscopy.
2. Describe the functions of the fluoroscopic unit.
3. Explain the difference between static and fluoroscopic images.
4. List the applications for fluoroscopy in veterinary medicine.

APPLICATIONS

The application of the information in this chapter is relevant to the following areas:

1. Fluoroscopic real-time scanning and imaging in small and large animals.

Very shortly after the discovery of x-rays, scientists wanted to see moving images. Thomas Edison is credited with discovering the fluoroscope in the United States in 1896. Because Roentgen had patented the discovery of x-rays only in November of that year, Edison worked quickly to patent his new device before the end of the year.

The primary function of fluoroscopy is to provide dynamic real-time imaging of anatomical structures. Static images are very useful, but certain activities within the body enhance the diagnostic process if the veterinarian is able to view the activities as they happen. This is also true of fluoroscopically guided orthopedic surgery. Obtaining static images and processing them as the surgery progresses is very time-consuming, whereas anatomy may be imaged quickly in real time with fluoroscopy. Today the fluoroscope is connected to a radiographic camera, and a static image can be obtained without interruption of the dynamic examination.

Fluoroscopic Equipment

The fluoroscopic generator is virtually identical to a radiography unit. In fact, many veterinary units that are purchased from human hospitals have a fluoroscopy panel on the control.

The kilovoltage (kV), milliamperage (mA), and time values are the same. The difference is an added panel that allows the operator to select "fluoro." When the "fluoro" mode is selected, the unit switches to a low mA (2–5) and a high kilovoltage (100–120). The time is not independently selected because the image is created in real time and time is controlled by the veterinarian.

A foot switch (Figure 12-1) operates as the exposure switch, and x-rays are generated continuously if the switch is depressed. There is a timer on the unit that alerts the operator at a preset time (1, 2, or 5 minutes). It is important to remember that the milliamperes-seconds (mAs) is a function of mA × Time. If the mA value is 3 but the operator

extends the exposure time to 1 minute, the resulting dose to the patient is 3 × 60 sec or 180 mAs. Patients can receive radiation burns from a fluoroscopy unit if it is too close to the skin and remains in exposure mode too long.

The image intensifier monitor looks very much like a television monitor and is the display for the dynamic images.

The Image Intensifier

The image detector on a fluoroscopy unit is an image intensifier. Originally units were supplied with a cassette holder, and individual exposures were possible, but with the advent of digital imaging, there was no longer a need for these holders. Now if a single exposure is required it can be retrieved from the bank of dynamic images and stored in a separate folder. This improvement reduces the radiation exposure for the patient, because single static images are unnecessary.

The image intensifier (Figure 12-2) is an electronic device. This unit receives the remnant radiation exiting from the patient and converts it into a visible light image of high intensity.

An input phosphor receives the x-rays emitted from the patient and converts them into visible light. This unit is roughly 18 in × 18 in (43 cm × 43 cm) and is mounted at one end of the C-arm in a large installed unit.

On a portable C-arm, the image intensifier input phosphor is much smaller and is often circular, 15 in (38 cm) in diameter or even less. The phosphor material that is commonly used is cesium iodide (CsI). The function is similar to the conversion of x-rays in general radiography. The light is directed to a photocathode, which is bonded onto the input phosphor with a very thin, transparent adhesive layer. The photocathode is usually composed of a very thin layer of cesium and antimony. It responds readily to stimulation and emits light in direct proportion to the amount of x-rays it receives. This process is known as photoemission.

The image intensifier is approximately 20 in (50 cm) long but is slightly shorter in the C-arm configuration. The light

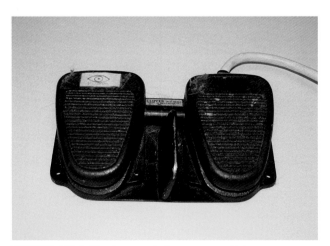

FIGURE 12-1 The foot switch (exposure switch) has two options. One side is a single exposure switch, and the other pedal is used for continuous exposure (fluoroscopy).

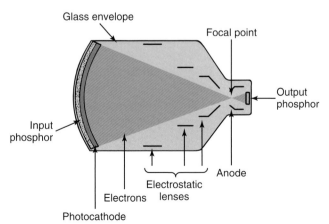

FIGURE 12-2 The image intensifier converts the remnant radiation from the patient into a bright visible light pattern.

is focused within the intensifier by means of a potential difference across the tube, so that the electrons produced by the photoemission are accelerated to the anode.

The electrons are now emitted from the photocathode to the anode of the image intensifier tube by photoemission. This is similar to the way the x-rays were emitted from the cathode of the x-ray tube by the process of thermionic emission.

The anode is a circular plate that attracts the electrons and passes them through a hole in its middle to the output phosphor. It is here that the electrons interact and produce light. The output phosphor is usually zinc cadmium sulfide.

The large image from the input phosphor has now been reduced to a small image at the output phosphor. It has been intensified by the electron optics as it has been miniaturized. The electronic method of focusing the electrons must be very precise because the image is maintained throughout these optical changes.

Each photoelectron that arrives at the output phosphor produces 50 to 75 times as many light photons as were necessary to produce it at the input phosphor. Hence the name "image intensifier."

C-Arm Configuration of the Fluoroscopy Unit

The original fluoroscopy units were mounted on a radiographic table and they were exceptionally large and unwieldy. They required a motor drive just to move the unit over the table to examine the patient from head to toe. In the 1960s a portable configuration was developed. It was and still is a two-part unit, with the x-ray tube and image intensifier mounted in a "C" configuration and the monitors and recording devices on a separate cabinet (Figure 12-3A). The C-arm is the most common veterinary fluoroscopy unit (Figure 12-3B). Most units in veterinary hospitals are purchased from human hospitals, and because their use is limited to surgical procedures in human hospitals they are usually in excellent condition (if somewhat cosmetically compromised). They are mounted on wheels and are portable if somewhat awkward to move about. Such a unit can be stored in a separate room and brought into the radiography room or surgery when required. The components are fairly rugged and withstand the bumps and shocks of uneven flooring and the loading and unloading on and off elevators.

The Fluoroscopy Table

One factor that is often overlooked is the table upon which the patient will lie for the fluoroscopic procedure. The tabletop must be free of obstruction above and below and must be radiolucent. The radiation will travel through the patient and the tabletop, and the configuration must be accessible so that either the x-ray tube or the image intensifier can be placed beneath the table.

An important consideration is the radiation absorption of the tabletop. A steel stretcher would act as a radiation

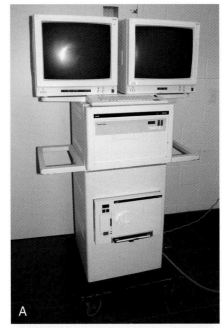

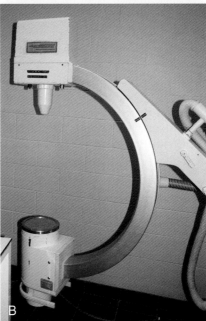

FIGURE 12-3 A, The two monitors are mounted on a rolling cabinet with the video recording devices below. **B,** The C-arm configuration of the x-ray tube above and the image intensifier below.

filter, absorbing a considerable amount of radiation and filtration would flatten the image. With a wooden tabletop, the rings and lines of the wood grain would be imprinted on the image, obscuring detail and reducing resolution. The best table is custom made of 1-inch (2.54-cm) squared tubular steel. The table top is a composite material that is completely radiolucent. The pattern may be extrapolated from the images in the text or from the diagram provided on the online learning (Figure 12-4).

The tabletop may be ordered through an imaging supplier. The table frame can be constructed by any welding

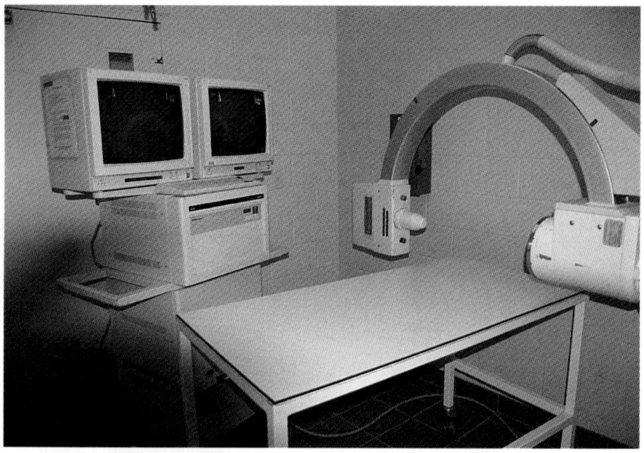

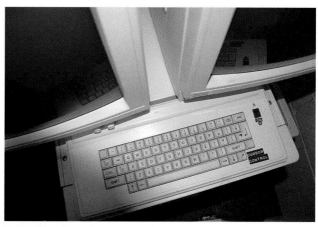

FIGURE 12-4 The C-arm positioned horizontally. The table is a sturdy construction with the support rails situated so that the x-ray tube can move beneath it unobstructed. This x-ray tube is a stationary anode tube.

FIGURE 12-5 The computer keyboard mounted beneath the two monitors.

shop. The outside dimensions are 56 in × 26 in (142 cm × 66 cm) outside dimensions. The bracing of the legs can be at a 45-degree angle to each leg or it can be in the form of rails, as shown in the image (Figure 12-4). The length of the image intensifier should be taken into consideration when the rails are mounted because it must be convenient to move the C-arm during surgery from the vertical position to the horizontal position (Figure 12-4). The table in Figure 12-4 was manufactured so that the x-ray tube fits below it, and the image intensifier is positioned above the patient. A surgical drape was custom made to completely encase the image intensifier. (The radiation penetrates the drape.)

Radiation Dose and Service Considerations

On a standard human hospital–installed unit, the x-ray tube is a high-end rotating anode tube. It must have a high heat capacity in order to withstand the long exposure times that are common in fluoroscopy. One method that is used to reduce the radiation dose to the patient is to pulse the exposures so that the radiation switches on and off at a predetermined rate. The image on the monitor is not affected because it is preprogrammed to react to a continuous stream and to ignore the pulses.

The x-ray tubes on a C-arm have a stationary anode (Figure 12-4), and particular care should be taken to limit the exposure times so that the tube does not overheat. Each unit is supplied with an anode cooling chart manual and x-ray tube specifications.

If a used unit is purchased from a hospital, all of the equipment manuals and the service manuals must be supplied. These will give a history of any problems that have arisen as well as a wiring diagram for any future service. Each C-arm, like any automobile, is upgraded and changed year to year, with major changes occurring at regular intervals, depending on the manufacturer. The wiring diagrams from 1 year are not necessarily relevant the following year even if they are produced by the same manufacturer.

Often this information may be obtained from the Internet, but not always.

The Monitor Tower

Two monitors are mounted on a cart and are usually positioned about eye level (5 feet 5 in [165 cm]) (Figure 12-3A). Older models of C-arms had only one monitor; however, the double monitor serves a useful purpose. One monitor presents the static image, and the second monitor shows the real-time dynamic image. During a surgical procedure, a prosthetic device or a catheter may not be in quite the right position. The surgeon may then hold the image on the left monitor, move the device under real-time imaging, and compare the two images.

A computer keyboard (Figure 12-5) and picture archiving and communications system (PACS) are mounted beneath the monitors. These are linked to the hospital radiology information system (RIS). The patient's information may be keyed in at the monitors or may be available through the RIS. The system may also allow measurements to be calculated or positional angles to be determined on the monitor.

The Procedure

The animal is placed on the table and wheeled into position between the x-ray tube and the image intensifier. The configuration is movable around the patient, so the tube can move from the dorsoventral/ventrodorsal position to the lateral configuration easily without the requirement to move the patient.

Dark Adaptation

The images on the fluoroscopic screen are not in color and may be dim in comparison with the routine images read on the illuminator. The veterinarian must allow his or her eyes to become accustomed to the dim light of the room (dark adaptation) before starting the procedure.

The human eye is not very sensitive to dim light. The rods and cones within the eye must adapt to changes in illumination. The rods are sensitive to low light levels, whereas cones are most efficient at 100 lux and greater. Cones, however, have greater ability to perceive fine detail, and so the eye must be allowed to undergo dark adaptation in order to see the image on the image intensifier most efficiently. Full dark adaptation for the average human eye takes about 15 minutes. The easiest method of dark adaptation is the use of dark sun glasses.

Archiving the Images

Once the image is configured at the output phosphor, it may be viewed in several different modes.

Just as an image detector in radiography displays an image, it can be digitized and sent to various recording units. Typically, the dynamic image is stored on a hard drive attached to the unit. Because the image is actually a series of still images, just like those in a movie camera, individual "spot films" may be extracted from the "movie." If a particular pathology is demonstrated the images may be started, fast forwarded, reversed, and then stopped and captured.

If the pathology is of sufficient interest, the images may be posted to a website and discussed by many veterinarians from anywhere in the world.

Individual images may also be printed on a laser printer, such as the one illustrated in Chapter 9.

Applications in Veterinary Medicine

Real-time imaging is useful as a surgical tool in equine radiography for a review of the equine legs; however, because the images are not as sharp as in radiography, it is more useful in the orthopedic surgery suite. Fracture reduction is enhanced by real-time imaging in the large and small animal hospital, as is placement of catheters, stents, and endotracheal tubes.

Contrast media studies commonly use fluoroscopy to image the function of the gastrointestinal system as well as narrowing or blockage of blood vessels in angiography studies. The form and function of the blood vessels can be studied with the use of a contrast medium, which is injected into the veins then concentrated and excreted by the kidneys.

Miniaturizing the C-Arm

In the early 1980s the miniature C-arm was developed (Figure 12-6). This unit was originally intended to be used in the emergency department of human hospitals to image the reduction of fractures and dislocations. It is light and very portable, and even though the image is comparatively low-resolution, (Figure 12-7) it is very useful for the purpose for which it was developed.

Shortly after it was introduced, it became a valuable tool in scanning equine legs and the joints of the extremities. It is not very powerful but it images the equine leg very well

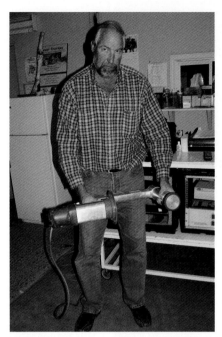

FIGURE 12-6 Dan McMaster, DVM, holds the XiTec Mini C-Arm (Xi-tec LLC, Connecticut, USA) to demonstrate its small size and portability. The x-ray tube port is beside his left thumb, and the image intensifier is in front of his right hand. The monitor cart is behind him.

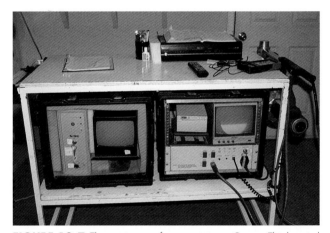

FIGURE 12-7 The monitor cart for two miniature C-arms. This hospital uses one unit and stores the other for backup. The video recorder is mounted on top of the cart. A small thermal printer is mounted beside the right-hand monitor.

and can demonstrate an area of trauma or pathology that should be examined further by radiography, computerized tomography, or magnetic resonance imaging.

SUMMARY

When Edison first used a zinc cadmium sulfide screen to examine a patient, he placed the screen directly over the patient and then looked down at the images, which he viewed as very pale yellow-green shadows. The image intensifier, which was developed in the 1950s and 1960s, is still a valuable diagnostic tool today and still uses Edison's zinc cadmium sulfide recipe.

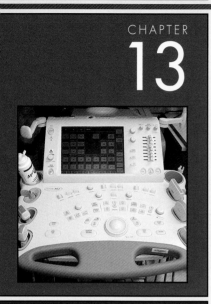

CHAPTER

13

Ultrasound

Robert Hylands, DVM

*A mind that is stretched by a new experience can never
go back to its old dimensions.*
—Oliver Wendell Holmes, Jr. American Author 1841–1935

KEY TERMS

Acoustic impedance
B-mode
Color-flow Doppler
Continuous-wave
  Doppler
Convex
Depth control
Gain control
Microconvex
M-mode
Multiplanar
  reconstruction
Phased array
Presets
Pulse-wave Doppler
Sector probe
Spatial resolution
Transducer

OUTLINE

LEARNING OBJECTIVES

When you have finished this chapter, you will be able to:

1. Understand the benefits of real-time ultrasound imaging.
2. Know the types of artifacts and limitations of ultrasonography.
3. Name the transducer types and their function.
4. Describe different image modes and their applications.
5. Understand the clinical applications for body systems.

APPLICATIONS

The application of the information in this chapter is relevant to the following areas:

1. Producing ultrasound images when advanced diagnostic imaging techniques are required.

Since its first introduction into veterinary medicine, the use of ultrasound as an indispensable imaging tool has grown to include a vast number of applications as the technology evolves. Ultrasound imaging (ultrasonography) not only advances our diagnostic capabilities but has also been proven to be safe. In almost 30 years of rigorous studies focusing particularly on prenatally exposed children, ultrasound has been found to have no associated health risks. Studies in 1982 and 1987 by the Bioeffects Committee of the American Institute of Ultrasound in Medicine (AIUM) first proclaimed that there were no biological effects on the patient or instrument operators at intensities typical of diagnostic ultrasonography. In 1998, the World Health Organization stated that ultrasound imaging was both a safe and effective modality. This chapter discusses basic principles in order to familiarize the technician with the goals of an ultrasound examination.

Ultrasonography and Plain Radiography

One of the defining characteristics of ultrasound is the benefit of real-time imaging. During a scan, a continuous stream of live, digitized data is obtained. From these data, video recordings can be saved, which then can be transferred into a *cine loop*. This capacity allows the area of interest to be visualized over a much more prolonged period as a continuous feed. Comparably, plain radiography catches the area of interest in the split second when the exposure is taken.

The advantage of real-time imaging is seen when we use ultrasound for cardiac studies. We can watch the movement and function of the heart and internal structures over the course of a cardiac contraction. Newer matrix probes can even take this a step further by instantly projecting the acquired data in multiple planes. These planes are reconstructed by computer and can allow visualization in a three-dimensional format. This, visualization, called multiplanar reconstruction (MPR), allows ultrasound to project an image similar to more advanced diagnostics such as magnetic resonance imaging and computerized tomography.

A second benefit to ultrasound is the ability to move the diagnostic probe in any direction or plane of the body required. Comparable radiography usually requires standardized positioning and orientation. Moving the ultrasound probe over the area of interest gathers a greater amount of information about the subject.

High-quality ultrasound instruments are able to manifest fine anatomical detail through the use of multiple, sensitive receptors in the ultrasound transducer (probe) (Figure 13-1).

Finally, as already mentioned, the safety precautions required for the use of ionizing radiation are *not* a factor in ultrasound. No protective gowns and gloves are required, and multiple people may be in the room during the ultrasound study. There are many other benefits to this modality, which we explore in this chapter, including the ability to visualize detailed pathology through tissue and fluid that can pose difficulty for radiographic imaging.

The Ultrasound Machine
Principles

The basic principle of the ultrasound machine is the production of sound waves by an ultrasound probe (also known as the transducer) and the return of that reflected sound wave. Sound waves enter the tissues and are reflected back to the probe differently, depending on the various tissue densities. The probe receives the reflected sound waves and then translates the information to the computer so that it can be read on the video screen by the operator.

The most important components of an ultrasound machine are the elements in the transducer. These elements

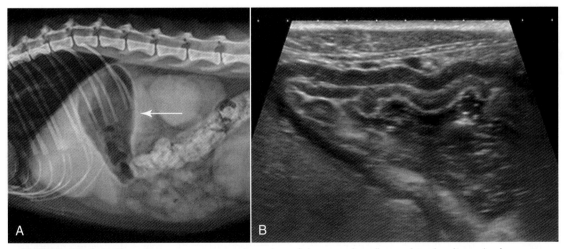

FIGURE 13-1 A, The *white arrow* represents the outline of the stomach wall on a lateral radiograph of a canine abdomen. Very little information about the wall thickness or health can be extrapolated from this image. B, A high-resolution image of the stomach wall acquired in a near-field ultrasound examination. In the ultrasound study, we can observe gastric motility and can visualize the detail of each anatomical layer of the stomach wall.

are predominantly made of piezoelectric ceramics. These materials have unique properties that allow them to change shape in the presence of an electrical current. When the ultrasound machine emits a desired frequency, strong but very short electrical pulses make the ceramics vibrate. This vibration causes the crystals within the ceramics to emit a mechanical vibration at a preset frequency. The sound frequency emitted is usually set anywhere between 2 and 18 megahertz (MHz) but can reach as high as 50 MHz in probes used for ophthalmic studies. The sound wave pulses can then be directed, steered, or focused to the desired depth as set by the ultrasonographer. Each of the crystals is connected to an individual circuit, known as an *element*, allowing them to be directed independently. It is this individual control of the crystals that allows them to be steered and focused through timing delays.

When mechanical energy from the returning sound waves makes contact with the transducer elements, they once again distort the shape of the individual ceramics, creating electrical energy that is released back to the machine to analyze. It is this electrical current that is digitized to create a diagnostic image.

Practicality

Modern ultrasound machines come in a variety of formats, including larger cart models, laptop units, and even hand-held portable devices. Each unique system offers different levels of image quality and software options. Many considerations affect the selection of an ultrasound machine for use in a veterinary practice. For example, machines may vary as to the available types and frequencies of their transducers, the computer processor speed, the quality of the viewing monitors, and many optional software applications. Some machines also vary according to whether they will support either a cardiac or a general imaging platform. Ideally, for small animal veterinary practices, a machine with dual-function capability would be the most beneficial.

Patient Preparation

Small animals may be examined by ultrasound in ventral recumbency on a padded trough, standing, or in lateral recumbency. Animals undergoing a cardiac study are often placed on a specialized cardiac table so that the transducer may be placed through a small cut-out opening on the "down" side of the patient's chest.

Large animals are usually examined in a standing position.

It is important that the patient remain still for an accurate ultrasound examination. Panting, struggling, and tensing up will decrease the diagnostic capabilities of the sonographer through reduced image resolution and clarity. Sedation is required to overcome these obstacles.

Sound waves do not travel through air; therefore, the probe must have direct contact with the skin surface. Ideally, fur is clipped away and alcohol is wiped on the skin to remove superficial fats. Finally, a coupling gel is applied to

Speed of sound through different mediums			
Air	330 m/s	Fat	1460 m/s
Lung	600 m/s	Water	1480 m/s
Skull bone	4080 m/s	Liver	5550 m/s
Muscle 1600 m/s			

FIGURE 13-2 A chart quantifying the different speeds, or velocities, for sound traveling through different media, or tissues within the mammalian body. It is these differences that help create contrast between tissues when the echo returns to the ceramic elements and results in varying electrical pulses.

the skin surface and to the surface of the probe to improve contact between them.

Sound Velocities and Acoustic Impedance

The ultrasound study depends on varying densities in the tissues that the sound beam passes through. The speed of the sound produced by the crystals is changed according to whether the tissue it is traveling through is more or less dense. This is illustrated by the following simple equation:

$$Z = pV$$

where Z is the acoustic impedance (or sound impediment), p is the density of the tissue, and V is the acoustic velocity. So the denser tissue (higher p) has more acoustic impedance (impediment).

Figure 13-2 summarizes the velocity of sound in different mediums and tissues. On the basis of these numbers, it is clear that the velocities through some tissues are very similar; note, for instance, those for fat and water. Although minute, the differences in velocity are still significant enough for the ultrasound unit to clearly differentiate between them. The resulting image quantifies the differences. It is the acoustic impedance that gives us the contrast between pixels in the image (Figures 13-3 and 13-4).

Gray Scale

Ultrasonography offers a much wider range of tissue densities through gray-scale levels than can be seen in plain radiographs (Figure 13-5). Typically, 256 shades of gray are incorporated into the display of an image obtained through ultrasound. This creates a much superior level of contrast than that with plain radiographs. The human eye can distinguish approximately 32-64 shades of gray (Figure 13-6).

Modes in Ultrasound Imaging

In ultrasound imaging, the echo data collected can be formatted into specific images that represent different interpretations of the characteristics of the tissues being evaluated. This section offers summaries of the individual characteristics of each mode.

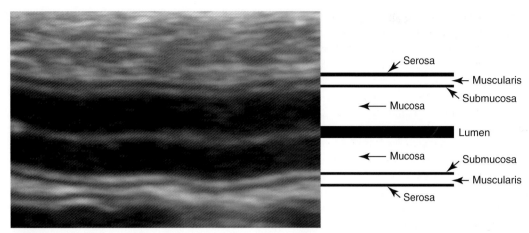

FIGURE 13-3 Ultrasound image showing a segment of the canine jejunum and its structural components. Acoustic impedance gives contrast to the anatomical layering of the intestines, allowing them to be visualized on ultrasound because the sound wave traverses different tissue densities at variable velocities. These variables lead to a different shade of gray representing each density. This can be very useful for identifying different types of intestinal pathology, because each type may be associated with changes in a different layer.

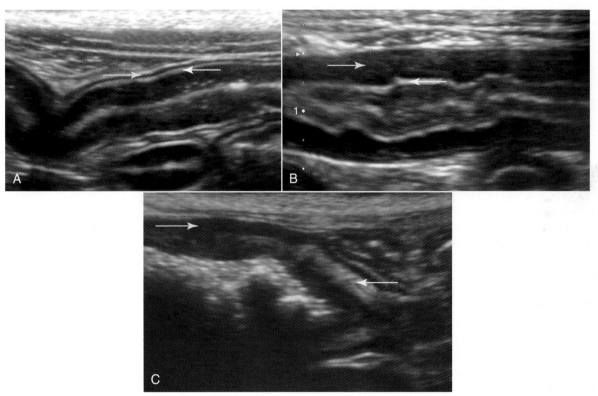

FIGURE 13-4 Three different sections of intestine found during an ultrasound examination. In each image, the *yellow arrow* shows the muscularis layer and the *white arrow* shows the mucosa. **A,** Normal layering of the jejunum. **B,** Intestinal lymphoma with a thickened and hypoechoic muscularis layer. **C,** Ulcerative colitis affecting both the mucosal and submucosal layers. Although ultrasonography on its own is not considered to give a histological diagnosis, the changes seen during an examination can often be shown to have a high correlation with known pathology as seen here.

B Mode

In B-mode ultrasound, the B is abbreviated to represent *brightness.* The returning echo intensity and speed to the transducer is interpreted and then transformed into a digitalized pixel within a two-dimensional image on screen. The pixel is either classified as hyperechoic (bright) or hypoechoic (dark).

The full spectrum of 256 shades of gray is used to create each pixel composed in an image. The spatial resolution (or distance) between pixels can be as low as 0.3 mm, depending

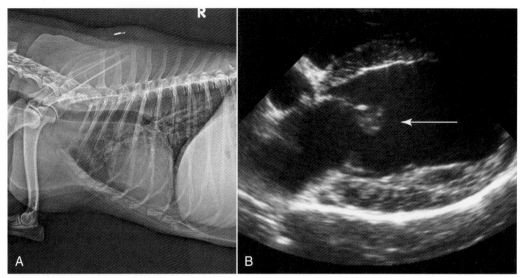

FIGURE 13-5 The heart represented in two separate modalities. **A,** A radiograph shows the heart as a homogeneous fluid density represented as a single shade of gray. **B,** The ultrasound image clearly shows inside the left ventricle, where the *arrow* points to a lesion on one of the mitral valve leaflets.

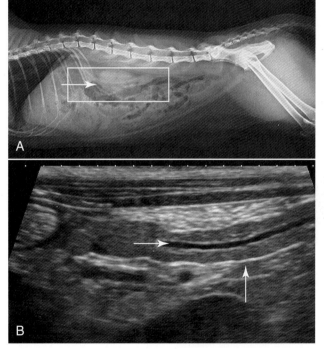

FIGURE 13-6 **A,** The area outlined by the *white box* in the abdominal radiograph delineates the space that is usually occupied by the pancreas. Note that the tissue's gray-scale limitations in plain radiographs do not allow visualization of the pancreas. **B,** Compare this with the significant difference in visualization of the pancreas (*vertical arrow*) relative to the surrounding tissues with ultrasound imaging. This is possible only because of the higher number of grays used to generate the ultrasound study. The detail is so sensitive that the pancreatic duct within the organ is also visualized (*horizontal arrow*).

on the type of transducer and the frequency used to perform the scan.

M Mode

M-mode ultrasound is motion mode. In this mode, a cursor line is set over an area of interest as imaged in B-mode. M-mode simultaneously creates a B-mode image (light and dark) while displaying the motion of the tissues over a two-dimensional scale. This creates a continuous waveform and plots at which each pixel intersects the cursor line.

M-mode ultrasound is particularly useful for evaluating the heart. Using this mode and plotting movement of each pixel of light and dark, we can determine the thickness and diameter of the ventricular wall through different stages of the cardiac cycle. We can measure cardiac dimensions and evaluate movement of the valvular leaflets within the ventricles.

Doppler

Doppler ultrasonography is used to image the flow of blood and other liquids as well as to measure their velocity.

Color-Flow Doppler

In color-flow Doppler imaging, the information collected is presented as a color overlay on top of a B-mode image. This application was first introduced in the mid-1980s. There are different gradients of superimposed color, depending on color map selections. In standard imaging, for instance, we track blood flow by using the color blue to show blood flow away from the transducer and the color red for blood flowing towards the transducer. This is best remembered by using the BART (blue away/red towards) acronym.

The addition of another type of more sensitive color mapping may add variances that detect abnormal turbulence within the normal laminar flow of blood (Figure 13-7).

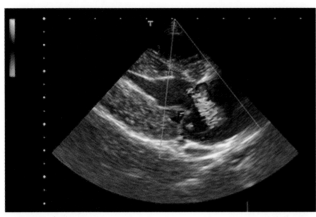

FIGURE 13-7 A color-flow ultrasound image of the left side of a heart demonstrating turbulence as the brightly colored area in the middle of the left atrium. Here it is caused by the abnormal flow of blood leaking from a mitral valve defect during systole. This is a mitral regurgitation "jet."

Power Color

Power color Doppler imaging is yet another form of color imaging that is very sensitive to the flow of blood but does not identify its direction. It is used predominantly to detect lower velocities in tissues where the directional flow is less important than detecting the flow itself. An example of this would be in evaluating the vascularity (blood vessel pattern) of a neoplastic mass.

Pulse Wave

As the name implies, pulse-wave Doppler (PW) imaging is produced by a transducer that alternates between sending and receiving sound signals. This alternation allows the area being analyzed to be set to within a very small sample volume, or "gated." The sampling or listening area can be set anywhere along a cursor line that transects the concurrent B-mode image. PW imaging can read blood flow velocities in the 0.4 to 0.6 m/s range, making it very useful for small peripheral vessels.

PW imaging can detect blood flow velocities up to a maximum of 1.4 m/sec. At these velocities, the probe reaches what is called a *Nyquist point*. These readings then inaccurately display inverse or flow reversal, making their true measurement impossible to quantify with any accuracy. At these velocities, continuous-wave (CW) measurements should be taken instead of PW (see later).

Continuous Wave

Continuous-wave Doppler imaging requires that the scanner have two different transducers or set of crystals built within it that work together. One set of crystals is continually sending out signals while the other set receives. This arrangement allows accurate measurements to be made during studies of the very-high-velocity blood flow found in many congenital heart diseases. It is, however, less accurate for selectively measuring flow at a certain depths, and it cannot be gated as can PW Doppler studies.

Harmonic Mode

The use of tissue harmonics helps to decrease ultrasound artifacts (see later) in very large or obese patients. In this mode, a single deep frequency or multiple deep penetrating frequencies are emitted into the body along with a harmonic overtone. The overall objective is to achieve deeper homogeneous penetration with fewer artifacts, because this mode utilizes software to filter the returning sound wave, removing echoes that may interfere with a clearer image.

Multiplanar Reconstruction

Multiplanar reconstruction (MPR) studies involve reconstructing images from various planes to allow simultaneous visualization on the monitor. Although multiplanar reconstruction has been the norm in both computerized tomography and magnetic resonance imaging studies for some time, it is a relatively new imaging format for the field of ultrasonography.

Three- and Four-Dimensional Modes

Although currently of limited practicality in veterinary medicine, both stationary three-dimensional and time-lapsed four-dimensional reconstructions are available in human ultrasonography. These modes are currently used primarily for human fetal, obstetrical, and cardiac valve imaging. As newer applications arise, these technologies will likely spread to veterinary use.

Knobology

Every ultrasound machine, regardless of manufacturer, has a common set of instrument adjustments that can modify both the performance of the machine and its image quality. These adjustments are made either mechanically (manipulating knobs and boards) or by contact on a software-driven touch screen.

Gain

The gain control, or gain adjustment, affects the brightness of the image. It affects the range of the gray scale used to format the image for that particular study. Most machines offer a choice of preformatted gray scale and colored maps to start as the base image for the gain. These are chosen according to the ultrasound study required. For example, cardiac studies do not require the full gray-scale range but instead use a high-contrast image in order to better define the edges of the cardiac musculature. Abdominal studies, on the other hand, benefit from a wide range of gray scale to better detect minor anatomical changes within an organ or tissue.

Depth

Every type and size of transducer has a set maximum and minimum depth at which it can send and receive sound waves. A common mistake during imaging of an area of interest is to set the depth control too high (deep). Although it may appear to give a better perspective of the tissue relative to the surrounding structures, such a setting inevitably wastes valuable pixels that could give finer organ detail. As a rule of thumb, one should limit the depth of the scan so that the area of interest fills the full monitor screen for closer analysis.

Time Gain Compensation

Time gain compensation (TGC) allows the operator to selectively adjust the gain at various depths. Echoes that return from deeper structures are more attenuated because they travel back through more tissues. This makes part of the far-field image appear darker. TGC adjustments allow one to compensate the gain to obtain a smooth gray-scale image throughout the full depth of the scan view. This adjustment is often done by manipulating a series of sliding tabs that affect the level of brightness at various depths.

Presets

Presets are preinstalled settings programmed by the manufacturer. The settings included with the machine's software are meant to facilitate and maximize the performance of a transducer depending on the type of study required. Selecting a preset for a cardiac study may affect such parameters as the sensitivity and range of the Doppler reading for either adults or neonates. Presets affect the dynamic range, gain settings, gray map selection, transducer frequency, number of focal zones, and depth of scan. Some machines may also allow the operator to modify these presets or create and save his or her own because personal preferences vary.

Focal Zones

Adjustments to the focal zones allow the ultrasound beam to converge more at a particular depth during the study. This maximizes the axial and lateral spatial resolution at the area of interest (see later definitions). This focal setting works best if selected within the near-field imaging parameter of a transducer. A maximum of only two focal spots should be used at a time even though some machines allow the operator to select up to five.

Frequency Selection

Individual transducers generate sound waves with a set range of frequencies based on the size of the piezoelectric ceramic crystals used within the ultrasound probe (see later transducer discussion). The frequency selection knob allows the operator to change the frequency within the range of frequencies allowed by that probe. The chosen frequency affects the maximum depth of penetration of the sound waves in the tissues. It is important to be aware that depth of penetrance is inversely related to frequency (the higher the frequency, the less the penetrance). The advantage of using higher frequencies is that they provide for better optimization of the spatial resolution of the area in question.

Optimization

Another option found on many newer machines is a single step adjustment that automatically optimizes the settings in order to obtain the best image. Choosing this setting affects the gain settings and the tissue harmonics to obtain the ideal image as the sound beam travels through a particular part of the body. Ultrasound manufacturers have different names for this option with the same end result. Optimization is meant to help operators with limited knowledge of individual settings and adjustments to quickly obtain the best possible image.

Transducers

As already discussed, the purpose of the ultrasound transducer (or probe) is to change electrical energy into mechanical energy (sound waves) that penetrate into the tissues and to receive the reflected sound waves, converting them back into electrical impulses that are then read by the computer. This is accomplished by piezoelectric crystal elements that can change shape and vibrate in response to electrical or mechanical stimulation (see also earlier principles discussion).

The greatest advancement in ultrasound imaging came in the early 1990s, when there was an explosion in the development of both high-speed digital electronics and powerful computer platforms that could support 20 to 30 billion operations per second. With the advent of the digitization of the systems, many fine adjustments to the processing software could be implemented, resulting in dramatic reductions in signal noise and artifacts. The numbers of elements on individual transducers can range from as low as 64 to more than 500 elements per transducer head. At the same time, improvements in the speed and quality of the receiving and processing card directly affected the image quality and resolution of the scan images for advanced studies.

Transducer Frequency

As mentioned previously, there is an inverse relationship between increasing the frequency output of a probe and the maximum depth that it can scan. This means that the higher the frequency of the transducer, the less it will penetrate (Figure 13-8).

Secondly, there is a direct relationship between increasing the frequency of a transducer and lateral spatial resolution. *Lateral spatial resolution* is the ability to distinguish between

Transducer Frequencies			
• Increasing frequency			
• Decreased penetration capability			
• But increases fine detail. Better spatial resolution.			
	Depth	Wavelengths	Max spatial resolution
3 MHz	20 cm	0.44 mm	0.76 mm
5 MHz	15 cm	0.31 mm	0.62 mm
7.5 MHz	10 cm	0.21 mm	0.42 mm
10 MHz	7 cm	0.15 mm	0.33 mm

FIGURE 13-8 Comparison of transducer frequencies with depths of penetration and levels of spatial resolution.

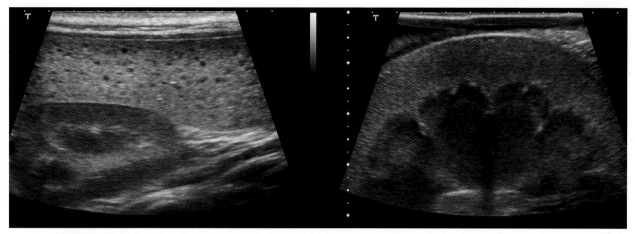

FIGURE 13-9 Spatial resolution is improved when a higher-frequency transducer is used in the near field. On the image on the *left* there is decreased detail over the transition point of the renal cortex to the medullary zone of the kidney. Contrast this to the image on the *right*, on which minute changes in the echogenicity of the transitional zone can be seen with greater clarity.

two objects or echoes that are adjacent to each other yet perpendicular to the sound wave and hence are influenced by the sound beam's width. The lateral resolution is best in the near field, (area closest to the transducer) where the sound beam is narrowest.

The *axial resolution* is the ability to differentiate between two structures along the beam's length and is equal to half of a pulse's length.

Choosing a Transducer

A typical small animal practice may require up to three or four different types of transducers, depending on the type of ultrasound studies being performed. For instance, a clinic that does both cardiac and abdominal scans needs more transducers than a clinic performing only general abdominal ultrasonography. In comparison, an equine practice devoted exclusively to lameness studies may require only a single high-frequency linear transducer to perform most tendon studies.

Because the frequency of wavelength at which that the ceramics are vibrating affect the spatial resolution within an image, higher-frequency transducers are required for detailed studies. Many higher-end ultrasound machines can reach frequencies of up to 18 MHz.

Transducers have single-frequency or multiple-frequency ranges on a single probe. In veterinary medicine, the wide range in both the sizes and weights of patients makes the use of single-frequency transducers difficult. The veterinary practice is advised to consider multiple-frequency transducers in order to purchase fewer transducers. Considering the high cost for the individual transducer, multiple-frequency transducers are more economical to the practice (Figure 13-9).

Markers

Each ultrasound probe is tagged with a marker, which may be in the form of an indentation, a raised surface, or an

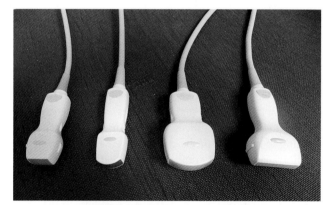

FIGURE 13-10 Various transducers.

illuminated "in use" light. This marker is associated with a similar identification tag on the upper left corner of the ultrasound screen. Orienting the marker on the transducer toward the marker on the screen assists in performing a standardized ultrasound examination.

In keeping with standardized convention, in a sagittal scan plane, the cranial aspect of the patient body should be displayed on the left side of the monitor, and when one is viewing transverse planes, the right side of the pet should be presented to the left of the screen as well. It is the marker icon represented on the screen, along with the reference point etched over the transducer, that helps the sonographer properly orient and record the scan.

Transducer Types

A wide variety of different kinds of transducer probes are available to veterinarians (Figure 13-10). The most commonly used in veterinary medicine are described here. Other types of probes include those used within endoscopes, esophageal probes, and endocavity probes used for obstetrics. The size, frequency range, and conformation of the actual footprint (the part of the probe that makes contact with the patient) vary among probes and among vendors as well.

Linear Transducer

The linear transducer design was one of the first probes to appear on the ultrasound scene. It has a flat contact surface or footprint. The earlier designs would only scan in a limited rectangular view of tissues directly beneath the probe. This resulted in many artifacts, such as side lobes (see later discussion of artifacts). With the advent of digital technology and the ability to focus the sound beam, the linear probe now has the added option of trapezoid imaging. This option keeps the high resolution of the linear probe and gives some of the broader advantages of the curvilinear probe (see later). Software changes have also resulted in a dramatic reduction in artifacts, and the faster processing time has improved the linear probe's capability. Because of these adaptive changes, linear probes have reemerged in popularity as ideal diagnostic tools for fine-detail imaging.

Convex Transducer

The convex transducer, also known as a sector probe or curvilinear probe, was first introduced in the late 1970s and early 1980s. At the time they exceeded the popularity of the linear probe because of their curvilinear shape, which offered a wider field of view at the sacrifice of spatial resolution (especially in human obstetrical studies). In some cases the footprint was too wide for small animal use. As the trapezoid imaging of the linear probe has improved and increased the detail available in the scans (discussed earlier), the convex and the linear probes have become almost equally popular. Many ultrasonographers use a convex probe for a general scan and then switch to a linear probe for higher-resolution inspections.

Microconvex Transducer

Although very similar to convex probes because of the curvilinear shape, the micro-convex transducer has a much reduced footprint size. This difference makes them more practical for smaller animal patients. This is especially true for intercostal studies where the distance between the ribs limits the probe's view and contact with the patient. The disadvantage of this size change is the reduced number of elements and the spread of the wide angle view which ends up sacrificing some degree of image quality. Micro-convex probes are particularly useful in smaller canines, felines, and exotic patients.

Phased Array Sector Transducer

Phased array transducers contain piezoelectric elements that are stimulated in complex timing sequences and controlled by circuitry to provide focus and sound beam steering at different depths simultaneously. In these types of transducers the crystals are electronically steered through firing time delays. They are most often used in cardiac studies, as they have the unique ability to offer a continuous-wave Doppler (CW) mode.

Matrix Transducer

The matrix transducer is the newest class of transducers and at this time is offered by only a select number of vendors. This type of transducer will likely replace many of the other probes as technology continues to improve and the size of the transducer becomes slightly more manageable. The probe offers the ability to scan in different planes at the same time (Figure 13-11) as a result of the high density of elements machined within it. The two-dimensional matrix allows the operator to create three-dimensional images of an area in question (e.g., heart valves). Unfortunately, cost has

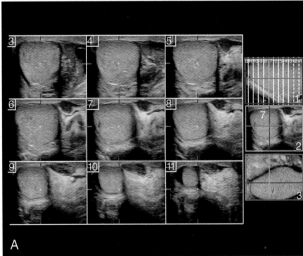

iSlice Epididymitis

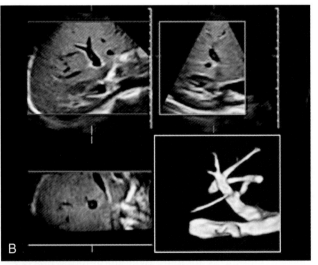

Volume imaging with the X6-1 transducer

FIGURE 13-11 These series of images represent two different methods of presenting cross sectional scans through an organ. The image to the left illustrates a collage of B mode photos taken through only one imaging plane representing the epididymitis. That on the right hand side is a frame grab that has hepatic reconstructions projected in 3 different planes all at the same time. It also includes a 3D volume image of vascular structures of the liver in the lower right hand side quadrant.

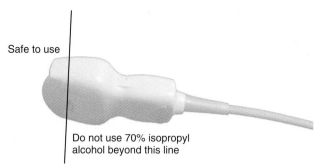

Safe to use

Do not use 70% isopropyl alcohol beyond this line

FIGURE 13-12 Proper cleaning of the ultrasound transducer.

limited the use of the matrix transducer in veterinary medicine at present.

For more example of probes check out the evolve website.

Transducer Care and Cleaning Guides

Each ultrasound transducer can be worth thousands of dollars when new ($3,000–16,000). Care must be taken in the handling of probes to avoid dropping or impacting them, which could damage the piezoelectric crystals.

After each use, the technician should wipe off any remaining acoustic gel found on the probe with either a dry or water-moistened *soft* cloth. Contaminated fluids on the transducer may be gently cleaned with either a 10% bleach solution, a glutaraldehyde-based disinfectant, or 70% isopropyl alcohol. The technician should check with the manufacturer's service manual, as not all companies recommend this. Required cleaning practices must be followed carefully to avoid warranty disruption.

Alcohol should *never* be used beyond 2 cm from the tip of the transducer because it can damage the housing joint seals (Figure 13-12). Alcohol should never be used on the transducer cables.

Probes used in endocavity procedures can be cleaned with a mild soap and water solution. Although transducers can be immersed for short periods, immersion is not recommended, and the connectors and distal cables should never be included. At no point should a transducer be autoclaved or gas-sterilized with ethylene oxide. Care should be taken also to avoid contact with gels that contain lotions, mineral oil, or lanolin.

Applications for Ultrasound

Bovine and Ruminant

In bovine and ruminant animals, ultrasound examination is predominantly used for reproductive work, such as follicle detection, pregnancy examination, and reproductive difficulties. Ultrasound-guided biopsies and monitoring with follow-up ultrasounds are also employed in these animals.

Equine

Two different disciplines exist in the equine world: sports medicine and reproduction. Ultrasound is invaluable in identifying both tendon and ligamentous strains and injuries. It is also particularly useful for monitoring progress as the horse improves and returns to normal with the prescribed therapeutics.

Fertility is also an important consideration in equine medicine. The use of ultrasound is the standard of care for following up on the early stages of gestation and fetal development.

Porcine

The main use for ultrasonography in pigs is to measure back fat levels found within animals for meat production.

Small Animals

The list of possible applications of ultrasound seems to be almost endless for small animal studies because the size of most patients is ideal for the types of frequency ranges available to the practitioner. The scope of studies is limited only by the imagination of the ultrasonographer.

Abdominal studies include all of the gastrointestinal system from the esophagus as it transverses the diaphragm, to the distal end of the colon including the rectum, which is imaged through the perineal area. Abdominal ultrasound studies also include the imaging of the liver, gallbladder, and biliary tree. The pancreas, spleen, kidneys, adrenals, and regional lymph nodes are routinely imaged and evaluated. For example, abdominal lymph nodes can be assessed with ultrasound for their level of inflammation and reactivity. The urinary bladder and excretory system up to the bony pelvic rim is also part of any examination, as are all of the components of both sexes' reproductive organs. The more distal structures can also be reached with more superficial scanning methods. The only major limiting factors are the obstructed views resulting from either bone densities or gas-filled organs.

Thoracic ultrasound studies in small animals include full cardiac examination with M-mode interpretations and Doppler velocity assessments. In emergency medicine, ultrasonography is the diagnostic modality of choice for assessing trauma and suspected abdominal bleeding.

Ultrasound Artifacts

Sound waves do not travel through air or bone. For this reason, there are situations in which a reflected sound wave may occur that interferes with the diagnostic scan. One of the most common examples of the reflection of sound waves occurs when the beam make contacts with air. The resultant artifact reflection is called *reverberation*. Common ultrasonographic artifacts are summarized here.

Comet Tail

The comet tail artifact (Figure 13-13) appears as a series of closely interspaced and intense reverberations or reflections that appear to look like the tail of a comet. They can occur with reflection of the sound wave off small reflector targets,

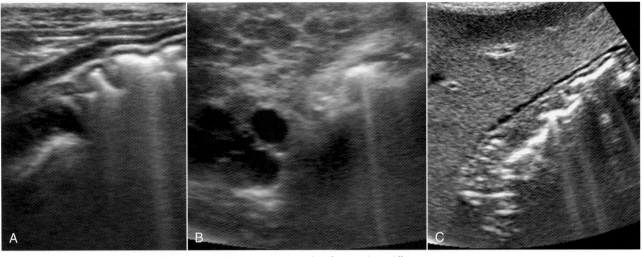

FIGURE 13-13 A to C, Comet tail artifacts in three different gastric images.

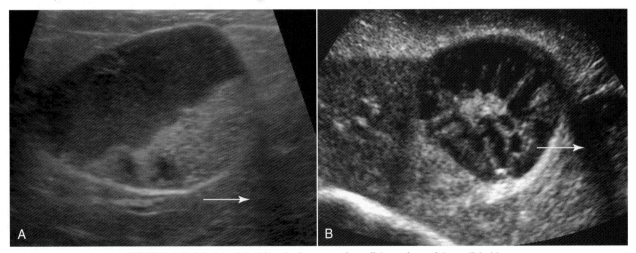

FIGURE 13-14 A and B, Edge shadowing artifact off the surface of the gallbladder.

such as air pockets in the gastrointestinal tract or metallic objects, like a foreign body or the tip of a biopsy needle. Figure 13-13 shows typical comet tails in three different gastric images.

Edge Shadowing

Edge shadowing is as a form of refraction, or redirection of the sound wave, as it passes through a fluid-tissue interface. It is associated with curved fluid-filled structures such as the gallbladder, urinary bladder, cysts, and even sometimes the kidneys. The phenomenon occurs in the far field of object (away from the entrance of the beam). It appears as a hypoechoic linear shadow that diverges from the surface of the curved structure.

Edge shadowing can occur when the incident angle of the sound beam hits the leading edge of a circular object (the near edge). The objects in question must be composed of different attenuation material, such as a liquid and solids side by side as in a cystic structure. Figure 13-14 shows edge shadowing off the surface of the gallbladder.

Acoustic Enhancement

Acoustic enhancement occurs when the sound beam travels through a weakly attenuating structure such as a bladder with fluid. The sound beams travelling through tissues *around* the bladder are slowed or attenuated, whereas the sound beams passing through the liquid will not have lost as much energy or intensity. When the sound beams hit the tissue at the far side of the bladder, the reflection will appear brighter (hyperechoic) than the surrounding tissues on the same plane. The resulting artifact appears as a distal enhancement (brighter on the far side of the structure) on B-mode imaging.

This predictable artifact is very useful in differentiating certain hypoechoic masses from cystic or fluid-filled structures. Figure 13-15 shows the increase in echogenicity in the

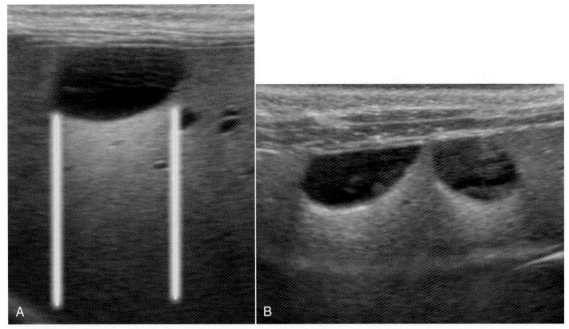

FIGURE 13-15 A and B, Acoustic enhancement is apparent in comparison with tissues around the gallbladder. The indicator lines in **A** outline the area of relative increase in echogenicity.

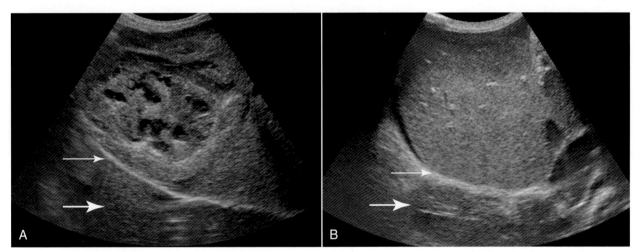

FIGURE 13-16 A and B, A mirror image of the liver (*large arrow*) is seen on the opposite side of the diaphragm (*small arrow*) from its normal place in the abdomen.

area outlined between the two white lines. This is consistent with acoustic enhancement.

Mirror Image

The strong reflective surface between the diaphragm and the air-filled lungs is a common place to observe a distinct mirror image of tissues in the abdomen (Figure 13-16). The sound beams reflected back from this interface are misinterpreted by the ultrasound machine, which then places a second image of the liver on the opposite side of the diaphragm. This artifact is important to recognize because an inexperienced ultrasonographer may interpret such an artifact as a diaphragmatic hernia, a thoracic mass, or even lung pathology.

Reverberation

Reverberation is due to repeated back-and-forth reflection of echoes trapped between two strong reflectors. The resulting effect appears like a bright veil similar to northern lights in the sky (Figure 13-17). It is principally seen in a superficially positioned gas-filled loop of bowel and within the stomach. The bright echo display makes it difficult to see anything distal to the artifact. The end result is that one cannot properly project an image of the opposing wall of the digestive tract.

Acoustic Shadowing

Acoustic shadowing (Figure 13-18) is the simplest of all of the artifacts to understand. When the sound beam contacts

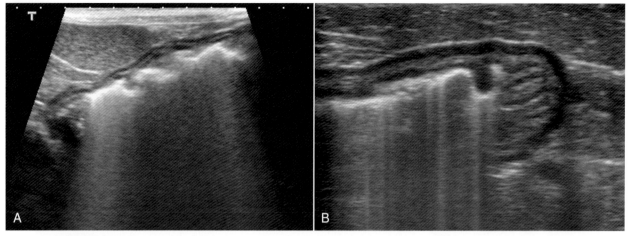

FIGURE 13-17 A and B, Reverberation due to repeated reflection of sound waves off gas in the gastrointestinal tract.

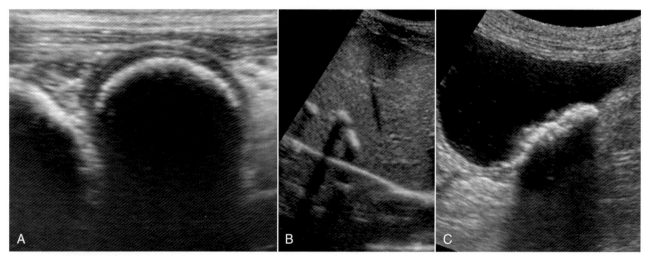

FIGURE 13-18 Acoustic shadowing as seen distal to a foreign body in the jejunum (A), stones in the biliary tree of the liver (B), and an aggregation of urinary bladder stones in the bladder (C). Note the dark shadowing below each dense structure.

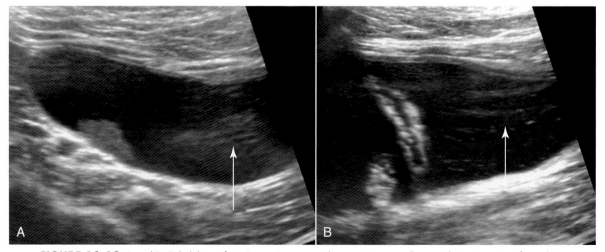

FIGURE 13-19 A and B, Side lobe artifacts (arrows) are secondary emissions usually seen during imaging of anechoic structures urinary bladder and gallbladder.

a highly attenuating surface, such as a urolith (bladder stone) or bone, most of the sound beam is either reflected away or absorbed. There is a lack of echo information distal to the dense object. The absence of data is displayed as a dark streak or shadow below the object, where the ultrasound beam has not penetrated. The shadow is lined up parallel to the direction of the emitting sound beam from the transducer.

Side Lobe

When a transducer is emitting sound beams, the majority are directed in a primary direction, but secondary lateral minor emissions are simultaneously created. These become more pronounced as a transducer is set at its upper threshold. These side lobe echoes (Figure 13-19) can be displayed on the monitor even if they did not originate from the principal or main sound beam. This artifact can be reduced by changing the position of the focal zone or by reducing the frequency of the transducer.

SUMMARY

The evolution of Ultrasound has progressed rapidly in the last several years and the future of this imaging modality is bright. This chapter has been a brief introduction to the science of imaging using sound.

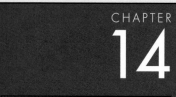

CHAPTER

14

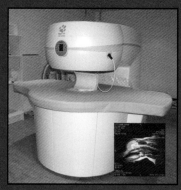

KEY TERMS

Atom
Echo time
Magnet
Magnetic field
Radio frequency
Repetition time
Resonance
Signal intensity
Specific absorption rate

Magnetic Resonance Imaging

Stephanie Holowka MRT(R), MRT(MR)

The world is your mirror and your mind is a magnet.
What you perceive in this world is largely a reflection of your
own attitudes and beliefs ...

—Michael LeBeuf - American Author and Mangement Professor - Univ. of New Orleans

OUTLINE

LEARNING OBJECTIVES

When you have finished this chapter, you will be able to:

1. Discuss the equipment necessary for magnetic resonance.
2. Understand the principles of magnetic resonance.
3. Know the MRI machine.
4. Describe how MRI is used in diagnosis.
5. List the safety issues in MRI.

APPLICATIONS

The application of the information in this chapter is relevant to the following areas:

1. Imaging using magnetism and resonance to determine pathology.

Magnetic resonance imaging (MRI) came into existence in the early 1980s. Its creation was based on the principles of magnetic spectroscopy—the use of a magnetic field and radio frequencies to determine the chemical makeup of a substance. The chemical makeup of a substance can be determined by which radio frequencies are emitted and which are received in response. MRI has become more and more common in human medicine and is now found in specialized veterinary centers as well (Figure 14-1). Because it shows the concentration of free-floating hydrogen molecules in tissue, it has much better subject contrast than computerized tomography (CT) scan and radiography. MRI is superior in demonstrating the brain, the spinal cord (Figure 14-2), and soft tissue structures such as the ligaments and cartilage in joints. MRI is also a desired modality in that it does not use any ionizing radiation in creating the images. This chapter gives an overview for understanding this fascinating and complex new technology.

Safety Notice

Magnets such as those used in MRI scanners are very dangerous machines, especially for untrained personnel (Figure 14-3). Anyone walking into a room with such a magnet must be screened for unsafe implants and any loose metal. The highest danger to staff and patients is the projectile effect—the launching of a metallic object into the magnet by the magnetic force. A person cannot predict how an object will project into a magnet. People have been severely injured or killed by such accidents. Only magnetically safe objects and people should be allowed to enter an MRI room. Only special stretchers, MRI-safe monitors, MRI-safe oxygen tanks, and so on, can be used in an MRI room. Every MRI site must have policies and procedures in place to ensure the safety of patients and staff.

Principles

To understand the workings of MRI, one has to start at the atomic level. All atoms have protons, neutrons, and electrons. The protons and neutrons are found in the center or core (nucleus) of the atom, and the electrons spin around on the outside. Every atom also spins and wobbles in space as well (Figure 14-4). This wobble (much like how a top wobbles) is called *precession*. Atoms join together create molecules. All atoms and molecules (as in anything electrical) exhibit the ability to show magnetic polarity or fields. When

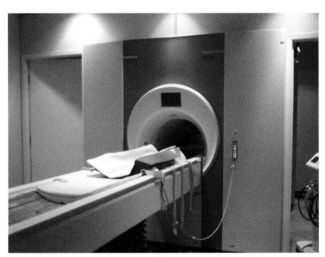

FIGURE 14-1 A magnetic resonance machine in a veterinary clinic. This is a high-field (1.5-Tesla) superconductor magnet. The machine was being prepared for a spine scan on a dog. It has the spine coil in place.

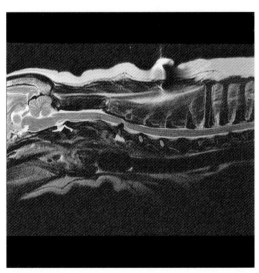

FIGURE 14-2 A sagittal T2-weighted MR image of a dog's spine. The scan shows that an intervertebral disc is bulging into the spinal canal and against the spinal cord. The compressed cord is brighter in that region, showing that it is swollen, or has edema.

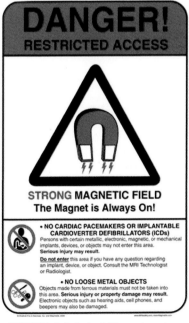

FIGURE 14-3 An MRI warning sign.

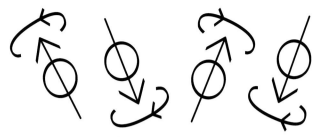

FIGURE 14-4 Atoms in their normal random positions, spinning and wobbling. *Arrows* represent the positions of their magnetic polarities.

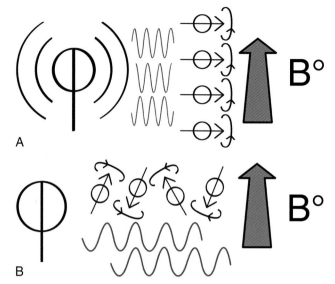

FIGURE 14-6 A, What happens in magnetic resonance imaging. A radio antenna emits radio waves in a resonant frequency that causes certain atoms to go into a higher energy state. The hydrogen atoms respond to this frequency by aligning their magnetism (*black arrows*) to 90 degrees from their original orientation (*blue arrow*) within the magnet. They also wobble or precess together. **B,** When the radio waves are turned off, the atoms return to their original magnetization state and their energy state back to equilibrium. The atoms give off radio waves, which are detected by the radio antenna.

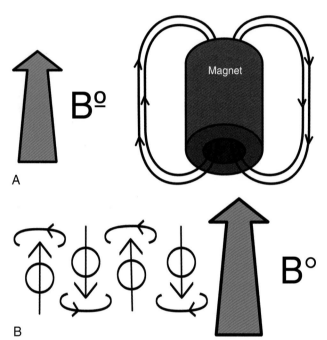

FIGURE 14-5 A, A magnet and its magnetic field. The total magnetic force is represented by B^0. **B,** What happens to atoms within a strong magnetic field. The atoms randomly align to their polarity, and B^0 represents the total magnetization of the atoms.

Magnet and Magnetism

A magnet is any object that exhibits a magnetic field or force. Magnetic force can be created in an object several ways. It can occur naturally in some substances, such as iron and malachite. It can be induced into an object; some metallic objects become magnetized if exposed to a strong magnetic field and as a result act as magnets. A magnet can be created by electricity. When an electrical current is applied through a series of copper windings, an electromagnet can be created. Magnetic force also exhibits polarity, in that there are two poles, north and south, like positive and negative in electricity. In magnetism, opposite poles attract each other and pull two magnets together. Like poles repel and push two magnets away from each other.

The imperial unit of measurement for magnetism is the gauss (G). For example, the earth has a magnetic field of 1 gauss. The most common measurement of magnetism is the metric equivalent, the tesla (T). 10,000 G = 1.0 T. The earth's magnetic field is 10^{-4} T. Tesla is the unit that people use in describing a medical magnet's field strength.

In medical MRI three types of magnets can be in use. There are permanent magnets. These consist of two slabs of magnetic material facing each other, and they tend to be lower field strengths—less than 0.3 T. There are electromagnets, or resistive magnets (Figure 14-7), created by an electrical charge applied through copper wire wrapped around a center. These also tend to be lower field magnets—less than 0.6 T. The most common medical magnets are called superconducting magnets. They are massive electromagnets made

placed in a magnetic field, they will respond according to their own polarity.

How Does MRI Work?

In a most basic description, one puts an animal or person into the magnet. All of the subject's molecules align on the basis of polarity and become magnetized (Figure 14-5). In performing a scan, a technologist applies a radio frequency tuned to the precessing frequency of hydrogen atoms (Figure 14-6A). The hydrogen atoms in the subject respond by resonating (or responding) into a higher energy state. They also change the angle of their magnetization and wobble together. The radio frequency is removed, and the molecules return to their normal energy state (Figure 14-6B). In doing so, they give off a radio frequency that the MRI scanner calculates into an image. The actual method is quite a bit more complicated, but this is the basic concept of MRI.

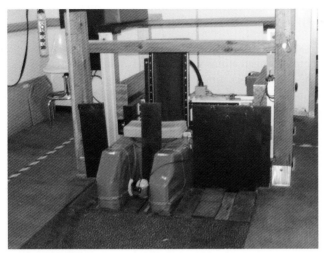

FIGURE 14-7 A resistive magnet MRI unit used to image horse legs. The magnet covers only a specific field of view. A white spherical phantom (in between the two blue magnets) is covered by a surface coil.

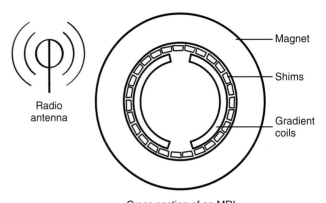

Cross section of an MRI

FIGURE 14-8 A basic overview of the components needed to make up a basic MRI machine. A superconducting magnet would have a vacuum and helium chambers outside the actual magnet assembly but within the casing of the machine.

of windings that are superconductive in very low temperatures. Liquid helium (the coldest substance available on earth, with a temperature very close to absolute zero [−273°C/−459°F]) is used to keep the magnet active.

> **POINT TO PONDER** For the use of a superconducting magnet, great consideration is made in terms of the construction of the room surrounding the magnet. Special ventilation ducts must be created for quenching the magnet, a process whereby the liquid helium vents out rapidly and shuts off the magnet by increasing the resistance across the windings. Liquid helium has an expansion ratio of 1-to-700 liters. There are at least 1000 liters of liquid helium in a superconductor magnet, so the total expanded volume would rapidly exceed the size of any MRI room. It is these magnets (1.0 T or more field strength) that are never turned off. The very strong magnetic field is always on, even when the machine is not taking pictures.

Aside from the magnet, many other parts make an MRI work (Figure 14-8).

Magnetic Shims or Shim Coils

Shims are pieces or plates of metal used to correct the magnetic field within the magnet. For an MRI unit to work properly, the main magnetic field of the bore must be entirely homogenous. Any alterations of the main magnetic field could result in distorted images.

Gradients

Gradients are coils or assemblies within the magnetic bore that enable the machine to create images in any plane. An incremented current is applied across the gradient (in an orientation chosen by the technologist), thus slightly varying the magnetic field in that direction. When the radio frequency is applied to the body, the variances in the frequency are calculated back to determine the "x-y-z" dimensions in space of each of the voxels of the image. The reconstruction method used to reconstruct images from the gradients is called two-dimensional Fourier transformation. It is the design of the gradients that allows MRI to create images in any plane—axial (or transverse), coronal, or sagittal.

Radio Antenna

The radio antenna used in the MRI machine is quite strong, in that it could be used for a radio station. The antenna sends and receives radio waves to and from the patient. Radio waves are part of the electromagnetic spectrum, as are light, microwaves, and x-rays (see Chapter 3, Figure 3-3). They are a form of energy but are not radioactive. Because the radio waves are important to the creation of images, MRI rooms have to be shielded with a Faraday cage against any external radio signals (see Evolve webside & Faraday cage). Outside radio waves can cause artifacts on the MR images.

Surface Coils

MRI machines are able to produce patient images from the main magnet (or body coil) itself; however, the radio signals received from smaller body parts have very poor resolution. Surface coils are devices that receive (and sometimes send) radio wave signals from a body part that is covered or contained by them (Figure 14-9). There are specialized coils for many body parts, including the brain, spine, shoulders, head and neck, and hocks. These coils are made or adapted to each vendor's scanner and are not usually interchangeable, because of the plug-in design for the coil, which is specific for each scanner. Typically, the smaller the coil, the better the image.

Use of surface coils depends on what needs to be seen. On a small dog brain scan, for example, one could use a chimney (human knee) coil because it may show a smaller field of view better than a human-sized head coil. Most superconductor magnets are designed for adult humans, and so other

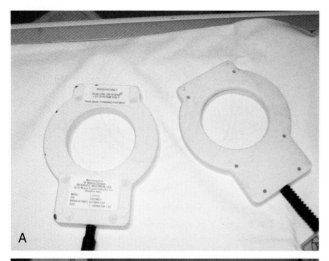

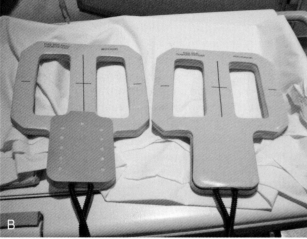

FIGURE 14-9 Surface coils are used to get better images of smaller structures in MRI. **A,** 3-inch coils. **B,** Cardiac coils. These coils demonstrate well any body part that can be contained within their dimensions.

sites, including veterinary, may have to make their own adjustments as to which coils are used. They may also have to create their own specialized coils. Coils and MRI technology are constantly advancing. Now many coils have multiple channels and settings to decrease the time of the scan and to increase the signal obtained from the body part. One rule to keep in mind with MRI is that any coil within the active scanner must be plugged in. Coils that are on the table but unplugged during a scan can be damaged or could burn a patient.

Computer

MRI scanners require computers to perform the reconstructions of the radio signals into images. The computers also enable the technologist to photograph, network, and manipulate MR images once formed. Unlike in CT, no raw data can be kept or stored with MRI. The images are acquired in their chosen field of view (like CT), matrix, slice thickness, and other factors. One cannot go back after a 5-minute MRI scan and change the resolution of the images as one can in CT.

Physics and Technique

As stated earlier, an MRI scanner uses radio waves to manipulate hydrogen atoms in and out of an excited energy state. The actual application of this technique is quite a bit more complicated, and whole books are written on the physics and progress of this technology.

The frequency used by MRI to produce images is based on a calculation called the Larmor equation. All atoms have the ability to respond to radio waves in a magnetic field. This ability is called the gyromagnetic ratio. The frequency applied in MRI is calculated by the following equation:

$$Wo = Y \times B^0$$

where Wo is the radio frequency, typically the tesla field strength; B^0 is the magnetic field, in typically Y is the ratio.

Medical MRI focuses on hydrogen, which also has the highest gyromagnetic ratio. The ratio for hydrogen is: 42.56 MHz $\cdot$ T^{-1} or MHz/T. In a typical medical MRI, the field strength is 1.5 T. Using the previous equation yields the typical frequency for medical MRI, as follows:

$$42.56 \text{ MHz/T} \times 1.5 \text{ T} = 63.8 \text{ MHz}$$

When this frequency is applied by the radio antenna in a medical 1.5-T MRI scanner, the hydrogen atoms respond (or resonate) into a higher energy level and change the direction of their magnetization in the scanner. When the radio frequency is stopped, the atoms return to their equilibrium or prior state within the magnet. Because the atoms were excited into a higher energy state, they give off energy upon return in the form of radio waves that are detected by the radio antenna. The actual change of magnetic direction of the atoms on the return gives off two types of signal. The first is called T1 decay, which is the direct magnetic movement of the center of the atom from its tipped position (90 degrees or whatever has been chosen) to its original state. The other is called T2 decay, the signal received from the spinning of the atom back into its original state. Tissues and molecules in the body have different responses with regard to T1 and T2 decay; this difference is what allows the MRI to show various tissues so well with all of the different settings.

The actual radio waves in these decayed signals are very small. During an MRI scan, the scanner applies the radio frequency in multiple pulses, which continue to "tip" the magnetic direction of the hydrogen molecules again and again. These repeated radio waves dramatically increase the radio signals received. One factor in an MRI technique is the time between the radio frequency pulses, which is referred to as TR or repetition time. A lower repetition time—699 milliseconds (ms) or less—shows the T1 decay response of the tissues. A higher repetition time—1500 ms or greater—shows the T2 decay response and changes the contrast of the images.

Another factor used in MRI is the echo time, or TE (in ms). This is the time between responses showing the maximum signal. As for TR, shorter TE times demonstrate the T1 response of tissues. Longer echo times show the T2 responses of tissues. MRI, like CT, shows images in slices. For an MRI, several slices are acquired in a single scan or sequence.

Signal Intensity and the Weighting of Images: T1 versus T2

In MRI, the various shades of gray seen in an image are referred to as signal intensities, not densities. If a part of the image is shown as bright or closer to white, it is described as having a high signal intensity. The reverse is true for anatomy seen in darker shades of gray; they are called low signal intensity. When looking at images from an MRI, people also refer to the T1 or T2 appearance of the tissues as *weighting*. The most typical comparison are tissues that have opposite weightings—water and fat.

In a true T1-weighted image (TR < 699 ms, TE < 30 ms), cerebrospinal fluid (CSF) looks black (low signal intensity) (Figure 14-10A). Fat (and skin) look bright or white (high signal intensity). In a true T2-weighted image (TR > 2000 ms, TE > 80 ms) shows CSF as bright and skin as black (Figure 14-10B).

Signal-to-Noise Ratio

Many factors beyond TR and TE can be altered in MRI. Many can affect the quality, the resolution, and the amount of time it takes to obtain images. Technologists must take all these factors into account when entering a protocol for an MRI sequence. The goal in acquiring MRI images is to have a high signal-to-noise ratio. The higher the amount of signal, the better the pictures. Individually, Table 14-1 lists the effects of altering technical factors in MRI in a classic spin-echo image (see later discussion of sequences).

In radiography, one compromises radiation dose for resolution or image noise. In MRI, the tradeoff is between time and image resolution. A technologist may, for example, want thinner slices, which will drop signal, and therefore may have to increase the number of excitations, which doubles the time of a sequence.

TABLE 14-1	Effects of Altering Technical Factors in MRI		
TECHNICAL FACTOR ALTERATION	**INCREASE OR DECREASE**	**EFFECT ON SIGNAL-TO NOISE-RATIO**	**EFFECT ON IMAGE RESOLUTION**
Field of view	Decrease	Decrease	Increase
Pixel size	Decrease	Decrease	Increase
Bandwidth	Increase	Increase	Decrease
Number of excitations or acquisitions	Increase	Increase	Increase
Slice thickness	Increase	Increase	Decrease
Image matrix size	Increase	Decrease	Increase

Specialty Sequences

In MRI, specialty sequences can be used to image various parts of the body. It is possible to image blood vessels by MRI without the use of a contrast agent. A couple of sequences are able to capture the phases of moving blood, for example. These specialty sequences are called magnetic resonance angiography (MRA) or magnetic resonance venography (MRV), and they can show the anatomy of blood vessels. These volumetric sequences enable the anatomy to be reconstructed in three-dimensional images, which are typically called MIPS (maximum intensity projections) (Figure 14-11). Also, the naming of sequences varies from vendor to vendor. Charts are now available that translate these names from machine to machine. For example, "turbo spin-echo sequence" on one scanner is the same as "fast spin-echo" on another. A three-dimensional T1-weighted volume

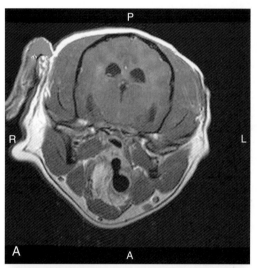

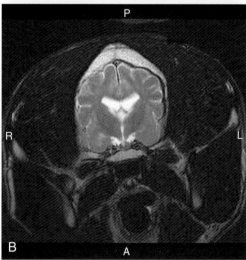

FIGURE 14-10 Coronal plane images on MR images of a dog's brain. **A,** A T1-weighted image. The cerebrospinal fluid in the ventricles is shown as black, and the skin and body fat are shown as white. **B,** A T2-weighted image. The T2 weighting can be identified from the longer TR and TE times listed as well as from the facts that the fat either is not visible or is black and the ventricles are bright with high signal intensity.

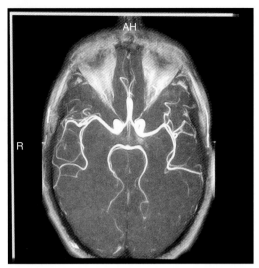

FIGURE 14-11 A noncontrast MR angiogram performed on a human patient. The vessels are visible as a function of the blood flow within them. It is reconstructed as a maximum intensity project (MIP) and viewed from inferior to superior view.

acquisition scan can be called "MPRAGE" by one vendor, "3D SPGR" by another, and a "FFE, or fast field-echo," by a third. MRI technologists must constantly learn and upgrade their knowledge about the physics and techniques of their scanning.

Another aspect of MRI that is available is the ability to suppress fat signal. This is desired in places where the fat may alter the ability to see pathology, such as the orbits and in soft tissue structures. The expression for this is *fat saturation*, for which various MRI methods can be used.

Contrast and MRI

MRI does require the usage of a contrast agent to highlight infection, tumors, or vascular disease. The contrast agent used in MRI is called gadolinium (Figure 14-12); various chemical formulas include this molecule. Gadolinium is a paramagnetic—meaning that it has partially magnetic qualities. It alters the T1 properties of tissues so that they enhance, or light up, in the picture. After contrast is injected into the patient, only T1-weighted sequences (with or without fat saturation) will show the enhancement of tissues. Because gadolinium is removed by the kidneys, it is very important that a subject's kidney function is assessed. In veterinary practice, because the patients are under general anesthesia when scanned, blood work assessing kidney function is always performed prior to the MRI. In humans, necrotizing systemic fasciitis (NSF), a very rare and irreversible complication, has occurred when gadolinium was given to patients with renal failure. In this condition, the skin and connective tissues permanently stiffen and retract, causing the patient to lose kidney function. For this reason, gadolinium is administered only to patients who have normal renal function.

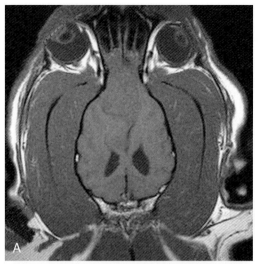

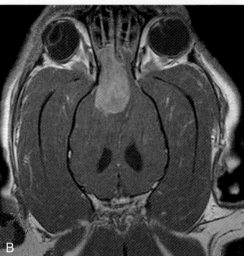

FIGURE 14-12 The change in how a tumor is seen when gadolinium contrast is administered. **A,** The T1-weighted image without contrast. **B,** The T1-weighted image with contrast. Usually tissues enhance because the contrast decreases the T1 contrast of the pathology.

Protocols

From this chapter, you have learned that there are many ways to scan a patient using MRI. Various surface coils and sequences can be used.

In a typical veterinary site, patients are accepted for MRI scans only when referred by specialists. The patient is prepared and evaluated prior to the MRI examination. These scans are not short in duration, each sequence typically lasting around 5 minutes or so and an entire scan of body parts taking 20 minutes or longer. For this reason, patients are always scanned after being anesthetized or sedated. The technologist or veterinarian chooses the most appropriately sized surface coils for the region to be covered. An MRI scan always starts with a low-quality, quick image called a *localizer*. The localizer allows the technologist to see the anatomy on MRI and to plan subsequent images. Most MRI sites have specific protocols for each body part, using multiple sequences in at least two planes.

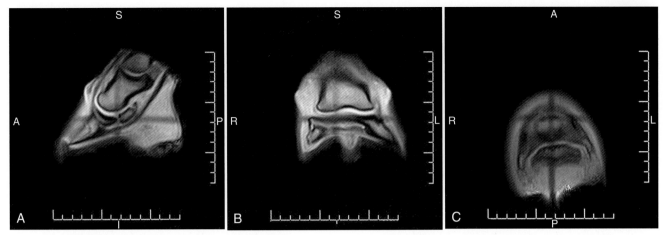

FIGURE 14-13 Quick images in coronal (**A**), sagittal (**B**), and axial (**C**) planes showing the position of the horse's leg within the scanner.

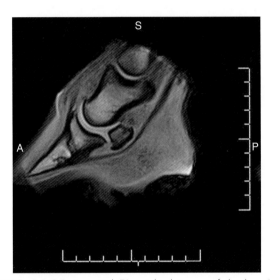

FIGURE 14-14 A sagittal T1-weighted image of the horse's left forefoot. Several images in a plane were acquired in multiple settings.

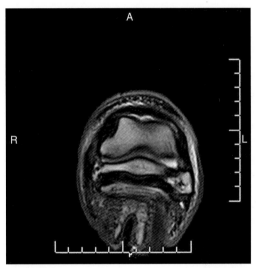

FIGURE 14-16 Axial T2-weighted image taken through the horse's forefoot. These images were acquired with the MRI unit shown in Figure 14-7.

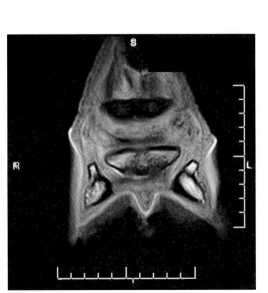

FIGURE 14-15 Coronal T1-weighted image through a horse's forefoot.

MRI has a great advantage over other modalities. It has excellent subject contrast, in that the soft tissues are better seen than even with CT. The images are also acquired in any plane or angle that the technologist may desire (Figures 14-13 through 14-16).

Further Safety Considerations

As described previously, MRI uses a high–field strength magnet to produce images, so the safety of patients and staff is of utmost importance. The most dangerous aspect of MRI is the projectile effect, whereby an object launches into a magnet. Injuries and deaths have occurred from such accidents. MRI applies radio frequencies to the entire body of the patient. Implanted devices, such as pacemakers and certain aneurysm clips, cannot go near the magnetic field, which might move them. Another risk of implanted metal is heating with possible burning of the patient. All implants must be screened for MRI safety with use of the written checklist or form given to anyone planning to enter the MRI room.

Another safety concern in MRI is the ability of the patient's body to dissipate heat from the interaction of the magnet and radio frequencies. Specific absorption rate (SAR) is a calculation made on the basis of the mass of the patient. Every written scan sequence in MRI lists the potential SAR value for the patient. This is much more significant in higher–field strength magnets (>3 T) than with the weaker ones. MRI machines are also acoustically very noisy. Many MRI scans produce noise in excess of 60 to 90 decibels (dB). Ear shielding (ear plugs or head phones) is necessary for patients and anyone staying in the MRI room during a scan.

The static MRI field is not considered a risk for pregnant personnel. However, a pregnant woman should not remain in the room while a scanner is in use.

Further policies should be made within MRI departments in planning for emergencies. For situations such as fire, magnet quench, flood, and cardiac arrest, normal screening procedures cannot apply, because it is impossible to rapidly screen everyone and every object entering the room to deal with an emergency.

SUMMARY

This chapter has given an overview on the modality of magnetic resonance imaging. MRI uses a high magnetic field strength and radio waves to create images. It should be performed only by trained individuals. For further reading, consult the bibliography of this chapter.

Nuclear Medicine

Lois Brown, RTR (Cdn/USA), ACR, MSc

*To raise new questions, new possibilities, to regard old problems
from a new angle, requires creative imagination and marks real
advance in science.*

—Albert Einstein, German-born theoretical physicist, 1879–1955

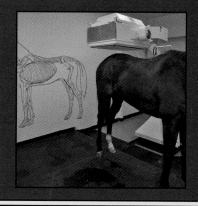

LEARNING OBJECTIVES

When you have finished this chapter, you will be able to:

1. Understand the science of nuclear scintigraphy.
2. Know the etiology that indicates scintigraphy.
3. Define the term isotope and its use in nuclear scintigraphy.
4. Know the protocol for equine studies.
5. List the use of other isotopes for small animal studies.
6. Understand radiation protection in nuclear medicine.

APPLICATIONS

The application of the information in this chapter is relevant to the following areas:

1. Diagnosis of skeletal trauma and pathology using an auxiliary diagnostic approach.

In the first section of this book, we spoke of the atom, the elements, and isotopes. A quick review is in order here because it is these isotopes that are used extensively in nuclear scintigraphy (Figure 15-1).

The Atom and Radioactivity

Each atom consists of three basic components: the electrons, which we manipulate in radiography, and protons and neutrons, which are contained in the nucleus. It is the neutrons which we will discuss now.

A stable atom such as helium, the second atom in the periodic table, has two protons, two neutrons, and two electrons. The protons determine the characteristic of the element. If the number of neutrons differs in a substance, it is an isotope of the element. Barium, a contrast medium with which we will are familiar, has seven naturally occurring isotopes.

> *POINTS TO PONDER* Atoms that have the same atomic number but different atomic mass numbers are isotopes. Isotopes can occur naturally but also may be artificially produced in a laboratory.

Radioactivity describes atoms that are in an abnormally excited state characterized by an unstable nucleus. To reach stability these atoms spontaneously emit particles and energy to transform themselves into other atoms. This process is called radioactive disintegration or radioactive decay. The method of determining the activity of a radioisotope involves establishing how long it takes for the isotope to decay to half of its original radioactivity. This is called its half-life. The atoms involved in this process are called radionuclides. An atom with any rearrangement of the nucleus is called a nuclide; therefore, the atoms with nuclei that undergo radioactive decay are radionuclides.

In the 1940s and 1950s, a scientific branch of imaging was developed to examine radionuclides with respect to medical diagnosis. It was already known that infection produces heat, tumors attract cellular activity, and trauma causes an increase in blood supply around the wounded area. It was speculated that if a radioactive source was introduced within the patient either by swallowing or by injection, that source would gravitate to the area supplied by the most blood or with the highest cellular activity. The radiation emitted as the radionuclide decayed could then be imaged on a detection device that was connected to a camera. The substance ingested or injected must be nontoxic, other than the amount of radiation introduced, and it had to be capable of being excreted through the urine or via the bowels.

One other criterion that was very important to this study was the half-life of the radionuclide. The half-life is described as the length of time necessary to reduce the intensity of the radiation emitted by half. In medicine it is important that a radionuclide administered to a person or animal must decay within a relatively short period so that the patient is not a radiation hazard to itself or to people working in the area.

The Isotopes and Designations

The most common radionuclides used in veterinary medicine today are iodine I 131 and technetium Tc 99m. Iodine I 131 is mainly used to treat hyperthyroidism in felines and is not used for imaging. Technetium Tc 99m is used for nuclear scintigraphy, particularly in equine studies.

The quantity identifier for the radiation emitted by the isotopes is the curie (Ci), named after Marie and Pierre Curie, a husband and wife team who did very early research into radiation.

The amount of radioisotope used for each examination is measured in millicuries (mCi).

The hospital or clinic that uses radioisotopes must be registered with the local Atomic Energy Board. In Canada, it is the Canadian Nuclear Safety Commission (nuclearsafety.gc.ca). In the United States, It is the U.S. Nuclear Regulatory Commission (www.nrc.gov). Internationally, it is the International Atomic Energy Agency (www.iaea.org) that provides information regarding the regulations for various countries.

The Science of Nuclear Medicine

Nuclear scintigraphy is the science of diagnosis by means of radioisotopes. The patient is injected with a radionuclide, and the nuclear medicine camera detects the emission of the radioactivity from the patient.

Nuclear medicine is a very effective way to localize pathology or the results of trauma because the radioisotope is carried to the area with the most active blood supply. Certain isotopes are more readily attracted to certain types of tissue. Technetium Tc 99m is attracted to bone. Iodine I 131 is attracted to the thyroid gland.

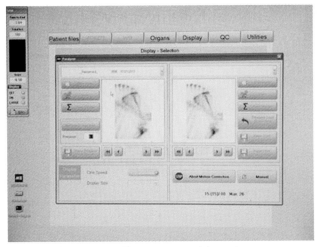

FIGURE 15-1 The progression of the nuclear scan.

In nuclear medicine, the patient is the emitter and the detector is the camera. This imaging is just the opposite of radiography, in which the x-ray tube is the emitter and the detector is the image receptor. Nuclear medicine demonstrates function of a tissue or an organ whereas radiography demonstrates the form of the anatomy.

Indications for Imaging with Nuclear Medicine

A subtle, severe, or multifocal lameness in horses may be very difficult to diagnose (Figure 15-2). When radiography does not demonstrate the abnormality, a very effective option is a nuclear scan. Bone scans can also be used to monitor the healing process of fractures. They are also significant tools in a prepurchase examination of a horse.

In the equine patient, some of the areas of concern are quite large and difficult to image via the traditional methods of imaging—computerized tomography (CT), magnetic resonance imaging (MRI), and radiography. Nuclear medicine scanning can rule out abnormalities in these areas or identify pathology or the evidence of trauma (see Figure 15-2). The animal does not have to be anesthetized to undergo the study.

Procedure

The horse is injected with 160 to 180 mCi technetium 99m, which has an affinity for localization in bone. After a certain period of time, the horse is brought to the camera, which is very large and has a room of its own (Figure 15-3). The horse's body is brought within the field of range of the camera, which detects the emission of radiation known as gamma photon bursts from the horse and records the activity on a computer. The camera is moved around by a gantry system.

An area of osteoblastic activity indicates accelerated metabolism within the bones, which will result in an indication of higher radiation emitted. It is termed a "hot spot."

Phases of a Bone Scan

The vascular phase is not commonly used in horses unless a thrombosis is suspected. In this phase, the camera is positioned over the horse while the isotope is being injected. The course of the isotope can then be traced as it moves through the circulatory system. The radionuclide is spread fairly thin at this phase.

The soft tissue phase (Figure 15-4) occurs approximately 5 to 10 minutes after injection. It detects the pooling of the nuclide and demonstrates tendons and ligaments in the equine lower limb.

The bone phase is the final phase as the nuclide is distributed throughout the bone (Figure 15-5). This phase is usually

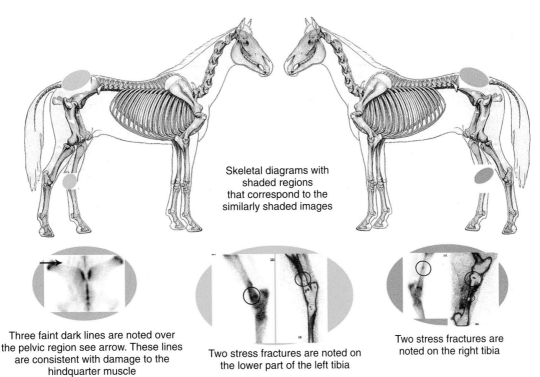

Skeletal diagrams with shaded regions that correspond to the similarly shaded images

Three faint dark lines are noted over the pelvic region see arrow. These lines are consistent with damage to the hindquarter muscle

Two stress fractures are noted on the lower part of the left tibia

Two stress fractures are noted on the right tibia

FIGURE 15-2 A case of multifocal lameness. This young horse had a history of being "off" in the hind end. Nuclear medicine studies revealed four stress fractures (2 right and 2 left hind) and muscle damage over the hindquarters (*arrow*).

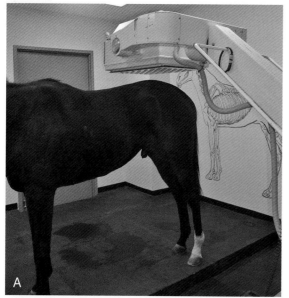

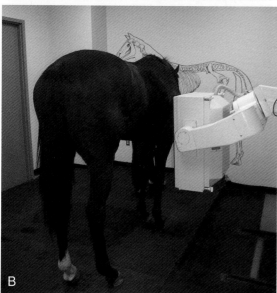

FIGURE 15-3 A and B, A horse stands quietly while the gantry is moved into various positions.

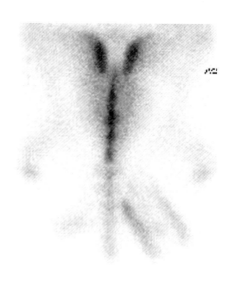

FIGURE 15-4 Exertional rhabdomyolysis. An example of post-traumatic demonstrated in the soft tissue phase.

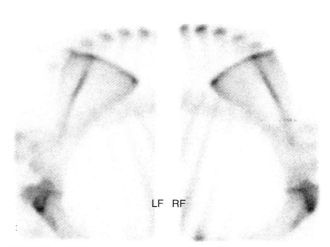

LF RF

FIGURE 15-5 Normal scans of the right and left scapulae. The bone phase of the scan reveals a normal set of scapulae in this case.

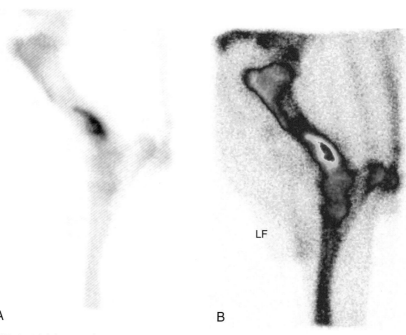

A

LF

B

FIGURE 15-6 A left humerus fracture (A) becomes more evident when color represents the location of the injury (B).

performed 2 to 3 hours after the injection to ensure that the maximum amount of nuclide has gathered at the point of interest.

For the safety of the handlers regarding radiation exposure, the horse is then hospitalized for 48 hours in order for the isotope to decay. The half-life of technetium Tc99m is about 6 hours, and it must go through several half-lives before the animal can be safely handled.

The Images

Because the images are demonstrating function and not anatomy, they are plotted out on the computer as a series of dots. These dots indicate radioactive bursts emitted from the horse. The structure of the anatomy is visualized so that the area of interest is easily identified. Newer cameras count the radiation bursts and display the results in color. The color red indicates high activity, and blue indicates low activity (Figure 15-6).

The following sections demonstrate normal and abnormal bone activity in horses and are identified as such. Please visit the Evolve website associated with this text to see more images.

Diagnosis

The veterinarian reading the scan compares the images from the left and right sides of the horse in order to make a diagnosis. Some areas of high activity are normal for certain breeds. Certain areas in young horses (the epiphyseal growth plates) should be highly active, and this is one reason why comparisons are essential. If one growth plate is not as active as the other, this finding could be a cause for concern (Figures 15-7 and 15-8).

Radiation Protection

Nuclear medicine studies take place only in an approved site where radiation safety is assured (Figure 15-9). The patient is the radiation emitter, and the half-life of the radioisotope must be taken into consideration when patient care and length of stay are issues. The half-life of technetium Tc 99m is 6 hours, but that means that the patient is emitting half of the original strength of the isotope. The typical equine protocol is to retain the horse at the hospital or clinic for a minimum of 24 hours and more typically for 48 hours.

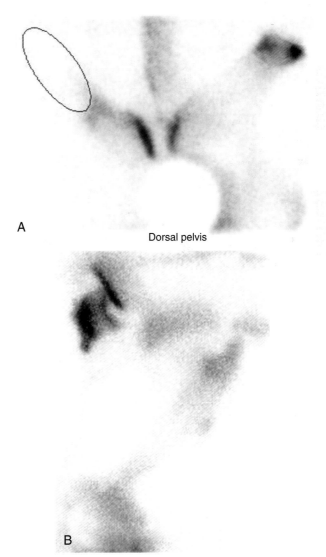

A

Dorsal pelvis

B

FIGURE 15-8 A particularly serious fracture of the pelvis. This horse was discovered in the stall in the morning refusing to bear weight on the left hind leg. **A,** The *oval* area indicates the portion of the pelvis that is missing. **B,** The lateral view shows a tuber coxae fracture with displacement.

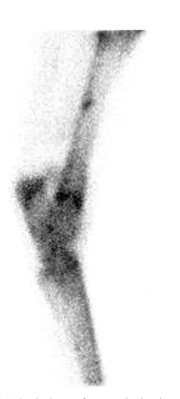

FIGURE 15-7 Right tibial stress fracture. The heightened activity in this scan demonstrates a fracture, whereas absence of activity could signify tissue necrosis.

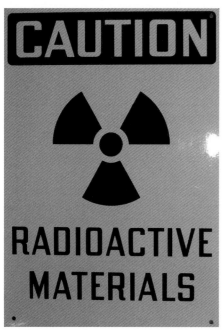

FIGURE 15-9 A legal door sign indicating the presence of radioactive sources. In some countries the sign would read "Danger–RadioHazard Materials."

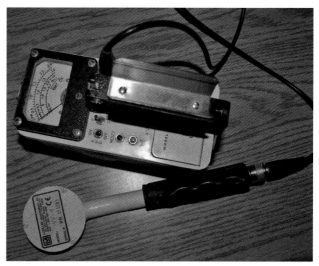

FIGURE 15-11 A Geiger counter is set to measure in kilocounts/minute (Kc/min).

When the radioisotope has been injected into the horse, its body, as well as its waste products, are radioactive. The waste products must be retained in a lead-lined container in a designated area for 48 hours. The staff handling the horses must wear lab coats, latex gloves, disposable boots, and dosimeters because of the risk of effluent contamination. The scan room and the camera should be scanned with a survey meter (Figure 15-10) prior to each examination to ensure that there is no contamination between examinations. The room is scanned at the start of the examination with a Geiger counter to establish a baseline. Fluorescent lights and concrete may emit a certain amount of radiation, which will be included in the count of a sensitive gamma camera (Figure 15-11).

SUMMARY

From the very early days of searching for a method to evaluate areas of heightened activity within the anatomy of their patients, scientists now not only can search the form of the pathology but also can evaluate the function. This ability is particularly valuable in equine studies, in which often the structures are so large that routine radiographs do not demonstrate the extent and inaccessible trauma and pathology.

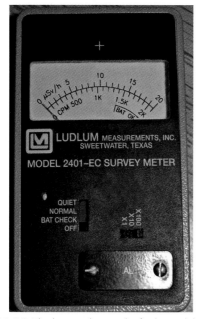

FIGURE 15-10 The horse is kept at the facility until the dose count on this dosimeter is below 4 microsieverts/hour. Usually the count is less than 1 after 48 hours.

CHAPTER

16

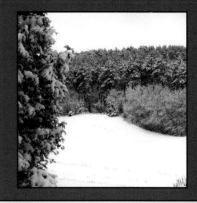

Radiation Protection: How X-rays Affect Cells

Research is to see what everybody else has seen, and to think what nobody else has thought.

—Albert Szent-Gyorgyi, Hungarian Scientist, 1893–1986

OUTLINE

KEY TERMS

Distance
DNA molecules
Fluoroscopy
Gonadal shields
Half-life
International Commission on Radiological Protection (ICRP)
Linear energy transfer
Mitosis
National Council on Radiation Protection and Measurements (NCRP)
Non–radiation worker
Organogenesis
Radiation dosimeter
Radiation worker
Radioactive decay
Radioactive disintegration
Radiography
Radionuclides
Secondary radiation
Shielding
Stochastic effects
Time

LEARNING OBJECTIVES

When you have finished this chapter, you will be able to:

1. Understand radiation risks.
2. Describe radiation and DNA.
3. Discuss radiation exposure and radioactivity.
4. Describe radiation protective apparel.
5. Know the laws and regulations regarding radiation protection.

APPLICATIONS

The application of the information in this chapter is relevant to the following areas:

1. Protecting the hospital or clinic staff from scattered and primary radiation.
2. Protecting the patients and their owners from radiation dose.

This chapter discusses the various methods of radiation protection and the means by which veterinary healthcare workers can ensure they are protected from excess amounts of radiation. Within the veterinary facility, the workers are educated regarding radiation protection. It is the law in most countries that, during the initial interview for any prospective employee, the employer must discuss the fact that the clinic uses radiation in the diagnosis of patients.

Radiation doses to workers within the veterinary facility must be reduced to a level as low as reasonably achievable (ALARA). This is a universal principle. It is very easy to become lax in the strict standards set out in the law because radiation in the radiography room is invisible. Protecting the staff and the patients from excess amounts of radiation over the course of a career is vital.

Wilhelm Roentgen first discovered the unknown, invisible ray, which he called the "X" ray, in 1896. He was doing experiments on the newly discovered cathode tube ray. Roentgen was a careful scientist, and because of his caution, he was one of the few pioneers in this new field of research who did not die from radiation-induced carcinoma. The safeguards that Roentgen used in his research are still in use today, and it is these methods that we examine.

Radiobiology

The human body is roughly 80% water. It is this radiation interaction that primarily affects the human body. When a radiation disaster strikes at a nuclear plant anywhere in the world today, the many precautions that have been put into effect since the radiation disasters known as Hiroshima, Nagasaki, and Chernobyl are very effective in preventing radiation illness and death.

In diagnostic imaging, the amounts of radiation are potentially damaging. However, at the levels of use and the amounts that are produced even in a typically busy hospital, the doses are very low. The effects of such amounts of radiation are stochastic in nature because they are delivered intermittently over long careers.

Because the human body is primarily a liquid, the radiation targets the DNA within the body. This is the most vulnerable area. The cell is particularly vulnerable during cell division. Radiation is nonselective. It affects the area of the cell upon which it arrives. DNA molecules and particularly the nucleus of the DNA may be affected by the disintegration

of the side rails of the double helix. Three things may occur when the DNA is affected by radiation:

1. The cell may display no immediate effects but damage may have occurred internally that will affect the individual later, when mitosis (cell division) occurs.
2. Cell damage may be obvious, with portions of the DNA compromised.
3. Cell death may occur from the "hit," severely damaging the molecule.

Diagnostic radiation workers (see later definition) are not as concerned about the massive cell damage that occurs with radiation therapy doses and nuclear disasters.

The main concern in diagnostic imaging is latent effects. To produce these latent effects, the radiation dose over time must be substantial. There are at present no recorded cases of death after diagnostic x-ray exposure. Early radiation workers did develop malignancies after radiation exposure before implementation of the safety precautions that are in effect today.

The principal effects experienced by radiation personnel consist of radiation-induced malignancy and genetic effects. Most late effects are called stochastic effects.

Radiation Exposure

Some photons travel so quickly that they still have enough energy after penetrating the patient to be absorbed by the atoms they encounter and then produce radiation from the atoms within the anatomy of the patient. If their energy is great enough, they activate the atoms within the patient to produce photons, which are then emitted from the patient. This effect is called secondary and/or scattered radiation.

It is the secondary radiation and scattered radiation that is uncontrolled and can affect the attendant healthcare worker.

Radioactivity

Certain atoms exist in an abnormally excited state characterized by an unstable nucleus. The nucleus is typically unstable as a result of an imbalance of neutrons and protons with reference to the number of electrons encircling the atom. To reach stability, the nucleus of the atom spontaneously emits particles and energy (decays), and transforms itself into another atom with a stable and proper ratio.

This process is called radioactive disintegration or radioactive decay. The atoms that emit particles and energy in order to become stable are called radionuclides. The radionuclides may be in the forms of solids, liquids, or gases. Radioisotopes are administered to patients by injection, inhalation, or oral consumption (See Chapter 15 Nuclear Medicine).

Isotopes are variants of atoms of a particular chemical element that have differing numbers of neutrons. If the isotope is radioactive it is called a *radioisotope*. Radioisotopes may be produced artificially in machines such as particle accelerators and nuclear reactors. For example, seven radioisotopes of the element barium have been artificially produced within nuclear reactors.

Radioisotopes were also produced naturally during the formation of the earth, and because they are very slow to decay, they are still emitting radiation today. An example is uranium, which ultimately decays to radium, which in turn decays to radon. Other isotopes, such as Carbon (C14), are produced continuously in the upper atmosphere by the action of cosmic radiation.

Each radioisotope has its own pattern of decay. The energies of particles or waves emitted have unique characteristics that can be associated with that specific radionuclide. The decay rate of a radionuclide is called its half-life. A half-life is the amount of time it takes for half of the radioactive atoms to disintegrate or decay into a stable form.

Intensity of Radiation

All types of radiation have the ability to penetrate tissue and transfer energy. This ability is called linear energy transfer (LET); the term is used to describe the amount of energy imparted to the target. In radiography, LET is a measure of the rate at which energy is transferred from ionizing radiation into soft tissue.

The higher the value of the LET, the greater the amount of energy being transferred to soft tissue per interaction. If large amounts of energy are transferred rapidly, the ability of the particle to penetrate is reduced because the energy decreases rapidly. However, this also means that the risk of potential damage to the target material is increased because the energy is absorbed into the tissue.

Alpha and beta particles have high LET with low penetrability. These are commonly the secondary and scattered radiations from which the healthcare worker requires protection. X-rays and gamma rays have low LET with higher penetrability. This means that their ability to travel through matter is high, producing less immediate effects on the tissue through which they pass. X-rays and gamma rays are produced in the radiography department.

The patient's body absorbs the photons of radiation according to the density of the tissue exposed to the x-ray beam. Bone is much denser than soft tissue or fat. Bone efficiently absorbs the radiation reaching it and therefore prevents the image receptor from being exposed. This explains why bony areas are white on the image; fat or air, which is radiolucent, allows the radiation to penetrate through it to the image receptor and shows up as black or dark areas on the image receptor.

Learning how to optimize the images by varying the settings on the machine is discussed in Chapter 6. It is important to note that the higher the kilovoltage (kV), the higher the scattered and secondary radiation and, thus, the potential risk to the x-ray worker. When a technique chart is developed, the kilovoltage should be optimized to penetrate the body part and the milliamperes-seconds (mAs) value should be set to provide the correct density on the film.

Methods of Protection

Once Roentgen had discovered the potential of the "X-ray," its value to medicine was immediately recognized. Very shortly thereafter, the detrimental effects of radiation were also identified.

The science of health physics develops protocols to protect healthcare workers, x-ray radiation workers, patients, and the general public. The three cardinal rules for radiation protection are time, distance, and shielding. Reducing the time of exposure, increasing the distance between the source of the radiation and the subject, and placing a shield or barrier between the subject and the source are the three primary methods for reducing exposure. This chapter examines each of these methods.

Protection from radiation is important for any individual. Particular attention should be paid to an individual male or female who has the ability to reproduce. This group includes all males of any age and all females prior to menopause.

One consideration that must be emphasized is that of the protection of the pregnant healthcare worker. Research indicates that the severity of the response of the fetus to radiation is related to both dose and time. The time from the 2nd to the 10th week of pregnancy is the most critical, as that is the period of major organogenesis. Because it is quite possible that a female may not yet be aware that she is pregnant, protection of any female of childbearing years is essential.

Time

RULE: *Exposure = Exposure Rate × Exposure time*

Meters to measure the rate of exposure are called *dosimeters*. They measure radiation dose. The radiation dose measured over time results in a given amount of exposure.

When a radiograph is produced, the technician lowers the exposure time to a minimal amount in order to reduce potential motion on the resulting image. This is much the same as when a photographer exposes a film; the faster the exposure time, the sharper, or clearer, the image because of reduced motion.

In order to ensure that the image has the correct density, the technologist must compensate for this reduced time by ensuring that all the other parameters that contribute to the image are optimized.

During fluoroscopy (real-time imaging), the veterinarian is trained to pulse the exposure rather than leaving the exposure on continuously. Doing so limits the time of the exposure and thus the dose to the patient as well as to any staff member who must restrain the patient.

A 5-minute reset timer notifies the veterinarian exactly how much exposure time has elapsed during each procedure. Many facilities note the time elapsed for each procedure on the patient's chart, so that if a question arises regarding the examination, the dose calculation may be completed easily.

Distance

In order to be specific regarding the intensity of radiation (Figure 16-1) at a particular point (distance) away from the source, one must know the following three things:

- The intensity of the radiation at its source (focal point)
- The distance of the object from the source (D2)
- The calculated distance (D1) (or the distance at which the intensity is to be calculated)

For example, if I sit one foot away from a lamp the intensity of the light reaching me is X. If I move to 2 feet from the source (2X), the intensity of the light reaching me is now decreased to one fourth ($\frac{1}{4}$) of its original value.

Shielding

RULE: *Positioning a shield or barrier between the healthcare worker and the radiation source greatly reduces the level of radiation exposure.*

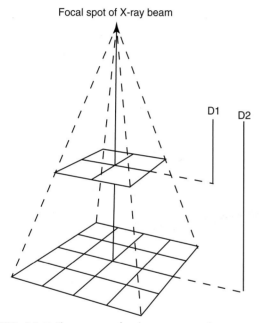

Focal spot of X-ray beam

D1   D2

FIGURE 16-1 The intensity of radiation is inversely proportional to the square of the distance (D1 and D2) of the object from the source.

Ideally the operator exposes the image while standing behind a shield or barrier. In some cases doing so is not possible because the veterinary patient must be restrained and is not anesthetized.

Shielding material is usually defined with reference to the thickness of lead. Other construction materials may be used, but they are commonly calculated according to their comparison with lead. For example, at 100 kV of energy, 2.20 centimeters of concrete is equal to 0.79 mm of lead. Large sheets of lead may be purchased for construction. The minimum thickness is usually 0.79 mm.

Calculations for the shielding of x-ray rooms are beyond the scope of this text. Legally in every country, the barriers (walls, ceiling, floor, and doorways) must be designated radiation barriers. The maximum amount of radiation that may affect these barriers over the course of time must be calculated to ensure that the appropriate protection is installed prior to the first exposure of the imaging equipment. The necessary calculations may be carried out only by radiation-trained personnel or a medical radiation physicist. The calculations for each barrier must be submitted to the appropriate legal authority and approved by that authority (Figure 16-2).

If the equipment in the room is changed by either upgrading or downgrading, a new set of plans must be submitted. If the adjoining areas of the facility are changed, a new set of calculations must be submitted. Any room containing an x-ray generator must be designated with the appropriate legal signage (Figure 16-3).

Radiation-Protective Devices

Shielding material, when used to protect the patient, is usually in the form of leaded aprons and/or gonadal shields (Figure 16-4). The leaded aprons are typically measured as to their effectiveness at 125 kV of radiation. Leaded gloves and thyroid protectors must be worn by the healthcare workers who are present in the room during the examination. Leaded glass goggles are also available to protect the lenses of the eyes. Movable leaded barriers are available as

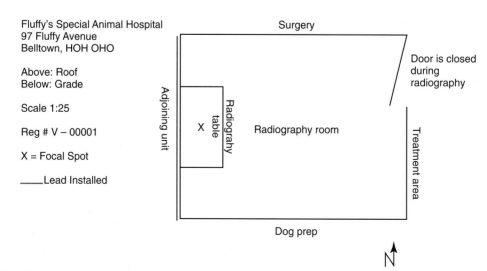

Fluffy's Special Animal Hospital
97 Fluffy Avenue
Belltown, HOH OHO

Above: Roof
Below: Grade

Scale 1:25

Reg # V – 00001

X = Focal Spot

_____ Lead Installed

Surgery

Door is closed during radiography

Adjoining unit

Radiograhy table

X

Radiography room

Treatment area

Dog prep

N

FIGURE 16-2 A sample floor plan designating the barriers of the radiography room and the installation of lead.

CAUTION X-RAYS

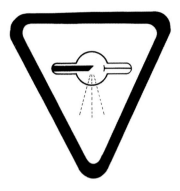

ATTENTION RAYONS X

FIGURE 16-3 This is an example of a legal door sign warning of the potential of radiation in the room behind it. The image denotes an early x-ray tube.

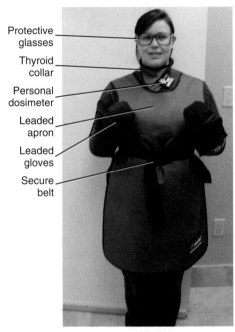

Protective glasses
Thyroid collar
Personal dosimeter
Leaded apron
Leaded gloves
Secure belt

FIGURE 16-4 Radiation-protective wear. The apron is secured across the shoulders with a hook-and-loop (Velcro) band so that it will remain in place while the technician is positioning a patient.

added protection in imaging rooms where the workers are exposed to a higher amount of radiation than their colleagues.

Use and Care

The lead used in aprons, gonadal and breast shields is usually manufactured in thin sheets that are then layered together to achieve the correct amount of radiation protection. The sheets of lead are very thin and must be handled with respect in order to last effectively for many years. The following guidelines help achieve that goal:

- Aprons should be hung up by the shoulders when not in use.
- Aprons should not be folded or creased under any circumstances.
- Aprons should be cleaned regularly with warm water and a mild soap.

The leaded apron should fit correctly. It should have a method to secure it on the wearer's shoulders so that it does not fall off the shoulder during use. Simply adding a strap with a piece of hook-and-loop (Velcro) to the shoulder units of the apron will ensure that it stays in place when the healthcare worker bends forward. If the apron is worn during fluoroscopy, it should wrap around the technologist's back. In this way, protection is ensured while the technologist is in the room during continuous radiation.

Thyroid collars should always be worn in conjunction with the leaded apron. They should be treated with the same care as the leaded aprons.

If a patient must be supported during an imaging procedure, the x-ray worker should stay as far away from the source of the radiation as possible. Whenever possible, a non–radiation worker (see later definition) should be asked to help the patient. Participation of non–radiation workers should be rotated throughout the shift so that no one is continuously exposed to radiation.

POINTS TO PONDER The following is an example of a specification under the Radiation Safety Act in Canada. It is similar to the NCRP and ICRP regulations for the rest of the world
SPECIFICATIONS REGARDING PROTECTIVE DEVICES— OCCUPATIONAL HEALTH AND SAFETY ACT
REGULATION 861/90, SECTION 16, PARAGRAPHS 1–8
Radiographic and Fluoroscopic leaded aprons must provide attenuation equivalent to at least 0.5 mm of lead at 150 kV. The lead equivalency must be permanently marked on the apron.
NOTE: Most leaded aprons are rated at 125 kV. To meet this standard, an extra layer of lead needs to be added to the basic apron.

6.3.1: Radiographic and fluoroscopic leaded aprons must provide attenuation equivalent to at least 0.5 mm of lead at 150 kV. The lead equivalency must be permanently marked on the apron.

6.3.2: Gonadal shields must have a lead equivalent thickness of 0.25 mm and should have a lead equivalency of 0.50 mm at 150 kV. Contact type gonad shields must be of sufficient size and shape to exclude the gonads completely from primary beam radiation.

6.3.3: Protective gloves must provide attenuation equivalent to at least 0.25 mm of lead at 150 kV. This protection must be provided throughout the glove, including the fingers and the wrist.

POINTS TO PONDER There are many different shapes and designs of protective mitt or glove. The important factor is to ensure that the hands and fingers are covered during the radiation exposure.

Further Methods to Reduce Radiation Exposure to the Healthcare Worker

Equipment to restrain and/or immobilize the patient during any imaging procedure should be available in each imaging suite. Such equipment includes radiolucent foam blocks (Figure 16-5), cloth restraints, and tie-downs. The patient should not be held in place by any person unless the person is fully clothed in protective apparel and is shielded from the direct beam by accurate collimation.

Radiation Monitoring Equipment and Dose Limits

Healthcare workers who are regularly required to work within imaging departments or who may be exposed to radiation during the course of their work are required to wear a personal radiation dosimeter (Figure 16-6).

Types of Dosimeters

Several companies supply personal dosimeters. Typically, they all work on the same principle. They are called *thermoluminescent dosimeters*. They register a charge over time if they are exposed to radiation. The important feature of these dosimeters is that they maintain that charge for the duration of time required by the facility.

The radiation protection officer or his or her designate replaces the dosimeters at specific time intervals in order that they may be read.

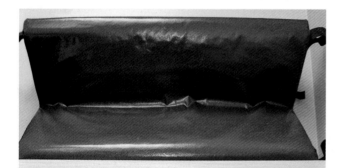

FIGURE 16-5 Foam block used to assist in positioning patients.

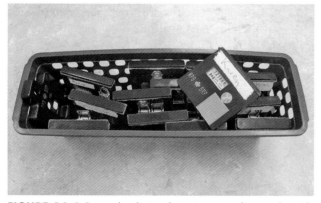

FIGURE 16-6 Personal radiation dosimeters are to be stored outside the radiography room.

Other dosimeters may be used in certain departments to measure personnel exposure for a specific period or a specified use.

The rules of use (see next section) apply to all dosimeters.

Use of Dosimeters

When a healthcare worker is issued a dosimeter, his or her personal information is required by the facility to which the service is registered. This process enables the dosimetry service to combine reports from other employers in order to calculate total exposure for an annual reading. If the worker is employed at more than one site, he or she must wear a different dosimeter at each site. In this way incidents can be tracked to a specific site.

The dosimeter:
- must not be taken home.
- must be stored in a location where it is not likely to be exposed to radiation.
- must not be stored where it will be exposed to heat and/or sunlight.
- must be worn only at the site to which it is registered.
- should be worn attached to the thyroid collar outside the apron by a worker who regularly restrains patients.
- must never be shared with another worker.
- must not be worn on a jacket or lab coat, which might then be removed and hung in a radiation area.

If the dosimeter is to be worn during fluoroscopic examinations, a second dosimeter should be worn attached to the thyroid collar outside the apron. These dosimeters must be clearly marked and must never be exchanged.

Visitors and new staff must be provided with personal dosimeters, and service personnel working on x-ray equipment should also wear personal dosimeters.

Each facility is responsible for posting the results of the dosimetry readings as they are received. Reports should be kept as a medical record according to the protocol of the facility.

Recommended Dose Limits for Radiation Workers and Non–Radiation—OHSA Section 10, and the Schedule (R16–18)

Specified dose limits apply to both non–radiation workers and radiation workers. There is no dose discrimination between men and women of reproductive capacity. Once pregnancy has been confirmed, the woman's fetus should be protected from x-ray exposure of all types.

X-ray radiation worker dose limits specifically apply only to irradiation resulting directly from their occupation and do not include radiation from medical diagnosis and background radiation. Dose limits for non–radiation workers are considerably higher than those for radiation workers, because radiation workers wear protective garments over the most sensitive areas of their anatomy.

The International Commission on Radiological Protection (ICRP) specifies the allowable doses and should be consulted for further information (www.icrp.org).

Legislation Regarding Radiation Doses to the Healthcare Worker

DISCLAIMER: *This section refers specifically to the protection of the healthcare worker regarding radiation safety. It is the responsibility of the radiation worker to read the entire act in terms of context prior to making a claim against any employer or section of this text. Each country provides legal direction specific to radiation workers within their borders. It is the responsibility of the individual worker to be familiar with these legal directions*

The radiation worker is defined as an individual who "could be exposed to radiation from man-made sources during their work." The non–radiation worker includes the rest of the population.

The doses allowed for the radiation worker assume that the individual has been supplied with and is wearing protective devices on the parts of his/her body that would be susceptible to radiation damage (e.g., leaded aprons, thyroid collar).

The Occupational Health and Safety Acts (Canada/Usa and International)

The Occupational Health and Safety Acts specify that it is the employer's responsibility to ensure that the healthcare worker is protected against any excessive radiation exposure. There are several sections that refer specifically to the radiation protection of the healthcare worker.

In these sections the numbers refer specifically to the Canadian Act but similar references can be found in the NCRP and ICRP documents.

The "director" referred to in the Act refers to the director of the Occupational Health and Safety Branch of the regulatory body of the country.

Section 8 (11)

A health and safety representative has the power to review any and all testing procedures which in any way affect the occupational, biological, chemical, or physical health and safety of any worker.

The employer must provide information regarding any potential or existing hazards to any worker.

Section 9 (18)

A health and safety committee has the power to identify hazardous situations in the workplace and make recommendations to establish monitoring programs, which will improve the present status of safety to the workers.

The committee will designate a member representing workers who shall monitor the testing procedures to ensure the safety of the workers.

Section 25 (1)

An employer shall ensure that equipment, materials, and protective devices are provided, in good condition, to the workers and that they are used as proscribed.

An employer must appoint a competent safety officer who will supervise the handling, storage, use and disposal of any article, device, equipment, or a biological, chemical, or physical agent. The safety officer will prepare and post a written health and safety report post it in a conspicuous location and review and maintain it annually.

Section 26

(1) An employer shall keep and maintain records of all handling, storage, and use of any hazardous biological, physical, and chemical agent. The local legal authority, must be notified if any of these agents are introduced into a facility and all records must be posted conspicuously.

(2) Standard limiting of exposure of a worker to these agents must be observed and a medical surveillance program must be established and maintained. Medical examinations and training programs must be available for workers as may be prescribed.

(3) If a worker must undergo a prescribed medical test relating to this act the employer must pay the regular or premium salary, the costs of the medical examination, and a reasonable travel cost respecting the prescribed tests.

Section 27

(1) A supervisor shall ensure that a worker is instructed in the use of the protective devices and that he/she uses or wears these devices appropriately.

(2) The supervisor must advise the worker of any potential of actual danger of which he/she may be aware and take every precaution to protect the workers under his advisement including providing written instructions regarding any unusual circumstance concerning dangers in the workplace.

Section 28

(1) The worker shall observe all the provisions of the Health and Safety Act of the country in which he/she is employed. Report to the supervisor any defect in any of the measures provided to ensure the safety of the workers.

(2) No worker shall remove any protective device required by the regulations or by his/her employer without providing adequate temporary protection. No worker shall engage in any act which would render the protective devices installed to be ineffective or nonexistent.

Section 31

(1) Every person who supplies any equipment shall ensure that the equipment is in good condition and complies with the safety measures outlined in this Act.

Section 33

(1) Where a biological, chemical, or physical agent is used in a workplace the local legal authority must be notified and shall decree whether the use is prohibited, limited, or subject to the safety conditions outlined in his/her directive.

Section 41

(1) A distributor must provide clear written instructions as to the use of any hazardous physical agent that he/she manufactures or designs to be used in the workplace.

(2) Where an employer has a thing described in subsection (1) in the workplace, the employer must ensure that the workers are aware of any potential hazard and that they are thoroughly instructed as to the proper use and maintenance of the thing.

(3) The employer must post prominent notices identifying and warning of the hazardous physical properties of the thing in the place in which the thing is to be used or operated.

(4) Notices must be written in English and whatever appropriate languages are prescribed.

Section 42 (1–4)

The employer must insure that any worker operating any hazardous or potentially hazardous equipment receives proper training and that the training is reviewed by a health and safety committee representative for the workplace. This training shall be reviewed and upgraded annually if appropriate.

The annual review may be more frequent if the workplace health and safety committee deems it to be necessary and if there is a change in the workplace circumstances that may affect the health and safety of the worker.

Regulation Respecting X-ray Safety (Reg 861/90)

This is a regulation written under the Canadian Occupational Health and Safety Act that refers specifically to the safety of the x-ray worker and the general public that may be affected by ionizing radiation.

Section 4

Except as permitted by The Healing Arts Radiation Protection Act, an X-ray source shall not be operated for the irradiation of a worker.

Section 9

(1) All employers of x-ray workers shall, at the time of employment:

[a] Inform the worker of their employment as an x-ray worker

[b] Inform the worker of the dose limits (these are specific to each jurisdiction and should be posted)

[c] Inform any female worker of the dose limits to pregnant x-ray workers if appropriate

(2) All employers shall maintain a list of all x-ray workers within their employ.

Section 10

(1) All dose equivalents received or that may be received by any worker shall be As Low As Reasonably Achievable (ALARA) and in any case:

[a] An x-ray worker shall not receive a dose in excess of the allowable annual limits.

[b] Any worker who is not an x-ray worker shall not receive a dose in excess of the allowable annual limits.

Section 12

(1) An employer shall provide each X-ray worker an accurate suitable personal dosimeter.

(2) The worker shall use the personal dosimeter as instructed by the employer.

(3) The employer must ensure that the personal dosimeter is read regularly and that the results are communicated to the worker.

(4) The employer shall review the doses to the workers and verify that no worker exceeds the doses outlined in Subsection 3. A health and safety inspector must be notified if the workers' dose exceeds the legal limit.

(5) The records of the worker's doses must be maintained for a period of three years.

Section 13

If a worker exceeds the allowable dose the employer shall investigate the cause and shall communicate the process of the investigation and the outcome and corrective measures taken to ensure compliance with the legal authority in that jurisdiction.

Section 14

Where an accident, failure of equipment, or other incident occurs which may result in a worker receiving a dose in excess of the annual limits the employer shall immediately notify the local legal authority and the joint health and safety committee by whichever means is the fastest. The employer must then, within forty-eight hours of the incident, send to the local legal designate a written report of the circumstances of the accident of failure.

Designated Competent Person with Respect to the X-ray Equipment; His/Her Duties

DISCLAIMER: *The following duties outlined are a summary only of the responsibilities of a radiation protection officer. A complete outline of these responsibilities is to be found in Regulation 861/90, section 8.*

In each facility the owner of the radiation emitting equipment or source must either assume the duties of the designated competent person or assign those duties in writing to an officer designate. That individual will assure that the directives of the appropriate government body are carried out. Further duties will include the training of the staff of the facility regarding radiation protection. He/she will also ensure that appropriate measures are in place to protect the patients and members of the general public who visit the clinic.

It is recommended that the equipment in a veterinarian's office should be tested every 2 years. This testing will include

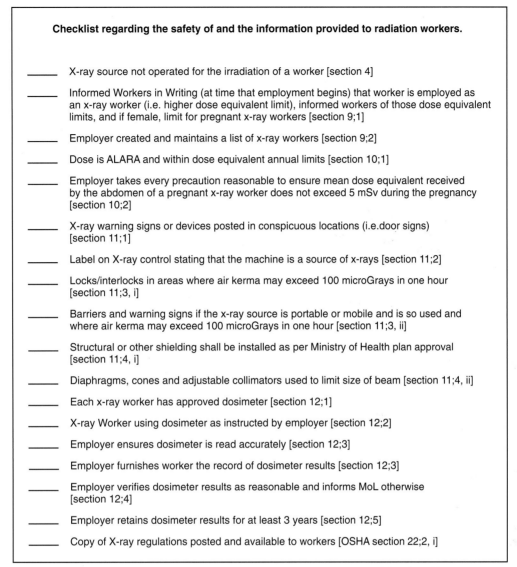

Checklist regarding the safety of and the information provided to radiation workers.

_____ X-ray source not operated for the irradiation of a worker [section 4]

_____ Informed Workers in Writing (at time that employment begins) that worker is employed as an x-ray worker (i.e. higher dose equivalent limit), informed workers of those dose equivalent limits, and if female, limit for pregnant x-ray workers [section 9;1]

_____ Employer created and maintains a list of x-ray workers [section 9;2]

_____ Dose is ALARA and within dose equivalent annual limits [section 10;1]

_____ Employer takes every precaution reasonable to ensure mean dose equivalent received by the abdomen of a pregnant x-ray worker does not exceed 5 mSv during the pregnancy [section 10;2]

_____ X-ray warning signs or devices posted in conspicuous locations (i.e.door signs) [section 11;1]

_____ Label on X-ray control stating that the machine is a source of x-rays [section 11;2]

_____ Locks/interlocks in areas where air kerma may exceed 100 microGrays in one hour [section 11;3, i]

_____ Barriers and warning signs if the x-ray source is portable or mobile and is so used and where air kerma may exceed 100 microGrays in one hour [section 11;3, ii]

_____ Structural or other shielding shall be installed as per Ministry of Health plan approval [section 11;4, i]

_____ Diaphragms, cones and adjustable collimators used to limit size of beam [section 11;4, ii]

_____ Each x-ray worker has approved dosimeter [section 12;1]

_____ X-ray Worker using dosimeter as instructed by employer [section 12;2]

_____ Employer ensures dosimeter is read accurately [section 12;3]

_____ Employer furnishes worker the record of dosimeter results [section 12;3]

_____ Employer verifies dosimeter results as reasonable and informs MoL otherwise [section 12;4]

_____ Employer retains dosimeter results for at least 3 years [section 12;5]

_____ Copy of X-ray regulations posted and available to workers [OSHA section 22;2, i]

FIGURE 16-7 Checklist for a typical facility in Canada. ALARA, as low as reasonably achievable; MoL, Ministry of Labour; OSHA, Occupational Safety and Health Act.

but is not limited to accuracy of kilovoltage, half-value layer, milliampere linearity, reproducibility, timer accuracy, and collimator accuracy.

In addition to the responsible user of the diagnostic facility, there must be a radiation protection (safety) officer delegated to act as advisor regarding all matters directly connected to the radiation protection aspects of the facility during initial stages of construction, installation of equipment and during subsequent operations.

The specific duties of the radiation protection officer are outlined in the Act. They include the provision of determination of the responsibility and monitoring of radiation doses emitted by the equipment and received by both personnel and patients.

Jurisdiction over Ionizing X-ray Radiation in Ontario Medical Facilities

Every jurisdiction must abide by very specific laws and regulations regarding radiation and the personnel who work with ionizing radiation. It is vital that each worker be familiar with the laws governing his or her workplace. The following is an example of the laws in effect in Ontario, Canada. The appropriate websites for other jurisdictions are listed at the end of this chapter.

1. Ministry of Health X-ray Inspection Service
   a. Healing Arts Radiation Protection Regulation
2. Ministry of Labour Radiation Protection Service
   a. Occupational Health and Safety Act

3. Canadian Nuclear Safety Commission
4. Radiation Protection Bureau
   a. Health Canada–Safety Code 20A

Veterinary Facilities Inspection Checklist

Figure 16-7 provides a checklist for a typical facility. It is available on the Evolve website for any facility to download and post.

SUMMARY

In this chapter we explored the regulations that have been put into effect to protect radiation workers, non–radiation workers, and patients undergoing radiographic examination from harmful doses. Protective apparel and its use and care have been discussed. The world of the radiation worker is much safer today than it was when the early pioneers were exploring this exciting new field. It is their discoveries that we build upon as we learn about new and fascinating challenges in the field of Roentgen's rays.

Websites Regarding Radiation Safety

General site for additional radiation safety training. *www.X-rayfocus.info/*.

Occupational Health and Safety Act. *www.e-laws.gov.on.ca/DBLaws/Statutes/English/900o1_e.htm*.

X-Ray Safety Regulation. *www.e-laws.gov.on.ca/DBLaws/Regs/English/900861_e.htm*.

Health Care and Residential Facilities Regulation. *www.e-laws.gov.on.ca/DBLaws/Regs/English/930067_e.htm*.

International Commission on Radiological Protection. *www.ICRP.org*.

National Council on Radiation Protection and Measurements. *www.NCRPonline.org*.

U.S. Nuclear Regulatory Commission, Radiation information Regarding Disposal of Nuclear Waste. *www.NRC.gov/waste.html*.

PART TWO

Radiographic Positioning and Related Anatomy

In the following positioning chapters these objectives will be stressed:

Describe the proper radiographic positioning techniques for all anatomic areas of small, large, and exotic animals so that for each position you are able to demonstrate:

- The normal views and protocol.
- Where you measure.
- Where you center the beam.
- The collimation and the peripheral boundaries.
- How you ensure that the patient is properly positioned.
- Important anatomy, concerns and idiosyncrasies.

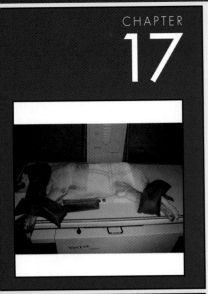

Overview of Positioning

In the end we will conserve only what we love;
we will love only what we understand; and we will understand
only what we have been taught.

—Baba Dioum, Senegalese poet and environmentalist, 1908—

LEARNING OBJECTIVES

When you have finished this chapter, you will be able to:

1. Understand the proper anatomical positioning terminology used in veterinary radiography.
2. Indicate the common rules for radiographic projections that are used when identifying and radiographing animals.
3. Apply the various principles of nonmanual restraint and animal handling so that the patient does not need to be manually restrained when being radiographed.
4. Describe standard safety procedures that should always be followed when any radiograph is taken.
5. Describe patient preparation that should be completed prior to the taking of a radiograph.
6. Describe the advantages and disadvantages of the various positioning aids available.
7. Know the required views.
8. List positioning guidelines to ensure production of good quality diagnostic radiographs.
9. Explain how the three important principles of radiation safety are used to protect the radiographer.
10. Describe when and how dividing the cassette should be used.
11. Describe important issues for labeling and identifying an image.
12. Properly place a radiograph on the illuminator.
13. Using a checklist, determine whether a radiograph is diagnostic.

KEY TERMS

Caudal (Cd)
Caudocranial (CdCr)
Cranial (Cr)
Craniocaudal (CrCd)
Distal (Di)
Dorsal (D)
Dorsal plane
Dorsopalmar (DPa)
Dorsoplantar (DPl)
Dose creep
Lateral (L)
Lateromedial (LaM)
Medial (M)
Oblique (O)
Palmar (Pa)
Palmarodorsal (PaD)
Plantar (Pl)
Plantarodorsal (PlD)
Proximal (Pr)
Recumbent
Rostral (R)
Sagittal plane
Skyline
Transverse plane
Ventral (V)

TECHNICAL NOTE

To preserve space, the radiographs presented in this chapter do not show collimation. For safety, collimation should always be performed so that the beam is limited to within the plate edges. You should see a clear border of collimation on every radiograph. In some jurisdictions, it is the law.

Part two educates the radiographer on how to properly position animals with a focus on nonmanual restraint. Veterinary medicine is practically the only health science field in which the radiographer seems to feel the need to restrain the patient while the exposure is being made, although some jurisdictions prohibit manual restraint. With simple tools and common sense, most exposures can be completed without exposing the radiographer to direct or scatter radiation.

If proper positioning is to occur with nonmanual restraint, the patient should be immobilized either by chemical restraint (sedation or general anesthesia) and/or positional devices. Please refer to a good anesthetic text for possible chemical agents. Overt manual restraint should be minimized. Even if chemical restraint is contraindicated, common behavior, restraint, and positioning principles can be applied to minimize radiographer exposure.

The canine patient usually responds to a calm, authoritative approach, whereas a feline patient resists too much restraint. If manual restraint is necessary, the radiographer must take all the precautions necessary to minimize being exposed to ionizing radiation. The welfare of both the patient and the radiographer should be kept in mind during the production of accurate diagnostic radiographs.

If manual restraint cannot be avoided, minimal safety procedures should be followed. All personnel in the radiographic suite during exposure must be shielded properly with the appropriate leaded apparel. (See Chapter 16 for proper manual restraint and shielding guidelines). As is also stressed in the chapter on safety, judicious adherence to distance, protection, and time helps minimize radiation exposure to the restrainer.

It is also essential that one is familiar with normal anatomy of the species and the proper terminology. A basic understanding of what is normal assists in producing diagnostic radiographs for accurate interpretation and diagnosis by the veterinarian.

Positional Terminology

It is important to understand the correct terminology. Most associations still use the *Nomina Anatomica Veterinaria* as the point of reference. The American College of Veterinary Radiology (ACVR) terms are also shown in Figures 17-1 and 17-2. The basic terms used are listed in Box 17-1.

BOX 17-1	Positional Terminology	
Dorsal (D)	Caudal (Cd)
Ventral (V)	Rostral (R)
Lateral (L)	Palmar (Pa, P)
Medial (M)	Plantar (Pl, P)
Left (L/Le)	Oblique (O)
Right (R/Rt)	Distal (Di)
Cranial (Cr)	Proximal (Pr)

Rules of Positioning

There are a few rules to keep in mind (based on ACVR) (see Figure 17-1):

1. Radiographic projections are named according to the direction in which the central beam anatomically enters the body part, followed by the area of exit of the x-ray beam.
2. Many projections require combinations of basic directional terms to accurately describe the point of entrance and point of exit. It is recommended that these terms be combined in a consistent order to increase standardization of the nomenclature. With the use of an overhead vertical beam, the position in which a:
   a. Patient is lying on its back (dorsal recumbency), is called VD *(ventrodorsal)*. The beam goes in the ventral (V) portion—the abdomen—and exits on the dorsal (D)aspect or the back (see Figure 17-2).
   b. Patient is lying on its abdomen (ventral recumbency), is called DV *(dorsoventral)*. The beam goes in the *dorsal (D)* portion—the back—and exits on the *ventral (V)* aspect or the abdomen.

> **TECHNICIAN NOTES** Remember that according to etymological rules, when you combine two terms, the combination of the root and the combining vowel (generally "o") is used.

3. For lateral recumbency, the image is labeled according to the side the patient is lying on. Thus, in a right lateral image, the patient is lying on its right side. The right limb in this case would be the side against the image receptor Technically a right lateral radiograph is properly referred to as a Le-RtL. Conventionally for ease of description, only the area of exit is included (Right lateral).
4. The terms *right* and *left* are not used in combination with other terms and should precede any other terms (e.g., right lateral).
5. The terms medial (M) and lateral (L) should be subservient (go second) when used in combination with other terms (e.g., dorsomedial).
6. On the head, neck, trunk and tail, the terms rostral (R), cranial, (Cr) and caudal (Cd) should take precedence (go first) when used in combination with other terms (e.g., caudoventral).

Limb Terminology

1. Cranial (Cr) and caudal (Cd) refer to the portion of the limb proximal to the carpus and tarsus.
2. The descriptors dorsal (D), palmar (Pa), and plantar (Pl) are used for that portion of the limb distal to and including the carpus and tarsus.
3. Palmar (Pa) is used in reference to the forelimbs, whereas plantar (Pl) refers to the hind limbs.
4. In describing the limbs, the terms dorsal, palmar, plantar, cranial, and caudal should take precedence when used in combination with other terms. Example: dorsoproximal.

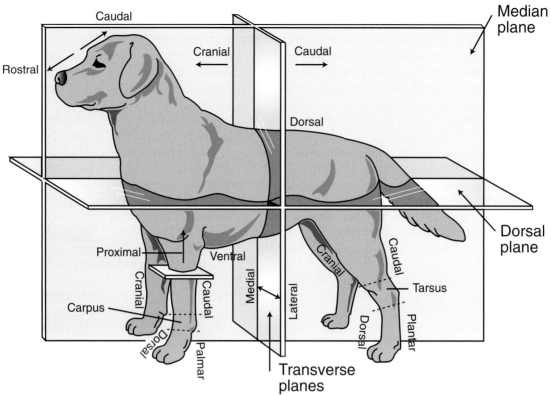

FIGURE 17-1 Correct anatomic directional terms.

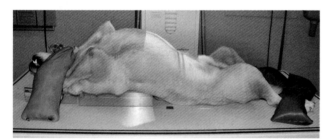

FIGURE 17-2 Patient lying in ventrodorsal recumbency. The beam enters the abdomen and exits out the back.

5. The term oblique (O) is added to the names of those projections in which the central ray passes obliquely (not parallel) to one of the three major directional axes—mediolateral (ML), dorsopalmar/dorsoplantar (DP) or craniocaudal (CrCd) through the body part. They are named in the same manner as the standard views. The term oblique is generally used in reference to limbs.
   a. Thus, in a dorsomedial-palmarolateral oblique (DM-PaLO) image of the carpus, the beam enters the dorsomedial aspect of the carpus and exits the palmarolateral aspect of the carpus (Figure 17-3).
   b. Technically, if this view was made by positioning the x-ray tube 60 degrees medially from the dorsal side, the designation would be D60°M-PaLO. This is discussed further in the large animal chapter (26).
6. In those views requiring a combination of directional terms, a hyphen should be inserted to separate the point

of entry and point of exit, for example, dorsoproximal-palmarodistal (DPr-PaDi) of a horse front digit. This means that the beam comes from the front of the foot and exits at the back of the foot. The plate is placed at the back of the foot.
7. The tangential or skyline views require no special designation because the point of entry to point of exit method describes these views concisely; for example, palmaroproximal-palmarodistal (PaPr-PaDi) in reference to an equine forelimb navicular. The beam aims from top (proximo-) to bottom (disto-) at the back (palmar) of the foot.

Patient Positioning

The Patient
The comfort and welfare of the patient should be considered at all times. Patience is vital, especially with animals that cannot be sedated. Animals are often put in positions that they are not familiar with, but if they feel secure patients will tolerate abnormal poses. To minimize anxiety, animals should be handled in a slow, quiet manner in a darkened room. Most animals respond to a calm, soft voice and gentle stroking. Do not underestimate the value of a muzzle. This often distracts the patient as well as being a "technician saver." The combination of patience with mild sedation and strategically placed positional aids, generally produce highly diagnostic radiographs. Quick, loud movements and severe restraint usually result in a frightened, tense, and even

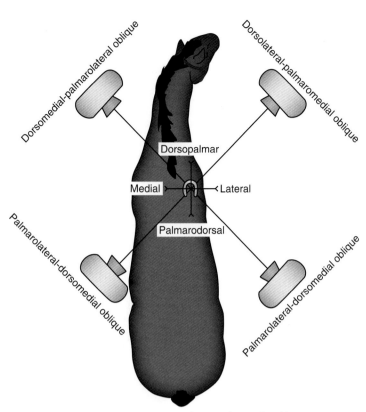

Dorsomedial-palmarolateral oblique

Dorsolateral-palmaromedial oblique

Dorsopalmar

Medial ◁▷ ◁ Lateral

Palmarodorsal

Palmarolateral-dorsomedial oblique

Palmarolateral-dorsomedial oblique

FIGURE 17-3 Correct anatomic directional terms for oblique views.

aggressive patient. Cats especially do not respond to over-restraint.

The rotor noise (spinning of the rotating anode) of the x-ray tube often startles animals. Consider starting and releasing the rotor switch when working with patients that exhibit signs of anxiety just prior to taking the radiograph, so the patient becomes accustomed to the noise.

To prevent retakes make sure that proper exposure factors are used and that the patient is properly positioned. Use a collimator, limiting the field of view to cover only the area of interest plus the peripheral borders (Figure 17-4). This practice not only further protects the patient and positioner from scatter radiation, but also increases the radiographic contrast.

Always wear protective equipment if you must hold the patient or be in the room when an exposure is made. For film/screen systems, use a fast combination to lessen the milliamperage and exposure time needed. Minimize dose creep in digital radiology.

Carefully plan and complete as much technical preparation for the exposure as possible prior to positioning the patient on the table, to minimize the length of time the patient is being restrained. This includes measuring the patient, setting the exposure technique on the machine console, positioning the cassette, making the label (if needed), gathering positional aids, and donning any protective gear. Proper preparation may mean being able to temporarily step away from scatter radiation for at least the canine lateral views, even without chemical restraint.

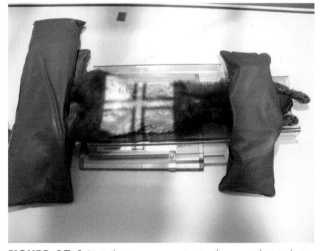

FIGURE 17-4 Limit the image receptor to the area that is being radiographed to prevent unnecessary radiation and excess scatter.

> **TECHNICIAN NOTES** Always remember the safety rules of time, distance, and shielding when working with x-rays.

Patient Preparation

The patient should be clean and free of any debris. If the hair coat of the patient is wet or full of debris, confusing artifacts can appear on the radiograph. Collars, harnesses, and leashes of any sort, especially those made of metal, should be

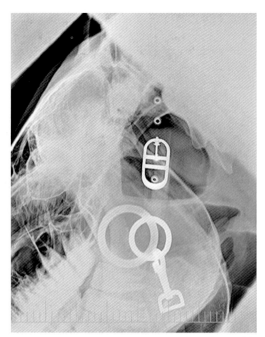

FIGURE 17-5 It is important to remove any object that could interfere with the image. The harness was not removed from this horse's head prior to exposure.

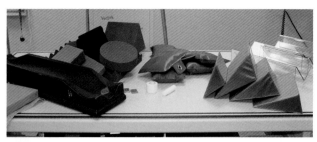

FIGURE 17-6 Positioning devices available for nonmanual restraint.

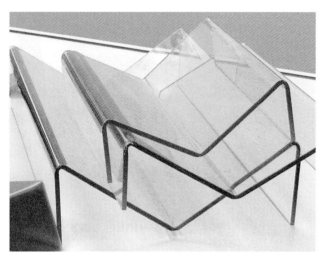

FIGURE 17-7 Acrylic troughs.

removed (Figure 17-5). Unless there is a definite medical reason for leaving them in place, remove bandages, splints, and casts before radiography. Pedal radiography of the horse may require removing the shoe and cleaning the frog of the foot, to minimize any artifacts that may obscure an area of interest. For radiography of the small animal abdomen, the gastrointestinal tract must be free of ingesta and fecal material. A cathartic such as an enema or a laxative may be indicated to remove the obstructive material. A more detailed discussion of patient preparation for abdominal study is in Chapter 25.

> **TECHNICIAN NOTES**   Always measure the animal in the position it is to be radiographed.

Human Safety

Positioning Aids

To assist in the positioning of the patient, devices such as sandbags, foam blocks and wedges, wood blocks, and a radiolucent trough can be used (Figure 17-6). Tape is essential; gauze, rope, bungee cords, and compression bands are also useful positioning aids. Any reusable aids should be waterproof, washable, and stain resistant as well as easy to store.

Positioning devices are commercially available. Prepared sandbags are generally prefilled with clean silica sand, permanently sealed, and often made of vinyl or nylon with plastic linings. Other material, such as bean bags, which are filled with polyester beads, can also be used; however, they do not offer the same support as sand. Sand and bean bags are radiopaque so should not be in the field of interest.

Commercial foam, available in various shapes and sizes, are generally covered in washable heavy vinyl covers.

Triangular and rectangular foam blocks are the most common. Foam tends to produce an air density shadow, and if not properly covered, to absorb and retain liquids that may be radiopaque when dry. Depending on what they are covered with, foam blocks may also leave density shadows on the processed radiograph.

U- and V-shaped troughs are essential to maintain a patient in dorsal recumbency. Generally they are clear plastic or vinyl-covered. The plastic/acrylic ones are radiolucent, lightweight, and easy to clean (Figure 17-7). U-shaped troughs offer good head support. Those with acrylic rods can be used to maintain the shape of the skull. When using troughs for abdominal or thoracic radiographs, ensure that the entire field of view is either on or off the trough; otherwise the radiograph will likely have distortion, artifacts or asymmetry. If using for areas such as the pelvis, keep the trough fully outside the collimated area for the same reasons.

Tape, gauze, and compression bands are extremely effective. Adhesive tape can be used to extend and hold limbs, rotate limbs, secure the patellae and femurs for a hip dysplasia view, widen the space between toes, temporarily secure a head out of the field of view, and so on (Figure 17-8). Rope and gauze, using a half hitch or variation (placing the end through the loop and then around the object) can be tied to the table if the patient is heavily sedated or anesthetized, or held by a person who can then back away from both the primary beam and scatter

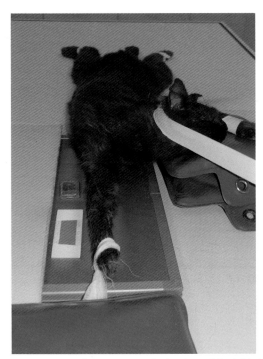

FIGURE 17-8 Use of tape to secure the head out of the field of view.

radiation. A wooden spoon can be used to keep a cat's head out of the field of view. Compression bands and hook-and-loop tape (Velcro) can be applied. Clothes pegs/pins for cats, a commercially available cat scruffer (see Figure 17-17) or nylon towel clamps, applied to the dorsal neck region (a feline behavior principle that the queen uses with her kittens) is also effective.

Your own devices can be made at a fraction of the cost of the commercially available positioning devices. Sandbags can easily be sewn and filled with sand. Empty sealable bags that can be filled with sand are also available. If you are making your own out of canvas (jean legs work well), make sure to use very narrow stitching. Fabric sand bags are not easily disinfected, so before each use, wrap them in disposable plastic. Most fabric stores sell foam that can be cut into desired shapes with a scalpel blade or electric knife. Covering the bags and wedges is essential for disinfection between patients and for keeping the devices dry so as to minimize radiographic artifacts.

With these devices, and sedation if necessary, minimal manual restraint can be used. Any nonmanual restraint used must always focus on the safety and comfort of the patient. The devices should be quickly applied and released and should never compromise the patient.

Positioning aids can give the patient the illusion that it is being held. Strategically placed sandbags or compression devices over the neck and limbs, judicious use of tape, a dimly lit room, calm deliberate movements, and a gloved hand placed over the head and held until the rotor is depressed, may keep patients, especially dogs in lateral recumbency, calm long enough for the restrainer to step back at least 6 feet. The moment the rotor is depressed, slip your hand out of the glove, leaving it over the animal's head so the patient

assumes that you are still there. Keep talking to the patient as you quietly step back. Move forward as soon as the radiograph has been taken. Another person should be depressing the exposure buttons on the console; if you are using the foot pedal, step back as far as possible. Increasing your distance from the beam drastically reduces your exposure.

If there is no alternative but to restrain a patient, it is imperative to look away from the field of view and lean back as far as possible while taking the radiograph. At no point should any part of your body be in the field of view. Protective equipment protects you from scatter radiation, not from the primary beam.

Acrylic tubes, stockinette material, pillowcases, paper bags, and plastic containers can also be strategically used for positioning of exotic animals. Please see Chapter 27 for more detail.

Equine radiographers are less likely to practice nonmanual restraint because of perceived physical safety for both the handler and the horse. However, every effort should be made to practice the three essential components of radiation safety.

> **TECHNICIAN NOTES** Have everything ready prior to taking the exposure. This includes measuring the animal, turning on the machine, setting the main voltage calibration if required, having proper source-image distance, using a grid or not, and setting the exposures. Have the cassettes or plates ready. Positioning devices should be close at hand, but any objects or distractions should be removed.
>
> The patient should be clean, have no artifacts in the area of interest, and be chemically restrained if possible.

Required Views and Positioning Guidelines

Here are some guidelines that assist in producing good-quality images:

- Two views of each anatomical area taken at right angles to each other are the minimum recommended exposures. You are trying to visualize a three-dimensional body on two-dimensional image, so details will be missed if two perpendicular views are not taken (Figure 17-9). There may be exceptions if the patient is debilitated, in trauma or if positions other than the lateral will cause undue stress to the animal. A horizontal beam radiograph could then be considered (Figure 17-10).
- If you position the area of interest closest to the image receptor, there will be a reduction in distortion and less magnification of the area under examination (Figure 17-11).
- When radiographing a limb, especially in immature or older patients, consider imaging the opposite corresponding limb to allow the pathological structure of one limb to be compared with the normal anatomy of the other.
- When tabletop technique is used, an image receptor can be divided to image more than one view and thus limit the number of films utilized (Figure 17-12). Place a lead sheet over half of the cassette to prevent exposure while the other side is being radiographed. The image

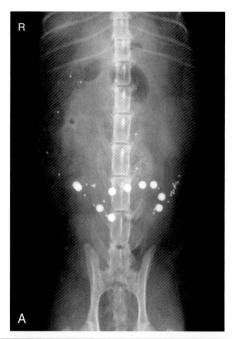

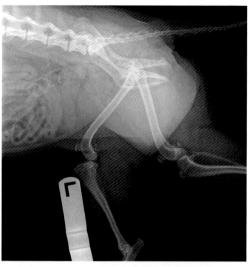

FIGURE 17-11 Note the difference in magnification between the left limb, which is closer to the plate, and the opposite right limb, which is raised from the image receptor. Also note that the bone edges are not as defined on the right limb.

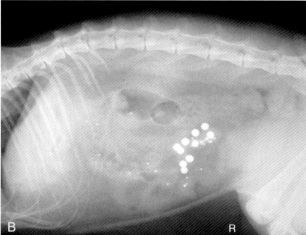

FIGURE 17-9 A and **B,** It would be difficult to determine exactly where the barium-impregnated polyurethane spheres (BIPS) are positioned without the two perpendicular views. Note the proper placement for viewing of radiographs.

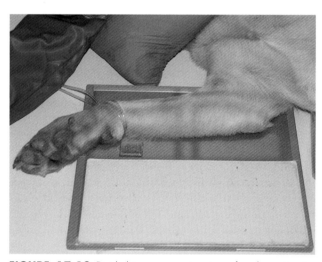

FIGURE 17-12 Divided image receptor view of a dog extremity. Through the use of a lead shield, both views can be exposed on one plate. The receptor is not divided when a grid is used.

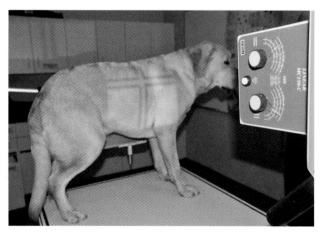

FIGURE 17-10 Horizontal beam of a dog in a standing lateral view.

receptor should still be collimated to only that half so that scatter and secondary radiation will not cause unnecessary fogging of the image. Lead sheets, which can be purchased from most x-ray supply companies, are usually supplied in preselected sizes, or larger sheets can be purchased and cut to the desired size. The lead should be at least 2 mm thick. If a lead sheet is unavailable, a lead glove can be placed over the area to be shielded.

- When using tabletop technique, place a nonslip pad under the cassette to keep it from slipping.
- When two separate views will be positioned on a radiograph, both views should be facing the same direction. For limbs, this would mean that the toes are facing the same side of the cassette; for the skull, the nose is in the same direction on each view.

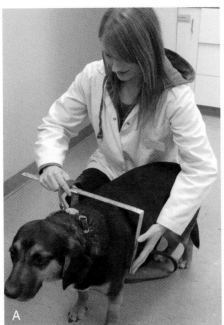
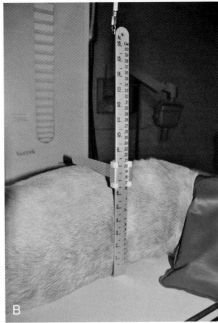

FIGURE 17-13 **A,** Measuring with a caliper in this position may lead to extra tissue thickness. **B,** Calipers are properly used when the patient is measured lying in the radiographic view to be projected.

- In general, the central ray should be centered directly over the area of interest. If there is a known lesion, however, it is important to center the beam directly over this area, especially to visualize fracture healing in limbs or spinal lesions. If the central ray is not directly over the area of interest, distortion and misdiagnosis may occur.

- The measurement for any anatomical region is generally taken over the thickest part. This practice ensures that all regions of the area of interest will be penetrated with sufficient exposure factors. A caliper is used to measure the anatomical area of interest so that proper exposures can be made. This is an inexpensive device that measures part thickness in centimeter increments (See Figure 17-13).

- The patient should be measured while in the same position used for the radiograph; if the animal is measured while standing, for example, the tissue thickness measurement will be greater than when the animal is recumbent, especially for soft tissue studies (Figure 17-13A). If there is a large difference in tissue thickness between the cranial and caudal borders, which is not uncommon in the abdomen and thorax of a deep-chested dog, two separate exposures may need to be taken. A compromise is best made if there is only a small difference in tissue density.

- Use an image receptor that is large enough to cover the body area being radiographed. Specific anatomy must be included for each anatomical area. For example, all radiographs of long bones (humerus and femur) should include the shaft of the bone as well as the joints both distal (Di) and proximal (Pr) to the bone. For joint radiography, the central ray must be centered over the joint space, and the beam should include a portion of the long bones distal and proximal to the joint. This is further expanded in Chapters 20 and 21.

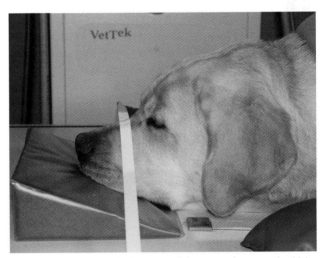

FIGURE 17-14 The thickest part of the area of interest should be toward the cathode, which is usually to the right side of the tube head.

- Have the thickest part of the area of interest toward the cathode side so that the strongest rays can assist in proper exposure (Figure 17-14).

Image Identification

Identification (ID) of the radiographs is important both for legal purposes and for knowledge that the radiographs belong to the patient in which you are interested. Please see Chapter 5 on image receptor imaging for further specific information. Be sure that each radiograph contains the following information: names of the owner and patient, date of examination, and the name of the clinic. Additional helpful

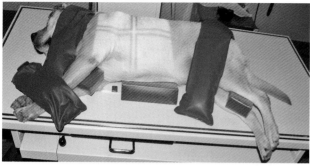

FIGURE 17-15 The patient is in right lateral recumbency, lying on the right side. Note that the marker is placed cranially and ventrally.

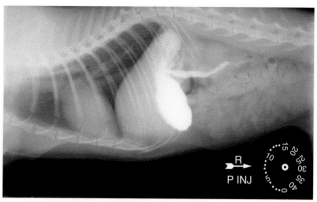

FIGURE 17-16 This radiograph of the feline patient lying on its right side is taken at 7 minutes after administration of contrast agent.

information includes age, breed, and sex of the patient but this can be written instead in the radiography log.

Positioning markers (right, left, front, hind) should be used so that the radiographs may be correctly interpreted. This is especially true for equine radiographs of areas distal to the carpus and tarsus or symmetrical anatomical areas such as a skull. By convention, for limbs, place markers laterally (as opposed to medially) for DP, CrCd or CdCr, and oblique radiographs. Place the markers cranially for lateral radiographs. In DV or VD views, place the appropriate L or R marker on the correct side of the patient. When a lateral projection of the body is taken, the marker should indicate the side that is down on the table or cassette. Thus an R would indicate a patient lying in right lateral recumbency. The marker or label would generally be placed cranially and ventrally in lateral recumbency (Figure 17-15).

When a special procedure is performed, such as a gastrointestinal contrast study that is part of a series, time elapsed or order taken is also important. This designation can be made on the lead tape label, or specialized time clocks can be used in which it is easy to adjust the time lapse (Figure 17-16). Gravity markers that indicate that a patient is standing are also available, although not frequently used.

TECHNICIAN NOTES Quickly go through a mental checklist such as this one *before* pushing the exposure button:
Are the settings correct?
Is the plate/cassette/machine/grid in position?
Is the thickest part toward the cathode if applicable?
Are the markers, and ID (if using) in the proper location and away from relevant anatomy?
Do you have the correct body part and view?
Is the patient properly centered? Are the borders correct?
Is the image receptor collimated?
Is the patient properly prepared, positioned, and restrained so that the image will be parallel to the image receptor and both are perpendicular to the beam.
Is the patient in the correct phase of respiration?

Viewing Radiographs

To assist in understanding normal radiographic anatomy, you should always view radiographs on the illuminator in the following manner (see Figure 17-9):

Lateral radiographs: The cranial part of the animal is to your left.

Dorsoventral/ventrodorsal radiographs: The cranial part of the animal points up and the animal's left side is on your right (as if you are going to shake its paw).

Lateral or oblique radiographs of the limbs: The proximal part of the limb points up and the cranial or dorsal aspect of the limb is to your left.

DP/PD/CrCd/CdCr radiographs: The proximal end of the extremity is at the top of the illuminator

Consistency is important. When labeling film radiographs, consider how the labels and markers are positioned so that they can easily be read when the radiographs are viewed in the proper positions.

Radiographic Checklist

Before submitting the radiographs to the veterinarian, you should ask yourself the following questions to ensure that you have optimal diagnostic and legal radiographs:

- Is the image labeled and legible?
- Are positional lead markers present?
- Do you have good exposure with appropriate contrast and density?
- Is your image properly centered?
- Are the appropriate borders included, and is there evidence of collimation?
- Is the body part properly positioned, with no rotation?
- Is there no evidence of a human exposure, such as a glove?
- Is the film properly developed (if applicable)?
- Have artifacts been kept to a minimum to prevent interference with the image?

If the answer is no to any of these questions, consider the next two:

- Is the image diagnostic?
- Does the image need to be repeated?

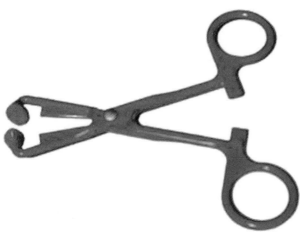

FIGURE 17-17 Commercially available cat scruffer.

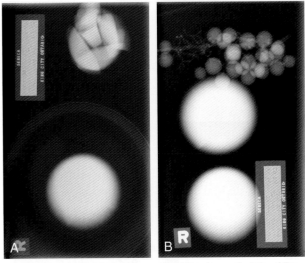

FIGURE 17-18 Mystery radiograph. What do you think the different objects are?

Bibliography

American College of Veterinary Radiology (ACVR): *Radiology 2—Equine*, 2009, ACVR. http://www.quia.com/files/quia/users/medicinehawk/2407-Vet/Radiology-2.pdf.

Aspinall V, Cappello M: *Introduction to veterinary anatomy*, London, 2009, Butterman-Heineman.

Colville T, Bassert J: *Clinical anatomy and physiology for veterinary technicians*, St. Louis, 2008, Elsevier.

Done SH, Goody PC, Stickland NC, Evans SA: *Color atlas of veterinary anatomy, the dog and cat*, London, 2009, Mosby.

Douglas SW: *Principles of veterinary radiography*, London, 1980, Bailliere Tindall.

Dyce KM, Sack WO, Wensing CJG: *Textbook of veterinary anatomy*, ed 4, St. Louis, 2010, Saunders.

Evans H, de Launta A: *Guide to the dissection of the dog*, ed 7, St. Louis, 2010, Saunders.

Faber TL: *Radiographic imaging and exposure*, St. Louis, 2009, Elsevier.

Han C, Hurd C: *Practical diagnostic imaging for the veterinary technician*, ed 3, St. Louis, 2005, Mosby.

Lavin L: *Radiography in veterinary technology*, ed 3, St. Louis, 2007, Saunders.

Morgan JP: *Techniques of veterinary radiography*, Ames, Iowa, 1993, Iowa State University Press.

Owens JM, Biery, DN: *Radiographic interpretation for the small animal clinician*, St. Louis, 1999, Ralston Purina.

Radiology of the equine limbs. (n.d.). http://www.quia.com/files/quia/users/medicinehawk/2407-Vet/Radiology-2.pdf.

Reid CF, Bathurst NW: *Large animal radiography nomenclature*, 1995, University of Pennsylvania School of Veterinary Medicine. http://cal.vet.upenn.edu/projects/larad/names/name.htm.

Romich J: *An illustrated guide to veterinary medical terminology*, Clifton, NY, 2009, Delmar Cengage Learning.

Ryan G: *Radiographic positioning of small animals*, Philadelphia, 1981, Lea & Febiger.

Sirois M: *Principles and practice of veterinary technology*, ed 3, St. Louis, 2011, Mosby.

Sirois M, Anthony E, Mauragis D: *Handbook of radiographic positioning for veterinary technicians*, Clifton Park, NY, 2010, Delmar Cengage Learning.

Smallwood JE, Shively MJ, Rendano VT, Habel RE: A standardized nomenclature for radiographic projections used in veterinary medicine, *Vet Rad* 26:2-9, 1985.

Thrall DE: *Textbook of veterinary diagnostic radiology*, ed 4, St. Louis, 2002, Saunders.

Thrall DE: *Textbook of veterinary diagnostic radiology*, ed 5, St. Louis, 2007, Saunders.

Ticer J: *Radiographic technique in small animal practice*, Philadelphia, 1984, WB Saunders.

Tighe M, Brown M: Mosby's comprehensive review for veterinary technicians, ed 3, St. Louis, 2008, Mosby.

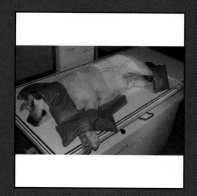

TECHNICAL NOTE

To preserve space, the radiographs presented in this chapter do not show collimation. For safety, always collimate so that the beam is limited to within the image receptor edges. You should see a clear border of collimation on every image. In some jurisdictions, use of collimation is the law.

Small Animal Abdomen

By three methods we may learn wisdom: first, by reflection, which is noblest; second, by imitation, which is easiest; and third by experience, which is the bitterest.

— Confucius, Chinese philosopher, 551–479 BCE

OUTLINE

LEARNING OBJECTIVES

When you have finished this chapter, you will be able to:

1. Properly and safely position a dog or cat for the two common abdominal views, with an emphasis on where to measure and center, where the borders are, and how to properly position, so that the body part is parallel to the image receptor and both are perpendicular to the central ray.
2. Understand the other views that may need to be completed as alternatives.
3. Identify normal radiographic abdominal anatomy.

Positioning for the abdomen is relatively straightforward, but visualization can be difficult owing to its similarity in densities and the presence of multiple organ systems. There are subtle differences in tissue density of the abdomen, with significantly less natural contrast than found in the thorax. The abdomen depends on the gas within the gastrointestinal (GI) tract and the fat in the peritoneal and retroperitoneal areas for contrast. Contrast media are often required to visualize differences.

Radiographic Concerns

- Appropriate kilovolt peak (kVp) and milliampere-seconds (mAs) should be used to differentiate the various shades of gray between organs and structures (generally use a higher kVp for the abdomen and thorax which provides more shades of grey, and a lower mAs (for shorter exposure and thus less motion artifacts). Because of the difference in thickness between the chest and caudal abdomen, deep-chested dogs exhibit a marked difference in density between the cranial and caudal halves of the abdomen. This is especially evident in the ventrodorsal (VD) view. Two separate exposures measured at the thickest part of each site may be needed. If there is only a minimal difference in anatomical thickness, a compromise can be made. Using the same technique with digital radiography may be possible for the full abdomen of such dogs.
- The two positions commonly viewed are the right or left lateral and ventrodorsal (Box 18-1). It is important to be consistent so that abnormalities can quickly be spotted. Contrast studies and other situations may also require further views.
- If a right lateral view is used, the animal is lying on its right side. Technically the correct terminology is left-right lateral (Le-RtL), if one considers, "point of entrance of the beam to point of exit;" however, this term is not generally used.
- Take advantage of the heel effect (the thickest part toward the cathode) to help reduce density differences, especially in the VD or DV views.
- Use a 14 in × 17 in image receptor for large dogs. A very large dog will likely require two radiographs-measure at the respective cranial and caudal abdomen.
- A grid must be used if the measurement exceeds 11 cm, to prevent scatter that causes fogging, which further decreases the contrast.
- To help prevent motion artifacts, use as high a milliamperage setting as possible, to produce the shortest exposure setting.
- Take the radiograph at the end of expiration, when a brief pause often occurs.

BOX 18-1	Protocol for Abdominal Radiography

Routine Views
Right or left lateral
Ventrodorsal

Optional Views
Dorsoventral
Lateral decubitus
Modified lateral/lateral oblique

- To minimize intestinal artifacts and prevent misdiagnosis, fast the patient (if possible) about 12 hours before and administer a cleansing enema about 3 to 4 hours prior to taking a radiograph, to clear the intestinal tract of fecal matter. This preparation is more important for contrast studies. See Chapter 25.
- To minimize radiation exposure to the personnel restraining a patient, nonmanual restraint should be utilized whenever possible. Use of a sedative or tranquilizer may be needed. The use of nonmanual restraint is illustrated in most of the following positions. Try to give the patient the illusion that it is being held by appropriate use of sandbags, tape, and so on. For further suggestions, please see Chapter 17.
- Abdominal compression may be utilized to reduce the thickness of the anatomical part. Compression moves an underlying organ to improve the visualization of a suspected lesion, as well as reducing the thickness which decreases scatter radiation. Remeasure the patient after compression has been applied, and use this new thickness to obtain the new kVp.

> **TECHNICIAN NOTES** Measure the animal in the position in which it is to be imaged.

> **TECHNICIAN NOTES** Have everything ready prior to taking the exposure. This includes measuring the animal, turning on the machine, setting the main voltage calibration if required, having proper source-image distance, and setting the exposures. Have the image receptors ready. Positioning devices should be close at hand, but remove any objects or distractions not utilized, to minimize scatter radiation.
>
> The patient should be clean, should have no artifacts in the area of interest, and should be chemically restrained if possible.

Positions

Lateral

Positioning

Place in: Right lateral recumbency. This tends to be the conventional position.

Head: Keep in a natural position; hold appropriately with a sandbag over the neck. Be careful not to restrict breathing.

Forelimbs: Pull cranially and sandbag. Place a small foam pad between the forelimbs to help eliminate rotation of the cranial abdomen.

Hind Limbs: Pull together caudally and sandbag, to prevent superimposition of the femoral muscles, which can mask portions of the urinary bladder and prostate. Place a foam pad of suitable thickness between the femurs to help eliminate rotation of the caudal abdomen and pelvis.

Sternum: Elevate with wedged sponges so the sternum is at the same plane as the thoracic vertebrae.

Comments and Tips

- Place any ID or markers on the ventral aspect of the abdomen.

- Ensure that the sternum and spine are on the same plane and parallel to the image receptor; the central ray is perpendicular to both.

- Expose immediately at the end phase of expiration. During expiration there is maximum amount of space for the abdominal contents as the lungs contract and the diaphragm relaxes.

- Focal radiographs using gentle pressure with a compression paddle such as a wooden spoon or plastic paddle may effectively isolate organs such as the kidneys in a VD position.[2] Remember to remeasure the patient because the decreased thickness will allow for a lower kVp and thus more contrast.

- There is better longitudinal separation of the kidneys[1] in a right lateral view, and the spleen is more consistently identified. Left lateral is preferable in vomiting patients, because gas is moved to the pyloric antrum and can potentially highlight a foreign body.

- A left lateral view may also be required in contrast studies, after the administration of contrast media.

MEASURE: Caudal aspect of 13th rib—at the thickest area (unless interested in a specific region).

CENTRAL RAY: Canine: Over caudal aspect of 13th rib at level of L2-L3.

Feline: Two to three fingerbreadths caudal to 13th rib.

BORDERS: Collimate cranially from the caudal aspect of T7 (full diaphragm and heart apex) and caudally to the greater trochanter to include the coxofemoral joints.

TECHNICIAN NOTES Remember to go through your mental check list before pushing the exposure button. See Chapter 17.

TECHNICIAN NOTES To get maximum expiration:
- If the patient is panting, cup or blow on the nose to momentarily stop breathing.
- Put light pressure on the abdomen to facilitate expiration.
- Breathe with the animal for a few breaths to determine proper point of exposure. Have the rotor depressed (initial button of a two-step process) so that the moment breathing is paused the exposure can be taken.

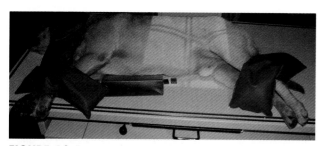

FIGURE 18-1 Proper positioning for the lateral abdomen view of a canine.

> **TECHNICIAN NOTES** Ways to determine whether the animal is properly positioned[3]:
>
> **Lateral View**
> * Rib heads are superimposed.
> * Intervertebral foramina are the same size.
> * Transverse processes are superimposed at the origin from the vertebral bodies.
> * Coxofemoral joints are superimposed.
>
> **Ventrodorsal View**
> * Spinous processes are aligned in the center of the vertebral bodies.
> * Rib and abdominal symmetry.
> * Wings of the ilium are symmetrical.
> * Obturator foramina are symmetrical.

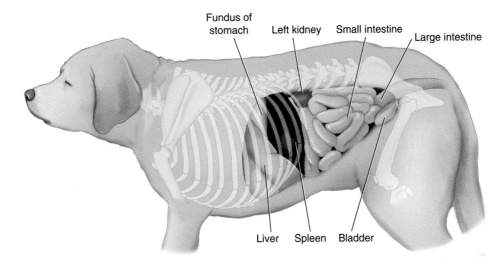

Fundus of stomach · Left kidney · Small intestine · Large intestine · Liver · Spleen · Bladder

FIGURE 18-2 Left to right lateral view of the abdomen showing major organs.

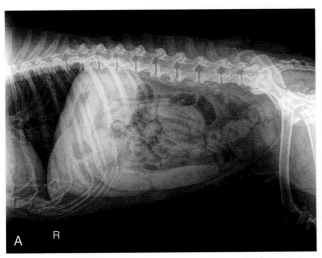
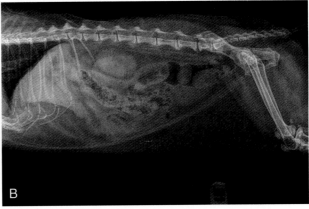

FIGURE 18-3 A, Right lateral radiograph of the abdomen of a dog. **B,** Right lateral radiograph of the abdomen of a 17-year-old DSH.

Ventrodorsal

Positioning

Place In: Dorsal recumbency. A trough may be needed-use clear plastic if possible, and place the device under the thoracic region, not the area being radiographed. This minimizes distortion and artifacts.

Head: Gently pull forward. If required, carefully position a sandbag over the head and neck, taking care not to restrict breathing.

Forelimbs: Extend forward with sandbags. If possible, position a sandbag just proximal to the elbows over the limbs. An alternative is either to tie each limb separately or to place a sandbag over each limb at the carpus and pull cranially.

Hind Limbs: Keep in a natural position, and place a sandbag over each limb.

MEASURE: Caudal aspect of the 13th rib at level of umbilicus (about L2-L3). The area of the liver is generally the widest part. If interested in another area measure that location.

CENTRAL RAY: Canine: Center on midline over caudal aspect of 13th rib at level of umbilicus (L3).
Feline: Two to three fingerbreadths caudal to 13th rib.

BORDERS: T9 vertebrae (diaphragm) cranially to the greater trochanter caudally to include the coxofemoral joints (pubic symphysis).

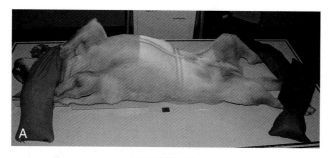

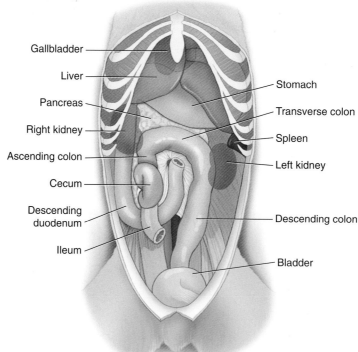

FIGURE 18-4 A, Proper positioning for the ventrodorsal abdomen view. B, Ventral anatomy of the abdomen.

Ventrodorsal—*cont'd*

Comments and Tips

- Place any ID or markers adjacent to the corresponding side of the abdomen.
- Ensure that the body is evenly positioned so that the two sides of the rib cage appear equidistant.
- Ideally a straight line should be imagined connecting the point of the nose with the caudal midline.
- Ensure that the sternum and spine are superimposed; image receptor and central ray are perpendicular to both.

- Expose immediately at the end phase of expiration (this ensures that the diaphragm is positioned cranially and is not compressing the abdominal contents).

> **TECHNICIAN NOTES** If radiographs of both the abdomen and thorax are required, complete both lateral views before imaging the ventrodorsal views. The positioning is the same for the lateral views of the two areas; only the central ray and borders change.

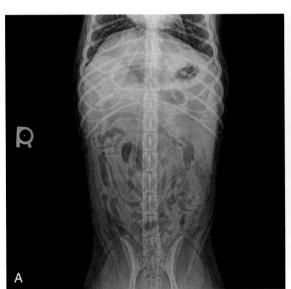
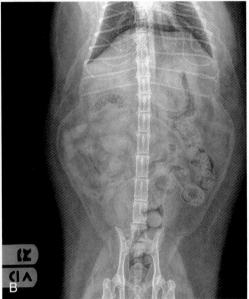

FIGURE 18-5 A, Ventrodorsal radiograph of the abdomen of a canine. B, Ventrodorsal radiograph of the abdomen of a 17-year-old feline.

Further Views

In case of injury, for gastric contrast studies, or with concern about fluid or free air, other views can be taken.

Dorsoventral

The DV view can be used in lieu of the VD view if the animal is compromised in the VD position or if an alternative view is needed for contrast studies.

Positioning

Place In: Ventral recumbency.

Head: Gently pull forward and carefully place a sandbag over the neck and head taking care not to restrict breathing.

Forelimbs: Extend slightly forward in a fairly natural position. Place sandbags over each elbow.

Hind Limbs: Keep in a natural position, and place a sandbag over each limb near the stifle.

MEASURE, CENTRAL RAY, BORDERS: Same as for the VD view.

Comments and Tips

- Place any identification or markers adjacent to the correct side of the abdomen.
- Ensure that the body is evenly positioned so that the two sides of the rib cage appear equidistant.
- Ideally a straight line should be imagined connecting the point of the nose with the caudal midline.
- Ensure that the sternum and spine are superimposed; the image receptor and central ray are perpendicular to both.
- Expose immediately at the end phase of expiration. During expiration there is a maximum amount of space for the abdominal contents as the lungs contract and the diaphragm relaxes.

> **TECHNICIAN NOTES** Collimate; ensure that labels/markers are included and that borders are visible for every image.

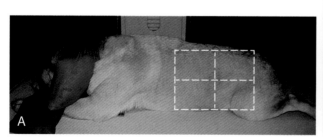
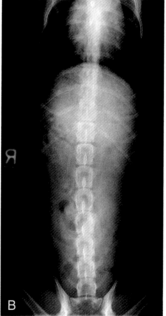

FIGURE 18-6 A, Dorsoventral positioning. **B,** Dorsoventral radiograph of the abdomen of a canine.

Lateral Decubitus (Ventrodorsal View with Horizontal Beam)

The lateral decubitus should be considered if fluid or free gas is suspected, such as in evaluation of gas-capped fluid levels that may be found in an abscess or in a bowel loop, or if the animal will be harmed if placed in an alternate position. Small amounts of fluid may not be identified radiographically.

Positioning

Place In: Right lateral recumbency on a thick foam pad or equivalent (to allow the dependent portion of the abdomen to be in the field of view).

Head: Keep in a natural position and hold appropriately with a sandbag over the neck taking care not to restrict breathing.

Forelimbs: Pull cranially and sandbag. Place a small foam pad between the front limbs to help eliminate rotation of the cranial abdomen.

Hind Limbs: Pull and sandbag caudally to prevent superimposition of the femoral muscles that can mask portions of the bladder and prostate area. Placing a foam pad of suitable thickness between the femurs helps eliminate rotation of the caudal abdomen and pelvis.

Sternum: Elevate the ventral abdomen with wedged sponges so the sternum is at the same plane as the thoracic vertebrae.

Comments and Tips

- The position is described according to the side of the patient closer to the table (i.e., right decubitus if the patient is in right lateral recumbency). Place the image receptor vertically behind the patient.
- The horizontal beam will be directed ventrodorsally, entering the sternum and exiting the vertebrae.
- Expose immediately at the end phase of expiration; this helps ensure that the diaphragm is positioned cranially and is not compressing the abdominal contents.
- Ensure that the sternum and spine are on the same plane; the central ray and image receptor are perpendicular to both.
- If free gas is suspected, wait at least 5 minutes once in position prior to the exposure to allow dorsal collection of the gas.[4]

MEASURE, CENTRAL RAY, BORDERS: Proceed as for the ventrodorsal view.

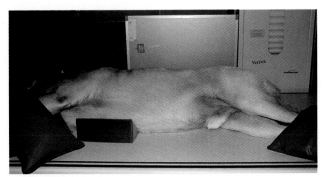

FIGURE 18-7 Positioning of a dog for lateral decubitus—ventrodorsal view with a horizontal beam. The patient is usually placed on a thick foam pad.

Modified Lateral and Lateral Oblique

If evaluation of the entire length of the urinary tract is of concern in a male, the hind limbs may mask the membranous and penile urethra[5] in a true lateral position. There are two alternatives that could be considered—the modified lateral and lateral oblique.

Modified Lateral
Positioning
Place In: Right lateral recumbency.

Head: Keep in a natural position, and hold appropriately with a sandbag over the neck. Be careful not to restrict breathing.

Forelimbs: Pull cranially and sandbag. Place a small foam pad between the forelimbs to help eliminate rotation of the cranial abdomen.

Hind Limbs: Pull the pelvic limbs cranially as far forward as possible without causing rotation of the body from the table. An appropriately sized foam pad placed between the femurs may help eliminate rotation of the pelvis. Place sandbags over the limbs.

Sternum: Elevate the ventral abdomen with wedged sponges so the sternum is at the same plane as the vertebrae. Have the central ray be perpendicular to both.

Comments and Tips
- Ensure that the pelvic limbs are not superimposed over the caudal aspect of the os penis.
- Expose immediately at the end phase of expiration.

Lateral Oblique
Positioning
Place in: Right lateral recumbency.

Head: Keep in a natural position and support appropriately with a sandbag over the neck.

Forelimbs: Pull cranially and sandbag.

Hind Limbs: Pull the dependent limb caudally and place a sandbag over the femur to keep in position. Raise the contralateral limb so that it is pulled dorsally and out of the field of view. A bungee cord or gauze tied around the tarsus and metatarsus and secured to the table, machine or sandbag will help keep the limb out of the field of view.

BOTH POSITIONS Measure: Over the ischium.

Central Ray: Over the cranial wing of the ilium unless the rectum is of interest; in that case have the central beam over the pelvis.

Borders: For a bladder, prostate, or caudal contrast study, include L4 and the caudal aspect of the rectum.

> 📎 **TECHNICIAN NOTES**   Remember to collimate to the area of interest and include the markers.

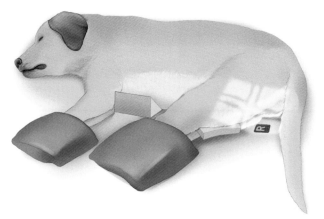

FIGURE 18-8 Positioning for a modified lateral view of a male for contrast studies. The hind limbs are pulled cranially as far as possible for evaluation of the membranous and penile urethra.

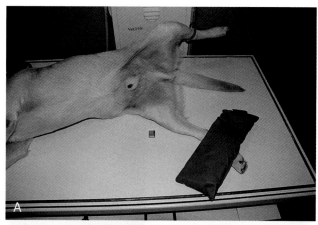

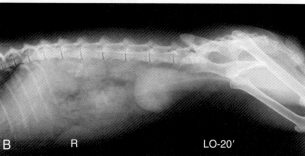

FIGURE 18-9 **A,** Positioning for lateral oblique view of the canine abdomen. Ensure that the pelvic limbs are not superimposed over the caudal aspect of the os penis. **B,** Lateral oblique radiograph of the abdomen of a feline patient during an excretory urography using iodine.

Modified Lateral and Lateral Oblique—cont'd

Comments and Tips

- Ensure that the pelvic limbs are not superimposed over the caudal aspect of the os penis.
- Expose immediately at the end phase of expiration.
- For male dogs, this view may be needed because on the ventrodorsal view there may be superimposition of the penis over the bladder.
- Oblique views can also be achieved by placing the patient in the VD or DV positions and rotating the body 15-30 degrees. This moves the esophagus, stomach, colon and urinary bladder away from the vertebrae to allow better visualization.
- The criteria for proper symmetry will not apply to the oblique views.

Note: Figure 18-10 shows the various positions of a Beagle during expiration, which is when the abdomen should be exposed. Figure 18-11 shows the positions during inspiration. Table 18-1 contains a summary of the radiographic anatomy discussed below in this chapter along with positional changes.

> **TECHNICIAN NOTES** Strategically used positioning aids give the patient the *illusion* that it is being held. A sandbag over the neck and limbs, and/or the use of tape is essential if the patient is not properly sedated.

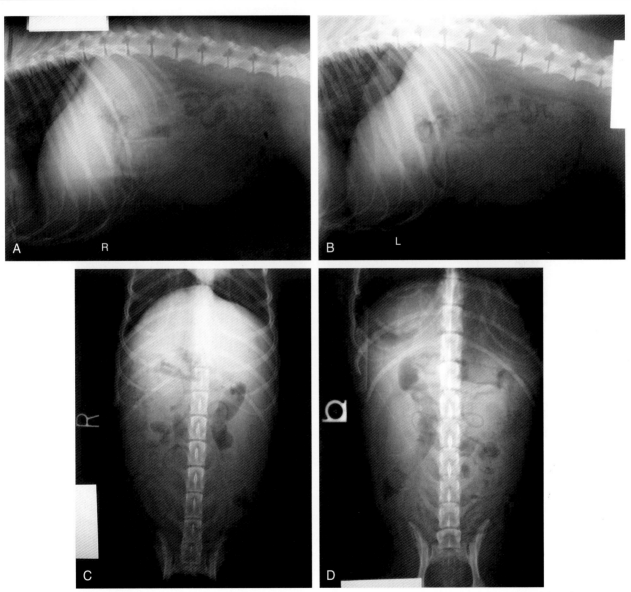

FIGURE 18-10 Radiographs showing the various positions of a Beagle during expiration. **A,** Right lateral. **B,** Left lateral. **C,** Ventrodorsal. **D,** Dorsoventral.

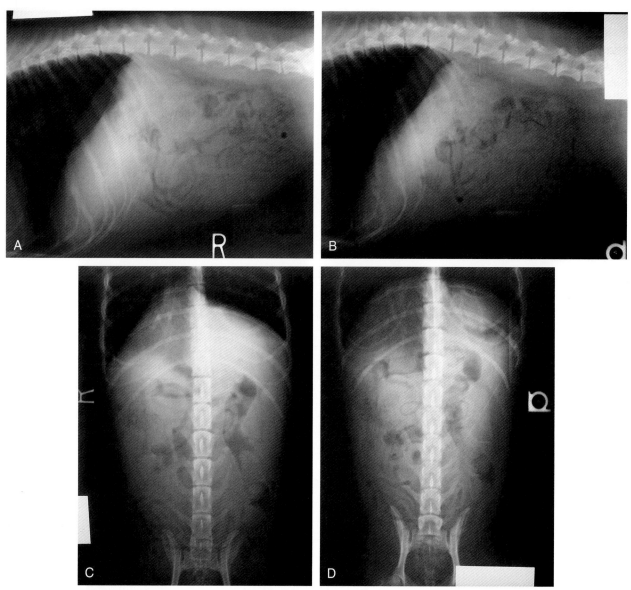

FIGURE 18-11 As a comparison to the suggested expiration during abdominal radiography, these radiographs show the various positions of a Beagle during inspiration. **A**, Right lateral. **B**, Left lateral. **C**, Ventrodorsal. **D**, Dorsoventral.

Normal Radiographic Anatomy of the Abdomen

Interpretation of abnormalities of the abdomen is beyond the scope of this text. Normal radiographic anatomy[6-17], is presented here so that the imager understands the implications of failure to properly position the patient: radiographic changes may be seen that are not attributable to disease processes or other findings. Also, the term "normal" may not be straightforward, because every organ or structure has particular normal findings, based on the shape, size, location, position, margins, number, and opacity, as well as being affected by superimposition of other tissues.

Paying attention to changes in the abdominal wall and extraabdominal soft tissue and bone structures can also aid

in the diagnosis. Variations depend on factors such as age and body condition, which can affect the interpretation of the peritoneum and retroperitoneal space. Fat in the abdomen serves as a contrasting opacity to help identify the structures. Thus you see various body images much better in a fat cat than in an emaciated one because of the various types of fat present. Fat types include subcutaneous fat, retroperitoneal fat, and fat within the falciform ligament ventral to the liver. If there is no body fat, such as in immature or cachexic patients, it will be hard to distinguish the peritoneal or retroperitoneal organs. Retroperitoneal and peritoneal fluid and gas also change the extent to which kidney and other organs are obscured.

Also keep in mind that not all normal structures that are present anatomically, are visible radiographically. The ureters,

TABLE 18-1	Radiographic Anatomy with Positional Changes
RADIOGRAPHIC ANATOMY	**POSITIONAL CHANGE(S)**

Right Lateral View (See Figures 18-3, 18-10A, 18-11A, 18-15A, and 18-16)

Fundus and body of the stomach	Gas-filled and in the dorsal and cranial aspects of the abdomen, caudal to the left crus of the diaphragm
The pyloric antrum	Soft tissue opacity ventrally, just caudal to the liver
Axis of stomach	Appears vertical
Liver	Appears larger than left; appears smaller in expiration.[18]
Left (upper) kidney	Appears more bean-shaped, is slightly magnified, and is caudal to the right kidney
Spleen	Distal extremity more noticeable in dogs but may not be seen as separate structure due to overlap of the liver
Crura of diaphragm where they cross	Appears parallel with right crus

Left Lateral View (See Figures 18-10B, 18-11B, and 18-15B)

The pyloric antrum and canal, and duodenum	Gas-filled
Stomach fundus and dorsal body	Fluid-filled and difficult to identify unless filled with contrast medium
Axis of stomach	Appears vertical
Liver	Appears smaller
Entire shadow of spleen	May be hidden under small intestines
Right kidney	Appears larger, is more bean-shaped, and is cranial to left kidney

Ventrodorsal View(See Figures 18-5, 18-10C, 18-11C, and 18-15C)

Body near midline, pyloric antrum, and descending duodenum	Gas-filled
The cardia, fundus and body	Partially fluid-filled and may be difficult to see
Axis of stomach	Appears horizontal
Diaphragmatic outline	Single "domelike" shadow with the right side slightly cranial
Ascending colon and cecum	On patient's right
Descending colon	On patient's left
Spleen	Left side, under liver; appears as small triangle caudal to fundus of stomach
Right kidney	Cranial to left kidney
Colon	Question-mark shape

Dorsoventral View (See Figures 18-10D, 18-11D, and 18-15D)

Fundus and cardia	Gas-filled and caudal to the left diaphragmatic crus
Ventral part of the body and the pyloric antrum	Difficult to see; filled with fluid
Ascending colon and cecum	On animal's right
Descending colon	On animal's left
Colon	Question-mark shape
Diaphragm (especially in deep-chested dogs)	Trilobed crura lateral to central cupula; diaphragm looks bumpy
Spleen	On left, under liver; appears as small triangle caudal to fundus of stomach
Right kidney	Cranial to left kidney

urethra, adrenal glands, pancreas, gallbladder, and mesenteric and rectal lymph nodes are examples of organs not normally seen on a radiograph. However, abnormalities such as enlargements and increased opacities, may cause such organs to become visible and may also cause variations in position of other organs.

This section offers a quick overview of the characteristic organs found in the abdomen of an animal. (Figure 18-12).

Mid-Abdomen, Liver, Spleen, Gastrointestinal Tract, and Pancreas[6,7,8, 9,16,17] (Figure 18-12, 13)

Liver[6,9]

The liver which is the largest organ in the body after the skin lies in the cranial abdomen between the diaphragm and stomach. Normal liver size is easier to assess on the lateral view but it does depend on subjective criteria and the

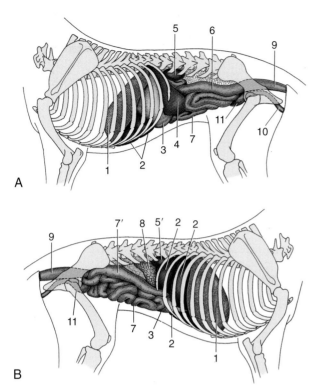

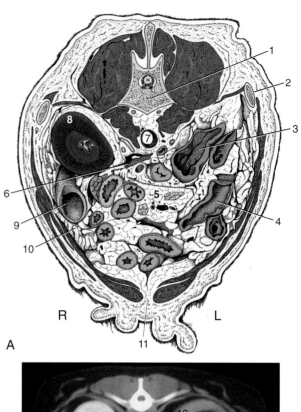

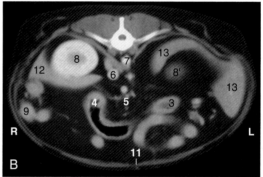

FIGURE 18-12 Visceral projections on the left (**A**) and right (**B**) canine abdominal walls. 1, Diaphragm; 2, liver; 3, stomach; 4, spleen; 5 and 5', left and right kidneys, respectively; 6, descending colon; 7, small intestine; 7', descending duodenum; 8, pancreas; 9, rectum; 10, female urogenital tract; 11, bladder.

FIGURE 18-13 A, Transverse section of the canine abdomen at the level of the first lumbar vertebra. **B,** Corresponding computerized tomography (CT) scan slightly more caudal than the section shown in **A**; the cat was lying on its back during the CT procedure. 1, First lumbar vertebra; 2, last rib; 3, descending colon; 4, transverse colon; 5, lymph nodes and blood vessels in mesentery, with the jejunum ventral to them; 6, caudal vena cava; 7, aorta, between crura of diaphragm; 8, right kidney; 8', cranial pole of left kidney; 9, descending duodenum and pancreas; 10, greater omentum; 11, linea alba; 12, liver; 13, spleen.

position of adjacent organs. The liver normally lies beneath the ribs, but the position is affected by the stage of breathing and the type of animal. The caudal margin of the liver is generally enclosed either within the rib cage or quite close to its caudal portion.

The margins of the liver are best evaluated on a lateral radiograph. The cranial margin of the liver almost parallels the contours of the dome-shaped diaphragm and is easily visualized, but the caudal margin may be difficult to see on the VD view. The liver in both the dog and the cat has four lobes (left, right, caudate, and quadrate). The left and right lobes are further divided into the medial and lateral sublobes.

There is superimposition between the lobes of the liver, between the liver and the diaphragm, and sometimes between the liver and the stomach; thus these areas are not always identifiable.

Gallbladder
In the dog and cat, the gallbladder is associated with the right liver lobes. Because of the overlapping, this organ which has the opacity of soft tissue, is not normally visible.

Spleen[6,9]
The normal spleen has no blunting or rounding of the edges. The head of the spleen (the proximal portion) is attached to the body and fundus of the stomach by the gastrosplenic ligament. The proximal extremity appears as a flattened triangular structure in the craniodorsal abdomen, is dorsal and caudal to the stomach, and is infrequently seen on a lateral radiograph. On a ventrodorsal radiograph the spleen is generally seen lateral to the fundic portion of the stomach, medial to the body wall, and craniolateral to the left kidney. The body and distal portion are mobile and can be found anywhere in the abdomen, depending on the size of the spleen—in the ventral abdomen to either left or right of midline.

In cats the spleen is relatively consistent in size with only the proximal extremity seen on the ventrodorsal views. Visualization of its distal extremity in the ventral abdomen of a cat in a lateral radiograph, usually indicates splenomegaly. In dogs there is more variation in the size of the spleen due to many factors, such as age and breed, as well as sedatives (e.g., barbiturates, phenothiazines) and other drugs that cause splenomegaly.

Esophagus[6]

The esophagus is usually not visible on neck and thoracic radiographs. However, it is sometimes seen on the lateral view of the thorax, either dorsal to the trachea when a small amount of air is present in its lumen, or between the aorta and the caudal vena cava when the esophagus is fluid filled[.].

Pharynx[6]

The pharynx is an air-filled cavity at the conjunction of the respiratory system and the alimentary tract. The soft palate is visible as a band of soft tissue between the nasopharynx dorsally and the oropharynx ventrally. The laryngeal cartilages are seen ventral and caudal to the pharynx. Often the pharyngeal side of the upper esophageal sphincter is also visible. The pharynx is best seen on a lateral view[.].

Stomach[6,8]

The stomach lies just caudal to the liver and cranial to the transverse colon. It is normally found within the rib cage, especially between meals, when the gastric contents are normally air and a small amount of fluid. Thus it is important to include part of the rib cage when taking radiographs of the abdomen. Food is seen in the stomach as a granular material of mixed (air, soft tissue, and mineral) opacity. The radiographic aspect of the stomach depends on the gastric content and the patient position. The stomach size and opacity vary according to the gastric contents, but generally, the size on a lateral view should not be more than two intercostal spaces. This organ is located at the level of about the 10th to 12th intercostal spaces. If it is radiographed after a meal, the stomach can be two to three times larger. In cats the cardia/body portions of an empty stomach look like circular soft tissue opacity 2 to 3 cm in diameter, located to the left of the midline and caudal to the liver.

The wall of the stomach with its rugal folds (gastric rugae) may be seen if the stomach is distended with gas or if it is empty. The rugal folds are most evident in the cardia and pyloric regions. However, the wall, as seen radiographically, may appear thicker than it really is, because of additional soft tissue opacities (gastric content). It is, therefore, difficult to assess the gastric (and intestinal) wall on survey radiographs.

The stomach can be divided into different portions—the cardia, fundus, body, pyloric canal, and pyloric antrum. The cardia lies just caudal to the diaphragm in the region of the esophageal hiatus. The fundus has a dome appearance at the left dorsal aspect of the stomach. The central located body is the largest portion of the stomach, lying between the fundus and pyloric portion. The pyloric portion is the distal third of the stomach that can be divided into the thin walled pyloric antrum (proximal two-thirds) and the

muscular pyloric canal (distal third) which contains a double sphincter.[7] In the right lateral position, the pylorus may appear as a soft-tissue opacity that can be misdiagnosed as a mass or foreign body. If there is any doubt, a left lateral view should be completed.

The long axis of the stomach (a line drawn connecting the fundus and the pylorus) varies depending on the stage of respiration, size of the liver, and degree of gastric filling. In the lateral view, the long axis of the stomach should lie approximately parallel to the caudal ribs, perpendicular to the vertebral column, or somewhere between, in a dog or cat. For the VD view of the dog, the cardia, fundus and body of the stomach, are situated to the left of midline while the pyloric portions are to the right of midline. The pylorus in the cat is closer to the midline and the stomach is more acutely angled.[7] In the lateral view, the axis appears almost vertical on the radiograph, whereas in the VD view the stomach has a horizontal appearance (Figure 18-14).

The gas or fluid pattern within the stomach is influenced by the volume and ratio of fluid to gas and the position of the patient. If one compares the stomach with a J shaped balloon in a transverse plane that is filled with water and air,

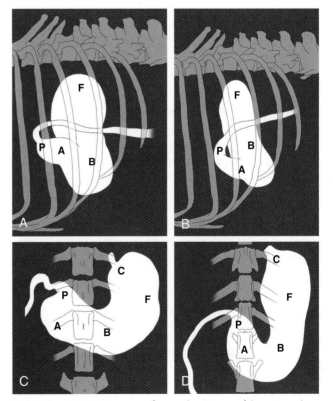

FIGURE 18-14 Diagrams of normal canine or feline stomach in lateral and ventrodorsal projections. **A,** Canine stomach in lateral recumbency. **B,** Feline stomach in lateral recumbency. The gastric axis is parallel with the ribs. **C,** Canine stomach in dorsal recumbency. The gastric axis is perpendicular to the spine, and the stomach is slightly U-shaped. **D,** Feline stomach in dorsal recumbency. The pylorus is located at the midline, and the stomach has more of an acute angle appearing J shaped. The major areas of the stomach are F, fundus; B, body; A, pyloric antrum; P, pyloric canal; C, cardia.

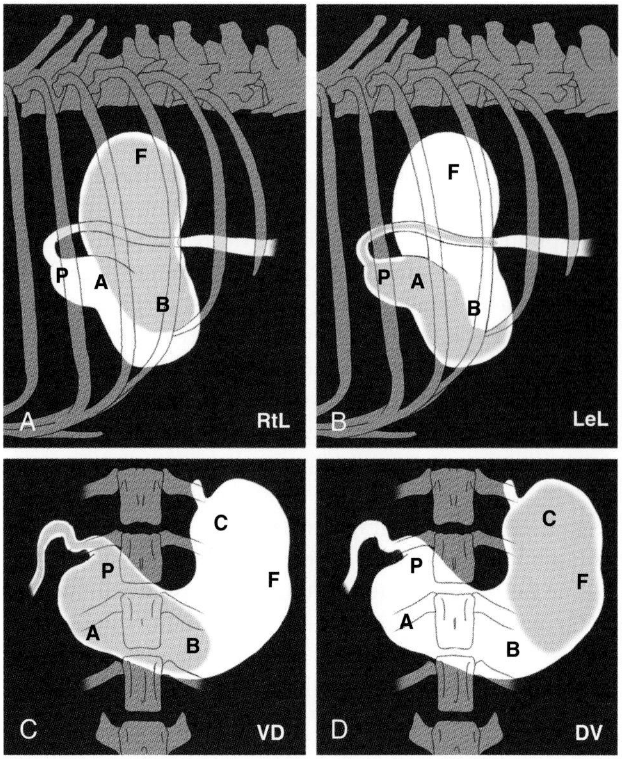

FIGURE 18-15 Effects of positional changes as shown in the canine stomach. **A,** Right lateral (RtL); gas is in the fundus (F) and dorsal body of the stomach (B). **B,** Left lateral (LeL); gas is in the main body, pyloric antrum (A) and canal (P), and duodenum. **C,** Ventrodorsal (VD); gas is in the pyloric antrum, body of the stomach, and descending duodenum. **D,** Dorsoventral (DV); gas is in the fundus and cardia (C).

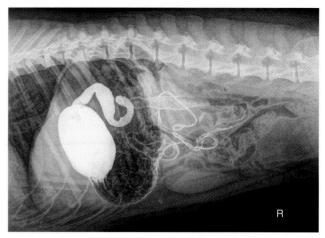

FIGURE 18-16 Right lateral radiograph showing the air in the fundus and body of the stomach and barium in the pyloric region and the duodenum. Further contrast studies can be found in Chapter 25.

one can see that the gas rises to the highest point and fluid moves into the gravity-dependent portion. Fluid gastric contents move to the dependent portion of the lumen and gas to the uppermost portion whether in a lateral or DV/VD position (Figure 18-15). In the right lateral view, the gas rises to the uppermost body and fundus, which are on the patient's left side (Figure 18-16). In the left lateral view, gas is in the pylorus, which is on the patient's right side. In the VD view, the gas is in the body near the midline and pyloric antrum, so when the position is a DV view, the gas rises to the cardia and the fundus.[6,8]

> **TECHNICIAN NOTES**   To remember the location of the gas in the stomach: For the DV view, think of "Da fundus" (D being the first letter of DV and Da sounding like "the").

Small Intestine[6,16]

The small intestine is found in the mid-abdomen. The diameter should be no wider than twice the width of a rib in a dog and "twice the height of the central portion of the L4 vertebral body" in the cat.

There are three parts: the duodenum, jejunum, and ileum. The duodenum originates at the pylorus, courses cranially

1 to 2 inches then caudally along the right body wall to the level of L5-L6. It then courses cranially as a midline structure when viewed in the VD position. The duodenum is described as having a proximal duodenal flexor, a descending duodenum, a caudal duodenal flexor, and an ascending duodenum.

In dogs, depressions of mucosa are seen in the duodenum; they are called "pseudo-ulcers" because they mimic the appearance of ulcers. The duodenum of the cat is often visualized as segmented because of the muscular (peristaltic) activity, which gives it an almost "string-of-pearls" appearance (See Figure 25-12).

The jejunum is in the mid-abdominal region and is easier seen if there is fat in the mesentery, omentum, or the falciform ligament, and if there is gas in the bowel. The ileum, which is the terminal portion of the small bowel, enters the colon at the ileocolic junction to the right of the midline. In the VD position, the ileum is normally at the dorsal portion of the abdomen at the level of L4.

Large Intestine[6,17]

The large intestine is about 16 inches in length in a 40-lb dog and is larger in diameter than the small intestine. It consists of the cecum and the colon, which has ascending, transverse, and descending components. In the ventrodorsal/dorsoventral position, the colon looks like a question mark.

In the lateral view, parts of the colon may either be superimposed over the stomach, just caudal to the left crus of the diaphragm, or over the cardia of the stomach.

The cecum of the dog is generally found to the right of midline in the VD view, adjacent to L2-L4, and in the central abdomen for the lateral view. It has a corkscrew or curved appearance in dogs and is often gas-filled. In the cat the cecum is not usually seen because it is very small. In contrast studies, it appears as a single V-shaped pouch entering the colon.

The ascending colon is to the right of midline and is found dorsally. The ascending colon is often indented along the medial wall adjacent to the cecum, at the site where the ileum enters the ascending colon. This is known as the ileocolonic sphincter. The transverse colon appears circular in configuration and lies caudal to the stomach. In the lateral view, the transverse colon can often be mistaken for a mass lesion. The descending colon generally lies adjacent to the left body wall, but it may change position to either the midline or the right side in the mid- and distal regions, especially if the animal is obese, the intestine is full of fecal matter, or the urinary bladder is distended.

The rectum is located in the pelvic canal.

Pancreas[6,7]

A normal pancreas is not visualized radiographically. Even pancreatitis may not show any radiographic abnormalities but may cause organ displacements. The right limb of the pancreas lies adjacent and caudal to the caudal margin of the stomach. The left portion is medial to and beside the descending duodenum. Ultrasonography is a better tool to identify a diseased pancreas.

Evaluation of the Urogenital System, Adrenal Glands, and Abdominal Lymph Nodes

Kidneys[6,11]

The kidneys are soft-tissue opacities found in the retroperitoneal space. Canine kidneys are elongated, and feline kidneys are short and round. In the dog the right kidney is usually found between T12 and L2, and in the cat between L1 and L3. The left kidney position, which can be more variable, is between L2 and L4 in the dog and L3 and L5 in the cat. Normal kidney size is generally judged in the VD view with the use of L2 as a comparison. In the dog, the normal kidney should be $2\frac{1}{2}$ to $3\frac{1}{2}$ times the length of L2, and in the cat, 2 to 3 times. However, this observation is a guideline only, because there are variations with factors such as age, size, sex and blood pressure. The kidneys may be displaced caudally by a full stomach or cranially by an enlarged uterus.

Both kidneys are usually identifiable on the feline radiograph. The left kidney is seen in most dogs with normal body condition, but only the caudal pole of the right kidney can be seen on a lateral radiograph and the organ is usually not seen at all in the VD radiograph. On the right lateral radiograph, the left kidney will be displaced from its dorsal position; it may be in the mid-abdomen and is often more visible than on a left lateral radiograph, especially in cats and obese dogs, in which there is more perirenal and retroperitoneal fat.

The margins of the kidneys should be smooth and of homogenous soft-tissue opacity. If a unilateral renal lesion is suspected, place the abnormal kidney in the upper position. It will be more "bean-shaped" because the upper kidney rotates on the longitudinal axis. This rotation allows that region, which is well covered with fat, to be presented tangentially to the x-ray beam. The increased object-film distance makes it appear more magnified as well.

Adrenal Glands[6,7]

Normal adrenal glands are not generally visualized on the radiograph, being better viewed on ultrasound and CT scanning. They are located in the retroperitoneal space just craniomedial to each kidney.

Urinary Bladder[6,12]

The urinary bladder is found in the caudoventral abdomen ventral to the rectum and descending colon. In the dog, the caudally facing neck of this pear-shaped organ is cranial to the pubis. In the cat, the bladder is more rounded and slightly more cranial.

A distended bladder may displace abdominal viscera cranially and the descending colon to right. An empty urinary bladder may not be visible, but if it contains urine, it may be seen on either the left or right side or centered on the midline.

Uterus and Ovaries[10]

The uterus and ovaries are not normally visualized on survey radiographs, although the body of the uterus may sometimes be visible between the bladder neck and colon in obese animals. The uterus is usually visualized only if it is abnormally large or gravid. Fetal skeletons become visible at approximately 42- to 45 days of gestation.

Urethra and Ureters[6,11,13]

Neither the urethra or the ureters are visible on a radiograph without contrast media. The female urethra is shorter and wider than that of the male. The male urethra is long and thin. The canine male urethra consists of three parts while the feline urethra has two parts. The ureters are in the retroperitoneal space and if injected with contrast media should not be larger than 2 to 3 mm.

Prostate Gland and Testicles[6,14,15]

The prostate is found in the pelvic canal and is not visible radiographically in the cat. In older dogs it may lie within the abdomen, as it may in young dogs when pulled cranially by a full urinary bladder. The prostate diameter in the dog should be no greater than two-thirds the width of the pelvic inlet on the VD view. The testicles are not normally evaluated with conventional radiography.

Abdominal Lymph Nodes

Abdominal lymph nodes are not normally visualized but may be seen if there is a considerable increase in size or a change in opacity. Ultrasound is an excellent modality to evaluate lymph nodes (see the description in Chapter 13).

NOTE

For information on alternate modes of imaging, please see Sections 3 and 4 in Part One. Further images available on line.

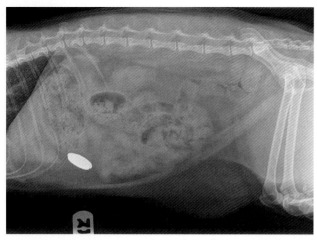

FIGURE 18-17 Mystery radiograph. What is the abnormal radiodense material, and where do you think it is located?

KEY POINTS

1. The lack of natural contrast inherent in the abdomen necessitates particular attention to appropriate exposure factors to ensure that proper diagnosis can be made.

2. As with other body areas, correct positioning and technique are required for proper interpretation. This includes where to measure and center, what to include, and how to ensure that the positioning shows proper symmetry.

3. The normal positions for the abdomen are the right lateral and ventrodorsal.

4. Because of a lack of inherent contrast in the abdomen, proper positioning is essential to minimize misdiagnosis. Knowledge of normal radiography assists in ensuring that perfect radiographs are presented for diagnosis.

5. Not all abdominal organs are visible radiographically, so other modalities such as ultrasound, magnetic resonance imaging (MRI), and computerized tomography (CT) may be required to view the abdomen as well as to further augment diagnosis of visible radiographic structures.

References

1. Lavin L: *Radiography in veterinary technology*, St. Louis, 2007, Saunders, p 231.
2. Thrall DE: *Textbook of veterinary diagnostic radiology*, ed 5, St. Louis, 2007, Saunders, p 627.
3. Thrall DE: *Textbook of veterinary diagnostic radiology*, ed 4, St. Louis, 2002, Saunders, p 489.
4. Morgan JP: *Techniques of veterinary radiography*, Ames, Iowa, 1993, Iowa State University Press, p 270.
5. Thrall DE: *Textbook of veterinary diagnostic radiology*, ed 4, St. Louis, 2002, Saunders, p 626.
6. Thrall DE: *Textbook of veterinary diagnostic radiology*, ed 4, St. Louis, 2002, Saunders, Chapter 36.
7. Thrall D: *Textbook of veterinary diagnostic radiology*. St. Louis, 2002, Saunders, Elsevier, Chapter 38.
8. Thrall DE: *Textbook of veterinary diagnostic radiology*. St. Louis, MO, 2007, Saunders, Elsevier, Chapter 45.(stomach).
9. Thrall DE: *Textbook of veterinary diagnostic radiology*, ed 4, St. Louis, 2002, Saunders, Chapter 39.
10. Thrall DE: *Textbook of veterinary diagnostic radiology*, ed 4, St. Louis, 2002, Saunders, p 642.
11. Thrall DE: *Textbook of veterinary diagnostic radiology*, ed 4, St. Louis, 2002, Saunders, Chapter 40.
12. Thrall DE: *Textbook of veterinary diagnostic radiology*, ed 4, St. Louis, 2002, Saunders, Chapter 41.
13. Thrall DE: *Textbook of veterinary diagnostic radiology*, ed 4, St. Louis, 2002, Saunders, Chapter 42.
14. Thrall DE: *Textbook of veterinary diagnostic radiology*, ed 4, St. Louis, 2002, Saunders, Chapter 43.
15. Thrall DE: *Textbook of veterinary diagnostic radiology*, ed 4, St. Louis, 2002, Saunders, Chapter 44.
16. Thrall DE: *Textbook of veterinary diagnostic radiology*, ed 4, St. Louis, 2002, Saunders, Chapter 46.
17. Thrall DE: *Textbook of veterinary diagnostic radiology*, ed 4, St. Louis, 2002, Saunders, Chapter 47.
18. Owens JM, Biery DN: *Radiographic interpretation for the small animal clinician*, St. Louis, 1999, Ralston Purina.

Bibliography

Aspinall V, Cappello M: *Introduction to veterinary anatomy*, London, 2009, Butterman-Heineman.

Colville T, Bassert J: *Clinical anatomy and physiology for veterinary technicians*, St. Louis, 2008, Elsevier.

Done, SH, Goody PC, Stickland NC, Evans SA: *Color atlas of veterinary anatomy, the dog and cat*, London, 2009, Mosby.

Dyce KM, Sack WO, Wensing CJG: *Textbook of veterinary anatomy*, ed 4, St. Louis, 2010, Saunders.

Evans H, de Launta A: *Guide to the dissection of the dog*, ed 7, St. Louis, 2010, Saunders.

Han C, Hurd C: *Practical diagnostic imaging for the veterinary technician*, ed 3, St. Louis, 2005, Mosby.

Owens JM, Biery DN: *Radiographic interpretation for the small animal clinician*, St. Louis, 1999, Ralston Purina.

Romich J: *An illustrated guide to veterinary medical terminology*, Clifton, NY, 2009, Delmar Cengage Learning.

Ryan G: *Radiographic positioning of small animals*, Philadelphia, 1981, Lea & Febiger.

Sirois M: *Principles and practice of veterinary technology*, ed 3, St. Louis, 2011, Mosby.

Sirois M, Anthony E, Mauragis D: *Handbook of radiographic positioning for veterinary technicians*, Clifton Park, NY, 2010, Delmar Cengage Learning.

Smallwood JE, Shively MJ, Rendano VT, Habel RE: A standardized nomenclature for radiographic projections used in veterinary medicine, *Vet Rad* 26:2-9, 1985.

Ticer J: *Radiographic technique in small animal practice*, Philadelphia, 1984, WB Saunders.

Tighe M, Brown M: *Mosby's comprehensive review for veterinary technicians*, ed 3, St. Louis, 2008, Mosby.

Small Animal Thorax

A good head and a good heart are always a formidable combination.

—Nelson Mandela, South African anti-apartheid activist and President, 1918—

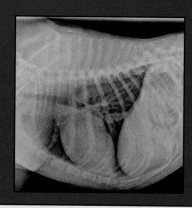

KEY TERMS

OFD
Orthogonal
Parenchyma
Positional Terminology

TECHNICAL NOTE

To preserve space, the radiographs presented in this chapter do not show collimation. For safety, always collimate so that the beam is limited to within the image receptor edges. You should see a clear border of collimation on every radiograph. In some jurisdictions it is the law.

LEARNING OBJECTIVES

When you have finished this chapter, you will be able to:

1. Properly and safely position a dog or cat for the common thoracic views with an emphasis on where to measure and center the beam, where the borders are, and how to properly position so that the body part is parallel to the image receptor and both are perpendicular to the central ray.
2. Be familiar with views that may need to be completed as an alternative.
3. Identify normal thoracic radiographic anatomy.

Thoracic radiography is a common diagnostic procedure in small animal practice, with specific indications including suspicion of heart disease, pneumonia, or neoplasia (primary or metastatic) and treatment or disease follow-up.

High-quality images require proper positioning, with emphasis on accurate centering of the x-ray beam, collimation, and appropriate patient positioning. If there is displacement of the x-ray beam or rotation of the patient, marked changes in thoracic anatomy may occur.

As with other body positions, there should be a minimum of two orthogonal views: either a lateral view or a VD/DV view. If pneumonia is suspected, both lateral views (a right and left) are recommended in addition to a ventrodorsal view. If cardiac disease is suspected, either a right or left lateral, and dorsoventral views are recommended. For a metastasis examination, both lateral views (right and left) and a ventrodorsal or dorsoventral view are recommended. On rare occasions, a further view to consider is the dorsoventral or ventrodorsal oblique view, made at 20 to 30 degrees from center. This angle moves the area of interest away from the spine or cardiac shadow and may help identify rib lesions or pulmonary lesions in the hilar region.

The protocol and patient preparation are the same for both dogs and cats (Figure 19-1). Make sure the patient has a clean, dry hair coat, and remove collars or leashes. A thick hair coat, especially the matted hair of cats, can cause prominent artifacts. Animals are best sedated or anesthetized to avoid manual restraint.

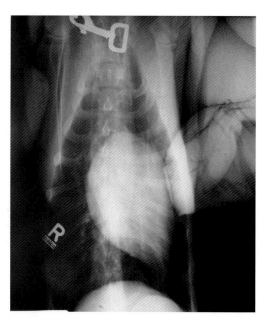

FIGURE 19-1 Make sure the patient has a clean, dry hair coat, and remove collars or leashes. Artifacts on this radiograph include the marker, sandbags, and leash clip.

Radiographic Concerns

- Because of the massive shoulder muscles, use the heel effect to advantage by having the thickest part toward the cathode.
- The thorax is best imaged radiographically with a long contrast scale, obtained with higher kilovoltage peak (kVp) and lower milliampere-seconds (mAs). Once the mAs has been determined, use the highest mA and shortest time possible to minimize respiratory motion artifacts.
- Underexposure may lead to an incorrect diagnosis of interstitial opacification.
- Overexposure or images taken with oversaturated digital systems can hide subtle lung lesions or lead to false diagnosis of pneumothorax.
- Grids may not be required until thorax measurement exceeds 15 cm.
- If a mediastinal mass or pleural fluid is suspected, increase the kVp exposure by 10% to 15%.
- The full lung field needs to be included, from the cranial thoracic inlet to the most caudodorsal lung field.
- If a dog is too large to allow full inclusion of the lung field on one image, each view may have to be divided into cranial and caudal sections.
- Exposure should be taken at peak inspiration to maximize lung contrast by increasing aeration of the lung field. There is also greater separation of the cardiac silhouette and diaphragm at peak inspiration, especially in the lateral view.
- Panting is not uncommon. Holding the patient's mouth shut as the pre-exposure button is depressed and then releasing at the time of exposure, may assist in having the dog take a deep breath.
- Sedated and overweight animals often do not ventilate as fully as nonsedated animals, leading to possible misinterpretation of an alveolar pattern or interstitial pattern.
- If the patient is connected to the anesthetic machine, positive ventilation can be applied to synchronize inspiration with the exposure time.
- Because of the increased opacity of the dependent lateral lung, the lateral view appears more opaque than the VD/DV views.
- Keep in mind that any image is only an instantaneous picture of the thorax a particular point in time.

> **TECHNICIAN NOTES** Always measure the animal in the position in which it is to be imaged.

> **TECHNICIAN NOTES** Strategically used positioning aids give the patient the *illusion* that it is being held. A sandbag over the neck and limbs, and/or the use of tape is essential if the patient is not properly sedated. Keep talking to it in a low, calm voice.

Positions

Table 19-1 lists the protocol for thoracic radiography.

Lateral Thorax

> *TECHNICIAN NOTES* The thorax is inside the rib cage, so include the full rib cage on the image.

Personal preference dictates the lateral view used. Most right-handed imagers prefer that the patient be lying on its right side, producing a right lateral view. Technically the correct terminology is left-right lateral view if one considers "point of entrance to point of exit"; however, this term is not generally used (Figures 19-2 and 19-3).

The left lateral can be taken in addition to or instead of the right lateral. A left lateral view makes distinguishing between right and left cranial lobe pulmonary vessels as well as determining relative vessel size, easier (Figures 19-5 and 19-6).

Lesions are best identified if they are away from the image receptor both because of the aeration of the upper lobes, which helps enhance contrast, and because of the slight magnification with the increased object-film distance (OFD).

Radiographs should be taken at maximum inspiration. However, radiographs taking during expiration may aid in detection of small amounts of pleural fluid or pneumothorax as well as in the diagnosis of tracheal or bronchial collapse.[1]

Positioning

Place in: Right to left lateral recumbency.

Head: Keep in a natural position. Hold appropriately with a sandbag over the neck so as not to restrict breathing.

Forelimbs: Pull as far cranially as possible without rotating the thorax. Place a small foam pad between the forelimbs to help eliminate rotation of the thorax, and support with a sandbag.

Hind Limbs: Pull together caudally; place a small foam pad between the limbs if needed, and support with a sandbag.

Sternum: Elevate with wedged foam pads so it is at the same plane as the thoracic vertebrae to eliminate rotation.

MEASURE: Caudal border of the scapula over the thoracolumbar (TL) spine.

CENTRAL RAY: At the caudal border of the scapula, between the fifth and sixth ribs (at the strongest heartbeat).

BORDERS: Cranial point of the scapulohumeral articulation (thoracic inlet) to the first lumbar vertebral body.

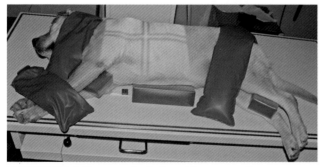

FIGURE 19-2 Positioning for the lateral thorax view. Place positioning devices appropriately to eliminate rotation of the thorax. The marker should be placed cranially and ventrally. It can be placed under the foam pad.

TABLE 19-1	Protocol for Thoracic Radiography
VIEW	**PROTOCOL**
Routine	Right and/or left lateral
	Dorsoventral or ventrodorsal
Optional	Lateral decubitus view
	Alternate lateral views with a horizontal beam:
	Standing lateral
	Lateral recumbent view
	Dorsoventral or ventrodorsal 20 to 30 degrees oblique
	Dorsoventral—thoracic inlet view
	Expiratory radiographs

Continued

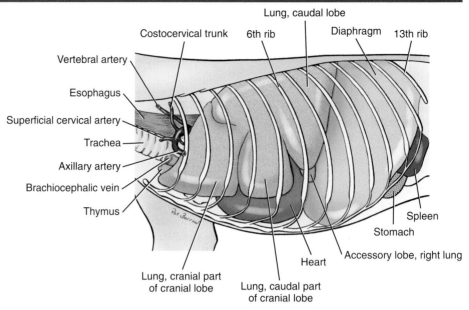

FIGURE 19-3 Diagram of the left thoracic viscera within the rib cage of this left-to-right lateral view.

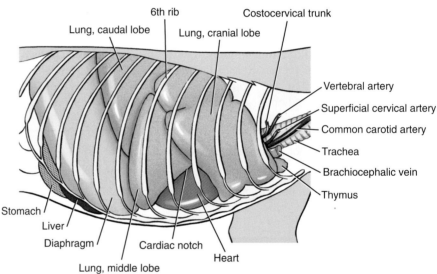

FIGURE 19-4 Diagram of the right thoracic viscera within the rib cage of this right-to-left lateral view.

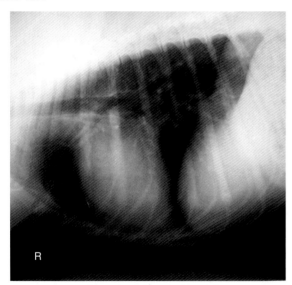

FIGURE 19-5 Radiograph of the right lateral thorax in inspiration. The thorax is inside the rib cage. In a normal average dog, the heart measured at the base, is about 2½ to 3½ times the width of an intercostal space, depending on the breed. In comparison with the left lateral view, the heart base appears more conical or oval on the right lateral view.

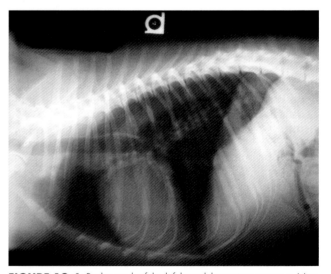

FIGURE 19-6 Radiograph of the left lateral thorax in inspiration. Note that on the left lateral view, the apex of the cardiac silhouette is displaced from the sternum, making the overall cardiac shape appear more rounded than on the right lateral view.

Lateral Thorax—cont'd

Comments and Tips

- Place any identification (ID) or markers on the ventral aspect of the abdomen near the axilla.
- Ensure that the sternum is parallel to the table and at the same level as the vertebrae, and that the beam is perpendicular to both.

- Expose immediately at full inspiration.
- The forelimbs need to be pulled as far cranially as possible to prevent any superimposition of the brachium muscles over the lung field.

> **TECHNICIAN NOTES** Inspiration is required to inflate the lungs and provide better contrast between the soft tissues of the thorax and air in the lungs.
> To obtain maximum inspiration from the patient:
> - Breathe with the patient, and depress the rotor of a two-step system at the point of either expiration or partial inspiration (depending on the patient's respiratory rate). Press the second button at maximum inspiration.
> - If the patient has an endotracheal tube (ET), squeeze the anesthetic bag or use an Ambu bag (bag valve mask).
> - If the patient is not sedated and will tolerate it, administer a puff of air in its face either by blowing or using an Ambu bag, and then watch for maximum inspiration.

> **TECHNICIAN NOTES** Quickly go through your mental check list *before* pushing the exposure button; the checklist includes but is not limited to the following items:
> - Settings correct
> - Image receptor/grid in position
> - Proper location of markers and ID (if using at this stage)
> - Correct body part and view
> - Properly centered
> - Borders correct and collimated
> - Thickest part to the cathode
> - Patient properly prepared, positioned, and restrained so the thorax will be perpendicular to the central ray and parallel to the image receptor
> - Full inspiration

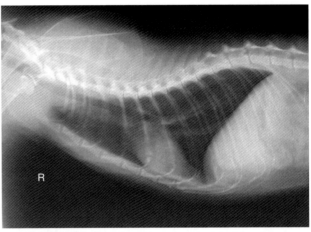

FIGURE 19-7 Right lateral radiograph of the feline thorax.

Dorsoventral Thorax

The DV thorax view is the best position for the heart, which will lie in a more natural position. The view offers better evaluation of the caudal pulmonary arteries and vein as well as the caudal lobar vessels. The DV view is also helpful for evaluating pneumothorax.[2]

Positioning

Place In: Ventral recumbency in a radiolucent V-trough if needed.

Head: Gently pull forward and carefully place a sandbag over the neck and head so it is not in the field of view. The chin can be supported on a pad to keep the cervical vertebrae at the same plane.

Forelimbs: Extend cranially. Slightly supinate the paws so that the elbows are together and the scapulae lie lateral to the lung field. Place sandbags over the limbs to maintain position.

Hind Limbs: Keep in a natural position, and sandbag.

Comments and Tips

- Place any identification or markers near the axilla in the collimated area.
- Ensure that the body is evenly positioned so that the two sides of the rib cage appear equidistant.
- Ideally, a straight line should be imagined connecting the point of the nose with the caudal midline.
- Ensure that the sternum and spine are superimposed; the central ray perpendicular to both.
- Expose immediately at full inspiration.
- If the limbs cannot be supinated, the forelimbs can be positioned with the elbows lateral to the thoracic inlet. This is easier but the scapulae will be superimposed over the lung field.

MEASURE: Over the caudal border of the scapula or at the highest point.

CENTRAL RAY: Midline at the caudal margin of the scapula or between the fifth and sixth ribs.

BORDERS: Cranial point of scapulohumeral articulation (thoracic inlet) to the first lumbar vertebral body.

> **TECHNICIAN NOTES** A common mistake is to center too far caudally. Center directly over the heart, and include cranially from the shoulder joint.

> **TECHNICIAN NOTES** Ways to determine whether the animal is properly positioned[3]:
>
> **Lateral View**
> Rib heads are superimposed
> Intervertebral foramina are the same size
> Transverse processes are superimposed
> Ribs over the heart are superimposed
>
> **DV/VD View**
> Sternum and spine are superimposed
> Ribs and thorax are symmetrical

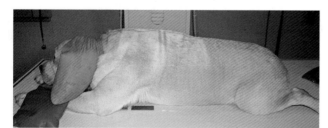

FIGURE 19-8 Positioning for the dorsoventral thorax view. This view is better than the VD for the heart, which lies in a more natural position.

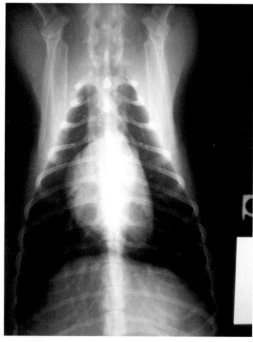

FIGURE 19-9 Dorsoventral radiograph of the thorax in inspiration. Include from the shoulder joint to the first lumbar vertebra. The right side of the heart appears more rounded than in a VD position. The diaphragm generally only has one convex shape (the cupula) projecting into the thorax in the DV.

Ventrodorsal Thorax

The VD thorax view is suggested for images of the lung, ventral pulmonary fields, caudal mediastinum, accessory lung lobes, and caudal vena cava. Changes in the descending aorta and great vessels are more noticeable in the VD than in the DV, and the accessory lung lobe is better aerated to allow for more accurate assessment of the caudal mediastinal or for accessory lobe pathology. In severely ill animals, a ventrodorsal view may cause compression of remaining functional lung fields.

Positioning

Place In: Dorsal recumbency in a radiolucent V-trough if needed.

Head: Pull gently forward. Carefully position a sandbag over the head and neck, being sure not to restrict breathing.

Forelimbs: Extend cranially with the nose between them. Secure with sandbags. If a sandbag is positioned proximal to the elbows over the limbs, the head and neck can also

MEASURE: Over the caudal border of the scapula.

CENTRAL RAY: Midline at the caudal margin of the scapula or between the fifth and sixth ribs.

BORDERS: Cranial point of the scapulohumeral articulation (thoracic inlet) to the first lumbar vertebral body.

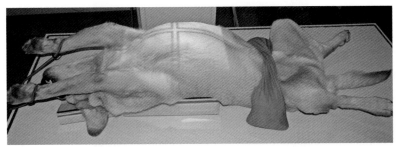

FIGURE 19-10 Positioning of the ventrodorsal thorax is generally suggested for views of the lung. The forelimbs are pulled cranially.

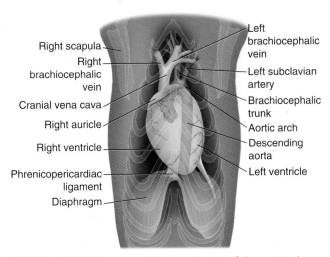

FIGURE 19-11 Diagram of the ventral view of the canine thorax showing the heart.

Right scapula
Right brachiocephalic vein
Cranial vena cava
Right auricle
Right ventricle
Phrenicopericardiac ligament
Diaphragm
Left brachiocephalic vein
Left subclavian artery
Brachiocephalic trunk
Aortic arch
Descending aorta
Left ventricle

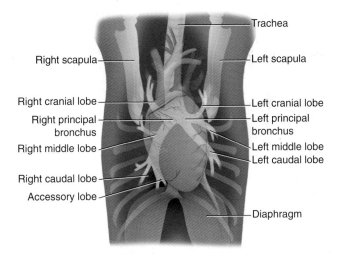

FIGURE 19-12 Diagram of the ventral view of the canine bronchial tree in the ventrodorsal position.

Right scapula
Right cranial lobe
Right principal bronchus
Right middle lobe
Right caudal lobe
Accessory lobe
Trachea
Left scapula
Left cranial lobe
Left principal bronchus
Left middle lobe
Left caudal lobe
Diaphragm

Continued

Ventrodorsal Thorax—cont'd

be held in place. An alternative is to either tie each limb separately or to place a sandbag over each limb at the carpus.

Hind Limbs: Keep the hind limbs in a natural position and support with sandbags.

Comments and Tips

- Place any identification or markers adjacent to the appropriate side of the thorax near the axilla.
- Ensure that the body is evenly positioned so that the two sides of the rib cage appear equidistant.

- Ideally a straight line should be imagined connecting the point of the nose with the caudal midline.
- Ensure that the sternum and spine are superimposed; the central ray perpendicular to both.
- Expose immediately at full inspiration.

> **TECHNICIAN NOTES** With exceptions, generally consider the DV position to image the heart and the VD position to image the lungs.

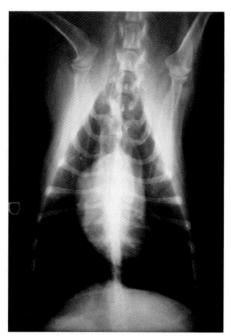

FIGURE 19-13 Ventrodorsal radiograph of the thorax in inspiration. The cardiac silhouette appears more elongated in the VD than the DV because of increased object-film distance (OFD). The cardiac apex shifts to the left laterally and dorsally.

Other Views

Lateral Decubitus View (Ventrodorsal View with Horizontal Beam)

The lateral decubitus view can be obtained to verify fluid or free air, or for a patient that would be compromised if placed in the VD or DV position. The decubitus view can be helpful if fluid is to be removed from an area to identify a mass. Sharp fluid lines will be noticed in horizontal beam radiographs only if there is a free fluid–free gas interchange.[4] Position as for lateral recumbency.

Positioning

Place In: Right lateral recumbency on a thick foam pad or equivalent (to allow the dependent portion of the thorax to be in the field of view).

Head: Keep in a natural position, and hold appropriately with a sandbag over the neck.

Forelimbs: Pull as far cranially as possible without rotating the thorax. Place a small foam pad between the forelimbs to help eliminate rotation of the thorax, and support with a sandbag.

Hind Limbs: Pull together caudally; place a small foam pad between the limbs if needed and support with a sandbag.

Sternum: Elevate with wedged foam pads so the sternum is at the same plane as the thoracic vertebrae.

Comments and Tips

- Place the image receptor vertically behind the patient.
- The position is described according to which side of the patient is closer to the table (i.e., right decubitus if it is lying on its right side).
- Place the marker ventrally near the axilla.
- The horizontal beam will be directed in a ventrodorsal direction, entering the sternum and exiting the vertebrae.
- Expose immediately at full inspiration.
- Ensure that the sternum and spine are on the same plane.
- If free air is suspected, keep the patient in position at least 5 minutes prior to exposure to allow dorsal collection of the air.[5]

> **TECHNICIAN NOTES** Collimate, ensuring that labels/markers are included and borders are visible for every image.

MEASURE: The caudal border of the scapula over the TL spine.

CENTRAL RAY: At the caudal border of the scapula, between the fifth and sixth ribs.

BORDERS: Cranial point of the scapulohumeral articulation (thoracic inlet) to the first lumbar vertebral body.

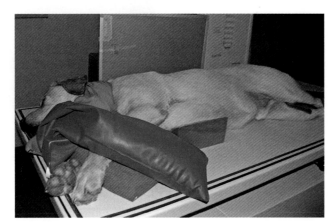

FIGURE 19-14 Positioning for the lateral decubitus view (ventrodorsal view with horizontal beam). The beam enters as for a VD. The patient is best raised with a foam pad.

Alternate Views with a Horizontal Beam

Alternative views with a horizontal beam can be used to verify the location of fluid or free air or for a patient that would be compromised if placed in a VD or DV position with a vertical beam. If free air is suspected, keep the patient in position at least 5 minutes prior to exposure to allow dorsal collection of the air.[5]

Standing Lateral View
Positioning
Have the patient in a natural standing position. There will be superimposition of the shoulder musculature over the cranial lung field. See Figure 19-15.

Comments and Tips
- Place the image receptor vertically behind and close to the patient, using a positioner if needed.
- The beam will be directed horizontally through the patient laterally.
- Expose immediately at full inspiration.
- The position is described as a standing right or left lateral, with the marker placed cranial to the axilla within the collimated area indicating the side against the image receptor.
- Use gravitational markers such as a Mitchell marker.

Dorsoventral Decubitus View
Positioning
Place In: Ventral recumbency on a thick foam pad or equivalent. Use a radiolucent V-trough if needed.

Head: Gently pull forward, and carefully place a sandbag over the neck and head so as not to impede the field of view. The chin can be supported on a pad.

Forelimbs: Extend cranially, and place sandbags over each limb for support.

Hind Limbs: Keep in a natural position, and support with a sandbag.

Comments and Tips
- Place the image receptor vertically behind the patient.
- Place the marker cranial to the axilla indicating the side closer to the image receptor within the collimated area.
- Use gravitational markers such as a Mitchell marker.
- The beam will be directed horizontally through the patient laterally.
- Expose immediately at full inspiration.
- Ensure that the body is evenly positioned so that the sternum and vertebrae are superimposed; the image receptor and central ray are perpendicular to both.
- Ideally a straight line should be imagined connecting the point of the nose with the caudal midline.

MEASURE: Caudal border of the scapula over the TL spine.

CENTRAL RAY: At the caudal border of the scapula, between the fifth and sixth ribs. Use a horizontal beam.

BORDERS: Cranial point of the scapulohumeral articulation (thoracic inlet) to the first lumbar vertebral body.

> **TECHNICIAN NOTES** For the dorsoventral decubitus view, position as for the dorsoventral view. Use a horizontal beam directed to the vertically placed image receptor for this alternative lateral view.

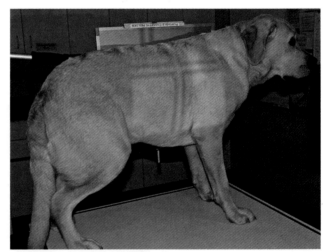

FIGURE 19-15 Positioning for a standing lateral view with a horizontal beam and the use of a portable cassette holder.

Dorsoventral Thoracic Inlet View[5]

To see the thoracic inlet without superimposition of the shoulder musculature. This position can be used for contrast studies of the esophagus to note the thoracic inlet.

Positioning

Place In: Ventral recumbency in a radiolucent V-trough if needed.

Forelimbs: Extend cranially in a natural position and place a sandbag over the limbs.

Hind Limbs: Keep in a natural flexed position.

Head: Hyperextend the head so that the nose is pointing up and caudal; secure with tape to keep in position.

Comments and Tips

- Place any identification or markers in the collimated area.
- Ensure the body is evenly positioned so that the both sides of the ribcage appear equidistant.
- Ensure that the sternum and spine are superimposed.
- Expose at expiration.
- The imaging technique should be decreased because of decreased tissue density.

MEASURE: Place the calipers between the ventral thoracic inlet and sternum just caudal to the limbs.

CENTRAL RAY: Over the thoracic inlet at a 45-degree craniocaudal angle. The beam will be directed ventrally to the neck.

BORDERS: Cranial point of the scapulohumeral articulation (thoracic inlet) to the caudal border of the scapula.

Patient Positioning Changes and Anatomy Concerns

A change in patient position as well as the phase of respiration does change the radiographic appearance (Figures 19-16 and 19-17, Table 19-2). These changes are more prominent in medium and larger dogs and less so in cats and small dogs.

Normal Thoracic Anatomy

The four basic anatomic regions of the thorax are generally considered to be the extrathoracic region, the pleural space, the pulmonary parenchyma, and the mediastinum, including the heart and great vessels.

Extrathoracic Structures

The extrathoracic region encompasses the thoracic skeleton, soft tissue of the thoracic wall, and diaphragm, and includes the following structures: sternum, vertebral bodies, ribs, costochondral junction, shoulder joints, humerus, scapula, crura and cupula of the diaphragm, diaphragm and cranial abdomen.

Supporting Structures

The thoracic wall is composed of skin, fat, subcutaneous and intercostal muscle, parietal pleura, blood vessels, nerves, and lymphocytes. The chest wall is formed by the rib cage. The dog generally has 13 pair of ribs, 9 of which are sterna.[6] Asymmetry is not abnormal as is the occasional finding of 12 or 14 pairs of ribs. On a lateral radiograph the first 3 or 4 ribs are almost vertical, and the remaining ribs slope increasingly caudoventrally from the rib head to the costochondral junction in the mid- to caudal thoracic spine. On

a DV/VD view, the first few ribs appear perpendicular to the spine.

The ribs themselves are relatively narrow, with wider intercostal muscles between them, and are lined internally by the parietal pleura. Costal cartilages (Figure 19-19) at first continue in the same direction as the bony ribs but then bend forward almost at right angles to form the rib "knees." The costal cartilages of an immature animal are radiolucent. As an animal ages, variable degrees of calcification of the costal cartilages and the costochondral junctions occur. Chondrodystrophic breeds, such as the Dachshund, Corgi, Pekingese, Lhasa Apso, and Beagle, show prominent and enlarged costochondral junctions.

The wall is supported by 9 sternebral segments and intersternebral disc spaces ventrally. The elongated manubrium is the most cranial sternebral segment, and the xiphoid process that extends to the level of the falciform fat is the most caudal sternebral segment.[4] The intervertebral and intersternebral discs are fibrocartilaginous joints. Costal cartilages from the first nine ribs insert at the intersternebral disc space. The remaining costal cartilages insert near the xiphoid process or on the preceding rib's costal cartilage. The costal cartilages of dogs and cats may mineralize early in life. They generally course in a caudodorsal-to-cranioventral direction from the costochondral junction to the sternum.[4]

Soft Tissues

Normally the soft tissues are homogenous in opacity.[4] Pedunculated soft tissues such as nipples, papillomas, and engorged ticks may be misdiagnosed as pulmonary modules. Marking the areas with a metal marker or barium may differentiate these artifacts. Nipple shadows are generally bilateral and within one intercostal space of each other in opposite lung fields on the DV or VD view. Folds of skin and fatty

Inspiration   **Expiration**

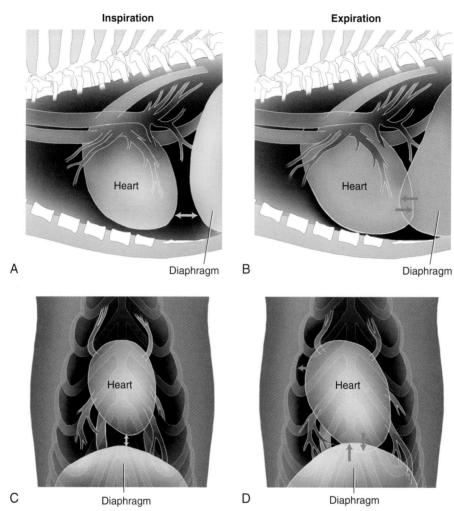

FIGURE 19-16 A, During inspiration in a lateral view, the heart appears smaller and the vessels appear more elongated. There is increased distance from the apex of the heart to the diaphragm, and less sternal contact. The intrathoracic portion of trachea widens, and the lungs appear more inflated and less radiopaque. B, During expiration, the heart appears larger and the lung lobes smaller and more radiopaque. There is increased sternal contact of the right side of the heart and superimposition of the apex over the diaphragm with dorsal elevation of the trachea. C, During inspiration in either the ventrodorsal (VD) or dorsoventral (DV) view, the heart appears smaller and the vessels appear more elongated. There is increased distance from the apex to the diaphragm. D, During expiration in either the VD or DV view, the heart appears larger. There is increased sternal contact on the right side. The diaphragm is superimposed on the caudal cardiac border. The lungs appear more radiopaque.

masses ventral to the sternum (especially noted on the lateral radiograph) also cause artifacts (Figure 19-20).

Cranially the thorax is limited at the thoracic inlet by structures such as the cervical trachea and caudal cervical vertebrae of the ventral neck region. The thoracic vertebral bodies form the dorsal part of the thoracic wall, and the forelimbs the lateral. The diaphragm is positioned caudally.

Diaphragm
The diaphragm is the muscular partition between the thoracic and abdominal cavities. It has a muscular part that divides into three sections according to where it is attached and a small V-shaped tendinous center. The right and left crura are formed from the lumbar muscle part and attached to the bodies of the third and fourth lumbar vertebrae. The

cupula attaches to the sternum and is the most cranial convex portion of the diaphragm that extends into the thorax. The intercrural cleft, along with the crura and cupula, are the only portions of the diaphragm visible on a radiograph because of the opacity of the nearby structures. The adjacent lung fields allow most of the thoracic surface to be visible.

The dependent crus will be displaced cranially to the contralateral crus while it is in lateral recumbency. Normally the crus intersects the spinal column at about T11-T13, but this position does vary with respiration by up to two vertebral body-lengths. The crura can appear to be separated by as much as $2\frac{1}{2}$ vertebral lengths if the patient is slightly rotated, or if the x-ray beam is not centered over the mid- or cranial thorax. Changing the position and the central ray also changes the appearance of the diaphragm to a single,

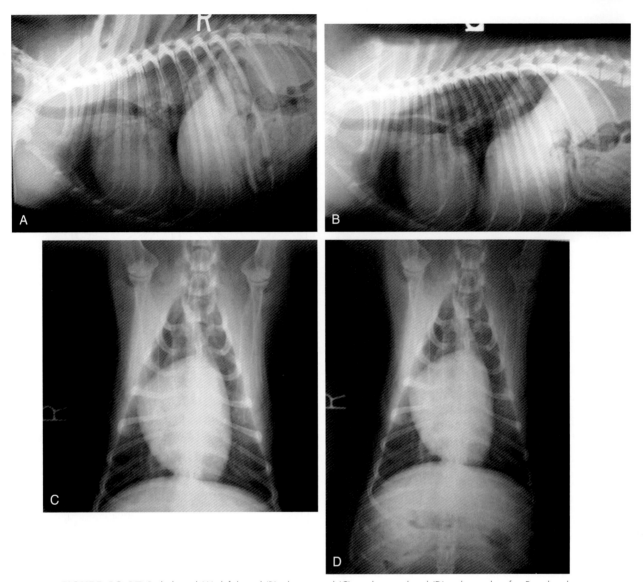

FIGURE 19-17 Right lateral (**A**), left lateral (**B**), dorsoventral (**C**), and ventrodorsal (**D**) radiographs of a Beagle taken during expiration. Note that the heart is slightly rounder in the lateral views in expiration. There is more contact with the diaphragm in all views and greater radiopacity of the lungs in these thoracic views than in corresponding views in Figures 19-5, 19-6 19-9, and 19-13 of the same Beagle in inspiration.

double or triple separately domed structure,[4] depending whether the cupula, crura, or all three structures are noted. See Table 19-2 for specific changes due to positional and respiratory changes. Feline diaphragmatic structures are not as defined because of the small thoracic size. In the DV or VD, in extreme inspiration and respiratory stress, small symmetrical projections may be seen along the thoracic diaphragmatic surface.[4]

Pleural Space

The pleura is composed of a visceral portion covering the lungs and a parietal portion lining the chest wall covering the cranial surface of the diaphragm (Figures 19-21 and 19-22). The pleural space normally contains a small amount of fluid that is not visible on a radiograph because the lungs are in contact with the parietal pleura of the chest wall. The

fluid is continually produced and absorbed, so a net accumulation does not occur. In older patients pleural thickening, especially evident on a left lateral radiograph between the right caudal and right middle lung lobes, is generally insignificant.[4]

Pulmonary Parenchyma and Lungs

Each lung is divided into lobes by the branching pattern of the principal bronchus into lobar bronchi. The principal left lung bronchus divides into a proximal common bronchus, which separates into the left cranial and left caudal lobes, and a distal bronchus which branches to the left caudal lobe, giving the radiographic appearance of three lobes on the left side (see Figure 19-3). The principal right lung bronchus divides into the right cranial, right middle, right caudal, and accessory lung lobe bronchi (see Figure 19-4).

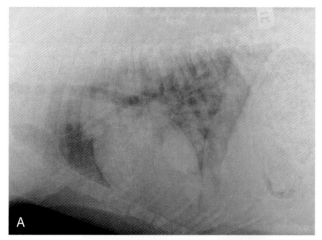

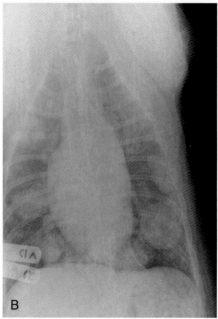

FIGURE 19-18 Right lateral (**A**) and ventrodorsal (**B**) radiographs showing metastatic lungs. At least two views are required to see the extent of the metastasis.

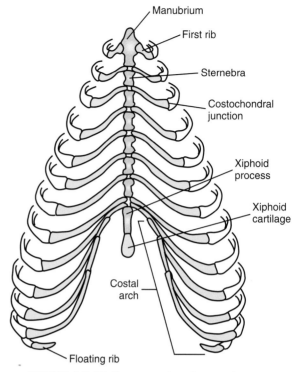

FIGURE 19-19 Canine costal cartilages and sternum.

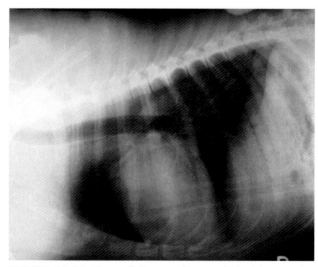

FIGURE 19-20 The parallel horizontal lines are folds of skin. Nipples, papillomas, or fatty masses can also cause artifacts.

The pulmonary parenchyma consists of three structures normally visualized on routine thoracic radiographs. They are the walls of the airways to the level of the secondary divisions of the bronchi, the pulmonary arteries and veins, and the connective tissue or lung interstitium, all of which are better visualized during inspiration.[4] Because of the difference in opacities, the pulmonary vessels are best identified in the hilar area of the lung fields. The pulmonary arteries and veins cannot be differentiated on the caudal aspect of the lateral radiograph. The bronchi are evident radiographically only if the walls are thickened or calcified. Calcification of the bronchial wall is common and insignificant in middle-aged and old dogs. It causes an increase in bronchial wall opacity but not thickness. The pulmonary vessels have a wider diameter when closest to the heart. Toward the periphery of the body, their diameter decreases and the vessels begin to branch. In general the size of the pulmonary artery

should match that of the corresponding pulmonary vein at the same level.[4]

Mediastinum

The mediastinum is the space between the lungs and is formed by the parietal pleura of the right and left hemithoraces and contains the trachea, esophagus, heart, aorta and its major branches, thoracic duct, lymph nodes, and nerves (See Figure 19-22). The mediastinum is the potential space between the right and left pleural sacs that divides the thorax into right and left sides. The

TABLE 19-2 Effect of Positional Changes and Phase of Respiration on Thoracic Radiographs

POSITION	HEART	DIAPHRAGM	OTHER	INSPIRATION	EXPIRATION
Right lateral (see Figures 19-2, 19-5, 19-7, 19-16AB, 19-17A)	More "conical" or oval—the cardiophrenic ligament prevents the heart from moving to dependent portion of pleural cavity	Diaphragmatic crura parallel to each other—the right crus will be more cranial.	May be air in the fundus of the stomach behind the left diaphragmatic crus. More difficult to assess the size of pulmonary arteries and veins because there is overlap between the right and left cranial lobe pulmonary vessels.	Heart appears smaller. Vessels appear more elongated. There is increased distance from the apex of the heart to the diaphragm. Less sternal cardiac contact because the lungs extend to the sternum. The lungs appear larger and more inflated. Intrathoracic portion of trachea widens and the cervical portion of the trachea narrows. The diaphragm is displaced cranially. In extreme inspiration, the diaphragm is more vertical and the shape moves from convex to straight.	Heart appears larger, and lung lobes smaller and more radiopaque. Increased sternal contact of the right side of the heart. Superimposition of apex over the diaphragm. Dorsal elevation of trachea. Intrathoracic portion of the trachea narrows, and cervical portion widens.
Left lateral (see Figure 19-4, 19-6, 19-16AB, 19-17B)	The apex of the cardiac silhouette is displaced from the sternum, making the overall cardiac shape appear more rounded	The left crus is more cranial. The right and left crura diverge from each other ventrally to dorsally (appear to cross).	The fundic portion is caudal to the left crus. Easier to determine vessel size and to distinguish between right and left cranial lobe pulmonary vessels. Caudal vena cava silhouettes with right crus, usually caudal to the left crus.	Same as for right lateral.	Same as for right lateral.

Continued

TABLE 19-2	Effect of Positional Changes and Phase of Respiration on Thoracic Radiographs—cont'd			
POSITION	**HEART**	**DIAPHRAGM**	**OTHER**	**INSPIRATION**	**EXPIRATION**
Dorsoventral (DV) (see Figures 19-9, 19-16CD, 19-17C,)	Cardiac shape more oval owing to upright position. Cardiac silhouette often displaced to the left by the cranially displaced diaphragm (left side looks almost straight). The cranial and right borders are rounded—appearance of lop-sided egg. In dogs with deep chests, the heart may appear more rounded than oval because of upright orientation.	Diaphragm displaced cranially—generally has only one convex shape (the cupula) projecting into the thorax. There are clear left and right crura with medially located cupula. Especially noted in deep-chested patients.	Better visualization of the caudal lobar pulmonary vessels and bronchi—more magnified and perpendicular to the beam. Accessory lung lobe region is less aerated owing to cranial diaphragm placement. Superimposition of cardiac silhouettes, great vessels, trachea, and esophagus.[1] Vertebrae appear more magnified.	Heart appears smaller. Vessels appear more elongated. There is increased distance from the apex to the diaphragm. DV radiographs produced during deep inspiration show the apex of the heart nearer to the midline.	Heart appears larger. Increased sternal contact on the right side. The diaphragm superimposes the caudal cardiac border. The lungs appear more radiopaque.
Ventrodorsal (VD) (see Figures 19-13, 19-16CD, 19-17D)	The cardiac silhouette is more elongated (increased OFD). Minor changes in size and shape not as accurate in VD because of magnification. Cardiac apex shifts to the left laterally and dorsally. In dogs with deep and narrow chests, the heart may appear more rounded than oval because of upright orientation (see Figure 19-13).	Right and left diaphragmatic crura and the cupula project into the thorax.	Changes of descending aorta and great vessels are more noticeable. Accessory lung lobe region is better aerated and is elongated between the cardiac silhouette and diaphragm. Pulmonary arteries sometimes superimposed over the heart.	Same as for DV.	Same as for DV.

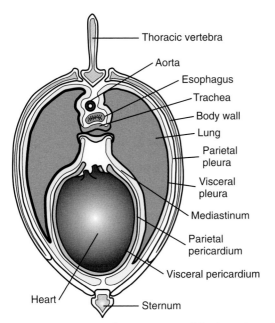

FIGURE 19-21 Diagram of a cross section of the thorax through the heart, showing contents.

Labels in figure:
- Thoracic vertebra
- Aorta
- Esophagus
- Trachea
- Body wall
- Lung
- Parietal pleura
- Visceral pleura
- Mediastinum
- Parietal pericardium
- Visceral pericardium
- Heart
- Sternum

mediastinum can be divided into cranial, middle, and caudal parts. It can also be divided dorsally and ventrally by a dorsal plane through the tracheal bifurcation. The cranial portion is wider dorsally and is that part lying cranial to the heart that includes the trachea as well as a number of soft tissue structures that cannot be distinguished from one another because of silhouetting. Most of the cranial mediastinum is superimposed on the spine in VD/DV views.

Heart and Cardiac Silhouette

The heart occupies two thirds of the middle mediastinum. The caudal vena cava ventrally and the descending aorta dorsally, are the prominent features of the caudal mediastinum. The esophagus and other structures of the dorsal middle mediastinum are not normally evident on the radiograph[4] (Figure 19-23). The cardiac silhouette is composed of the pericardium, great vessels (ascending aorta, aortic arch, and main pulmonary artery), heart, and the blood within the heart (Figure 19-24). Because the tissues are homogenous (appear gray on the radiograph), differentiation between the tissues requires the use of contrast media or imaging with alternative modalities.

For evaluation of the cardiac silhouette, thoracic conformation and other factors need to be considered. In dogs, the heart is generally located between the third rib and the sixth intercostal space (which corresponds to the most cranial attachment of the diaphragm). Empirically, if the normal heart is measured in a lateral position at the largest diameter (usually the base), it is found to be about 3 to 3½ times the width of an intercostal space. This relationship does vary with differences in thoracic conformation, age, whether the heart is in systole or diastole on the image, and phases of

respiration, among other factors. In deep narrow chested dogs, the heart appears more vertical and narrower, and is about 2½ intercostal spaces, whereas in shallow wide chested dogs, the heart appears more rounded, with more sternal contact, and measures about 3½ intercostal spaces in width. The right side of the heart appears enlarged and more rounded with the apex directed toward the left.

In cats, the maximum diameter of the heart is two to three times that of the intercostal space. The cardiac silhouette extends from the third or fourth rib to the sixth or seventh rib. The long axis of the heart forms more of an acute angle with the sternum, resulting in more sternal contact than in dogs. As a cat ages the cardiac silhouette becomes more horizontal.

Excessive fat accumulation around the heart in both dogs and cats can result in a double silhouette appearance, with the cardiac silhouette being found within the fat-expanded silhouette.[4] Fluid or tissue in the pericardial space or the mediastinum immediately adjacent to the heart also contributes to the overall size and shape of the cardiac silhouette.[4]

A rule of thumb is that the base-to-apex length of the cardiac silhouette on the lateral radiograph is usually 60% of the DV height of the thoracic cavity.[4] Another system of cardiac measurement to account for differences in breeds has been developed. Known as the *vertebral heart scale method of evaluation*, it determines heart size by measuring the lengths of the long and short axes of the heart and scales them against the lengths of the vertebral bodies that lie dorsal to the heart beginning with T4. Refer to the reference for a further description (Figure 19-25).[7]

Another method to help determine abnormalities of the heart and vessels, is to consider superimposing the face of a clock on the cardiac silhouette (Figure 19-26). In the cat, the left atrium forms the heart border from 2 o'clock to 3 o'clock. In the dog, the left atrium is not visible in this area and does not make up the heart border. The left ventricle forms the left heart border from 2 o'clock to 5 o'clock in the dog and from 3 o'clock to 5 o'clock in the cat. The main pulmonary artery makes up the heart border but is not normally seen as a separate structure. When evident, it is noted on the VD or DV views at the 1 o'clock position.[3]

Vessels

The aorta arises from the base of the heart between the pulmonary trunk to the left and the right atrium (See Figures 19-23 and 19-24). It passes to the right, first craniodorsally and then, arches dorsally and follows the vertebrae toward the diaphragm.[6] On the lateral radiograph, the predominant arch is noted. The aortic arch is not visible within the cranial mediastinum at the cranial heart border. The descending aorta is superimposed over the heart extending caudally and medially. The left lateral border of the aorta can be seen to the left of the adjoining vertebral columns.

The cranial vena cava passes ventral to the trachea, to the right of the brachiocephalic trunk and is in contact with the esophagus on the left side (See Figure 19-11).

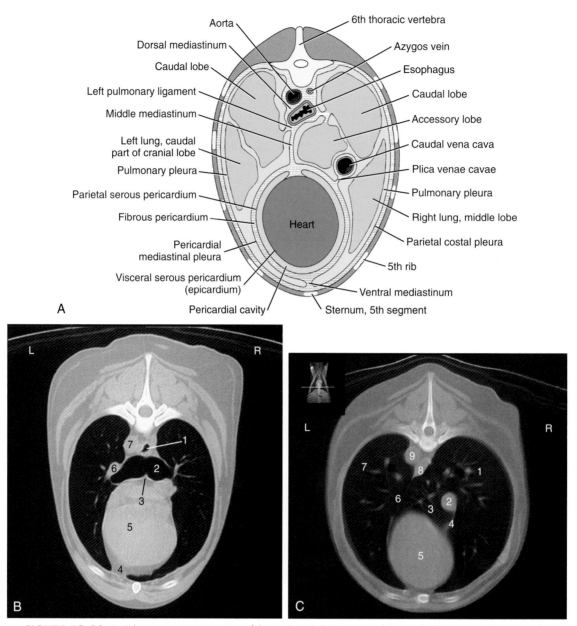

FIGURE 19-22 A, Schematic transverse section of thorax through the heart, caudal view. **B,** Computerized tomography (CT) scan at mid-thorax. 1, Esophagus; 2, right principal bronchus; 3, carina of trachea; 4, ventral mediastinum–phrenicopericardial ligament; 5, heart; 6, left pulmonary artery; 7, aorta. **C,** CT scan at caudal thorax. 1, Right caudal lobe; 2, caudal vena cava; 3, accessory lobe; 4, plica venae cavae; 5, heart; 6, caudal mediastinum; 7, left caudal lobe; 8, esophagus; 9, aorta.

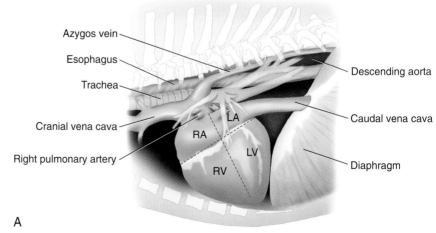

FIGURE 19-23 Anatomy of the canine heart and vessels A.

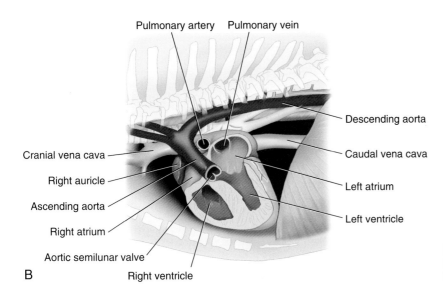

Pulmonary artery   Pulmonary vein

Descending aorta

Cranial vena cava

Caudal vena cava

Right auricle

Left atrium

Ascending aorta

Left ventricle

Right atrium

Aortic semilunar valve

B

Right ventricle

FIGURE 19-23, cont'd Left- to right-lateral view B. Right to left lateral view A, atrium; L, left; R, right; V, ventricle.

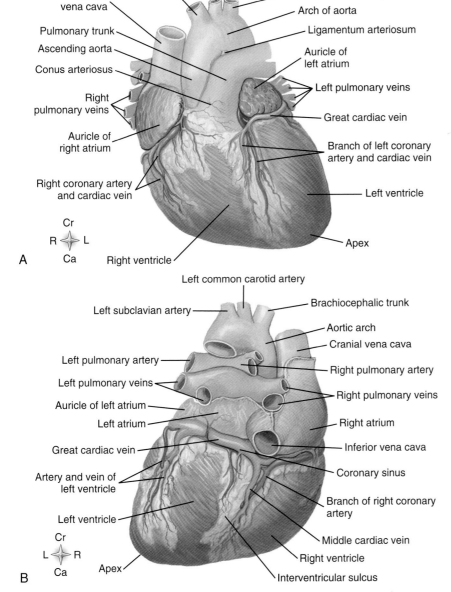

Left common carotid artery

Brachiocephalic trunk

Cranial vena cava

Left subclavian artery

Arch of aorta

Pulmonary trunk

Ligamentum arteriosum

Ascending aorta

Conus arteriosus

Auricle of left atrium

Right pulmonary veins

Left pulmonary veins

Great cardiac vein

Auricle of right atrium

Branch of left coronary artery and cardiac vein

Right coronary artery and cardiac vein

Left ventricle

Cr

R ✦ L

Ca

Apex

A   Right ventricle

Left common carotid artery

Left subclavian artery

Brachiocephalic trunk

Aortic arch

Cranial vena cava

Left pulmonary artery

Right pulmonary artery

Left pulmonary veins

Right pulmonary veins

Auricle of left atrium

Left atrium

Right atrium

Great cardiac vein

Inferior vena cava

Artery and vein of left ventricle

Coronary sinus

Branch of right coronary artery

Left ventricle

Cr

L ✦ R

Ca

Middle cardiac vein

Apex   Right ventricle

B   Interventricular sulcus

FIGURE 19-24 Diagrams of the heart and great vessels. **A,** Ventral view. **B,** Dorsal view.

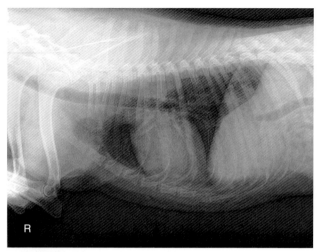

FIGURE 19-25 Heart size can be measured with use of the vertebral heart scale, which measures the lengths of the long and short axes of the heart and scales them against the length of the vertebral bodies that lie dorsal to the heart beginning with T4. In this image, the vertebral heart scale is 19.5[7].

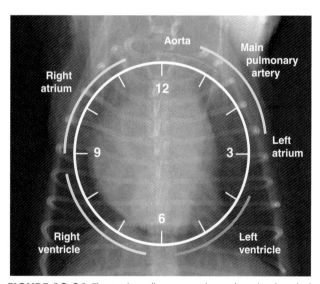

FIGURE 19-26 The cardiac silhouette can be evaluated with a clock face analogy.

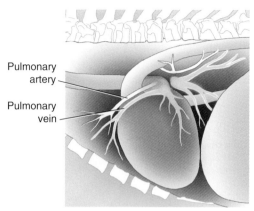

FIGURE 19-27 In the lateral radiographic projection of the normal canine thorax, it is difficult to differentiate pulmonary arteries from the veins. The artery is always dorsal to the vein in the cranial lung lobes.

Lateral View of the Mediastinum

The heart can be divided by drawing two lines perpendicular to each other (see Figure 19-23A). There is a cranial waist at the junction of the cranial vena cava and the right atrium, and a caudal waist at the atrioventricular groove, at the junction of the left atrium and left ventricle. Regardless of the recumbent position of the patient, the right atria and ventricles are always positioned more cranially then the left.

The aorta is seen superimposed over the right atrium, with the aortic arch extending caudodorsally to form the descending aorta. The main pulmonary artery is not visible on the lateral view, but the right pulmonary artery is often viewed on end as it leaves the main pulmonary artery just ventral to the carina. The pulmonary veins are most visible caudal to the heart apex as they enter the left atrium.[1] In lateral projections of the cranial lobe, the bronchus separates the arteries and veins. The arteries are dorsal and the veins ventral to the bronchus. The right cranial lobar artery and vein are best seen in left lateral recumbency, because the contralateral right lung is better inflated. Right lateral recumbency causes more superimposition of the right and left pairs of cranial lobe vessels.[4]

Dorsoventral/Ventrodorsal Views of the Mediastinum

In DV/VD views, the width and length of the thoracic cavity are increased, as indicated by placement of the diaphragmatic cupola (dome) caudal to the mid-T8 vertebral body. The caudolateral lung fields are caudal to T10. If there is collapse of the intrathoracic trachea, the exposure should be made at expiration.

In DV/VD views in the cat, the left atrium, left ventricle, right ventricle, and right atrium, form the cardiac border. In the dog, the main pulmonary artery forms the portion of the heart instead of the left atrium, because the latter is not visible in this view.[1] The normal heart at its widest point is about two thirds the width of the thoracic cavity, although this does vary with chest confirmation, age, systole or diastole, and phase of respiration, among other factors. Another

The caudal vena cava is variable in size, depending on the cardiac cycle and the phase of respiration. It spans the gap between the right atrium and the diaphragm and provides a very conspicuous feature on lateral radiographs.

The pulmonary arteries are sometimes seen superimposed over the heart originating from the main pulmonary artery. In DV/VD views, the left pulmonary artery extends beyond the heart at about 4 o'clock, and the right pulmonary artery is found at about 8 o'clock. The respective pulmonary veins enter the left atrium over the heart base medial to the respective pulmonary arteries. The peripheral pulmonary arteries and veins should have the same sizes and shapes (Figure 19-27).

rule of thumb is that the cardiac silhouette should not exceed 50% of the pleura-to-pleura diameter at the ninth intercostal space.[4]

The heart is found mainly in the left hemithorax on the DV especially, because of its left displacement by the cranial excursion of the diaphragm.

In both the DV and VD views, the arteries and veins are better compared in the caudal lobes. The pulmonary artery is lateral to the pulmonary vein with the associated bronchi between. There is improved pulmonary inflation in the DV view, and the caudal lobar vessels and bronchi are more perpendicular to the x-ray beam than in the VD view.

Other Structures

Esophagus, Trachea and Thymus, Larynx, and Pharynx

The esophagus enters the thoracic cavity to the left of the trachea, but in the cranial mediastinum it is found in a median position, dorsal to the trachea, although it does change position. The esophagus is generally not noted in the middle mediastinum on radiographs. Sometimes air can be seen in the esophagus, especially on a left lateral view, at the level of the base of the heart. Contrast agents such as barium allow visualization of the esophagus. See chapter 25 on contrast studies.

The air-filled trachea is found in the cranial mediastinum. The position of the trachea ventral to the esophagus at the level of the aortic arch produces a caudally open angle that is prominent on lateral radiographs.[6] In DV or VD radiographs the trachea is normally located to the right of the midline and typically enters the thoracic inlet, at or just to the right of, midline.[4]

The tracheal rings are cartilaginous and radiolucent in a young animal but do calcify as an animal ages. At the hilum, dorsal to the heart base, the trachea bifurcates into the right and left bronchi.

At the third rib, the trachea is generally considered to be about three times the diameter of that rib; alternatively, the height of the trachea should be half that of the thoracic inlet.[6]

In dogs less than a year old, the thymus can be seen in the ventral portion of the cranial mediastinum in both the DV and VD radiographic views. It is situated between the left and right cranial lung lobes and stretches from the thoracic inlet to the pericardium. When visualized, the thymus is usually curved and triangular, like a sail, convexly extending

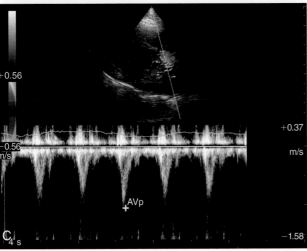

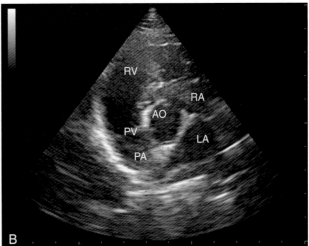

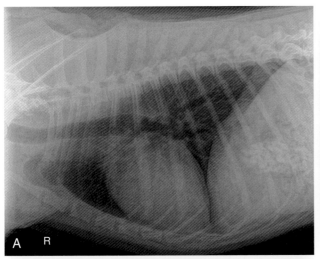

FIGURE 19-28 The heart as seen with three separate imaging modalities. **A,** Right lateral radiograph showing the heart as being relatively homogenous. A minimum of two orthogonal views is required for proper diagnosis. **B,** An ultrasound scan shows the right-sided short axis of heart chambers and vessels. Greater diagnostic information is available. *AO,* aorta; *LA,* left atrium; *PA,* pulmonary artery; *PV,* pulmonary vein; *RA,* right atrium; *RV,* right ventricle. **C,** Pulsed wave Doppler ultrasonograph (See chapter 13) evaluating blood flow across the aortic valve. There is a normal velocity across the valve (approximately 1 m/sec and a normal high resistance flow pattern). The flow of blood can be tracked:, *blue* indicates blood flowing away from the transducer, and *red* shows blood flowing toward the transducer (remember BART: blue away/red towards). Further color shows greater variances that detect abnormal blood flows.

from the midline, along the medial border of the left cranial lung lobe, into the left hemithorax.

On high-quality lateral radiographs, many laryngeal structures can be identified. On a VD view they are difficult to identify because of the overlying structures. In the lateral, the transverse basihyoid bone is generally quite evident, but because it is often projected on end, it may be mistaken for a foreign object. The pharynx is bordered by the base of the tongue and the retropharyngeal wall. It is divided by the soft palate into the nasopharynx and oropharynx, which extends to the level of the epiglottis.[4]

Figure 19-28 shows how the heart is visualized on a radiograph and two types of ultrasound images. See Chapter 13 for information on ultrasound.

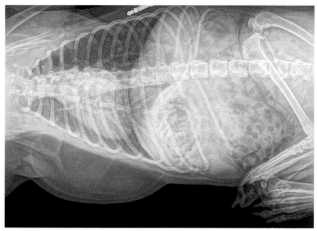

FIGURE 19-29 Mystery radiograph: What position could this patient be in? How can the position be more diagnostic?

KEY POINTS

1. Proper positioning and technique are essential for proper interpretation of thoracic images This includes where to measure and center, what to include, and how to ensure that the positioning shows proper symmetry.
2. Lateral and DV thorax views are generally completed for evaluation of the heart, whereas lateral and VD views are suggested for visualization of lung parenchyma.
3. Alternative views may be needed, depending on the suspected condition.
4. Lung lesions are best identified on a lateral view of the nondependent position(lesions in the left lung will be more noticeable in right lateral recumbency).
5. Measurement is made over the caudal border of the scapula, the central ray is over the heart, and the full rib cage should generally be included.
6. The exposure is generally taken at maximum inspiration unless the thoracic inlet is being examined.
7. A long scale of contrast, obtained by higher kVp and lower mAs, is suggested; underexposure or overexposure may lead to misdiagnosis.
8. Knowledge of normal radiography helps ensure that perfect images are presented for diagnosis.
9. A change in patient position, central ray, inaccurate positioning or phase of respiration, affects the radiographic appearance.
10. The four basic anatomic regions of the thorax are generally considered to be the extrathoracic region, the pleural space, the pulmonary parenchyma, and the mediastinum, including the heart and great vessels. Knowing the normal anatomy of these areas helps the technician take proper radiographs and, ultimately, the veterinarian make the correct diagnosis.
11. Other modalities such as ultrasound, magnetic resonance imaging (MRI), or computerized tomography (CT) are more diagnostic and may be required to properly view the thoracic anatomy or augment diagnosis of radiographically visible structures.

References

1. Owens JM, Biery DN: *Radiographic interpretation for the small animal clinician*, St. Louis, 1999, Ralston Purina.
2. Han C, Hurd C: *Practical diagnostic imaging for the veterinary technician*, St. Louis, 2005, Elsevier, Mosby.
3. Thrall DE: *Textbook of veterinary diagnostic radiology*, ed 4, St. Louis, 2002, Saunders.
4. Thrall DE: *Textbook of veterinary diagnostic radiology*, ed 5, St. Louis, 2007, Saunders.
5. Morgan JP: *Techniques of veterinary radiography*, Ames, Iowa, 1993, Iowa State University Press.
6. Dyce, KM, Sack, WO, Wensing, CJG: *Textbook of veterinary anatomy*, ed 4, St. Louis, 2010, Saunders.
7. Thrall DE: *Textbook of veterinary diagnostic radiology*, ed 5, St. Louis, 2007, Saunders. p 568.

Bibliography

Colville T, Bassert J: *Clinical anatomy and physiology for veterinary technicians*, St. Louis, 2008, Elsevier.

Done, SH, Goody PC, Stickland NC, Evans SA: *Color atlas of veterinary anatomy, the dog and cat*, London, 2009, Mosby.

Evans H, de Lahunta A: *Guide to the dissection of the dog*, ed 7, St. Louis, 2010, Saunders.

Han C, Hurd C: *Practical diagnostic imaging for the veterinary technician*, ed 3, St. Louis, 2005, Mosby.

Lavin L: *Radiography in veterinary technology*, St. Louis, 2007, Saunders.

Romich J: *An illustrated guide to veterinary medical terminology*, Clifton, NY, 2009, Delmar Cengage Learning.

Ryan G: *Radiographic positioning of small animals*, Philadelphia, 1981, Lea & Febiger.

Sirois M: *Principles and practice of veterinary technology*, ed 3, St. Louis, 2011, Mosby.

Sirois M, Anthony E, Mauragis D: *Handbook of radiographic positioning for veterinary technicians*, Clifton Park, NY, 2010, Delmar Cengage Learning.

Ticer J: *Radiographic technique in small animal practice*, Philadelphia, 1984, WB Saunders.

Tighe M, Brown M: *Mosby's comprehensive review for veterinary technicians*, ed 3, St. Louis, 2008, Mosby.

Small Animal Forelimb

How many legs does a dog have if you call the tail a leg?
Four. Calling a tail a leg doesn't make it a leg.
—Abraham Lincoln, U.S. President, 1809–1865

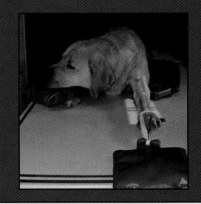

OUTLINE

LEARNING OBJECTIVES

When you have finished this chapter, you will be able to:

1. Identify the common positions and principles used to radiograph the pectoral limb.
2. Properly and safely position a dog or cat for the various common positions of the forelimb with an emphasis on where to measure and center the beam, where the borders are, and how to properly position so that the body part is parallel to the image receptor and both are perpendicular to the central ray.
3. Understand other views that may need to be completed as an alternative.
4. Distinguish and identify the normal anatomy found on a radiograph.

KEY TERMS

Caudocranial /
  craniocaudal
Flexed
Mediolateral
Oblique
Positional terminology

TECHNICAL NOTE

To preserve space, the radiographs presented in this chapter do not show collimation. For safety, always collimate so that the beam is limited to within the image receptor edges. You should see a clear border of collimation on every radiograph. In some jurisdictions, use of collimation is the law.

Imaging of the appendicular skeleton (Figure 20-1) is completed to detect fractures, pain, or lameness. A comparison with the opposite limb is often suggested in lameness of younger or older dogs. In this case a survey of both limbs from the shoulder joint to the elbow is recommended. Cats generally do not have developmental dysplasia of the bones and joints that leads to lameness; trauma is the most likely reason for imaging feline limbs.

> **TECHNICIAN NOTES**   Mentally place the patient in sternal recumbency for the distal portion of the limb and in dorsal recumbency for the proximal portion, and the positional terms will make sense.

Radiographic Concerns

In order to properly diagnose three-dimensional objects such as limbs, radiographic views that are perpendicular to each other are required. Therefore, in addition to a lateral (L) view, the patient is generally placed in dorsal recumbency to acquire a view of the proximal portion of the limb (shoulder, scapula, and humerus) or in sternal recumbency for the distal portion (elbow, radius and ulna, carpus, metacarpus, and digits) (Figure 20-2).

Along with the lateral, the common views are the caudocranial (CdCr) for the shoulder, scapulua and humerus; craniocaudal (CrCd) for the elbow, radius and ulna; and dorsopalmar (DP/DPa) for the carpus, metacarpus and digits (Table 20-1). The lateral view is relatively straightforward to image, but the CrCd/CdCr views can be challenging in dogs especially, because of the difficulty of keeping the bones parallel to the table to minimize geometric distortion. In cats, it is generally easier to obtain symmetry with CrCd/CdCr views.

Oblique positioning in both species is generally not used but may be useful for the elbow, carpus, metacarpus, or digits. The flexed view of the elbow and carpus may also be taken. If it is too painful for the patient to complete a perpendicular view to the lateral, use of a horizontal beam should be considered if the machine allows. Radiographs of the opposite limb are a valuable reference if there are any anatomical variant concerns, such as in physically immature patients.

The field of view for long bones generally includes the proximal and distal joints. For joints, the field of view is one third each of the long bones, proximal and distal to the joint. Along with ensuring that the required anatomy is included, it is also essential to achieve symmetry for proper diagnosis.

> **TECHNICIAN NOTES**   For long bones, the field of view includes the joints proximal and distal. For joints, include one third each of the bones proximal and distal.

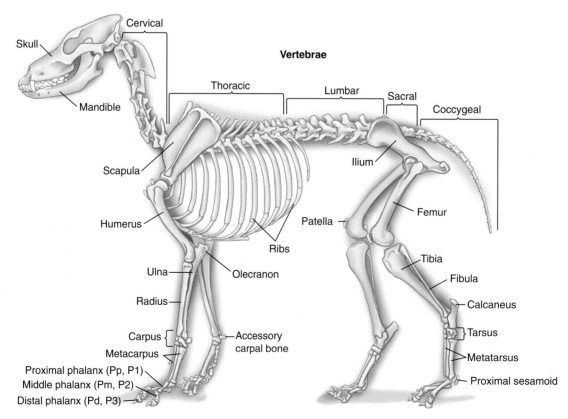

FIGURE 20-1 Canine skeleton.

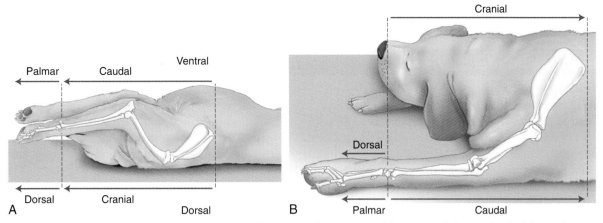

FIGURE 20-2 A, Patient in dorsal recumbency for the contralateral image of the proximal limb -scapula, shoulder, and humerus. The humerus would then be referred to as caudocranial (CdCr) in this position. The thorax is termed ventrodorsal in this view. **B,** For positioning of the distal forelimbs (elbow, radius/ulna, carpus, metacarpus, and digits), the patient is generally in sternal recumbency. Note that the terminology changes at and including the carpus. Thus in this position the elbow would be referred to as craniocaudal (CrCd) and the carpus as dorsopalmar (DP or DPa).

TABLE 20-1	Protocol for the Pectoral Limb Radiography	
ANATOMICAL LOCATION	**ROUTINE VIEWS**	**OPTIONAL VIEW(S)**
Shoulder	Lateral, caudocranial	Extended or flexed lateral
Scapula	Lateral, caudocranial	Lateral—dorsally placed
Humerus	Lateral, caudocranial	Craniocaudal
Elbow	Lateral, craniocaudal	Caudocranial (horizontal beam), extended or flexed lateral, obliques
Radius/ulna	Lateral, craniocaudal	
Foot: carpus, metacarpus, and digits	Lateral, dorsopalmar	Extended or flexed lateral, obliques

Except for the shoulder and scapula in some dogs, most projections are completed on the tabletop. A grid is not generally used because the tissue thickness of the forelimb is less than 11 cm, so it is important to collimate the field as tightly as possible to reduce scatter radiation. Doing so also helps achieve higher contrast, which is generally preferred for viewing bones.

When tabletop is used, both positions can be placed on the same image receptor if the size of the animal and body part allows. If the image receptor is split, point the toes of each view in the same direction, collimate tightly and use a lead shield to cover the side not being imaged, to prevent scatter radiation from affecting the contrast. Preparation other than having a clean hair coat is not required. Unless otherwise indicated, a vertical beam is used. Chemical restraint assists in extending the limb more fully, especially for the CdCr views. Emphasis in this book is placed on nonmanual restraint. Review the suggestions in Chapter 17 on techniques that can be used. For nonmanual restraint, it is essential to give the patient the illusion that it is being held with judicious use of sandbags, V-troughs, compression bands, tape, and so on. If splints and casts are not removed compensate with increased exposure factors. Use positioning devices in the field of view appropriately, because they may affect exposure or cause image artifacts.

> **TECHNICIAN NOTES** The label is placed at the dorsal or cranial aspect of the limb for lateral views and on the lateral aspect of the limb for the opposite views.
> Measure at the thickest part of the area to be radiographed.
> Always measure the patient in the position in which it is to be x-rayed.
> Always have the central ray at the area of interest—either the center of the bone or at the joint.
> Keep the bone parallel to the image receptor and the central ray perpendicular to both to minimize distortion.

Shoulder Joint

Lateral (Mediolateral) View

Positioning

Place In: Lateral recumbency with the affected limb down.

Head and Neck: Arch the head and neck dorsally, placing sandbags over the neck to keep the position, taking care not to restrict breathing.

Hind Limbs: Leave in a natural position and support with sandbags if needed.

Forelimbs: Pull the contralateral limb as far caudally as possible, and secure with a sandbag or tie the limb, to avoid superimposition. The affected limb should be extended downward and cranially, so it is ventral to the sternum. Support with a sandbag.

Comments and Tips

- Think of the head and limbs being in a T-shaped position—the head and contralateral limb forming the top of the T, and the affected limb its main stem.
  - The extension of the head and neck places the shoulder joint ventral to the sternum and air-filled trachea, and puts the trachea dorsal to the scapulohumeral articulation, separating the joint surfaces.
- The sternum will be slightly rotated from the thorax. Avoid overrotation of the thorax, which would place the shoulder joint in an oblique position and make evaluation of the articular surfaces of the shoulder joint difficult.[1]

MEASURE: At the level of the shoulder joint.

Extend the caliper to the point of the unaffected shoulder, but be careful not to include that limb.

CENTRAL RAY: Palpate the proximal head of the humerus and the glenoid of the scapula, and center at the scapulohumeral articulation.[5]

BORDERS: Proximal third of both the humerus and scapula.

> 📎 **TECHNICIAN NOTES**   Remember to go through your mental check list *before* pushing the exposure button. See Chapter 17.

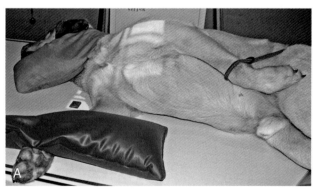

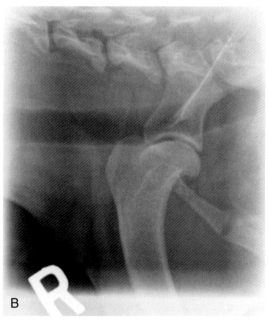

FIGURE 20-3 A, Positioning of the lateral projection of the shoulder joint and scapula. Think of the head and limbs as being in a "T"-shaped position—the head and contralateral limb form the top of the T and the affected limb the main stem of the T. **B,** Mediolateral radiograph of the shoulder joint.

Caudocranial View of the Scapula

Positioning

Place In: Dorsal recumbency in a trough or with the use of tape if needed. Foam pads can also be placed under the midthoracic and mid-abdominal regions.

Head and Neck: Push the head slightly laterally from the affected limb to avoid superimposition of the cervical spine over the joint.

Hind Limbs: Leave in a natural position and support with sandbags if needed.

Forelimbs: Tape and extend both forelimbs cranially, especially the affected limb. Use sandbags or tie the affected limb to the table, so that the humerus is almost parallel to the table.

Comments and Tips

- The patient should be maintained in a true ventrodorsal position.
- The dog's or cat's body and ribs should fall slightly away from the scapula to avoid superimposition on the scapula and to have the spine of the scapula perpendicular to the table.
- Avoid over-rotation of the humerus, which would produce an oblique shoulder joint.
- If the joints need to be compared, both can be included and the beam centered between the joints.

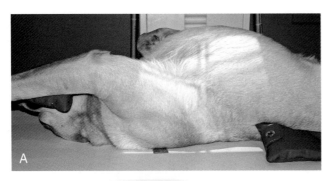

MEASURE: At the shoulder joint—at the level of the scapulohumeral articulation.
     Extend the calipers over the caudal cervical vertebral bodies but do not include the opposite limb.

CENTRAL RAY: Palpate the proximal head of the humerus and the acromion of the scapula at the center of the scapulohumeral articulation (shoulder joint).

BORDERS: Proximal third of the humerus and distal third of the scapula.

> **TECHNICIAN NOTES** Use a modified abdomen technique chart for the scapula, shoulder, and humerus. The bone chart produces images that are too dark, owing to the increased tissue measurement, and the thorax settings produce images that are too light.

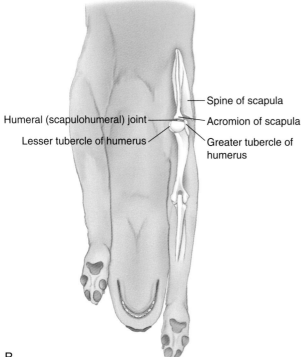

Spine of scapula
Humeral (scapulohumeral) joint
Acromion of scapula
Lesser tubercle of humerus
Greater tubercle of humerus

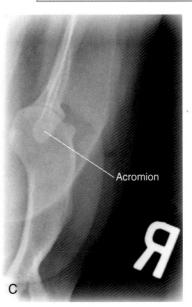

Acromion

FIGURE 20-4 A, Positioning of the caudocranial shoulder joint and scapula. B, Caudal view of the right shoulder joint and scapula. C, Caudocranial radiograph of the shoulder joint.

Scapula

Lateral (Mediolateral) View

Positioning (Figure 20-3A)

Place In: Lateral recumbency with the affected side down.

Head and Neck: Arch the head and neck dorsally, placing sandbags over the neck to keep it in position, taking care not to restrict breathing. This is like the T position as described for the scapula, with the head and contralateral limb forming the top of the T. The difference is that for this view, pressure is more forcibly applied to the affected limb to position the full scapula dorsal to the vertebral column.

Hind Limbs: Leave in a natural position and support with sandbags if needed.

Forelimbs: Pull the contralateral limb caudally and dorsally to avoid superimposition, and tie in place or use a sandbag. Grasp the affected limb below the elbow joint, keeping the joint extended so it cannot flex. Push the limb perpendicular to and dorsally toward the spine until the spinous processes can be seen bulging dorsal to the thoracic vertebral spinous processes. Use a heavy sandbag over the elbow to keep the limb in position.

Comments and Tips

- The goal is an unobstructed view positioning the scapula dorsal to the vertebral column. Pulling the opposite limb slightly rotates the thorax which further isolates the scapula dorsal to the body.
- This nonobstructed view allows good evaluation of the neck of the scapula.

Superimposition of the Scapula Over the Cranial Thorax

- If the patient is in pain or manipulation is not possible, the positioning is altered so that the affected limb is pulled caudally and ventrally; the upper limb is extended cranially.
- This places the body of the scapula over the radiolucent lung fields to allow visualization of the neck and body.

MEASURE: Dorsally at the cranial border of the scapula at about the site of the first vertebral body.

CENTRAL RAY: Center of the scapula.

BORDERS: Shoulder joint and caudal border of the scapula.

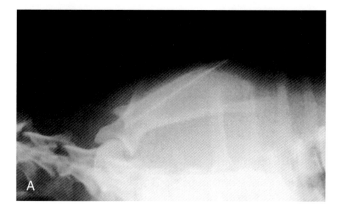

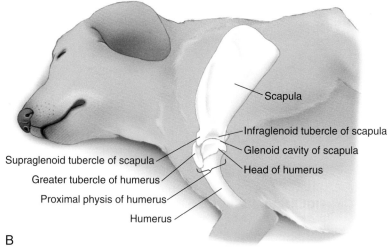

FIGURE 20-5 A, Mediolateral radiograph of the scapula, dorsal to the vertebral column. The affected limb should be pushed up more dorsally if the full scapula is to be above the thoracic spine. **B,** Medial view of the right shoulder joint and scapula.

Caudocranial View of the Scapula

Positioning

Position as for the shoulder joint. (See Figure 20-4A).

Place In: Dorsal recumbency in a trough or with the use of tape if needed.

Head and Neck: Push the head slightly laterally from the affected limb to avoid superimposition of the cervical spine over the joint. Place a sandbag over the neck if required, taking care not to restrict breathing.

Hind Limbs: Leave in a natural position and support with sandbags if needed.

Forelimbs: Tape and extend both limbs cranially, especially the affected limb. Use sandbags or tie the affected limb to the table so that the humerus is almost parallel to the table.

Comments and Tips

- Rotate the patient's sternum from the scapula about 10 to 12 degrees to avoid superimposition of the scapula and ribs, and to have the spine of the scapula perpendicular to the table.
- To find calcified bodies in the bicep brachii tendon, a skyline view of the shoulder may be required with the patient in sternal recumbency.

MEASURE: At the level of the scapulohumeral articulation so that the calipers are extended over the first thoracic vertebral body.

CENTRAL RAY: Center of the scapula.

BORDERS: Shoulder joint and caudal border of the scapula (about level of eighth rib).

TECHNICIAN NOTES Some terms relating to radiographic anatomy associated with bones[2]:

- Condyle—rounded projection on the bone for articulation with another bone.
- Diaphysis—the shaft of the long bone.
- Epicondyle—a projection of bone on the lateral edge above its condyle.
- Epiphysis—the end of the long bone, with each long bone having a distal and proximal epiphysis.
- Epiphyseal plate or growth plate—plate of cartilage at the junction of the proximal and distal epiphysis with the diaphysis that ossifies as the animal matures.
- Foramen—opening or passage into or through a bone.
- Fossa—hollow or depressed area on a bone usually filled with muscles or tendons.
- Trochlea—usually grooves in bone that allow tendons to act as pulleys.
- Tuberosity/trochanter/tubercle—protuberances on the bones usually for muscle attachment.
- A long bone is described as having a head, shaft and neck.

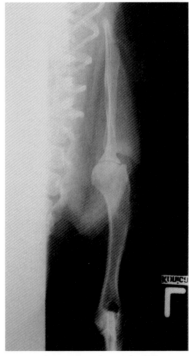

FIGURE 20-6 Caudocranial radiograph of the scapula, humerus, and shoulder joint.

Humerus

Lateral (Mediolateral) View

Positioning
Place In: Lateral recumbency with the affected limb down.
Head and Neck: Move the head and neck upwards, placing sandbags over the neck to maintain the position, taking care not to restrict breathing.
Hind Limbs: Leave in a natural position and support with sandbags if needed.
Forelimbs: Extend the contralateral limb caudally and secure it to avoid superimposition. The affected limb should be extended downward and cranially. Secure with a sandbag or tie.

Comments and Tips
* Larger dogs may require two views if there is a significant difference in tissue density between the elbow and the shoulder. Measure each area separately.

MEASURE: Toward the proximal humerus at the level of the scapulohumeral articulation (shoulder joint).

CENTRAL RAY: Midshaft of the humerus.

BORDERS: Proximal to shoulder and distal to the elbow joint.

> **TECHNICIAN NOTES** Collimate and ensure that labels/markers are included and that borders are visible for every image taken.

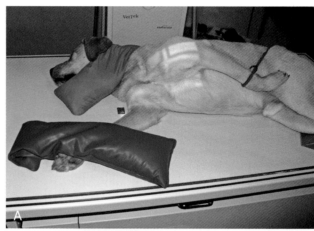

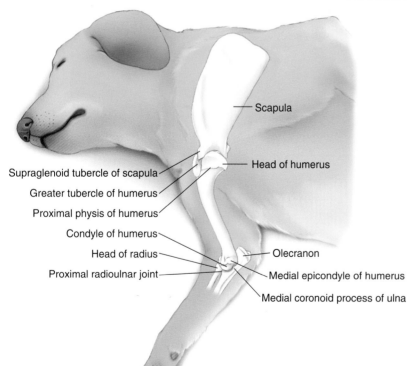

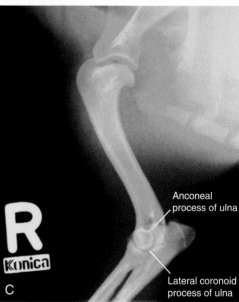

FIGURE 20-7 A, Positioning for the mediolateral view of the humerus. **B,** Medial view of the right humerus. **C,** Mediolateral radiograph of the humerus.

Scapula

Head of humerus

Supraglenoid tubercle of scapula

Greater tubercle of humerus

Proximal physis of humerus

Condyle of humerus

Head of radius

Proximal radioulnar joint

Olecranon

Medial epicondyle of humerus

Medial coronoid process of ulna

Anconeal process of ulna

Lateral coronoid process of ulna

R

Konica

Caudocranial View of the Humerus

Positioning

Place In: Dorsal recumbency in a trough or with the use of tape if needed.

Head and Neck: Keep the head and neck fairly parallel to the humerus, and secure with a sandbag if needed, taking care not to restrict breathing.

Hind Limbs: Leave in a natural position so that the spine is perpendicular to the table. Support with sandbags if needed.

Forelimbs: Tape and extend both forelimbs cranially, especially the affected limb. Use sandbags or tie the affected limb to the table, keeping the humerus almost parallel to the table.

Comments and Tips

* There is some distortion as a result of increased object-film distance (OFD). Pull the limb as cranially and as close to the image receptor as possible.

* This positioning may not be tolerated by patients with fractures or severe degenerative joint disease. Consider using a horizontal beam if required in these situations.

Horizontal Beam

* Center, measure, and include as for the caudocranial view.
* The patient is in opposite lateral recumbency with the extended affected side resting uppermost on a large sponge.
* The image receptor is positioned against the cranial aspect of the affected forelimb.
* The tube head is directed horizontally from the caudal aspect of the limb and perpendicular to the humerus and image receptor.
* In cats, it may be difficult to place the image receptor proximally enough to view the humeral head and the shoulder with a horizontal beam.

> **TECHNICIAN NOTES** Note that the actual positioning procedures are similar, with slight variations, for the lateral and caudocranial views of the scapula, shoulder, and humerus.

MEASURE: Midshaft toward proximal aspect; across at the level of T1.

CENTRAL RAY: Midshaft of the humerus.

BORDERS: Proximal to the shoulder and distal to the elbow joint.

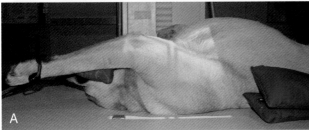

A

FIGURE 20-8 A, Positioning for the caudocranial view of the humerus. **B,** Caudal view of right canine humerus. **C,** Caudocranial radiograph of the humerus.

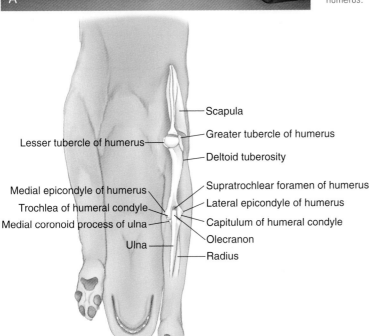

Scapula
Greater tubercle of humerus
Lesser tubercle of humerus
Deltoid tuberosity
Medial epicondyle of humerus
Supratrochlear foramen of humerus
Trochlea of humeral condyle
Lateral epicondyle of humerus
Medial coronoid process of ulna
Capitulum of humeral condyle
Ulna
Olecranon
Radius

B

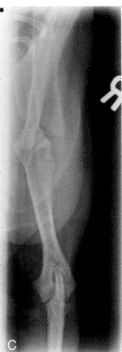

C

Craniocaudal View of the Humerus

Positioning

Place In: Dorsal recumbency in a trough or with the use of tape if needed.

Head and Neck: Keep the head and neck fairly straight, and secure with a sandbag if needed, taking care not to restrict breathing.

Hind Limbs: Leave in a natural position and support with sandbags if required.

Forelimbs: Extend the unaffected limb cranially and secure. The affected limb is flexed at the shoulder and pulled as far caudally as possible, so that the humerus is parallel to the table. Tie to the table or carefully place a sandbag over the limb. The unaffected limb is left in a natural position.

Comments and Tips

- Use the craniocaudal view when adequate extension of postoperative patients cannot be achieved for the caudocranial.
- The humerus is more nearly parallel to the table but there is increased OFD.
- Alternatively the patient can be placed in sternal recumbency with the limbs pulled forward. Extend the affected limb (Figure 20-9B).

TECHNICIAN NOTES For efficiency and ease of positioning ensure that the body parts that are not in the beam are positioned and secured first. Then position the area of interest.

MEASURE: Midshaft of the humerus toward the proximal aspect.

CENTRAL RAY: Midshaft of the humerus.

BORDERS: Proximal to the shoulder and distal to the elbow joint.

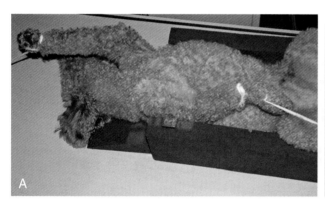
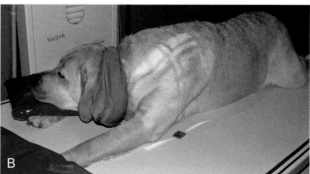

FIGURE 20-9 A, Positioning for the craniocaudal view of the humerus, in dorsal recumbency. **B,** Alternate positioning for the craniocaudal humerus view.

Elbow

Lateral (Mediolateral) Extended View

The lateral or mediolateral extended view of the elbow joint can show a fragmented process of the elbow joint.[3]

Positioning

Place In: Lateral recumbency with the affected limb down.

Head and Neck: Move dorsally, placing sandbags over the neck to keep in position, taking care not to restrict breathing.

Hind Limbs: Leave in a natural position and support with sandbags if needed.

Forelimbs: Extend the contralateral limb caudally and secure with ties or sandbag. Pull the affected limb cranially so that the elbow joint is in a 120-degree extended position. Depending on the animal, a small foam wedge can be placed under the metacarpus and/or the shoulder region.

Comments and Tips

- A small foam pad under the shoulder and distal region of the affected limb may help maintain lateral symmetry of the structures.
- A properly positioned extended elbow should show superimposition of the distal humeral condyles and a clear view of the olecranon.

TECHNICIAN NOTES Remember to always collimate as closely as possible.

MEASURE: Thickest part of the elbow at the distal humerus.

CENTRAL RAY: Palpate and center on the distal humeral condyles.

BORDERS: Proximal third of the radius/ulna to distal third of the humerus.

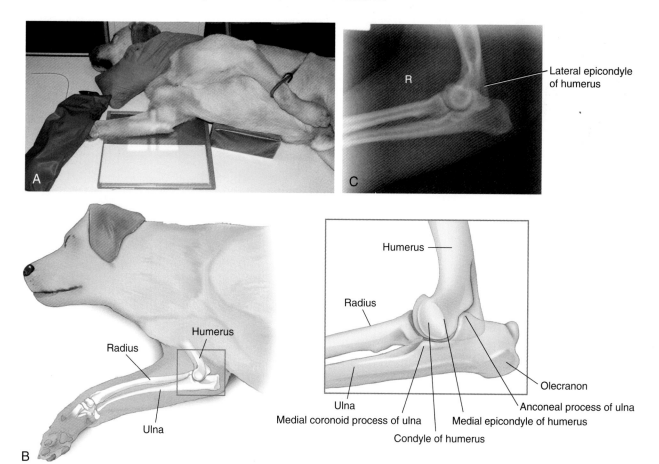

FIGURE 20-10 A, Positioning for the mediolateral view of the elbow joint. **B**, Medial view of the elbow joint. **C**, Mediolateral radiograph of the elbow joint.

Lateral Flexed (Mediolateral) View of the Elbow

The flexed 90-degree limb allows evaluation of the ulnar anconeal process and is indicated when an ununited anconeal process (failure of the anconeal process to unite with the ulna, resulting in a fracture through the growth plate) or when a fragmented coronoid or osteochondrosis, is suspected. Elbow dysplasia is seen primarily in young dogs of large breeds and can cause varying degrees of weight-bearing lameness and arthritis. Extreme flexion of the medial to lateral view is required if radiographs are being sent to the Orthopedic Foundation of Animals (OFA) for elbow dysplasia evaluation.[4]

Positioning

Place In: Lateral recumbency with the affected limb down.

Head and Neck: Move dorsally, placing sandbags over the neck to keep in position.

Hind Limbs: Leave in a natural position and support with sandbags if needed.

Forelimbs: Secure the unaffected limb caudally. Flex the affected elbow as much as possible by bending the limb dorsally and securing the paw under the head with sandbag or tape. Tape is preferred. Place tape on the metacarpal region, flex the limb, and fasten the tape on the lateral aspect of the metacarpus. Affix the tape to the table under the cranial cervical region.

Comments and Tips

- A sponge under the shoulder may prevent the flexed elbow from moving medially.
- The limb should be flat on the table in a true lateral position with no rotation.
- If the tape was secured on the medial aspect upward rotation would occur, causing the site of interest to be oblique.

> **TECHNICIAN NOTES**   Flexion assists in full examination of the joint.

MEASURE: At the distal humerus with the elbow in the flexed position.

CENTRAL RAY: Palpate and center on the humeral condyles.

BORDERS: Proximal third of radius/ulna to the distal third of the humerus.

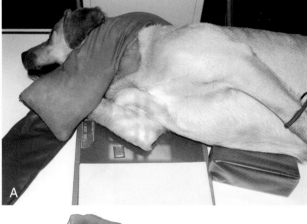

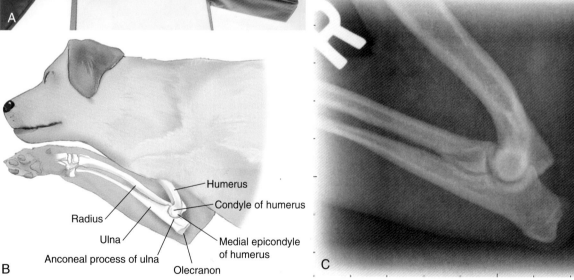

FIGURE 20-11 A, Positioning for the mediolateral flexed view of the elbow joint. **B,** Medial projection of the right flexed elbow. **C,** Mediolateral radiograph of the flexed elbow.

Craniocaudal View of the Elbow

Positioning

Place In: Sternal recumbency.

Hind Limbs: Leave in a natural position to keep the spine straight and support with sandbags if needed. A V-trough may be used for stability of the caudal portion of the body.

Forelimbs: Extend both front legs forward. Pull the unaffected limb, placing a small foam pad under the elbow to prevent rolling and rotation. Extend the affected forelimb and secure it with a sandbag at the distal portion or tie to the table or to a sandbag.

Head and Neck: Pull away from the affected limb and the beam. Support the head at a natural height with foam pads. Tape can be placed around the head to keep it out of the field of view.

MEASURE: Thickest part of the elbow at the distal humerus.

CENTRAL RAY: Palpate and center on the humeral condyles at the level of articulation.
Angle the beam distoproximally 10 to 20 degrees to visualize the joint surfaces if full extension is not possible.

BORDERS: Proximal third of the radius/ulna to distal third of the humerus.

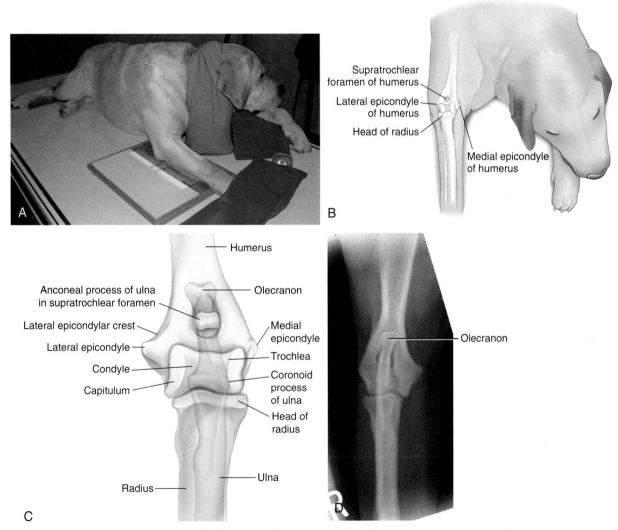

FIGURE 20-12 A, Positioning for the craniocaudal projection of the elbow joint. Putting a sponge under the opposite elbow and head helps keep the olecranon in true CrCd position. **B and C** Cranial views of the right elbow. **D,** Craniocaudal radiograph of the elbow joint.

Continued

Craniocaudal View of the Elbow —cont'd

Comments and Tips

- Symmetry is essential. Move the patient's body slightly until palpation reveals the olecranon of the ulna to be in the center of the joint. The olecranon should be positioned midway between the lateral and medial humeral epicondyles on the finished radiograph.
- The slight raising of the opposite limb helps place the olecranon between the humeral epicondyles. This keeps the radius and ulna parallel and the humerus at a slight angle to the tabletop.
- The paw of the affected limb is not flat on the table for a true craniocaudal elbow view.

Craniocaudal View with a Horizontal Beam

The CrCd elbow view could also be taken with a horizontal beam if required:

- Measure, center, and include as for the craniocaudal view:
  - **Measure:** At the distal humerus with the elbow in the flexed position.
  - **Central Ray:** Palpate and center on the humeral condyles.

- **Borders:** Proximal third of the radius/ulna to distal third of the humerus.
- The patient would be in lateral recumbency with the extended affected side uppermost, resting on a large sponge, and with the head hyperextended away from the x-ray beam.
- The image receptor is positioned against the caudal aspect of the upper forelimb.
- The tube head is directed horizontally from the cranial aspect of the limb and perpendicular to the elbow and the image receptor.

> **TECHNICIAN NOTES** For a true craniocaudal view, palpate the olecranon and make sure that it rests midway between the humeral epicondyles.

> **TECHNICIAN NOTES** Remember to place the label or marker cranial to the bone or joint for the lateral view and on the lateral aspect of the limb for the opposite views.

Oblique View of the Elbow

An oblique view may be needed to properly visualize the supratrochlear foramen of the humerus and the anconeal process of the ulna (Figure 20-13).

- Measure, center, and include as for the craniocaudal view:
  - **Measure:** At the distal humerus with the elbow in the flexed position.
  - **Central Ray:** Palpate and center on the humeral condyles.
  - **Borders:** Proximal third of the radius/ulna to distal third of the humerus.

- Support the patient and limb with foam pads and sandbags.
- Pull and support the affected limb as cranial as possible and rotate the elbow joint laterally about 30 degrees for the medial oblique (craniolateral-caudomedial oblique) view or position the olecranon towards the patient (medially) about 30 degrees for the lateral oblique (craniomedial-caudolateral oblique) view.
- Include only the structures making up the articulation.

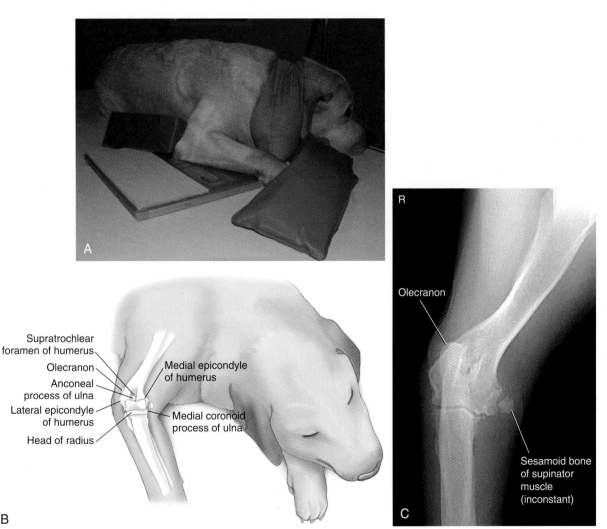

FIGURE 20-13 A, Positioning for an oblique projection of the elbow joint. This is the craniolateral-caudomedial (medial) oblique position. Ideally the limb should be pulled more cranially. **B,** Medial oblique view of the right elbow joint. **C,** Craniolateral-caudomedial (medial) oblique radiograph of the right elbow.

Radius/Ulna

Lateral (Mediolateral) View

Positioning

Positioning is the same as for the lateral extended elbow view:

Place In: Lateral recumbency with the affected limb down.

Head and Neck Move the head and neck dorsally placing sandbags over the neck to keep in position, taking care not to restrict breathing.

Hind Limbs: Leave in a natural position and support with sandbags if needed.

Forelimbs: Extend the contralateral limb caudodorsally and secure with a sandbag, or tie. Place the affected limb parallel to the edges of the image receptor or table and support with a sandbag. Slightly flex the carpus to avoid supination of the limb. Depending on the patient anatomy, a small foam wedge can be placed under either the metacarpal region or the shoulder region to keep a true lateral view of the elbow.

Comments and Tips

- Placing foam under the humerus and cranial thorax may help keep proper alignment.
- Make sure the image receptor is large enough to include both the proximal row of carpal bones and the proximal olecranon.
- If the distal portion of the radius and ulna is the area of interest, measure at the midshaft of the bone to minimize overexposure.

> **TECHNICIAN NOTES**   Note the similarity in positioning procedures for the elbow, radius and ulna, and foot.

MEASURE: Site of the distal humerus.

CENTRAL RAY: Midshaft of the radius and ulna.

BORDERS: Proximal to elbow joint and distal to carpal joint.

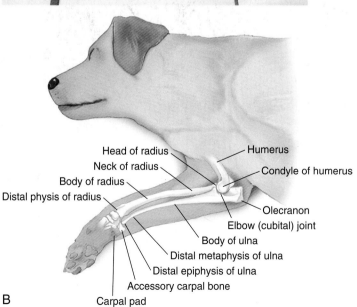

A

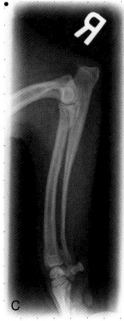

C

FIGURE 20-14 A, Positioning for the mediolateral projection of the radius and ulna. B, Medial view of the right radius and ulna. C, Mediolateral radiograph of the radius and ulna.

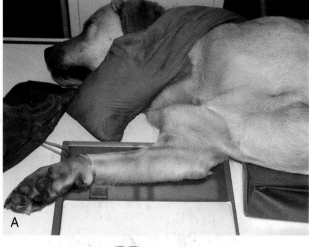

Head of radius
Neck of radius
Body of radius
Distal physis of radius
Humerus
Condyle of humerus
Olecranon
Elbow (cubital) joint
Body of ulna
Distal metaphysis of ulna
Distal epiphysis of ulna
Accessory carpal bone
Carpal pad

B

Craniocaudal View of the Radius/Ulna

Positioning

Positioning is the same as for the CrCd elbow view:

Place In: Sternal recumbency.

Head and Neck: Move away from the affected limb and beam. Support the head in a comfortable position with foam pads. Sandbags or tape can be placed around the head to keep it out of the field of view.

Hind Limbs: Leave in a natural position to keep the spine straight and support with sandbags if needed. A V-trough may be used for stability of the caudal half of the body.

Forelimbs: Place a small foam pad under the elbow of the unaffected limb to prevent rolling or rotation. Extend the affected forelimb and hold it with a sandbag or tie to the table or to a sandbag.

Comments and Tips

- Palpate to confirm that the olecranon is positioned midway between the humeral epicondyles for a true CrCd view of the radius/ulna.
- A thin foam pad placed between the point of the elbow and the image receptor may stabilize the elbow.
- Make sure that the image receptor is long enough to incorporate the carpus and elbow as well as the radius/ulna.
- If the distal portion of the radius and ulna is the area of interest, measure at the midshaft of the bone to minimize overexposure.
- A horizontal beam can also be taken to show the CrCd view of the radius and ulna (Figure 20-16).

MEASURE: Site of the distal humerus.

CENTRAL RAY: Midshaft of the radius and ulna.

BORDERS: Proximal to the elbow joint and distal to the carpal joint.

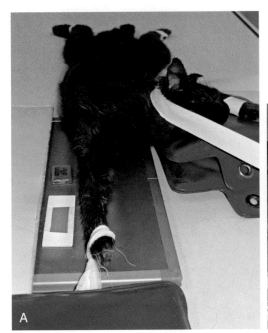
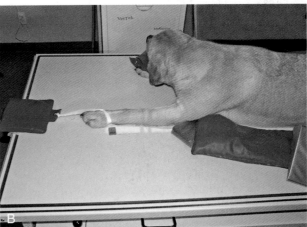

FIGURE 20-15 A, Positioning for the craniocaudal view of the feline radius and ulna. Tape can be used to keep the head out of the field of view. **B,** Positioning for the craniocaudal view of the canine radius and ulna.

Continued

Craniocaudal View of the Radius/Ulna—*cont'd*

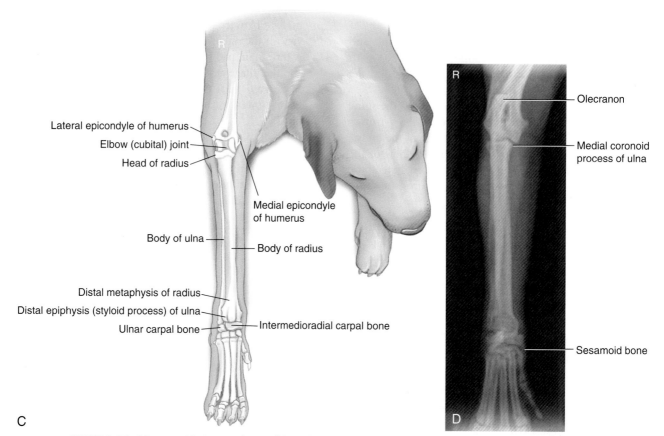

Lateral epicondyle of humerus

Elbow (cubital) joint

Head of radius

Medial epicondyle of humerus

Body of ulna

Body of radius

Distal metaphysis of radius

Distal epiphysis (styloid process) of ulna

Ulnar carpal bone

Intermedioradial carpal bone

C

Olecranon

Medial coronoid process of ulna

Sesamoid bone

D

FIGURE 20-15, cont'd C, Cranial view of the right canine radius and ulna. D, Craniocaudal radiograph of the right canine radius and ulna.

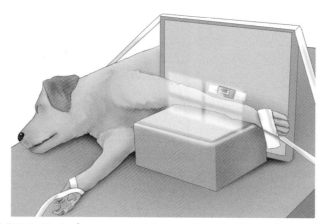

FIGURE 20-16 Positioning for a craniocaudal view of the radius/ulna utilizing a horizontal beam.

The Foot: Carpus, Metacarpus, and Digits

The carpus, metacarpus, and digits are typically radiographed in one view. If there is a particular area of interest, center and measure on this site. See Figure 20-24 for anatomy of the carpal joints of various species.

Lateral (Mediolateral) View of the Foot

Positioning

Place In: Lateral recumbency with the affected limb down.

Hind Limbs: Leave in a natural position and support with sandbags if needed.

Head and Neck: Move the head and neck dorsally, placing sandbags over the neck to keep the position, taking care not to restrict breathing.

Forelimbs: Extend the contralateral limb caudally, and secure with a sandbag. Extend the affected limb cranially, placing sandbags on the proximal portion of the limb. Tie or support the distal metacarpus to the table or a sandbag.

For the digits: Separate the digits to prevent superimposition. This is best completed by:

* Separately taping around the toenail of the lateral (fifth) phalanx and the medial (second) phalanx.
* Pull the lateral phalanx slightly cranially and laterally, and the medial phalanx slightly caudally and laterally.

Tape can also be put around the digit itself, or cotton can be placed between the toes, although the latter method does not separate the phalanges as effectively.

MEASURE: At the site of interest:
   Carpus: At the carpal joint.
   Metacarpus or phalanges: At the site of the phalangeal metacarpal articulation.

CENTRAL RAY: Centered on the area of interest:
   Carpus: Middle row of carpal bones.
   Metacarpus or phalanges: Center of the phalangeal metacarpal articulation.

BORDERS: Carpus: Proximal third of the metacarpus to distal third of the radius and ulna.
   Metacarpus or phalanges: Carpus proximally to the distal phalanges.

> **TECHNICIAN NOTES** The image receptor can be split to include both views on the image, if the grid is not used. Make sure that the toes point the same direction, collimate tightly and place a lead shield on the side not being imaged to prevent scatter radiation from affecting the contrast.

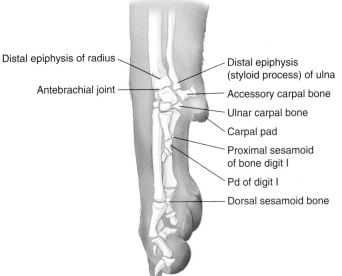

Distal epiphysis of radius
Antebrachial joint
Distal epiphysis (styloid process) of ulna
Accessory carpal bone
Ulnar carpal bone
Carpal pad
Proximal sesamoid of bone digit I
Pd of digit I
Dorsal sesamoid bone

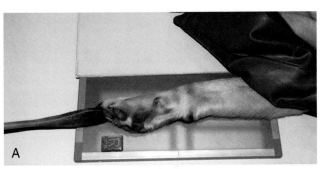

A
B

FIGURE 20-17 A, Positioning for the mediolateral projection of the canine carpus, metacarpus, and digits. Tape can also be used to secure the limb. **B,** Medial view of canine carpus, metacarpus, and digits.

Continued

Lateral (Mediolateral) View of the Foot—cont'd

Comments and Tips

- A wooden or plastic paddle supported with a sandbag can assist in positioning.
- The foot can be flexed by applying slight dorsal pressure to the digits.

For the Hyperextended Lateral View of the Foot[5]

- Hyperextend the carpus by bending the toes upwards
- Apply tape at the radius and ulna, and secure to the table laterally (Figure 20-18).

- Apply tape at the distal metacarpus/digits; extend the limb and secure the tape in the opposite direction of the tape on the radius/ulna.
- A wooden spoon can also be used to extend the toes anteriorly, provided that lateral counter-pressure is placed on the radius/ulna.
- This view helps determine distribution of joint involvement and lesions that might not be visible if the joint is not stressed.

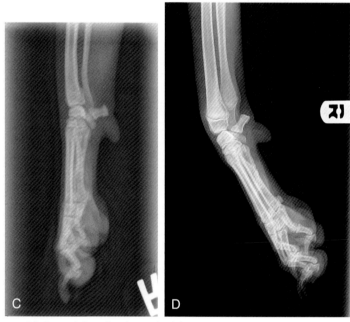

FIGURE 20-17, cont'd C, Mediolateral radiograph of the canine, metacarpus and digits. D, Flexed lateral radiograph of the carpus when pressure is applied to the dorsal surface of the digits.

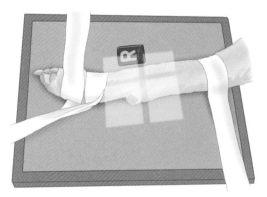

FIGURE 20-18 Position for the hyperextended lateral view of the carpus.

Lateral (Mediolateral) Hyperflexed View of the Carpus

Positioning

Place In: Lateral recumbency with the affected limb down.

Head and Neck: Move dorsally, placing sandbags over the neck to keep it in position, taking care not to restrict breathing.

Hind Limbs: Leave in a natural position and support with sandbags if needed.

Forelimbs: Extend the contralateral limb caudally, and secure with a sandbag. Extend the affected limb and hyperflex the carpus, by either:

- Taping a figure eight pattern around the metacarpus and radius and ulna (best).

- Keeping the carpus flexed by (1) bending the toes caudally toward the radius and ulna, (2) pushing a wooden or plastic paddle at the phalanges, and (3) securing with a sandbag.

Comments and Tips

- Do not extend the carpus beyond the patient's available range of motion.
- This position helps evaluate the carpal articulation when joint laxity is noted.

MEASURE: At the carpus joint while in the flexed position.

CENTRAL RAY: On the middle row of carpal bones.

BORDERS: Proximal third of the metacarpus, including the digits if desired, to distal third of the radius/ulna.

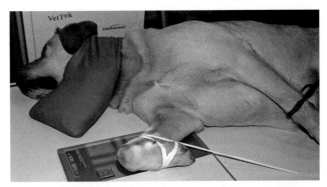

FIGURE 20-19 Positioning for the flexed mediolateral projection of the canine carpus, metacarpus, and digits.

Dorsopalmar View of the Foot

Positioning

Place In: Sternal recumbency.

Head and Neck: Displace and support the head laterally with foam pads, sandbags, or tape away from the affected limb and the beam.

Hind Limbs: Extend in a natural position to keep the spine straight and support with sandbags if needed. A V-trough may be used for stability of the caudal half of the body.

Forelimbs: Extend both forward. Secure the affected forelimb with a sandbag at the proximal portion. Tie the metacarpus/digits at the distal portion and secure the limb to a sandbag.

Comments and Tips

- Abduct the affected elbow slightly to straighten the carpus.
- If joint laxity of the carpus is present and evaluation of the joint space is required, stress can be put on the carpus if tape is applied to the midradius/ulna and the distal metacarpus. Pull in opposite directions, as for the extended lateral view of the carpus. (Figure 20-21).[6]

MEASURE: At the site of interest:

Carpus: Carpus joint.

Metacarpus or phalanges: Site of the phalangeal metacarpal articulation at the level of the middle phalanx.

CENTRAL RAY: Centered on the area of interest:

Carpus: Middle row of carpal bones.

Phalanges—third and fourth phalangeal metacarpal articulations.

BORDERS: Carpus: Proximal third of the metacarpals to distal third of the radius/ulna.

Metacarpus or phalanges: Carpus proximally to the distal phalanges.

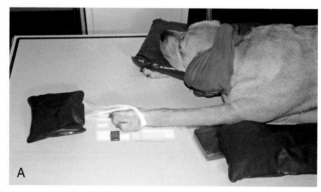

FIGURE 20-20 A, Positioning for the dorsopalmar projection of the canine carpus, metacarpus, and digits.

Dorsopalmar View of the Foot—*cont'd*

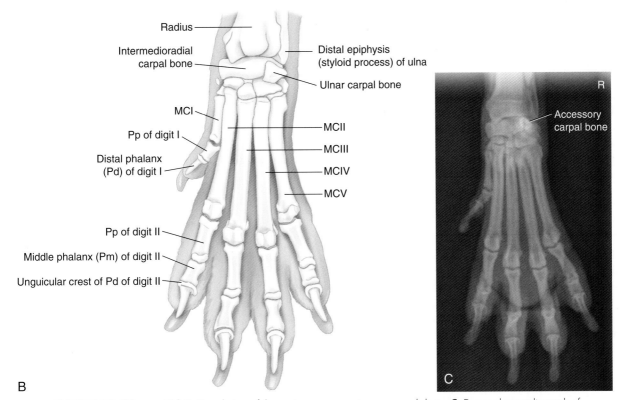

Radius

Intermedioradial carpal bone

Distal epiphysis (styloid process) of ulna

Ulnar carpal bone

MCI

Pp of digit I

Distal phalanx (Pd) of digit I

MCII

MCIII

MCIV

MCV

Pp of digit II

Middle phalanx (Pm) of digit II

Unguicular crest of Pd of digit II

R

Accessory carpal bone

B

C

FIGURE 20-20, cont'd B, Dorsal view of the canine carpus, metacarpus, and digits. **C,** Dorsopalmar radiograph of the canine carpus, metacarpus, and digits.

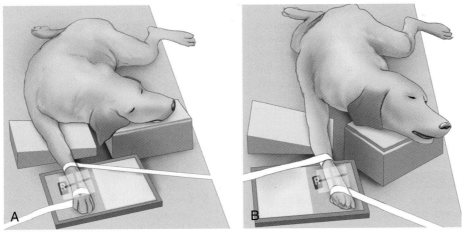

A

B

FIGURE 20-21 Stress radiographs of the carpus may be completed if joint laxity is to be determined. The position and pulling of the tape changes where pressure is applied on the carpus: **A,** Medial stress; **B,** lateral stress.

Oblique Views of the Foot

The two oblique views of the foot are the dorsolateral palmaromedial oblique (DLPMO)–medial oblique view and the dorsomedial palmarolateral oblique (DMPLO)–lateral oblique view (Figures 20-22 and 20-23).

Positioning
Place In: Sternal recumbency.
Head and Neck: Displace and support the head laterally, with foam pads, sandbags, or tape, away from the affected limb and beam.
Hind Limbs: Extend caudally in a natural position to keep the spine straight and support with sandbags if needed. A V-trough may be used for stability of the caudal half of the body.

Forelimbs: Extend both forward. Secure the affected distal metacarpus/digits and pull cranially.
- For the medial oblique view, rotate the elbow joint laterally and support it with tape and sandbag.
- For the lateral oblique view, rotate the elbow joint medially and support it with tape and sandbag.

Comments and Tips
- Rotate the elbow just enough so that the beam will enter the limb at 35 to 45 degrees from the mid-sagittal plane either laterally or medially.

MEASURE: At the site of interest:
  Carpus: Carpus joint.
  Metacarpus or phalanges: Site of phalangeal metacarpal articulation at the level of the middle phalanx.

CENTRAL RAY: Centered on the area of interest:
  Carpus: Middle row of the carpal bones.
  Phalanges: Third and fourth phalangeal-metacarpal articulations.
    For the lateral oblique view: center the beam 45 degrees medially from the mid-sagittal plane (Figure 20-22).
    For the medial oblique view: center the beam 45 degrees laterally from the mid-sagittal plane (Figure 20-23).

BORDERS: Carpus: Proximal third of the metacarpus to distal third of the radius/ulna.
  Metacarpus or phalanges: Carpus proximally to the distal phalanges.

> **TECHNICIAN NOTES** The beam is described as "point of entrance to point of exit," so for the DLPMO, the beam enters dorsally on the lateral side and exits at the palmar aspect on the medial side. The "point of exit" is where the image receptor is placed, which in this case is on the palmar side. Because the beam does not exit perpendicular to the midline, the view is called oblique. In this case it is a medial oblique because the beam exits medially. (This concept is further described in Chapter 26).

> **TECHNICIAN NOTES** Use positioning aids strategically to give the patient the *illusion* that it is being held. A sandbag over the neck and limbs, and/or the use of tape is essential if the patient is not properly sedated. Keep talking to your patient in a calm, low voice.

> **KEY POINTS**
> 1. For views perpendicular to the mid-sagittal plane, the dog or cat generally lies in dorsal recumbency for the proximal limb (scapula, shoulder, and humerus) and in sternal recumbency for the distal limb (elbow, radius/ulna, and foot).
> 2. Correct positioning and techniques are required for proper interpretation. This includes where to measure and center, what to include, and how to ensure that the positioning shows proper symmetry.
> 3. The label is placed cranially for the lateral projections and laterally for the perpendicular projection.
> 4. For a joint, include one third of the bones proximal and distal to it and for long bones, include the proximal and distal joints.
> 5. Keep in mind the similarity in positioning, with slight variations, between the proximal views (scapula, shoulder, and humerus) and also amongst the distal views (elbow, radius/ulna, and foot).

Oblique Views of the Foot—cont'd

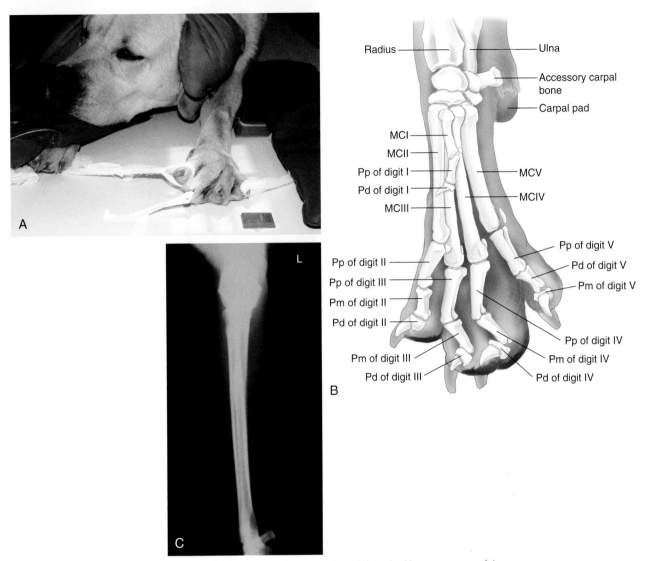

FIGURE 20-22 **A,** Positioning for the dorsomedial-palmarolateral (lateral) oblique projection of the canine metacarpus and digits with the digits separated. **B,** Dorsomedial-palmarolateral (lateral) oblique view of the canine carpus, metacarpus, and digits. **C,** Dorsomedial-palmarolateral (lateral) oblique radiograph of the canine radius and ulna.

Continued

Oblique Views of the Foot—*cont'd*

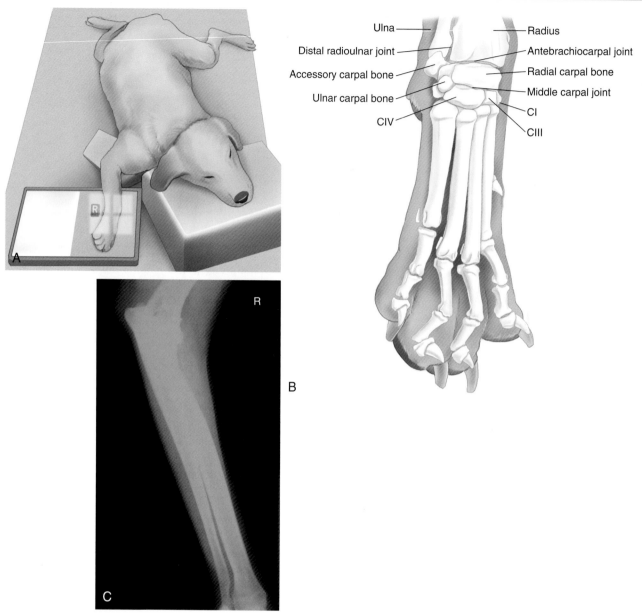

Ulna

Radius

Distal radioulnar joint

Antebrachiocarpal joint

Accessory carpal bone

Radial carpal bone

Ulnar carpal bone

Middle carpal joint

CIV

CI

CIII

FIGURE 20-23 **A,** Positioning for dorsolateral-palmaromedial (medial) oblique radiograph. **B,** Medial oblique radiographic anatomy of the canine carpus. **C,** Medial oblique radiograph of the canine radius and ulna.

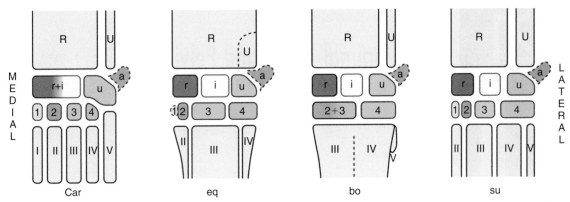

FIGURE 20-24 Schematic diagrams of the bones of the carpal skeleton in carnivore (Car), horse- (Eq), cattle (Bo), and pig (Su).

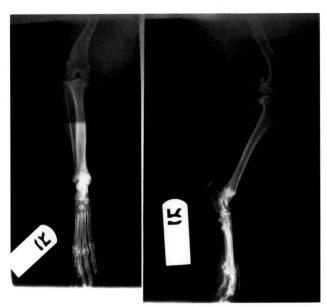

FIGURE 20-25 Mystery radiograph: Other radiographs from the same source have a similar appearance, with the variation in contrast on one section of the radiograph. What could some of the causes be?

References

1. Morgan JP: *Techniques of veterinary radiography*, Ames, Iowa, 1993, Iowa State University Press.
2. Aspinall V, Cappello M: *Introduction to veterinary anatomy*, London, 2009, Butterman-Heineman.
3. Han C, Hurd C: *Practical diagnostic imaging for the veterinary technician*, ed 3, St. Louis, 2005, Mosby.
4. Orthopedic Foundation for Animals: Application for Hip/Elbow Dysplasia Database, 2010. http://www.offa.org/pdf/hdedapp_bw.pdf.
5. Sirois M, Anthony E, Mauragis D: *Handbook of radiographic positioning for veterinary technicians*, Clifton Park, NY, 2010, Delmar Cengage Learning.
6. Ryan G: *Radiographic positioning of small animals*, Philadelphia, 1981, Lea & Febiger.

Bibliography

Colville T, Bassert J: *Clinical anatomy and physiology for veterinary technicians*, St. Louis, 2008, Elsevier.

Done, SH, Goody PC, Stickland NC, Evans SA: *Color atlas of veterinary anatomy, the dog and cat*, London, 2009, Mosby.

Dyce KM, Sack WO, Wensing CJG: *Textbook of veterinary anatomy*, ed 4, St. Louis, 2010, Saunders.

Evans H, de Launta A: *Guide to the dissection of the dog*, ed 7, St. Louis, 2010, Saunders.

Lavin L: *Radiography in veterinary technology*, St. Louis, 2007, Saunders.

Owens JM, Biery DN: *Radiographic interpretation for the small animal clinician*, St. Louis, 1999, Ralston Purina.

Ryan G: *Radiographic positioning of small animals*, Philadelphia, 1981, Lea & Febiger.

Thrall DE: *Textbook of veterinary diagnostic radiology*, ed 5, St. Louis, 2007, Saunders.

Tighe M, Brown M: *Mosby's comprehensive review for veterinary technicians*, ed 3, St. Louis, 2008, Mosby.

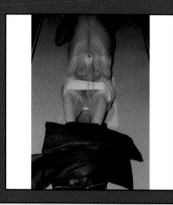

Small Animal Pelvis and Pelvic Limb

Adopt the pace of nature: her secret is patience.

—Ralph Waldo Emerson, American Essayist and Poet, 1803–1882

TECHNICAL NOTE

To preserve space, the radiographs presented in this chapter do not show collimation. For safety, always collimate so that the beam is limited to within the image receptor edges. You should see a clear border of collimation on every radiograph. In some jurisdictions, use of collimation is the law.

OUTLINE

LEARNING OBJECTIVES

When you have finished this chapter, you will be able to:

1. Identify the common positions and principles used to radiograph the pelvic limb.
2. Properly and safely position a dog or cat for the various common positions of the hind limb, with an emphasis on where to measure and center the beam, where the borders are, and how to properly position, so that the body part is parallel to the image receptor and both are perpendicular to the central ray.
3. Understand the other views that may need to be completed as an alternative.
4. Identify normal anatomy of the pelvis and hind limb found on a radiograph.

Imaging of the appendicular skeleton is completed to detect fractures, pain, or lameness. Imaging of the pelvis is generally performed to evaluate dysplastic or degenerative changes of the coxofemoral joints (Box 21-1). Fractures, joint-associated neoplasia, and arthritis are further reasons for radiographing not only the pelvis but also the femur, stifle, tarsus, metatarsus, and phalanges, which make up the remaining portion of the hind limb of the appendicular skeleton. The pelvis, the proximal portion of the pelvic limb, consists of the paired ilia, acetabula, pubis, and ischia.

As with other body parts, a minimum of two perpendicular views of the pelvis and pelvic limbs is required (Table 21-1). In addition to the lateral (L) view, the general rule for limbs, is to have the animal in dorsal recumbency for the proximal portion of the pelvis and limb (pelvis and femur) (Figure 21-1) and in sternal recumbency for the distal portion (stifle, tibia/fibula, tarsus, metatarsus, and digits) (Figure 21-2).

If we keep the normal positioning in mind, it is easy to remember what the views should be named. Thus the orthogonal view for the pelvis is the ventrodorsal (VD). The positioning for the femur would be referred to as the craniocaudal (CrCd). For views of the limb distal to and including the stifle the patient is in sternal recumbency, so the positions are referred to as caudocranial (CdCr) for the stifle, tibia and fibula. For views distal to and including the tarsus, the positions are termed plantarodorsal (PlD/PD).

BOX 21-1	Normal Coxofemoral Anatomy

There are breed variations that must be kept in mind, but generally:
- The cranial third of each coxofemoral joint space is equal in width.
- At least half of the femoral head should be positioned within the acetabulum.
- The angle of the femoral neck should be about 130 degrees.
- Femoral heads should be rounded and smooth; the fovea capitus is a normal flattened area on the femoral head.
- The femoral neck should be smooth with no proliferative remodeling changes.

TECHNICIAN NOTES Mentally place the patient in sternal recumbency for the distal portion of the limb and in dorsal recumbency for the proximal portion, and the terms will be easier to remember.

If it is too painful for the patient to complete the orthogonal view in sternal or dorsal recumbency, use of a horizontal beam should be considered if the machine allows. Further views, such as oblique positioning or flexed or extended

---

TABLE 21-1	Protocol for the Pelvis and Pelvic Limb Radiography	
ANATOMICAL LOCATION	**ROUTINE VIEWS**	**OPTIONAL VIEWS**
Pelvis	Lateral, ventrodorsal hip-extended	Ventrodorsal: frog-leg PennHIP*: compression, distraction
Femur	Lateral, craniocaudal	Caudocranial
Stifle	Lateral, caudocranial	Proximodistal (Skyline)
Tibia/fibula	Lateral, caudocranial	
Foot: tarsus, metatarsus, and digits	Lateral, plantarodorsal	Flexed and extended lateral, dorsoplantar, obliques

*Requires certification and training.

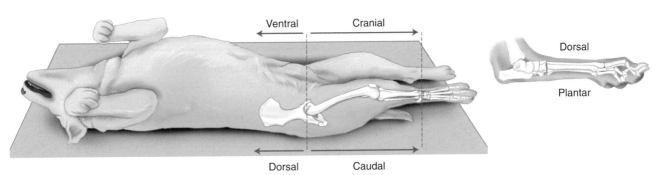

FIGURE 21-1 Patient in dorsal recumbency for the proximal portion of the contralateral image of the pelvis, acetabulum, and femur. In this position the femur is the craniocaudal (CrCd) view and the pelvis is ventrodorsal (VD) view. Though this view is not usually used for the foot, the digits would be termed dorsoplantar (DPl/DP) in this position.

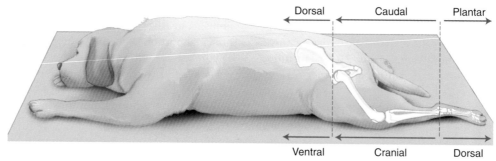

FIGURE 21-2 For positioning of the distal rear limbs (patella, tibia, fibula, tarsus, metatarsus, and digits), the patient is generally in sternal recumbency. Note that the terminology changes at and including the tarsus. Thus in this position the patella would be referred to as caudocranial (CdCr) and the tarsus as plantarodorsal (PID/PD).

lateral views, may facilitate diagnosis, depending on the body part or the condition. Radiographs of the opposite limb are a valuable reference if there are any anatomical variant concerns, such as in immature animals.

The field of view for a long bone generally includes the joints proximal and distal to the bone. For a joint, the field of view is one third each of the long bones proximal and distal to the joint.

> **TECHNICIAN NOTES**   For long bones, the field of view includes the joints proximal and distal. For joints, the field of view includes one third each of the bones proximal and distal.

Radiographic and Patient Concerns

A high-contrast film is desirable, with lower kilovoltage peak (kVp) and higher milliampere-seconds (mAs). Most projections of the pelvic limb are completed tabletop. A grid is not generally used because the tissue thickness is less than 11 cm, so it is important to collimate the field as tightly as possible to reduce scatter radiation. Doing so also helps achieve higher contrast, which is generally preferred for viewing bones. Most canine pelvis views require a grid because of the greater thickness. The Orthopedic Foundation of Animals (OFA) requires that for radiographic submissions, "film contrast should be such that the microtrabecular pattern of the femoral head and neck are readily seen. The dorsal-lateral margin of the acetabulum must also be visible."[1]

When tabletop is used, both positions can be placed on the same image receptor if the size of the patient and body part allows. If the image receptor is split, point the toes of each view in the same direction, collimate tightly and use a lead shield to cover the side not being imaged to prevent scatter radiation from affecting the contrast on that side. Preparation other than having a clean hair coat is not required. Unless otherwise indicated, a vertical beam is used.

Chemical restraint assists in extending the limb more fully to achieve the symmetry required for proper diagnosis.

Anesthesia or sedation that permits muscle relaxation is required for a good-quality diagnostic view of the ventrodorsal hip-extended pelvis. Emphasis as in other chapters, is placed on nonmanual restraint.

It is essential to give the patient the illusion it is being held, if a patient is not appropriately sedated. This can be accomplished by the judicious use of sandbags, compression bands, tape, constant talking to the patient, and so on. Review the suggestions in Chapter 17 on techniques that can be used to assist in obtaining high-quality radiographs with the use of nonmanual restraint. Use sandbags, foam pads, and other positioning devices appropriately to prevent artifacts. Splints and casts require increased exposure.

> **TECHNICIAN NOTES**   The label is placed at the dorsal or cranial aspect of the limb for the lateral views, and on the lateral aspect of the limb for the orthogonal views.
>
> Measure at the thickest part of the area to be radiographed.
>
> Always measure the patient in the position in which it is to be imaged.
>
> Center at the area of interest—either the center of the bone or at the joint.
>
> Keep the bone parallel to the image receptor and the central ray perpendicular to both to minimize distortion.

Pelvis

The ventrodorsal hip-extended and lateral views are the standard positions used to evaluate the small animal pelvis, especially in suspected trauma. The frog-leg position can be used when there is too much pain for the patient to tolerate a ventrodorsal hip-extended radiograph. The frog-leg view is also good for assessing the coxofemoral joint if there is suspicion of capital physeal or femoral neck fracture.[2]

The most common view for diagnosis of hip dysplasia (Box 21-2) is the ventrodorsal hip-extended projection, which has been adopted for coxofemoral joint certification

- There is increased width of the joint space.
- A shallow acetabulum is noted.
- There is flattening and deformity of the femoral head.
- Subluxation or luxation occurs.
- Secondary degenerative joint disease is noted:
  - There is subchondral bone sclerosis and/or exostosis on the rim of the acetabulum (specifically the dorsal cranial margin).
  - Proliferative remodeling degenerative changes can be seen on the femoral neck at the site of the joint capsule attachment.
- The angle of the femoral neck is less than 130 degrees (coxa vara) or more than 130 degrees (coxa valga).

by the OFA. Hip dysplasia is the abnormal development of the femoral joint, that results from a lack of conformity between the acetabulum and the femoral head. Hip dysplasia is a heritable disease manifested as hip joint laxity that leads to the development of osteoarthritis (OA). This polygenic and multifactorial disease is the most commonly inherited orthopedic disease in dogs. All breeds are affected, and in some cases more than 50% of the breed has canine hip dysplasia (CHD).

The ventrodorsal hip-extended view has been shown to tighten the joint capsule and the surrounding soft tissue, an effect that may mask evidence of joint laxity in mild to moderate hip dysplasia.[3] This finding has led to greater attention to dynamic pelvic radiographic studies such as the University of Pennsylvania School of Veterinary Medicine's Hip Improvement Program (PennHIP) to document the degree of laxity in coxofemoral joints.[2,4,5] PennHIP is discussed in this chapter.

Other radiographic stress techniques described in the literature do not require certification, such as the ventrodorsal view with limbs extended using a fulcrum positioning and the ventrodorsal view with limbs flexed for a distraction positioning.[2,6] These are not discussed in this chapter.

If exact duplicates are required for film radiography, two films can be placed in the cassette, and the kVp increased by about 10%. However, for optimum film quality, it is best to take two separate exposures.

In order for the radiographs to be eligible for OFA registration there must be permanent patient identification on the film emulsion. It could include lead letters, a darkroom imprinter, or radiopaque tape. The information required is the hospital or veterinarian's name, the date the radiograph was taken, and the registered name or number of the patient. Alternative authorized identification, further information, and forms can be found on the OFA's website (www.offa.org). Information regarding radiographic requirements for PennHIP can be found at http://research.vet.upenn.edu/pennhip. Because of the Digital Imaging and Communications in Medicine (DICOM) standards, digital radiographs already include all of the identifying information.

TECHNICIAN NOTES Have the thickest part of the pelvis toward the cathode to take advantage of the heel effect.

Ventrodorsal Hip-Extended View

Positioning

Place In: Dorsal recumbency. A V-trough can be used for the cranial portion of the body. If the pelvis is included there will be increased object-film distance (OFD) (Figure 20-3).

Head: Point forward and secure with a sandbag over the neck if needed, being careful not to restrict breathing.

Forelimbs: Pull the forelimbs cranially, and secure with a sandbag, or tie to the table.

Hind Limbs: The hind limbs should be positioned as follows:

- Have one person grasp each hind limb at the level of the metatarsus so the thumbs face each other on the medial aspect of the patient's limb.
- The femurs are rotated inward so that the patellae lie over the trochlear groove of the femurs and the femurs are parallel to each other and the long axis of the spine, and level with the table.
- At the back of proximal stifle, have another person place a piece of tape long enough so it can overlap to the lateral aspect of the opposite femur.
- Take each end of the tape and forcibly pull to the opposite limb at the level of the proximal stifle to ensure that the femurs are maintained in a medial rotation.

- Additional tape can be placed around the pelvis just cranial to the acetabulae.
- Slowly lower the limbs until a point of resistance is felt. Place a pad underneath the tarsus to maintain this level.
- It is best to also tape each limb individually at the metatarsus. Extend the limbs and secure with tape caudally, so that the two digits are even with each other.
- Place a sandbag over the distal portion of the limbs to further keep them level with the table.

Comments and Tips

- Sedation or anesthesia that permits muscle relaxation is required for proper positioning.
- To minimize any rotation of the body, make sure the nose is equidistant between the forelimbs and in line with the tail and that the sternum and vertebrae are superimposed.
- Palpate the greater trochanter of each femur to ensure the pelvis is symmetrical.
- Label appropriately. A positional marker should be included and placed at the cranial aspect of the pelvis.
- Keep the tail aligned with the spine.
- The dog must be 24 months old before the radiographs can be OFA certified.

MEASURE: Thickest part of the pelvis.

CENTRAL RAY: Midline at the caudal portion of the ischium.

BORDERS: The crest of the ilium (last two lumbar vertebrae) and to the distal patella.

> **TECHNICIAN NOTES** It is important to snugly secure the tape around the proximal stifles so that the femurs are parallel to each other and the patellae are superimposed over the centers of the femoral condyles. It is better to err on the side of having the tape be too snug.

> **TECHNICIAN NOTES** If the image shows that the obturator foramina are of unequal size, for the subsequent image, slightly lower the side of the pelvis that has the larger circular obturator foramen. This repositioning will result in the more true oval shape of each obturator foramen (big is up).

> **TECHNICIAN NOTES**
> - For the pelvis radiograph to be evaluated, make sure that:
>   - The radiograph is legally labeled and positional markers are included.
>   - The femurs are parallel to each other.
>   - The patellae are positioned over the centers of the femoral condyles.
>   - There is no rotation, so that the wings of the ilia, the sacroiliac joints, and the obturator foramina are equal in size and mirror images of each other.
>   - The entire pelvis, femurs, and stifles are included.

Ventrodorsal Hip-Extended View—*cont'd*

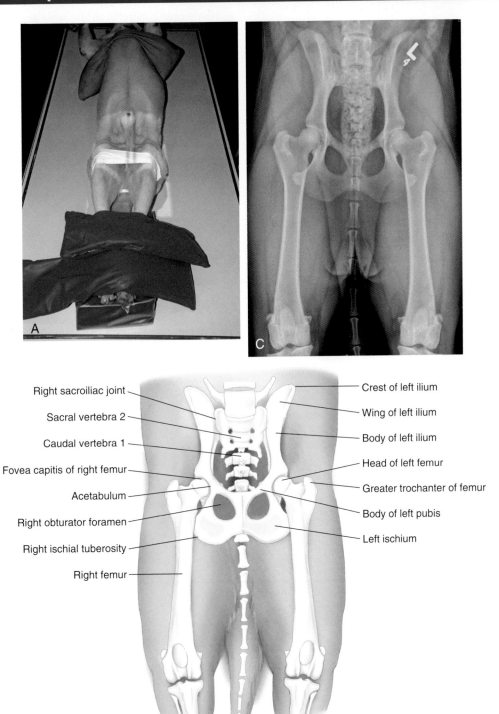

Right sacroiliac joint

Sacral vertebra 2

Caudal vertebra 1

Fovea capitis of right femur

Acetabulum

Right obturator foramen

Right ischial tuberosity

Right femur

Crest of left ilium

Wing of left ilium

Body of left ilium

Head of left femur

Greater trochanter of femur

Body of left pubis

Left ischium

FIGURE 21-3 **A**, Positioning for the canine ventrodorsal hip-extended projection. Tape or gauze can be placed around the metatarsus and pulled caudally to keep the limbs as parallel to the table as possible. With enough support in the sandbag, tape may not be necessary. **B**, Ventral view of the canine pelvis. **C**, Radiograph of a standard ventrodorsal hip-extended projection. Note that the femurs are parallel to each other, the patellae are positioned over the center of the femoral condyles, there is no rotation, and the entire pelvis, femurs and stifles are included.

Lateral View of the Pelvis

Positioning

Place In: Lateral recumbency with the affected leg down.

Head: Keep in a natural position and if needed support appropriately with a sandbag over the neck. Be careful not to restrict breathing.

Forelimbs: Pull the forelimbs cranially, and secure with a sandbag, or tie to the table.

Hind Limbs: Place a foam wedge between the hind limbs so that the pelvis is superimposed. Scissor the limbs so that the limb closest to the cassette is cranial and the contralateral limb is pulled caudally to differentiate the femurs. Place a foam pad under the uppermost limb so the femur is parallel to the table and sandbags over the distal portion of the limbs to keep them in place.

Comments and Tips

* To ensure symmetry, have the femoral heads, the ilial wings, and the transverse processes of the caudal lumbar vertebrae superimposed.
* The upper limb will be more magnified because of increased OFD.
* Separation of the limbs is particularly important if hip luxation is suspected.

MEASURE: At the level of the trochanter or the thickest part.

CENTRAL RAY: Greater trochanter of the femur.

BORDERS: Slightly cranial to the wing of the ilium to include at least one lumbar vertebrae, and caudally to the caudal ischium. Include one-third of the femur.

> **TECHNICIAN NOTES**   Remember to go through your mental checklist *before* pushing the exposure button: settings correct; image receptor/machine/grid in position; proper location of markers and ID (if using at this stage); correct body part and view; properly centered; borders correct and collimated; patient properly prepared, positioned, and restrained so that the pelvis or limb being imaged is perpendicular to the beam and parallel to the image receptor.

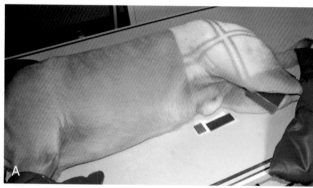

FIGURE 21-4 A, Positioning for the canine lateral pelvis projection. with the femurs superimposed. The legs are best scissored, but the wings of the ilia must be superimposed and parallel to the table. Place a foam pad under the upper limb so the unaffected femur is parallel to the table.

Lateral View of the Pelvis—*cont'd*

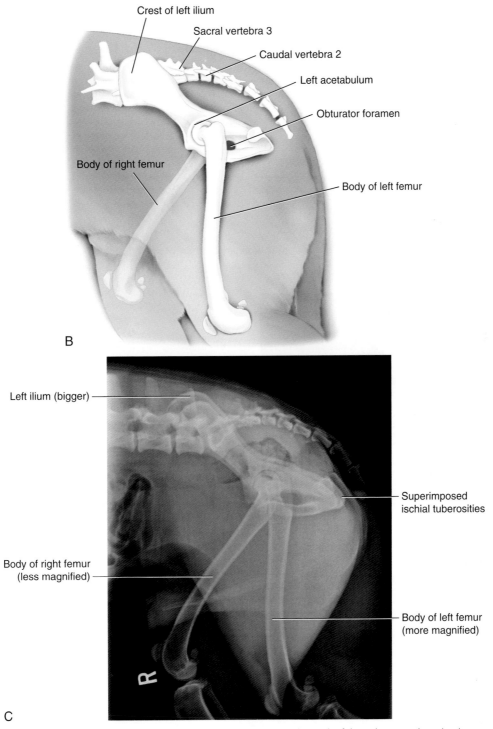

FIGURE 21-4, cont'd B, Lateral view of the pelvis. C, Radiograph of the right canine lateral pelvis.

Ventrodorsal Frog-Leg View

Positioning

Place In: Dorsal recumbency. A V-trough can be used for the cranial portion of the body, but do not include the pelvis to avoid increased object-film distance (OFD).

Head: Keep in a natural position with the nose pointing forward. If needed, support appropriately with a sandbag over the neck. Be careful not to restrict breathing.

Forelimbs: Pull the forelimbs cranially, and secure with a sandbag or tie to the table.

Hind Limbs: Leave the hind limbs in a naturally flexed position, which for most patients is 45 degrees to the spine.

In some larger dogs, it may be 90 degrees to the spine. Place a sandbag over the tarsal joints.

Comments and Tips

- Keep the limbs positioned identically to maintain symmetry.
- Place the marker and label at the caudal region.
- Locate the ischium by palpating for the right and left ischial tuberosity.

MEASURE: Thickest part of the pelvis or over acetabulum.

CENTRAL RAY: Midline at the caudal portion of the pubis.

BORDERS: The wings of the ilia to the caudal border of the ischium. Include at least one third of each femur.

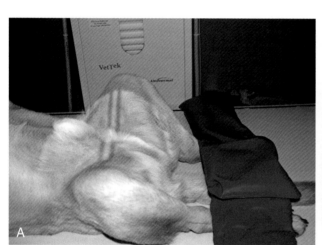

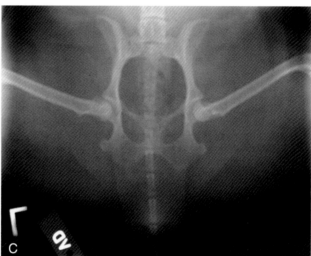

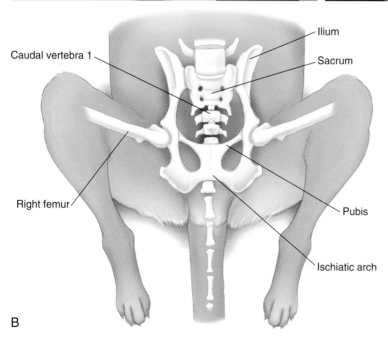

FIGURE 21-5 **A,** Positioning for the canine ventrodorsal frog-leg pelvis projection. **B,** Ventral view of the canine pelvis in a frog-leg position. **C,** Radiograph of the canine ventrodorsal frog-leg pelvis view.

(Labels in figure B: Caudal vertebra 1, Ilium, Sacrum, Right femur, Pubis, Ischiatic arch)

OFA Evaluation of Hip Dysplasia

Through the OFA, three board-certified radiologists independently evaluate the phenotype of the hips on a standard ventrodorsal hip-extended view. The seven possible categories are normal (excellent, good, fair), borderline, and dysplastic (mild, moderate, severe).

Excellent, good, and fair hip grades are within normal limits and are given OFA numbers. This information is in the public domain and is accepted by the American Kennel Club and the Canadian Kennel Club, for dogs with permanent identification (tattoo, microchip). The radiograph is reviewed and a report verifies the abnormal radiographic findings if radiographs reveal borderline, mild, moderate, or severe hip dysplasia grades. Dysplastic hip grades are not in the public domain, unless the owner has chosen the open database.

Other hip registries are maintained by the Fédération Cynologique Internationale (FCI; European), British Veterinary Association (BVA; UK), and the Verein für Deutsche Schäferhunde (SV; Germany); each has its own grading system.[1]

PennHIP Radiographs

PennHIP is a radiographic screening method that quantitatively measures canine hip joint laxity through the use of stress radiographs.

The PennHIP method measures joint laxity to determine how likely a dog is to develop canine hip dysplasia (CHD) and hip arthritis later in life.[7] Osteoarthritis (OA), also known as degenerative joint disease (DJD), is the hallmark of hip dysplasia. The degree of laxity in an individual dog, is also ranked, relative to others of the same breed. This allows the animals that have tighter hips within each breed, in which OA or CHD is less likely to develop, to be identified and to be considered suitable for breeding. The PennHIP method of evaluation is more accurate than the current standard in its ability to predict the onset of osteoarthritis.[4,8,9]

Radiographs taken by PennHIP-certified veterinarians and technicians are sent to the University of Pennsylvania School of Veterinary Medicine in Philadelphia for evaluation and storage in an ever-expanding database, that collects information on the etiology, prediction, and genetic basis of canine hip dysplasia. For quality assurance of the submissions to the database, veterinarians are required to be trained and certified. Qualified technical personnel are allowed to accompany the veterinarian to the training seminars and, like the veterinarian, may become certified to perform the procedure. Alternatively, a PennHIP-certified veterinarian may train technical staff in his/her practice, who may then submit quality assurance radiographs for the certification process (Figure 21-6).[10]

Radiographs

Three radiographs are part of the PennHIP evaluation. The first is the standard ventrodorsal hip-extended view, which has been described. The second is the distraction view, which requires specialized acrylic distractor rods to be placed between the hind limbs at the femoral heads. The rods act as a fulcrum at the proximal femurs (Figure 21-7), which lateralize the femoral heads when a small adduction force is applied. The third radiograph is the compression view, in which slight medial pressure is applied lateral to the greater trochanters. The distraction view and compression view are used to obtain accurate and precise measurements of joint laxity and congruity, respectively. The hip-extended view is used to obtain supplementary information regarding the existence of osteoarthritis of the hip joint. To circumvent the selection bias in databases with "voluntary" image submission, it is mandatory that all hip radiographs by PennHIP veterinarians be submitted for analysis and inclusion in the PennHIP database.[11,12]

For both the distraction and compression views, the patient's hips are in a neutral or standing orientation referred to as the "stance-phase" of weight bearing. This position is optimal for the measurement of hip joint laxity, which is the primary risk factor that predicts the development of DJD.

Measuring Hip Joint Laxity

The distraction radiograph measures to what degree the femoral head is displaced from the acetabulum. A distraction index (DI) formula is applied. The formula is used to take factors such as growth, dog size, and magnification into account. The distraction index ranges from 0 to 1, with 0 representing full congruency of the hip joint and 1 representing complete luxation.

The closer the DI is to 0, the less joint laxity present and the less likelihood for predisposition to degenerative joint disease or osteoarthritis. Hips scoring close to 1 are considered to be very loose and thus highly likely to develop hip dysplasia. A DI of 0.46 would mean that the femoral head comes out of the joint by 46% and is twice as lax as a hip that has a DI of 0.23 which is 23% out of the joint.[7]

Average DI does vary by breed. Because the dog is anesthetized or deeply sedated and is not weight bearing, the laxity as determined by the DI is actually passive hip laxity, as opposed to functional hip laxity, which to date is not measurable.[7] A report is sent indicating where the particular dog stands in relation to the average for the breed, expressed as a percentile. A percentile of 75 means that a dog's hips are tighter or better than about 75% of those in the breed. Dogs having hip laxity better than the respective breed average, are considered appropriate for breeding. PennHIP is not a pass/fail system. Dogs can be screened using PennHIP as early as 16 weeks of age. Dogs with DI values < 0.3 have very low "risk" for development of OA later in life.[7]

The compression view can be measured to show true depth and congruency of the hip joint. In conjunction with the distraction radiograph, objective laxity measurements are obtained. If there is a nonzero compression index, there is lack of complete congruity. This may be the earliest identifiable indication of incipient OA.[12]

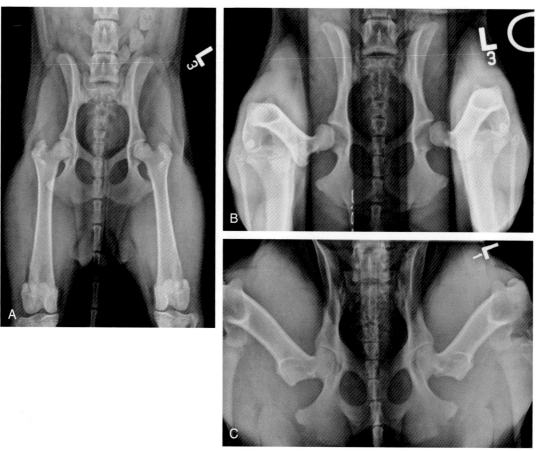

FIGURE 21-6 A, Radiograph of a ventrodorsal hip-extended projection with an Orthopedic Foundation of Animals (OFA) rating of "good." **B,** Radiograph of a PennHIP distraction projection with an index of 0.92 of the same dog shows marked laxity that is not evident on the ventrodorsal hip-extended view. The dark lines are caused by the air between the foam and acrylic rods. **C,** Radiograph of a PennHIP compression view.

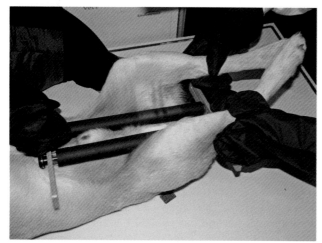

FIGURE 21-7 Positioning for the distraction view, utilizing the distractor rods with the limbs in a natural stance.

Further Comments

PennHIP as a hip screening system controls the quality of data entered into the database. Thus, training is necessary. The system also attempts to eliminate the selection bias by mandating that the images of every dog evaluated are submitted to the database, so that the breed-based ranking has a genuine value. For further information, view the PennHIP website (http://research.vet.upenn.edu/pennhip).[13]

> **TECHNICIAN NOTES**   All dogs have some degree of joint laxity—even Greyhounds and Borzois—so if you do not see any laxity, check the technique and the level of sedation.

Pelvic Limb Positions

Femur

Lateral (Mediolateral) View of the Femur

Positioning

Place In: Lateral recumbency with the affected leg down.

Head: Keep the head in a natural position, and support the neck with a sandbag. Be careful not to restrict breathing.

Forelimbs: Pull the forelimbs cranially, and support with a sandbag.

Hind Limbs: Flex the unaffected limb, abduct and pull laterally:

  Support the limb with a bungee cord or rope to the machine tube stand.

  Extend the affected limb and secure with a sandbag over the distal limb.

Comments and Tips

- The beam may have to be angled distoproximally if the upper limb is not out of the field of view.
- Be sure to palpate the femoral joint and ensure that the full affected limb will be radiographed.
- Abducting the affected limb eliminates superimposition of the proximal femur over the tuber ischium.
- Owing to the difference in thickness at either end of the femur, especially in thickly muscled dogs, two views may need to be taken (measure accordingly at each end).
- If preferred, a fluid bag can be positioned over the distal end to emulate soft tissue. This may prevent overexposure to the distal aspect. Measure at the proximal femur.[14]
- Position the patient so that the femoral head is pointing toward the cathode of the x-ray tube.

MEASURE: Mid-shaft of the femur (to compensate for the difference in tissue thickness at either end of the femur).

CENTRAL RAY: Mid-shaft of the femur.

BORDERS: The coxofemoral joint to the stifle.

> **TECHNICIAN NOTES**   To be more efficient, ensure that the body parts that are not in the beam are positioned and secured first. Then position the area of interest.

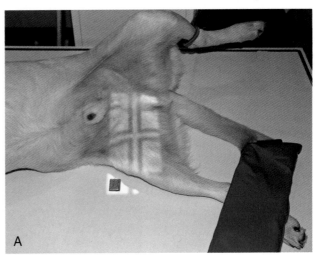

A

FIGURE 21-8 A, Positioning for the mediolateral view of the canine femur.

Continued

Lateral (Mediolateral) View of the Femur—*cont'd*

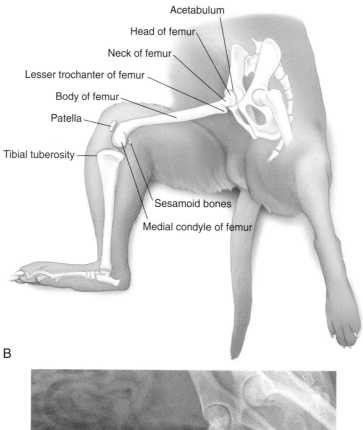

B

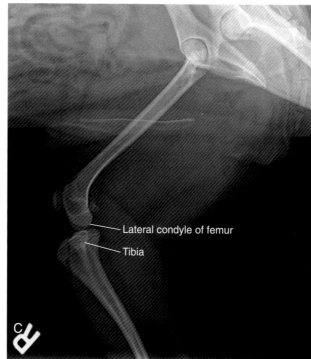

C

FIGURE 21-8, cont'd B, Medial view of the femur. C, Radiograph of the right canine mediolateral femur view.

Craniocaudal View of the Femur

Positioning

Place In: Dorsal recumbency in a V-trough or secure with the use of tape or a sandbag if needed. It is usually best if the patient can be positioned as for a ventrodorsal hip-extended view. Center on the affected limb.

Head: Keep in a natural position and if needed support appropriately with a sandbag over the neck. Be careful not to restrict breathing.

Forelimbs: Pull the forelimbs cranially, and secure with a sandbag, or tie to the table.

Hind Limbs:

Rotate both femurs inward so that the patellae lie over the patellar grooves.

Tape around the femurs just proximal to the stifle.

Place a sandbag over the distal portion of the limbs.

Place a small sponge under the tarsus to prevent rotation of the stifle.

Comments and Tips

- Complete extension is required, so ensure that the affected limb is well secured.
- Measure only the femur itself.

MEASURE: Mid-shaft of the femur.

CENTRAL RAY: Mid-shaft of the femur.

BORDERS: The coxofemoral joint to the stifle.

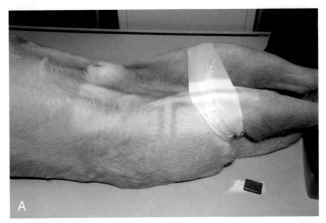

FIGURE 21-9 A, Positioning for the craniocaudal view of canine femur.

Continued

Craniocaudal View of the Femur—*cont'd*

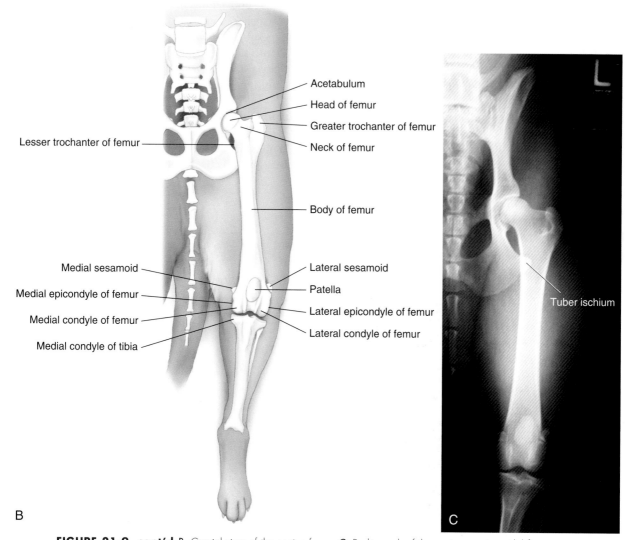

Acetabulum

Head of femur

Greater trochanter of femur

Neck of femur

Lesser trochanter of femur

Body of femur

Medial sesamoid

Medial epicondyle of femur

Medial condyle of femur

Medial condyle of tibia

Lateral sesamoid

Patella

Lateral epicondyle of femur

Lateral condyle of femur

Tuber ischium

B

C

FIGURE 21-9, cont'd B, Cranial view of the canine femur. **C**, Radiograph of the canine craniocaudal femur view.

Caudocranial View (Horizontal View) of the Femur

Positioning

Place In: Lateral recumbency with the affected limb uppermost and supported on a sponge.

Head: Keep in a natural position and if needed support appropriately with a sandbag over the neck. Be careful not to restrict breathing.

Forelimbs: Pull the forelimbs cranially, and secure with a sandbag, or tie to the table.

Hind Limbs: Position a cassette vertically against the cranial aspect of the affected limb. Extend the limb as much as possible, and support with a sandbag, or tie to a secure object.

Comments and Tips

- The horizontal beam is directed caudocranially.
- Complete extension is required. Ensure that the affected limb is well fastened.
- It is difficult to include the proximal portion of the femur and acetabulum with this position.

> **TECHNICIAN NOTES** Remember to place the label and markers on the cranial aspect of the limb for the lateral views and on the lateral aspect for the opposite views.

MEASURE: Mid-shaft of the femur.

CENTRAL RAY: Mid-shaft of the femur.

BORDERS: The coxofemoral joint to the stifle.

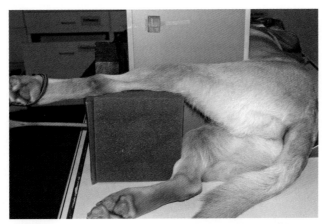

FIGURE 21-10 Positioning for the caudocranial (horizontal) view of the canine femur.

Stifle

Lateral (Mediolateral) View

Positioning

Place In: Lateral recumbency with the affected leg down.

Head: Keep in a natural position and support appropriately with a sandbag over the neck. Be careful not to restrict breathing.

Forelimbs: Pull the forelimbs cranially, and secure with a sandbag or tie to the table.

Hind Limbs: Flex the unaffected limb, abduct and pull laterally. Support the limb with a bungee cord or rope to the machine tube stand.

Extend the affected limb, keeping the stifle in a relatively natural position, and secure with tape or a sandbag over the distal limb.

Comments and Tips

- The unaffected limb needs to be extended only dorsally enough to be out of the field of view.
- Place a sponge pad under the affected tarsus so the tibia is parallel to the image receptor.
- In a true lateral view, there will be superimposition of the femoral condyles.

MEASURE: At the distal end of the femur.

CENTRAL RAY: Palpate and center on the indentation of the stifle joint (intercondylar fossa of the femur).

BORDERS: Proximal third of the tibia and distal third of the femur.

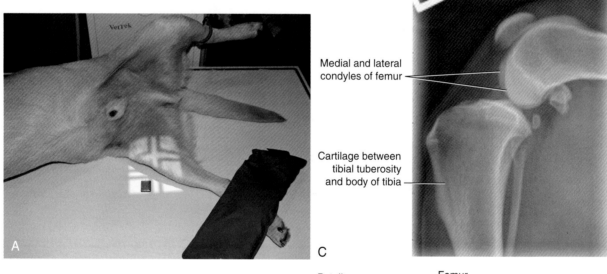

Medial and lateral condyles of femur

Cartilage between tibial tuberosity and body of tibia

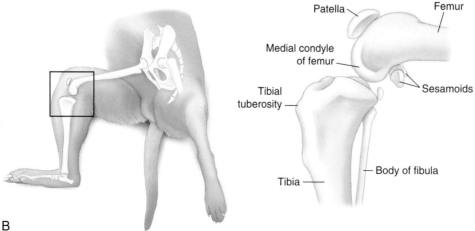

Patella

Femur

Medial condyle of femur

Sesamoids

Tibial tuberosity

Tibia

Body of fibula

FIGURE 21-11 A, Positioning for the mediolateral view of the canine stifle. B, Medial view of the canine stifle joint. C, Radiograph of the canine mediolateral stifle view.

Caudocranial View of the Stifle

Positioning

Place In: Sternal recumbency in a V-trough, or secure with sandbags if needed. (The cat will not likely need further support.)

Head: Keep in a natural position and support appropriately with a sandbag over the neck. Be careful not to restrict breathing.

Forelimbs: Pull the forelimbs cranially, and secure with a sandbag, or tie to the table.

Hind Limbs: Allow the unaffected limb to lie flexed, next to the body, and raise with a foam pad. Extend the affected limb and support with tape or a sandbag. Place a small sponge under the tarsus to prevent rotation of the stifle.

Comments and Tips

- It is essential that the affected limb rest on the patella.
- Raising the unaffected limb will help place the affected patella in the patellar groove. The body will be slightly rotated.
- Palpate the femoral condyles to ensure proper placement in the patellar groove.
- The x-ray tube head may need to be angled cranially about 10 to 15 degrees to create a "tunnel" view of the distal femur.

Positioning with a Horizontal Beam for the Caudocranial Stifle Joint

Place In: Lateral recumbency with the affected limb uppermost and supported on a sponge.

Head: Keep in a natural position and if needed support with a sandbag over the neck. Be careful not to restrict breathing.

Forelimbs: Pull the forelimbs cranially, and secure with a sandbag, or tie to the table.

Hind Limb: Position a cassette vertically against the cranial aspect of the affected limb and extend the limb as much as possible. Support with a sandbag, or tie to a secure object (See Figure 21-10).

Comments and Tips

The horizontal beam is directed in a caudocranial direction.

> **TECHNICIAN NOTES** Collimate, ensuring that labels and markers are included and borders are visible for every image.

> **TECHNICIAN NOTES** Strategically used positioning aids give the patient the *illusion* that it is being held. A sandbag over the neck and limbs, and/or the use of tape is essential if the patient is not properly sedated. Keep talking to it in a calm, low voice.

MEASURE: At the distal end of the femur.

CENTRAL RAY: On the stifle joint.

BORDERS: Distal third of the femur and proximal thirds of the tibia/fibula.

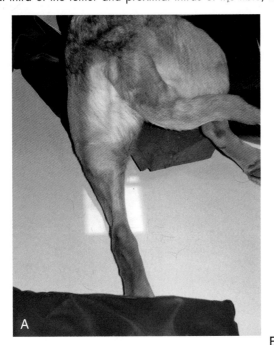

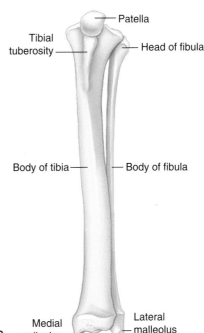

FIGURE 21-12 A, Positioning for the caudocranial view of the canine stifle. B, Caudal view of canine stifle joint.

Continued

Caudocranial View of the Stifle—*cont'd*

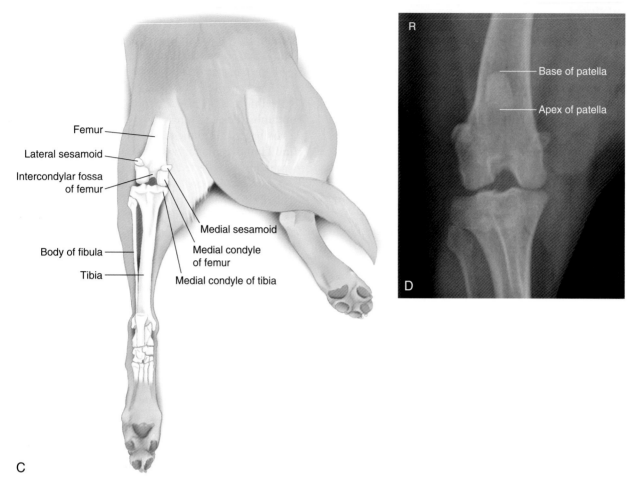

Femur
Lateral sesamoid
Intercondylar fossa of femur
Medial sesamoid
Body of fibula
Medial condyle of femur
Tibia
Medial condyle of tibia

C

R

Base of patella
Apex of patella

D

FIGURE 21-12, cont'd C, Caudal view of tibia and fibula. D, Radiograph of the canine caudocranial stifle view.

Proximodistal (Cranioproximal-Craniodistal) or Skyline View of the Stifle

Positioning

Place In: Sternal recumbency in a V-trough or secure with sandbags if needed. (The cat will not likely need further support).

Head: Keep in a natural position with the nose pointing forward and if needed support appropriately with a sandbag over the neck. Be careful not to restrict breathing.

Forelimbs: Pull the forelimbs cranially, and secure with a sandbag, or tie to the table.

Hind Limbs: Allow the contralateral limb to flex partially and position itself laterally. Flex the affected pelvic limb lateral to the caudal abdomen, with the foot flexed, to slightly elevate the patella. Rotate the pelvis toward the affected limb, keeping the femur perpendicular to the image receptor. Place a sandbag or sponge under the nonaffected limb to keep it slightly elevated (see Figure 21-13).

Comments and Tips

- It is essential that the affected limb rest on the tibia. A small foam pad may be placed beneath the patella for more comfort though there will be some object-film distance.
- Palpate the patella against the trochlea to determine the exact angle.

Positioning with a Horizontal Beam for the Skyline Stifle Joint (Patella)

Place In: Lateral recumbency with the affected limb uppermost and supported on a sponge.

Head: Keep in a natural position and if needed, support appropriately with a sandbag over the neck. Be careful not to restrict breathing.

Forelimbs: Pull the forelimbs cranially, and secure with a sandbag, or tie to the table.

Hind Limb: Completely flex the affected limb as much as possible. Secure with a sandbag over the tarsus and pelvis or tie a gauze or a cord around the metatarsus and fasten to the tube stand (see Figure 21-13B). Alternatively tape a figure-of-eight type bandage around the mid-tibia and femur to hold the stifle in place.

Comments and Tips

- Place the cassette against the cranial surface of the upper limb, and direct the beam in a craniocaudal direction.
- Because of decreased tissue thickness kVp will be less than a regular caudocranial stifle.

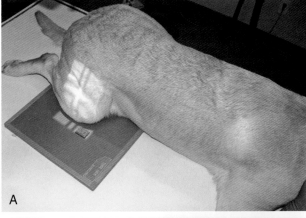

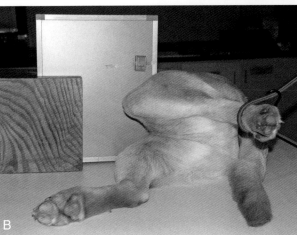

MEASURE: At the patella.

CENTRAL RAY: Over the patella angled 10 degrees in a craniocaudal direction.

BORDERS: Distal third of the femur and proximal thirds of the tibia/fibula.

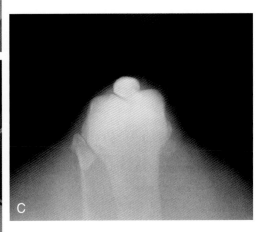

FIGURE 21-13 A, Positioning for the proximodistal view of the canine patella. **B,** Alternate positioning for the proximodistal view of the canine stifle joint (patella) using a horizontal beam. **C,** Radiograph of the canine proximodistal patella view, sometimes referred to as the skyline view.

Tibia and Fibula

Lateromedial View

Positioning

Place In: Lateral recumbency with the affected limb down.

Head: Keep in a natural position and if needed support appropriately with a sandbag over the neck. Be careful not to restrict breathing.

Forelimbs: Pull the forelimbs cranially, and secure with a sandbag, or tie to the table.

Hind Limb: Flex the unaffected limb, abduct and pull laterally, supporting the limb with a bungee cord or rope to the machine tube stand.

Extend the affected limb in a natural position, and either fasten the metatarsus with a sandbag, or tie or tape the metatarsus to the table or to a sandbag (Figure 21-14).

Comments and Tips

• Place a sponge under the tarsus to elevate it and to also prevent obliquity of the limb.

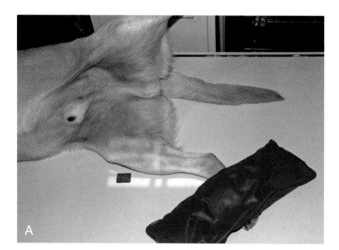

MEASURE: Mid-shaft of the tibia and fibula (to compensate for the difference in tissue thickness at either end).

CENTRAL RAY: Mid-shaft of the fibula and tibia.

BORDERS: The tarsus and the stifle.

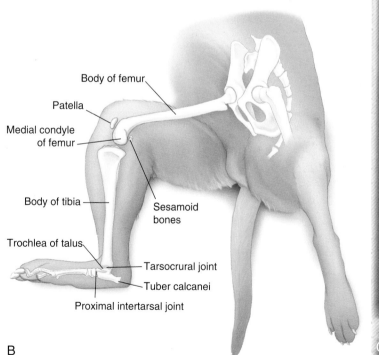

Body of femur

Patella

Medial condyle of femur

Body of tibia

Sesamoid bones

Trochlea of talus

Tarsocrural joint

Tuber calcanei

Proximal intertarsal joint

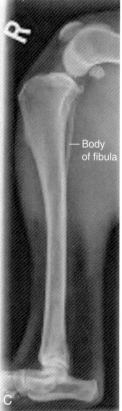

Body of fibula

FIGURE 21-14 **A,** Positioning for the mediolateral view of the canine tibia and fibula. **B,** Medial view of canine tibia and fibula. **C,** Radiograph of the canine mediolateral tibia and fibula view.

Caudocranial View of the Tibia/Fibula

Positioning

Place In: Sternal recumbency in a V-trough, or secure with a sandbag or the use of tape if needed. (The cat will not likely need further support.)

Head: Keep in a natural position and if needed, support appropriately with a sandbag over the neck. Be careful not to restrict breathing.

Forelimbs: Pull the forelimbs cranially, and secure with a sandbag, or tie to the table.

Hind Limbs: Allow the unaffected limb to lie flexed next to the body and slightly raise it with a foam pad. Secure the affected limb over the metatarsus with a sandbag, or tie or tape the metatarsus to the table or to a sandbag. Place a small sponge under the tarsus to prevent rotation of the stifle (Figure 21-15).

Comments and Tips

- It is essential that the affected limb rest on the patella. If you place a foam pad under the unaffected stifle, the raised limb will help place the affected patella in the patellar groove. The body will be slightly rotated.

Positioning with a Horizontal View for the Caudocranial Tibia and Fibula Projection

Place In: Lateral recumbency with the affected limb uppermost and supported on a sponge.

Head: Keep in a natural position and if needed support appropriately with a sandbag over the neck. Be careful not to restrict breathing.

Forelimbs: Pull the forelimbs cranially, and secure with a sandbag or tie to the table.

Hind Limbs: Position a cassette vertically against the cranial aspect of the affected limb and extend the limb as much as possible. Secure over the metatarsus with a sandbag, or tie or tape the metatarsus to a secure object.

Comments and Tips

- The horizontal beam is directed caudocranially.
- Complete extension is required, so ensure that the affected limb is well secured.

MEASURE: Mid-shaft of the tibia and fibula (to compensate for the difference in tissue thickness at either end).

CENTRAL RAY: Mid-shaft of the tibia and fibula.

BORDERS: The tarsus and the stifle.

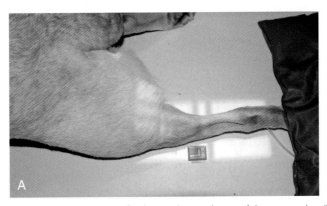

FIGURE 21-15 A, Positioning for the caudocranial view of the canine tibia/fibula.

Continued

Caudocranial View—*cont'd*

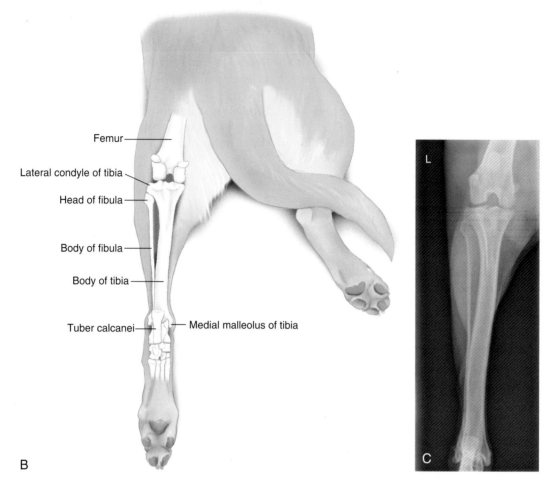

Femur

Lateral condyle of tibia

Head of fibula

Body of fibula

Body of tibia

Tuber calcanei

Medial malleolus of tibia

L

B

C

FIGURE 21-15, cont'd B, Caudal view of the canine tibia and fibula. C, Radiograph of the canine caudocranial tibia/fibula view.

The Foot: Tarsus, Metatarsus, and Digits

The tarsus, metatarsus, and digits are typically radiographed in one view. If there is a particular area of interest, center and measure on this site. See Figure 21-21 for the tarsal bones of various species.

Lateral (Mediolateral) Views of the Foot

Positioning

Place In: Lateral recumbency with the affected limb down.

Head: Keep in a natural position and if needed support appropriately with a sandbag over the neck. Be careful not to restrict breathing.

Forelimbs: Pull the forelimbs cranially, and secure with a sandbag, or tie to the table.

Hind Limbs: Abduct the unaffected limb, pull dorsally, and either secure with tape around the stifle and tarsus or support with a bungee cord to the x-ray tube stand.

Positioning for a Natural Lateral View of the Tarsus

Place the affected limb in a natural position, and secure with tape, gauze, or a sandbag (Figure 21-16A and B).

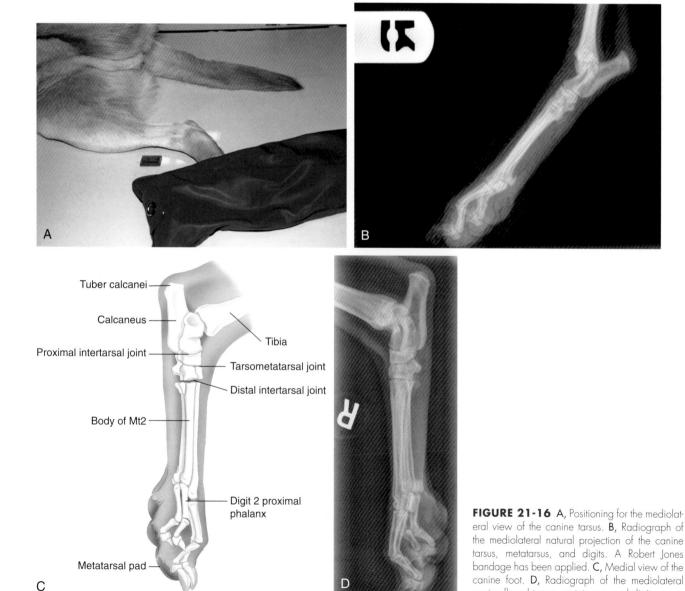

C

Tuber calcanei
Calcaneus
Proximal intertarsal joint
Tibia
Tarsometatarsal joint
Distal intertarsal joint
Body of Mt2
Digit 2 proximal phalanx
Metatarsal pad

FIGURE 21-16 A, Positioning for the mediolateral view of the canine tarsus. **B,** Radiograph of the mediolateral natural projection of the canine tarsus, metatarsus, and digits. A Robert Jones bandage has been applied. **C,** Medial view of the canine foot. **D,** Radiograph of the mediolateral canine flexed tarsus, metatarsus, and digits.

Continued

Lateral (Mediolateral) Views of the Foot—*cont'd*

Positioning for an Extended Lateral View of the Tarsus

Extend the affected limb fully by pulling away from the body, and secure with tape, gauze, or a sandbag. (Figure 21-17).

Positioning for a Flexed Lateral View of the Tarsus

Flex the affected foot at 90 degrees, and support with a paddle or sandbag. Alternatively, place a figure-of-eight tape around the distal tibia and proximal metatarsus, to achieve full flexion of the tarsus. Place tape at the distal metatarsus, and pull slightly cranially and laterally (Figure 21-18).

Positioning for a Lateral View of the Digits

- Separate the digits to prevent superimposition.
- This is best completed by separately taping around the toenail of the lateral (5th) phalanx and the medial (2nd) phalanx.
- Pull the lateral phalanx slightly cranially and laterally, and the medial phalanx slightly caudally and laterally.
- Tape can also be put around the digit itself.
- Cotton can be placed between the toes, though this alone does not separate the phalanges as effectively.

Comments and Tips

- As for all lateral limb positions, keep the label cranial to the joint or bone.

MEASURE: At the site of interest:
  Tarsus: At the tarsus joint.
  Metatarsus or Phalanges: On the joint.

CENTRAL RAY: Center on the area of interest:
  Tarsus: At the tarsus joint.
  Metatarsus or Phalanges: On the central bone.

BORDERS: Tarsus: Proximal third of metatarsus to distal third of the tibia and fibula.
  Metatarsus or Phalanges: Tarsus proximally to the distal phalanges.

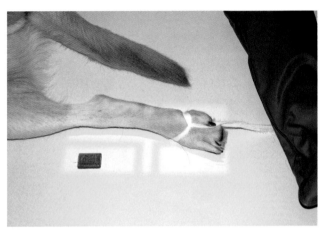

FIGURE 21-17 Positioning for the mediolateral extended view of the canine tarsus, metatarsus, and digits. The digits should be separated if they are of interest.

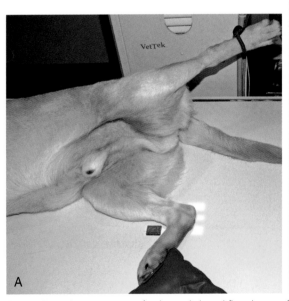

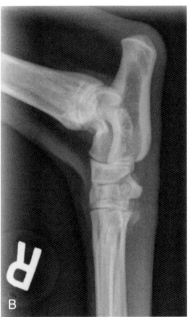

FIGURE 21-18 **A,** Positioning for the mediolateral flexed view of the canine tarsus. **B,** Radiograph of the mediolateral flexed canine tarsus view.

Plantarodorsal (PD) View of the Foot

Positioning

Place: The patient is placed in sternal recumbency in a V-trough or secured with the use of a sandbag if needed. (The cat will not likely need further support).

Head and Forelimbs: Secure the head and forelimbs with a sandbag or tie the limbs to the table.

Hind Limbs: Allow the unaffected limb to lie flexed next to the body. Extend the affected foot and support with a sandbag or tie at the metatarsus/digits and secure to the table or a sandbag.

Comments and Tips

- If you place a foam pad under the unaffected stifle, the raised limb will assist in keeping the calcaneus more centered. The body is slightly rotated.
- Palpate for the tibial tuberosity to obtain a true plantarodorsal view.
- A dorsoplantar view is not routinely completed. If this view is required, the patient can be in either dorsal recumbency with the limb extended or in sternal recumbency with the plantar aspect of the foot against the image receptor (See Figure 21-19D).

MEASURE: At the site of interest:
Tarsus: Tarsus joint.
Metatarsus or Phalanges: On the joint.

CENTRAL RAY: Center on the area of interest:
Tarsus: Tarsal joint.
Metatarsus or Phalanges: On the central bone.

BORDERS: Tarsus: Proximal third of metatarsus to distal third of tibia and fibula.
Metatarsus or Phalanges: Tarsus proximally to distal phalanges.

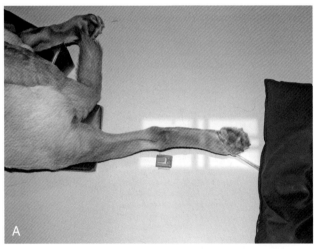

FIGURE 21-19 A, Positioning for the plantarodorsal view of the canine tarsus, metatarsus, and digits.

Continued

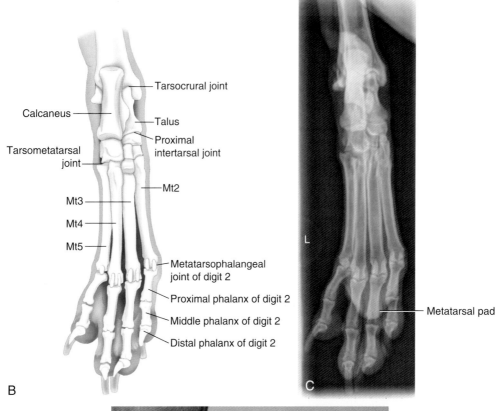

B

Tarsocrural joint

Calcaneus

Talus

Proximal intertarsal joint

Tarsometatarsal joint

Mt2

Mt3

Mt4

Mt5

Metatarsophalangeal joint of digit 2

Proximal phalanx of digit 2

Middle phalanx of digit 2

Distal phalanx of digit 2

C

L

Metatarsal pad

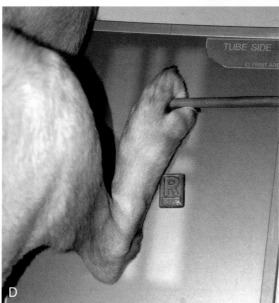

D

FIGURE 21-19, cont'd B, Plantar view of tarsus, metatarsus, and digits. C, Radiograph of the plantarodorsal view of the canine tarsus, metatarsus, and digits. D, Positioning for the dorsoplantar view of the canine metatarsus and digits. A dorsoplanar view taken in this position has less object-film distance than that with the patient in dorsal recumbency. This view can also be used for the skyline of the calcaneous.

Oblique Views of the Foot

The oblique views of the hind foot are the plantarolateral-dorsomedial (PLDMO)-medial oblique view and the plantaromedial-dorsolateral (PMDLO)-lateral oblique view (Figure 21-20).

Positioning

Place In: Sternal recumbency. A V-trough may be used for stability.

Head: Keep in a natural position and if needed support appropriately with a sandbag over the neck. Be careful not to restrict breathing.

Forelimbs: Pull the forelimbs cranially, and secure with a sandbag, or tie to the table if needed.

Hind Limb: Keep the unaffected limb in a natural position. Tie and secure the affected metatarsus/digits as far caudally as possible.

For the medial oblique view: No rotation of the pelvis or padding is needed under the unaffected limb because the foot is in an oblique position naturally.

For the lateral oblique view: Rotate and elevate the unaffected pelvic limb with a large sponge.

Comments and Tips

* If the machine is capable, the patient can be placed in a true plantarodorsal position and the tube head angled 10 to 15 degrees toward the medial side of the tarsus for the lateral oblique view, or 10 to 15 degrees toward the lateral side of the tarsus for the medial oblique view.

> **TECHNICIAN NOTES** The beam is always described as "point of entrance to point of exit." For the PMDLO the beam enters at the plantar aspect on the medial side and exits dorsally on the lateral side. The "point of exit" is where the image receptor is placed, which in this case is next to the dorsal surface. Because the beam does not exit perpendicular to the midline, the view is called an oblique. In this case it is a lateral oblique because the beam exits laterally. (This concept is further described in Chapter 26.)

> **KEY POINTS**
> 1. For views perpendicular to the midsagittal plane, the dog or cat generally lies in dorsal recumbency for the pelvis and the proximal limb (femur), and in sternal recumbency for the distal limb (stifle, tibia and fibula, and foot).
> 2. Correct positioning and technique are required for proper interpretation. This includes where to measure and center the beam, what to include, and how to ensure that the positioning shows proper symmetry.
> 3. The label is placed lateral to the limb for the perpendicular projections and at the cranial aspect for the lateral projections.
> 4. For joints, include one third each of the limbs proximal and distal, and for long bones, include the joints proximal and distal.

MEASURE: At the site of interest. Generally this view is for the tarsus:
Tarsus: Tarsal joint.
Metatarsus or Phalanges: Site of phalangeal metatarsal articulation at level of middle phalanx.

CENTRAL RAY: Center on the area of interest:
Tarsus: Tarsal joint.
Phalanges: Third and fourth phalangeal metatarsal articulations.
* For the medial oblique view: center the beam 45 degrees laterally.
* For the lateral oblique view: center the beam 45 degrees medially.

BORDERS: Tarsus: Proximal third of metatarsus to distal thirds of the tibia and fibula.
Metatarsus or Phalanges: Tarsus proximally to the distal phalanges.

Continued

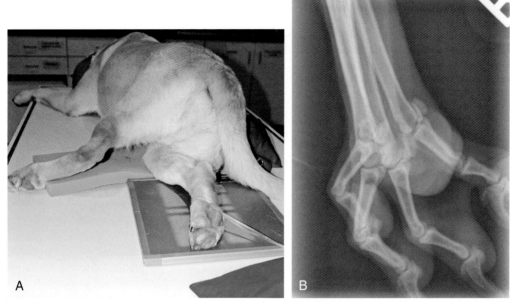

FIGURE 21-20 A, Positioning for the plantaromedial-dorsolateral (lateral) oblique view of the canine tarsus, metatarsus, and digits. B, Radiograph of an oblique canine tarsus, metatarsus, and digits view.

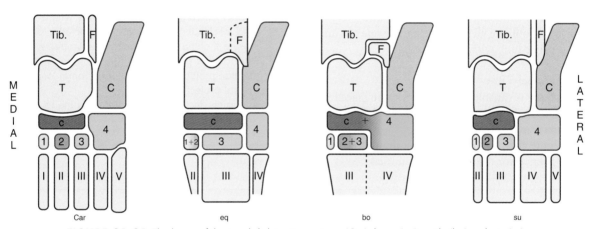

FIGURE 21-21 The bones of the tarsal skeleton in carnivore (Car), horse (eq), cattle (bo) and pig (su).

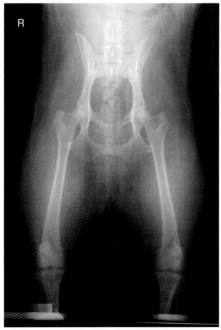

FIGURE 21-22 Mystery Radiograph: What has caused a density issue in this radiograph?

References

1. Keller G: *The use of health databases and selective breeding: a guide for dog and cat breeders and owners*, ed 5, 2006, Orthopedic Foundation of America. http://www.offa.org/pdf/monograph2006web.pdf.
2. Thrall DE: *Textbook of veterinary diagnostic radiology*, ed 5, St. Louis, 2007, Saunders.
3. Smith GK, Biery DN, Gregor TP: New concepts of coxofemoral joint stability and development of a clinical stress-radiographic method for quantitating hip joint laxity in the dog, *J Am Vet Med Assoc* 196:59-70, 1990.
4. Powers MY, Karbe GT, Gregor TP, et al: Evaluation of the relationship between Orthopedic Foundation for Animals' hip joint scores and PennHIP distraction index values in dogs, *J Am Vet Med Assoc* 237:532-541, 2010.
5. Verhoeven GEC, Fortrie RR, Duchateau L, et al: The effect of a technical quality assessment of hip-extended radiographs on interobserver agreement in the diagnosis of canine hip dysplasia, *Vet Radiol Ultrasound* 51:498-503, 2010.
6. Morgan JP: *Techniques of veterinary radiography*, Ames, Iowa, 1993, Iowa State University Press.
7. PennHIP—The University of Pennsylvania Hip Improvement Program: What is PennHIP? http://research.vet.upenn.edu/GeneralInformation/WhatisPennHIP/tabid/3232/Default.aspx.
8. Gold RM, Gregor TP, Huck JL, et al: Effects of osteoarthritis on radiographic measures of laxity and congruence in hip joints of Labrador Retrievers, *J Am Vet Med Assoc* 235:1549-1554, 2009.
9. Runge JJ, Kelly SP, Gregor TP, et al: Distraction index as a risk factor for osteoarthritis associated with hip dysplasia in four large dog breeds, *J Small Anim Pract* 51:264-269, 2010.
10. PennHIP—The University of Pennsylvania Hip Improvement Program: About PennHIP training courses. http://research.vet.upenn.edu/pennhip/Training/AbouttheSeminars/tabid/3248/Default.aspx.
11. PennHIP—The University of Pennsylvania Hip Improvement Program: Frequently asked questions. http://research.vet.upenn.edu/Default.aspx?TabId=3234
12. Smith GK, Karbe GT, Agnello KA, et al: Pathogenesis, diagnosis, and control of canine hip dysplasia. In Tobias KM, Johnston SA, editors: *Veterinary surgery: small animal*, St. Louis, 2011, Elsevier, pp 824-848.
13. PennHIP information courtesy of Drs. GK Smith and M Wallace, University of Pennsylvania.
14. Sirois M, Anthony E, Mauragis D: Handbook of radiographic positioning for veterinary technicians, Clifton Park, NY, 2010, Delmar Cengage Learning.

Bibliography

American College of Veterinary Radiology (ACVR): *Radiology 2—equine*, 2009, ACVR.
Aspinall V, Cappello M: *Introduction to veterinary anatomy*, London, 2009, Butterman-Heineman.
Colville T, Bassert J: *Clinical anatomy and physiology for veterinary technicians*, St. Louis, 2008, Elsevier.
Done SH, Goody PC, Stickland NC, Evans SA: *Color atlas of veterinary anatomy, the dog and cat*, London, 2009, Mosby.
Douglas SW: *Principles of veterinary radiography*, London, 1980, Bailliere Tindall.
Dyce KM, Sack WO, Wensing CJG: *Textbook of veterinary anatomy*, ed 4, St. Louis, 2010, Saunders.
Evans H, de Launta A: *Guide to the dissection of the dog*, ed 7, St. Louis, 2010, Saunders.
Faber TL: *Radiographic imaging and exposure*, St. Louis, 2009, Elsevier.
Han C, Hurd C: *Practical diagnostic imaging for the veterinary technician*, ed 3, St. Louis, 2005, Mosby.
Keller G: *The use of health databases and selective breeding: a guide for dog and cat breeders and owners*, ed 5, 2006, Orthopedic Foundation of America. http://www.offa.org/pdf/monograph2006web.pdf.
Lavin L: *Radiography in veterinary technology*, ed 3, St. Louis, 2007, Saunders.
Orthopedic Foundation for Animals: An examination of hip grading. 2010. http://www.offa.org/hd_grades.html.
Orthopedic Foundation for Animals: Application for Hip/Elbow Dysplasia Database. 2010. http://www.offa.org/pdf/hdedapp_bw.pdf.
Owens JM, Biery DN: *Radiographic interpretation for the small animal clinician*, ed 2, Baltimore, 1999, Williams & Wilkins.
PennHIP—The University of Pennsylvania Hip Improvement Program. 2010. http://research.vet.upenn.edu/pennhip/.
Powers MY, Karbe GT, Gregor TP, McKelvie P, Culp WT, Fordyce HH, Smith GK: Evaluation of the relationship between Orthopedic Foundation for Animals' hip joint scores and PennHIP distraction index values in dogs, *JAVMA* 237(5):532-541, September 1, 2010.
Romich J: *An illustrated guide to veterinary medical terminology*, Clifton, NY, 2009, Delmar Cengage Learning.
Ryan G: *Radiographic positioning of small animals*, Philadelphia, 1981, Lea & Febiger.
Sirois M: *Principles and practice of veterinary technology*, ed 3, St. Louis, 2011, Mosby.
Smallwood JE, Shively MJ, Rendano VT, Habel RE: A standardized nomenclature for radiographic projections used in veterinary medicine, *Vet Radiol* 26:2-9, 1985.
Smith GK, Karbe GT, Agnello KA, et al: Pathogenesis, diagnosis, and control of canine hip dysplasia. In Tobias KM, Johnston SA, editors: *Veterinary surgery: small animal*, St. Louis, 2011, Elsevier, pp 824-848.
Thrall DE: *Textbook of veterinary diagnostic radiology*, ed 4, St. Louis, 2002, Saunders.
Ticer J: *Radiographic technique in small animal practice*, Philadelphia, 1984, WB Saunders.
Tighe M, Brown M: *Mosby's comprehensive review for veterinary technicians*, ed 3, St. Louis, 2008, Mosby.

Small Animal Vertebral Column

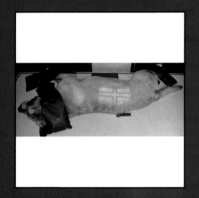

The best lightning rod for your protection is your own spine.

—Ralph Waldo Emerson, American Essayist and Poet, 1803–1882

TECHNICAL NOTE

To preserve space, the radiographs presented in this chapter do not show collimation. For safety, always collimate so that the beam is limited to within the image receptor edges. You should see a clear border of collimation on every radiograph. In some jurisdictions, use of collimation is the law.

LEARNING OBJECTIVES

When you have finished this chapter, you will be able to:

1. Know the common positions and principles used to radiograph the small animal vertebral column.
2. Properly and safely position a dog or cat for the various common positions of the spine, with an emphasis on where to measure, center the beam, where the borders are, and how to properly position, so that the body part is parallel to the film and both are perpendicular to the central ray.
3. Be familiar with other views that may need to be completed as an alternative.
4. Identify normal spinal anatomy found on a radiograph.

Most patients requiring spinal imaging have suffered spinal injuries and are presented with paresis or paralysis, either partial or complete. Another reason for radiography is chronic but progressive neurological changes, with suspected intervertebral disc disease being one of the more important indications. Common intervertebral discs protrusion sites are T12-T13, T13-L1, C2-C3, and C3-C4. Images are needed to see changes in the bone opacity, shape, and angulation of the vertebrae or vertebral column.[1] Survey radiographs do demonstrate many of the signs consistent with intervertebral disc protrusion, but definitive evidence should be obtained by myelography, computerized tomography (CT), or magnetic resonance imaging (MRI) prior to spinal decompression.[1]

Radiographic Concerns

Accurate imaging is important, because many of the imaging signs are subtle. Each of the vertebral segments and adjacent intervertebral discs needs to be examined, so proper positioning and attention to detail are important. General anesthesia should be used; otherwise false narrowing of the intervertebral disc spaces due to muscle spasm may occur.[2] Center the primary beam on the spine, and tightly collimate immediately adjacent to the spine to increase the detail and contrast. The directional and identification labels should be in the field of view, but be conscious of overlapping the label on important anatomy, especially in ventrodorsal views. If using, the label may have to be taped to the patient in lieu of being placed on the image receptor. For lateral views, place the label along the dorsum.

Choose a high-detail cassette/film combination if film is used. Low kilovoltage peak (kVp) and high milliampere-seconds (mAs) provide better radiographic contrast. The use of a grid further increases the contrast. The hair coat should be clean and dry. Remove the collar for any cranial views.

Having the anatomy parallel to the image receptor and perpendicular to the center of the beam is essential for accurate diagnosis. Tape placed along the spine may assist in proper alignment[3] (Figure 22-1).

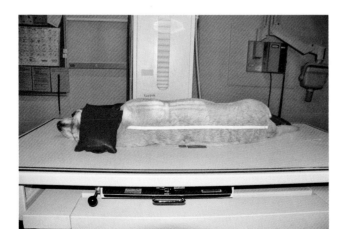

FIGURE 22-1 Placing tape along the vertebrae helps maintain correct alignment and position.

Use sponges or cotton padding to keep the spine parallel to the tabletop and to prevent body rotation. Sandbags can also be used on areas that will not be in the field of view. For patients without spinal cord injuries, pulling and supporting the front and hind limbs in opposite directions keeps the thoracolumbar vertebral column extended to a near-parallel position, as well as opening the intervertebral spaces.[4]

Use smaller cassettes and take multiple views, limiting the number of vertebrae examined so that the intervertebral disc spaces are more perpendicular to the central beam. Coned-down views give further high-quality images. The farther away the area of interest is from the central beam, the greater the geometrical variation and the more inaccurate the interpretation of that area.

The common views of this portion of the axial skeleton are the lateral (L) and ventrodorsal (VD) views of the cervical, thoracic, thoracolumbar, lumbar, lumbosacral, sacral, and caudal vertebrae. Generally it is more comfortable for right-handed radiographers to place the dog or cat in right lateral recumbency, but either side can be dependent. If the patient is compromised, ventrodorsal views can also be made using the horizontal cross-table beam with the patient in lateral recumbency. This is especially useful if vertebral body fractures are suspected. Dorsoventral (DV) views are not as accurate because of the increase in object-film distance

> **TECHNICIAN NOTES** To demonstrate the optical illusion of variation in spacing that occurs further from the central beam, evenly place a row of pennies about ½ inch" (1.5 mm) apart, along the center length of the image receptor. Take an x-ray and look at the image. On the resulting image notice how the spacing between the pennies appear to distort as they progress towards the outside edges of the film.

> **TECHNICIAN NOTES** In general, each vertebra is made up of a body (the denser ventral portion which is separated from bodies of adjacent vertebra by intervertebral discs), vertebral arch (located dorsal to the body), and various processes (the cranial and caudal articular processes, the dorsal spinous process and the lateral transverse process) (Figure 22-3, 22-11, 22-12, 22-16, 22-17).

> **TECHNICIAN NOTES** The vertebral column is divided into 5 regions—cervical (neck), thoracic (chest), lumbar (abdomen), sacral (pelvis) and caudal (tail-sometimes referred to as coccygeal). To refer to a particular vertebra, use abbreviations for the region followed by the number within the region, beginning at the cranial end. For example, T12 is the twelfth thoracic vertebra. The abbreviation for caudal vertebrae is Cd (though sometimes the tail vertebrae are called coccygeal and the abbreviation is Cy).
> The first letter designating each group, followed by the number of vertebrae in each group, is the vertebral formula. The vertebral formula for a dog and cat is $C_7T_{13}L_7S_3Cd_{6-20}$.

TABLE 22-1	Protocol for Spinal Radiography		
ANATOMICAL LOCATION	**ROUTINE VIEWS**		**OPTIONAL VIEWS**
Survey study:			
Large dog	Lateral		Ventrodorsal—center as for the lateral
	Center at C4, T6-T7, thoracolumbar, L4, lumbosacral		
Small dog	Lateral		Ventrodorsal—center as for the lateral
	Center at C4, T6-T7, L4, lumbosacral		
Cat (coned-down views where needed)	Lateral		Ventrodorsal—center as for lateral
	Center at T6-T7 or area of interest		
Cervical vertebrae	Lateral, ventrodorsal		Hyperextended or hyperflexed lateral, open-mouth ventrodorsal, coned-down views, oblique
	Center at C4		
Thoracic vertebrae	Lateral, ventrodorsal		Oblique, dorsoventral
	Center at T6-T7		
Thoracolumbar vertebrae	Lateral, ventrodorsal		Oblique
	Center at thoracolumbar junction		
Lumbar vertebrae	Lateral, ventrodorsal		Oblique
	Center at L4		
Lumbosacral vertebrae	Lateral, Ventrodorsal		Hyperextended or flexed lateral
	Center at lumbosacral junction		

(OFD). Also, it may be more difficult to obtain a parallel technique if the animal is in the DV position.

Hyperflexion and hyperextension views can further evaluate the caudal aspect of the lateral cervical and the lumbosacral vertebrae if the patient is chemically restrained and will not be traumatized by such handling.

Survey Study

Routine views include the lateral and the ventrodorsal projections of the various vertebral sections. Depending on the size of the dog, a full study is either four or five images of each orthogonal view. Cat studies of the vertebrae are often part of the whole body view. For both the dog and the cat, coned-down views are important for areas of interest. Because most feline patients requiring vertebral radiography likely present with spinal injury, sedation or general anesthesia and gentle handling are needed. Dynamic views of the vertebrae are not common in cats but can be completed.

Table 22-1 indicates where to center for the survey views. For further information on where to measure, and the borders, position, and comments, see sections on specific spinal areas and views. (Table 22-2)[1] gives information on the vertebral number and characteristics of the vertebrae of some common species.

Cervical Vertebrae

Lateral View

Positioning

Place In: Lateral recumbency.

Hind Limbs: Superimpose and place the pelvic limbs caudally; secure with a sandbag.

Forelimbs: Position and superimpose the forelimbs caudally; secure with a sandbag. A small foam pad can be placed between the limbs.

Head/Neck/Sternum: Elevate the nose using a sponge. Keep the head in a, true lateral position. Support the cranial area of the head with a sandbag, or secure it with tape. Place sponges under the sternum to achieve true alignment with the vertebrae.

Vertebrae: Use foam pads or cotton beneath the cervical vertebrae to keep them parallel to the table.

MEASURE: Across the shoulder at the level of C6 to ensure adequate penetration of the caudal cervical vertebrae. Overexposure may occur with the cranial cervical vertebrae. Coned-down views can be made of these areas.

CENTRAL RAY: C4.

BORDERS: Base of the skull to the spine of the scapula (just past the shoulder joint). Collimate tightly to the edge of the wings of the atlas and the center of the spine of the scapula.

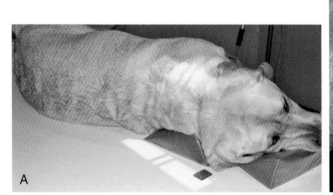

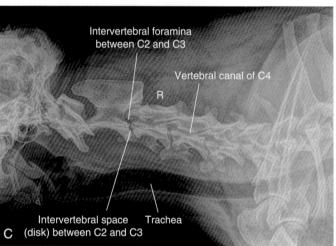

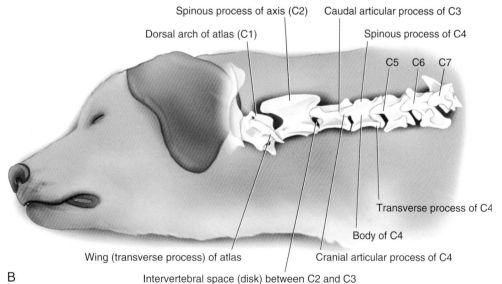

FIGURE 22-2 A, Positioning for the lateral view of the cervical vertebrae. B, Left-to-right lateral anatomy of the cervical vertebrae. C, Lateral radiograph of cervical vertebrae.

Continued

Lateral View—*cont'd*

Comments and Tips

- Keep the spine parallel to the table—the transverse processes of each vertebra should be superimposed on the image. A separate image of the cervicothoracic junction may be required to better evaluate this region.[1]
- The head must be in a true lateral position, because any obliquity of the head can change the position of the cranial cervical vertebrae.
- To see if the head is in a true lateral, draw an imaginary line between the medial canthi, and make sure this line is perpendicular to the table.
- Try to keep lateral positioning of the entire body even if radiographing only the cervical area. Too much or too little padding can cause false narrowing of the intervertebral discs.

- Do not overextend the limbs because doing so might cause rotation of the spine.
- Do not flex or extend the head. To help align the cervical vertebrae with the long axis of the image receptor, position the pelvis region dorsally.
- On the radiograph the transverse processes should be superimposed.
- Larger canine patients may have to be radiographed in two sections for the lateral and ventrodorsal cervical vertebrae:
  - *Radiograph 1:* Central ray at C2-C3; include from the base of the skull to C4; measure at C2-C3.
  - *Radiograph 2:* Central ray at C5-C6; include from C4 to the center of the spine of the scapula; measure at the level of C6-C7.

> **TECHNICIAN NOTES**   Strategically used positioning aids give the patient the illusion that it is being held.

> **TECHNICIAN NOTES**   Pulling the front limbs caudally prevents shoulder soft tissue from overlapping the spine.

> **TECHNICIAN NOTES**   Be extra careful when manipulating small breed dogs that present with apparent neck pain.

> **TECHNICIAN NOTES**   Quickly go through your mental checklist *before* pushing the exposure button: settings correct; image receptor/machine/grid in position; proper location of markers and ID (if using at this stage); correct body part and view; properly centered; borders correct and collimated; patient properly prepared, positioned, and restrained so the vertebrae are in the same horizontal plane as the sternum for the lateral and superimposed for the VD, and parallel to the image receptor. Both are perpendicular to the central ray.

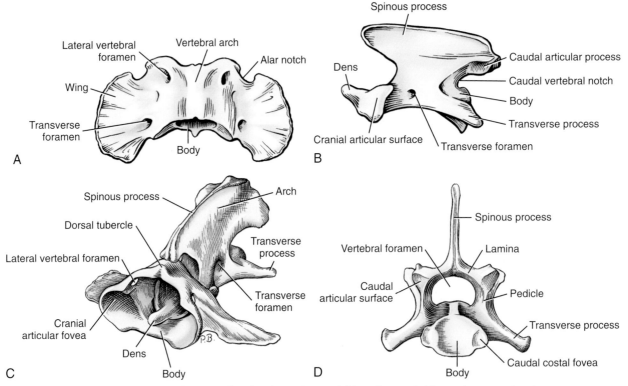

FIGURE 22-3 Cervical vertebrae. A, Atlas, dorsal view. B, Axis, left lateral view. C, Atlas, and axis articulated, craniolateral aspect. D, Seventh cervical vertebrae, caudal aspect.

Hyperextended Lateral View

Positioning

Place In: Lateral recumbency.

Hind Limbs: Superimpose and place the pelvic limbs caudally; secure with a sandbag.

Forelimbs: Position and superimpose the forelimbs caudally; secure with a sandbag. A small foam pad may be placed between the limbs.

Head/Neck/Sternum: Elevate and keep the nose level to the table, using a foam pad. Hyperextend the neck and head dorsally and caudally until resistance is met. Support the cranial area of the head with a sandbag, or secure with tape. Place foam pads under the sternum to achieve true alignment with the vertebrae.

Vertebrae: Use foam pad or cotton beneath the cervical vertebrae to keep each vertebra parallel to the table.

Comments and Tips

- For true hyperextension, all cervical vertebrae need to be extended dorsally.
- The head must be in a true lateral position, because any obliquity of the head can change the position of the cranial cervical vertebrae.

- To see if the head is in a true lateral: draw an imaginary line between the medial canthi, and make sure this line is perpendicular to the table.
- Try to keep lateral positioning of the entire body even if radiographing only the cervical area. Too much or too little padding can cause false narrowing of the intervertebral discs.
- Do not overextend the limbs, because doing so might cause rotation of the spine.
- If an endotracheal tube is present, be careful that the patient's breathing is not restricted at any point.
- Collimate tightly so that a coned-down view is obtained.
- The hyperextended and hyperflexed views (dynamic views) are useful during myelography to note any spinal cord impingement due to extradural changes associated with vertebral instability.[2]

> **TECHNICIAN NOTES** To align the cervical vertebrae with the long axis of the image receptor, position the pelvis region dorsally.

MEASURE: C3-C4 intervertebral space across the neck.

CENTRAL RAY: C3-C4 intervertebral space.

BORDERS: Base of the skull to the spine of the scapula (just past the shoulder joint).

Collimate tightly to the edge of the wings of the atlas and the center of the spine of the scapula.

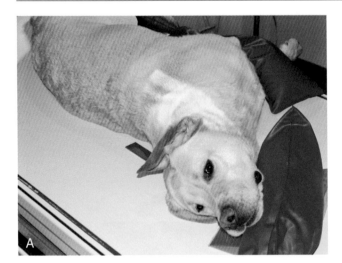

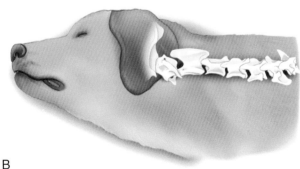

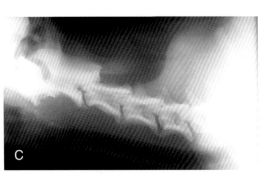

FIGURE 22-4 **A,** Positioning for the lateral view of the hyperextended cervical vertebrae. **B,** Left-to-right lateral anatomy of the hyperextended cervical vertebrae. **C,** Lateral radiograph of the hyperextended cervical vertebrae.

Flexed Lateral View of the Cervical Vertebrae

Positioning

Place In: Lateral recumbency.

Hind Limbs: Superimpose and position the pelvic limbs caudally; secure with sandbags.

Forelimbs: Position and superimpose the forelimbs ventrally and caudally, and secure with a sandbag. A small foam pad can be placed between the limbs.

Head/Neck/Sternum: Place tape or thin rope around the nose or canine teeth, and gently apply traction on the end so the neck and head are flexed. Pull the tape caudally between the forelimbs close to the body, and secure to a sandbag. If needed elevate the nose using a sponge. A sandbag can be placed dorsal to the nose to maintain the hyperflexed position. Place sponges under the sternum to achieve true alignment with the vertebrae.

Vertebrae: If needed, use sponges beneath the cervical vertebrae to keep the spine parallel to the table and at the same plane as the thoracic vertebrae.

Comments and Tips

- For true flexion, all cervical vertebrae need to be flexed.
- The head must be in a true lateral position, because any obliquity of the head can change the position of the cranial cervical vertebrae.
- Draw an imaginary line between the medial canthi, and make sure this line is perpendicular to the table.
- Try to keep lateral positioning of the entire body even if radiographing only the cervical area. Too much or too little padding can cause false narrowing of the intervertebral discs.
- Do not overextend the limbs, because doing so might cause rotation of the vertebrae.
- Be careful with hyperflexing the neck so as not to cause tracheal trauma or constriction of the endotracheal tube if present.
- Collimate tightly so that a coned-down view is obtained.

MEASURE: C3-C4 intervertebral space across the neck.

CENTRAL RAY: C3-C4 intervertebral space.

BORDERS: Base of the skull to the spine of the scapula (just past the shoulder joint).
    Collimate tightly to the edge of the wings of the atlas and the center of the spine of the scapula.

> **TECHNICIAN NOTES** Note that the positioning is fairly similar for most of the lateral views and for most ventrodorsal vertebral views.

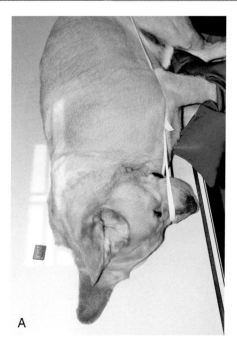

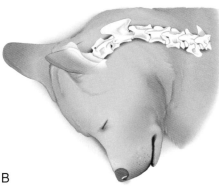

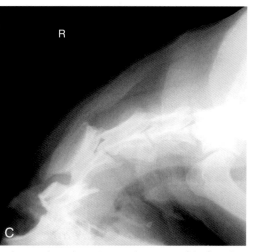

FIGURE 22-5 **A,** Positioning for the lateral view of the flexed cervical vertebrae. **B,** Lateral anatomy of the flexed cervical vertebrae. **C,** Lateral radiograph of the flexed cervical vertebrae.

Lateral Oblique View for the Odontoid Process

Positioning

Place In: Lateral recumbency (Figure 22-6).

Hind Limbs: Superimpose and place the pelvic limbs caudally; secure with a sandbag.

Forelimbs: Position and superimpose the forelimbs caudally; secure with a sandbag. A small foam pad can be placed between the limbs.

Head/Neck/Sternum: Use tape to keep the head in its natural oblique position.[5] Place sponges under the sternum to keep the sternum on the same plane as the thoracic vertebrae.

Vertebrae: Use padding to keep the cervical vertebrae lateral, and the head and C1 oblique.

Comments and Tips

- Position the ear pinnae laterally, and pull the tongue to avoid shadows on the radiograph.

MEASURE: C1 (for odontoid process).

CENTRAL RAY: C1 (for odontoid process).

BORDERS: Mid-skull to C4.

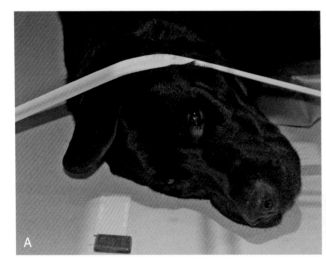

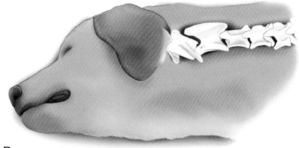

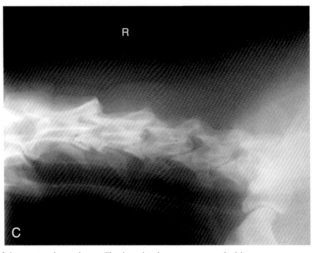

FIGURE 22-6 **A,** Positioning for the lateral oblique view of the cervical vertebrae. The head is kept in a natural oblique position and a wedge is placed under the sternum. **B,** A lateral oblique view of the cervical vertebrae. **C,** Lateral oblique radiograph of all the cervical vertebrae. For the odontoid process, center at C1.

Ventrodorsal View of the Cervical Vertebrae

Positioning

Place In: Dorsal recumbency in a V-trough or supported by tape or sandbag if needed.

Hind Limbs: Place the pelvic limbs in a neutral position, and secure with sandbags.

Forelimbs: Evenly position the forelimbs caudally, and secure with a sandbag.

Head/Neck/Sternum: Keep the head in a natural position as parallel to the table as possible. Secure with padding lateral to the head and neck. Keep the sternum superimposed over the vertebrae.

Vertebrae: Use padding beneath the rostral neck to keep the cervical vertebrae parallel to the table.

Comments and Tips

- Make sure that the sternum and vertebrae are superimposed and perpendicular to the image receptor, to minimize rotation.

- The nose should be in line with the base of the tail with the limbs positioned evenly.

- If there is an interest in the occipital bone, point the nose upward, and secure with sandbags lateral to the head and neck, so that there is no bone superimposition of C1-C2 with the occipital bone. As this is often the last view made, the endotracheal tube should be removed before the image is taken. An open-mouth view of the odontoid process can be made as described in Chapter 23.

- If the machine allows, angle the central ray slightly caudocranially to the table top so that it passes through the joint spaces.

> **TECHNICIAN NOTES** Remember to collimate tightly to the vertebrae. Place the label/marker on the dorsal aspect for the lateral views, and tape on the body or place on the table, in an area that will not obscure important anatomy, for VD views.

MEASURE: Level of C6 near the manubrium.

CENTRAL RAY: C4. Angle the beam in a slight caudocranial direction between the intervertebral space.

BORDERS: Base of the skull to the shoulder joint, with tight collimation laterally.

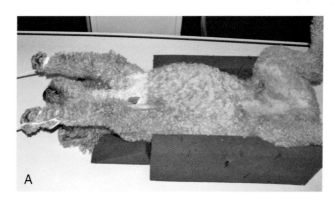

FIGURE 22-7 A, Alternate positioning for the ventrodorsal view of the cervical vertebrae. The forelimbs are usually pulled caudally.

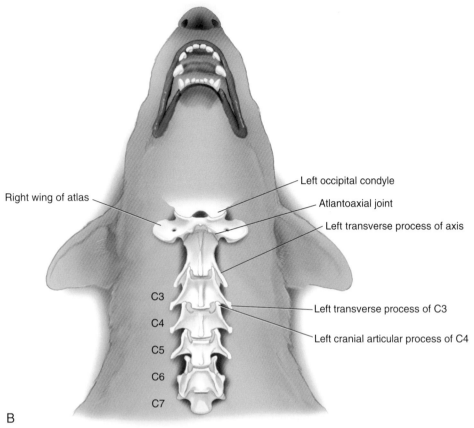

Left occipital condyle

Atlantoaxial joint

Left transverse process of axis

Right wing of atlas

C3

C4

C5

C6

C7

Left transverse process of C3

Left cranial articular process of C4

B

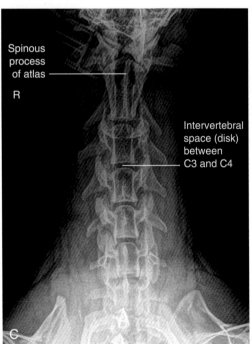

Spinous
process
of atlas

R

Intervertebral
space (disk)
between
C3 and C4

C

FIGURE 22-7, cont'd B, Ventrodorsal radiographic anatomy of the canine cervical vertebrae. C, Ventrodorsal radiograph of the cervical vertebrae.

Thoracic Vertebrae

Lateral View

Positioning

Place In: Lateral recumbency.

Hind Limbs: Superimpose and place the pelvic limbs caudally; secure with a sandbag. A small foam pad can be placed between the limbs.

Forelimbs: Superimpose and cranially position the forelimbs slightly; secure with a sandbag. A small foam pad can be placed between the limbs.

Head/Neck/Sternum: Keep the head in a natural position, and support the neck with a sandbag. If needed, use sponges under the sternum and between the limbs to achieve true alignment of the sternum and vertebrae.

Vertebrae: Use padding if needed to keep each thoracic vertebra on the same horizontal plane as the sternum. Using tape as in Figure 22-1, can assist with proper alignment.

Comments and Tips

- Try to keep lateral positioning of the entire body even if radiographing only the thoracic area. Collimate tightly.

- The pelvis should be positioned ventrally so that the thoracic vertebrae are aligned with the long axis of the image receptor. The reason is that in the mid- to caudal thoracic vertebrae region, dogs and cats have a natural area of kyphosis.[1]
- The ribs should be superimposed over each other so that the intervertebral spaces are better viewed, and the sternum should be at the same distance from the table as the vertebrae.
- Large dogs may require two separate views.

> **TECHNICIAN NOTES**   Placing padding under the nose and the natural curvatures of the spine (neck and lumbar regions) and between the limbs for the lateral positions, will keep the spine parallel and horizontal with the table/image receptor and perpendicular to the center ray.

MEASURE: Highest point of the mid-thorax.

CENTRAL RAY: T6-T7 or the caudal border of the scapula.

BORDERS: From C7 to L1 inclusive (shoulder joint to past the origin of last rib).

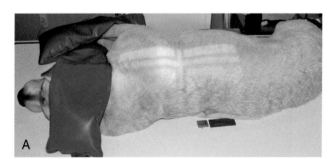

FIGURE 22-8 A, Positioning for the lateral view of the thoracic vertebrae.

Lateral View—*cont'd*

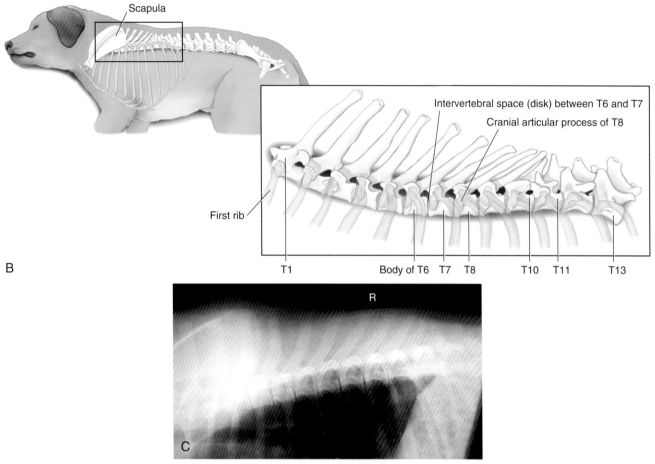

B

FIGURE 22-8, cont'd B, Left-to-right lateral anatomy of the thoracic vertebrae. C, Lateral radiograph of the thoracic vertebrae.

Ventrodorsal View of the Thoracic Vertebrae

Positioning

Place In: Dorsal recumbency in a V-trough or use sandbags if needed.

Hind Limbs: Equally place the pelvic limbs in a neutral position; secure with sandbags.

Forelimbs: Equally position the forelimbs cranially, and tie or secure with sandbags.

Head/Neck/Sternum: The head and neck are best positioned with the nose parallel to the table and equidistant between the limbs. Support with a sandbag being careful not to restrict breathing.

Vertebrae: Superimpose the sternum and vertebrae to minimize any rotation.

Comments and Tips

- Ensure that there is a straight line from the tip of the nose to the base of the tail to achieve rib symmetry on the radiograph.
- Large dogs may require two separate views.
- Symmetry of the normal patient is noted on a radiograph when the spinous processes are evident on the mid-vertebral body and the sternum is superimposed over the vertebrae.

> **TECHNICIAN NOTES** Image fewer vertebrae to prevent distortion.

MEASURE: T6-T7 or the caudal border of the scapula.

CENTRAL RAY: T6-T7 or the caudal border of the scapula.

BORDERS: C7-L1 (shoulder joint to past the origin of the last rib).

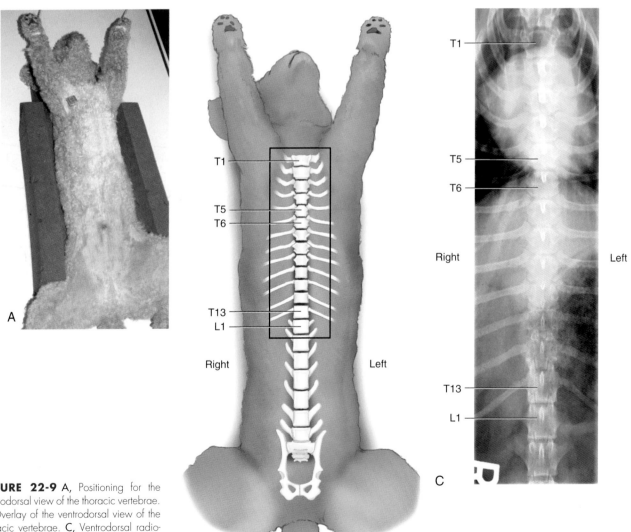

FIGURE 22-9 A, Positioning for the ventrodorsal view of the thoracic vertebrae. **B,** Overlay of the ventrodorsal view of the thoracic vertebrae. **C,** Ventrodorsal radiograph of the thoracic vertebrae.

Thoracolumbar Vertebrae

Lateral View

Positioning

Place In: Lateral recumbency.

Hind Limbs: Superimpose and place the pelvic limbs caudally; secure with a sandbag. A small foam pad can be placed between the limbs.

Forelimbs: Superimpose and cranially position the forelimbs slightly; secure with a sandbag. A small foam pad can be placed between the limbs.

Head/Neck/Sternum: If needed, use foam pads under the sternum to achieve true alignment of the vertebrae. Keep the head in a natural position, and support the neck with a sandbag being careful not to restrict breathing.

Vertebrae: Keep the thoracolumbar vertebrae on the same plane as the sternum. Using tape as in Figure 22-1 can assist with proper alignment.

Comments and Tips

- Try to maintain true lateral positioning of the entire body even if radiographing only the thoracolumbar area.
- Collimate tightly.
- The vertebrae should be limited to four on either side of the TL junction.
- The ribs should be superimposed over each other so that the intervertebral spaces are better viewed, and the sternum should be at the same distance from the table as the vertebrae.
- On the image:
  - The intervertebral foramina should be superimposed and they should be of equal sizes from the thoracolumbar junction towards the sacrum.

MEASURE: Highest point of the mid-thorax (mid-xiphoid).

CENTRAL RAY: T13-L1 intervertebral space.

BORDERS: Xiphoid to caudal portion of the last rib.

TECHNICIAN NOTES Keep these practical landmarks in mind as a general basis for the borders of all vertebrae: base of the skull, shoulder, origin of the last rib, and greater trochanter.

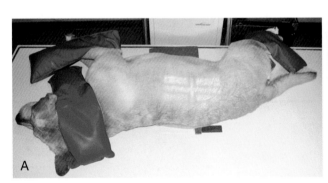

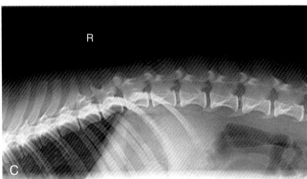

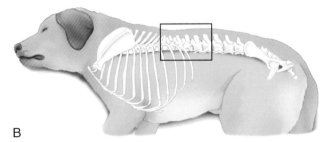

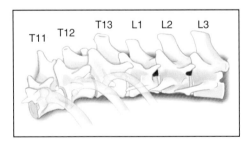

FIGURE 22-10 A, Positioning for the lateral view of the thoracolumbar vertebrae. B, Right-to-left lateral radiographic anatomy of the thoracolumbar vertebrae. C, Lateral radiograph of the thoracolumbar vertebrae. Limit the number of vertebrae on either side of the TL junction.

Continued

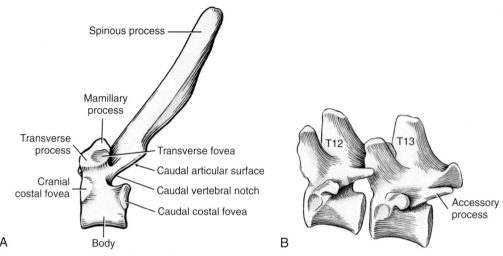

FIGURE 22-11 Left lateral views of the sixth thoracic vertebra (**A**) and 12th and 13th thoracic vertebrae (**B**).

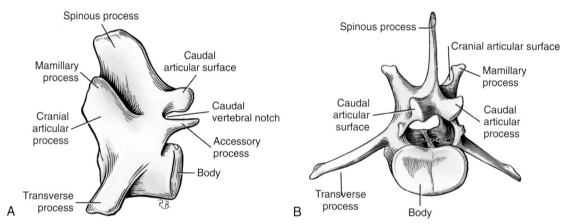

FIGURE 22-12 **A,** Fourth lumbar vertebra left lateral view. **B,** Fifth lumbar vertebrae, caudolateral view.

Ventrodorsal View of the Thoracolumbar Vertebrae

Positioning

Place In: Dorsal recumbency in a V-trough or use sandbags if needed.

Hind Limbs: Place the pelvic limbs in a neutral position; secure with sandbags if needed.

Forelimbs: Position the forelimbs cranially; tie or secure with sandbags.

Head/Neck/Sternum: The head and neck can be in a natural position. If needed, support with a sandbag being careful not to restrict breathing. The nose should be equidistant between both front limbs.

Vertebrae: Have the sternum and vertebrae superimposed to minimize any rotation.

Comments and Tips

• Ensure that there is a straight line from the tip of the nose to the base of the tail.

> **TECHNICIAN NOTES** Provide enough support with a trough, pads, or sandbags to prevent any rotation for ventrodorsal views. The spine and sternum must be in the same vertical plane and be perpendicular to the table and image receptor.

> **TECHNICIAN NOTES** Collimate tightly to include the transverse process and muscle mass, but do not include the fat and skin.

MEASURE: Highest point of the mid-thorax origin of last rib.

CENTRAL RAY: T13-L1 intervertebral space.

BORDERS: Xiphoid to the caudal portion of last rib.

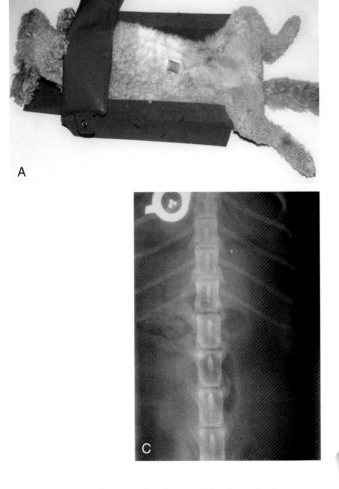

A

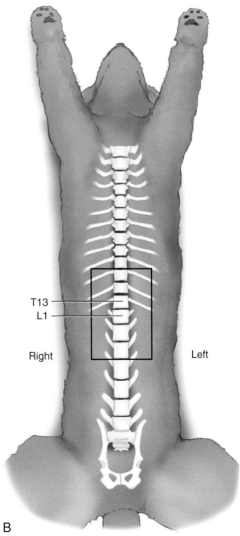

T13
L1

Right   Left

B

C

FIGURE 22-13 A, Positioning for the ventrodorsal view of the thoracolumbar vertebrae. B, Overlay of the ventrodorsal thoracolumbar vertebrae. C, Ventrodorsal radiograph of the thoracolumbar vertebrae.

Lumbar Vertebrae

Lateral View

Positioning

Place In: Lateral recumbency.

Hind Limbs: Superimpose and place the pelvic limbs caudally; secure with a sandbag. A small foam pad can be placed between the limbs.

Forelimbs: Superimpose and cranially position the forelimbs slightly; secure with a sandbag. A small foam pad can be placed between the limbs.

Head/Neck/Sternum: If needed, use foam pads under the sternum to achieve true alignment with the vertebrae. Keep the head in a natural position; support the neck with a sandbag being careful not to restrict breathing.

Vertebrae: Keep each lumbar vertebra parallel to the table and image receptor and on the same horizontal plane as the sternum. Using tape as in Figure 22-1, can assist with proper alignment.

Comments and Tips

- Try to maintain true lateral positioning of the entire body even if radiographing only the lumbar area.
- Collimate tightly.
- On the image:
  - The intervertebral foramina should be superimposed.
  - They should be of equal sizes from the thoracolumbar junction to the sacrum.
  - The transverse processes should be superimposed over each other. The view of this superimposition has been described as a "Nike swoosh."[1]

MEASURE: Level of L1.

CENTRAL RAY: Level of L4.

BORDERS: T12-S1 (cranial to origin of last rib to just before the greater trochanter).

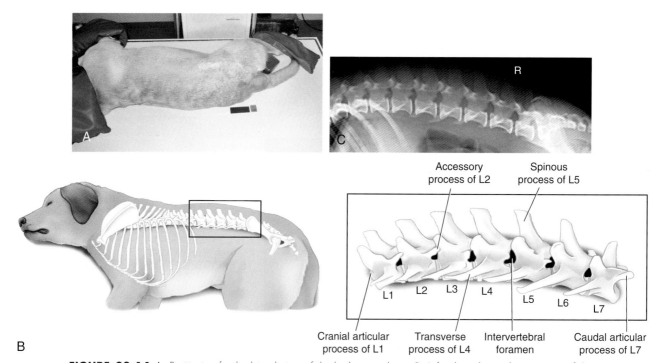

FIGURE 22-14 A, Positioning for the lateral view of the lumbar vertebrae. **B,** Left-right radiographic anatomy of the lateral lumbar vertebrae. **C,** Lateral radiograph of the lumbar vertebrae of a 19-year-old male, neutered French Bulldog. Note the calcification at T12-T13, L1-L2, and L3-L4. The transverse processes should be superimposed at their origins from the vertebral bodies, each pair appearing as one. This appearance has been described as a "Nike swoosh."

Ventrodorsal View of the Lumbar Vertebrae

Positioning

Place In: Dorsal recumbency in a V-trough or use sandbags if needed.

Hind Limbs: Superimpose and extend the pelvic limbs fully; secure with sandbags if needed.

Forelimbs: Position the forelimbs cranially, and secure with a sandbag if needed.

Head/Neck/Sternum: The head can be in a natural position. Support with a sandbag being careful not to restrict breathing. Have the nose equidistant between the forelimbs.

Vertebrae: Superimpose the sternum and vertebrae to minimize any rotation.

Comments and Tips

- Ensure that there is a straight line from the tip of the nose to the base of the tail.
- The transverse processes should be present and symmetrical on the image.
- Enemas are suggested before radiography of the lumbar and lumbosacral spine because feces can create artifacts.

MEASURE: Level of L1.

CENTRAL RAY: Level of L4.

BORDERS: T12-S1 (just cranial to both the origin of the last rib and acetabulum).

TECHNICIAN NOTES Extending the forelimbs and hind limbs and securing them, provide further support to help avoid rotation of the spine.

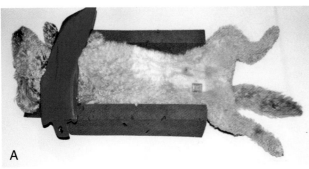

A

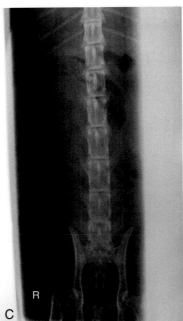

C

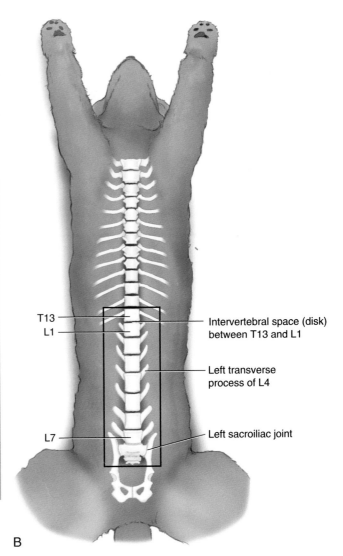

T13

L1

Intervertebral space (disk) between T13 and L1

Left transverse process of L4

L7

Left sacroiliac joint

B

FIGURE 22-15 **A**, Positioning for the ventrodorsal view of the lumbar vertebrae. **B**, Overlay of the ventrodorsal lumbar vertebrae. **C**, Ventrodorsal radiograph of the lumbar vertebrae.

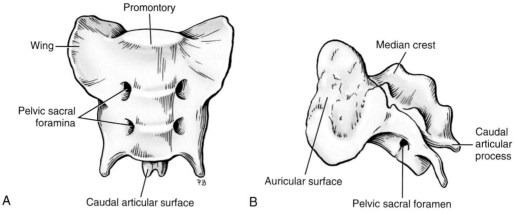

FIGURE 22-16 Sacrum. **A,** Ventral view. **B,** Left lateral view.

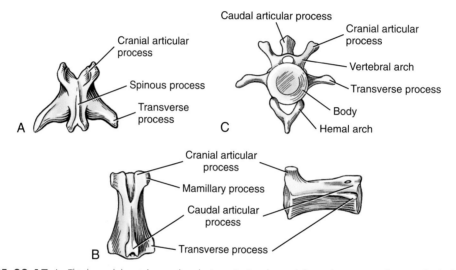

FIGURE 22-17 **A,** Third caudal vertebrae, dorsal view. **B,** Fourth caudal vertebrae, cranial view. **C,** Sixth caudal vertebra, dorsal (*left*) and lateral (*right*) views.

Lumbosacral Vertebrae

Lateral View—Natural Positioning

Positioning

Place In: Lateral recumbency.

Hind Limbs: Superimpose and pull the pelvic limbs into a fully extended position, with a foam pad between them; secure with sandbags. Ensure that the wings of the ilia are superimposed and parallel to the image receptor by placing padding under the upper limb.

Forelimbs: Superimpose and cranially position the forelimbs slightly; secure with a sandbag. A small foam pad can be placed between the limbs.

Head/Neck/Sternum: Use foam pads under the sternum to achieve true alignment with the vertebrae. Keep the head in a natural position; support the neck with a sandbag, being careful not to restrict breathing.

Vertebrae: Use padding to keep each lumbar vertebra parallel to the table and the image receptor.

Comments and Tips

- Use the pelvis technique chart to ensure adequate penetration.
- On the image:
  - The intervertebral foramina of the lumbar vertebrae should be superimposed and of equal sizes.
  - The transverse processes should be superimposed over each other to look like a "Nike swoosh."

MEASURE: Level of the lumbosacral junction or the highest point of the wings of the ilia.

CENTRAL RAY: Level of the lumbosacral junction (just caudal to the wings of the ilia).

BORDERS: L6 to the most cranial caudal vertebra (just cranial to the wings of the ilia to the femoral head).

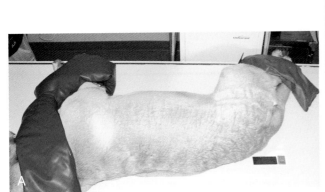

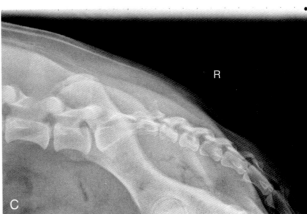

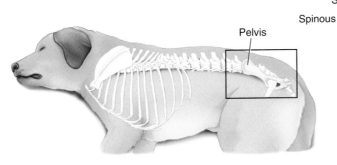

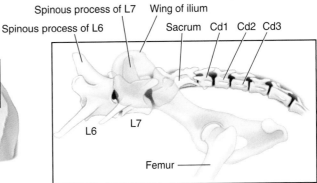

FIGURE 22-18 A, Positioning for the lateral view of the lumbosacral vertebrae. **B,** Overlay and radiographic anatomy of the lateral lumbosacral vertebrae. **C,** Radiograph of the lateral lumbosacral vertebrae.

Lateral View—Hyperextended View of the Lumbosacral Vertebrae

Positioning

Place In: Lateral recumbency.

Hind Limbs: Superimpose and hyperextend the pelvic limbs caudally toward the dorsum; secure with sandbags or tape. If needed, use sponges between the hind limbs to superimpose the wings of the ilia.

Forelimbs: Superimpose and cranially position the forelimbs slightly, and secure with a sandbag. A small foam pad can be placed between the limbs.

Head/Neck/Sternum: Keep the head in a natural position, and support the neck with a sandbag, being careful not to restrict breathing.

Vertebrae: Use padding if needed to keep each lumbar vertebra parallel to the table and image receptor.

Comments and Tips

- Use the pelvic technique chart to ensure adequate penetration.

MEASURE: Level of the lumbosacral junction or the highest point of the wings of the ilia.

CENTRAL RAY: Level of the lumbosacral junction (just caudal to the wings of the ilia).

BORDERS: L6 to the most cranial caudal vertebra (just cranial to the wings of the ilia to the femoral head).

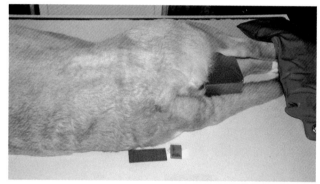

FIGURE 22-19 Positioning for the lateral view of the lumbosacral vertebrae—hyperextended view.

Lateral View—Hyperflexed View of the Lumbosacral Vertebrae

Positioning

Place In: Lateral recumbency.

Hind Limbs: Superimpose and hyperflex the pelvic limbs toward the sternum; secure with sandbags or tape. If needed, use sponges between the hind limbs to help superimpose the wings of the ilia.

Forelimbs: Cranially extend the forelimbs; secure with a sandbag. A small foam pad can be placed between the limbs.

Head/Neck/Sternum: Keep in a natural position and support with a sandbag if needed, being careful not to restrict breathing. Elevate the sternum so it is on the same plane as the vertebrae.

Vertebrae: Use padding if needed to keep each lumbar vertebra parallel to the table and image receptor.

Comments and Tips

Use the pelvic technique chart to ensure adequate penetration.

> **TECHNICIAN NOTES** Collimate, ensuring that labels/markers are included and that borders are visible, for every image.

MEASURE: Wings of the ilia.

CENTRAL RAY: Level of the lumbosacral junction (just caudal to the wings of the ilia).

BORDERS: L6 to the most cranial caudal vertebra (just cranial to the wings of the ilia to the femoral head).

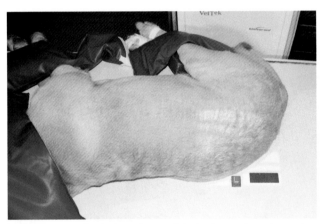

FIGURE 22-20 Positioning for the lateral view of the lumbosacral vertebrae—hyperflexed view.

Ventrodorsal View of the Lumbosacral Vertebrae

Positioning

Place In: Dorsal recumbency in a V-trough or use sandbags if needed.

Hind Limbs: Partially extend the pelvic limbs equally in a normal position, and secure with sandbags if needed. The pelvic limbs may be externally rotated.

Forelimbs: Position the forelimbs cranially, and secure with a sandbag.

Head/Neck/Sternum: The head can be in a natural position. Support with a sandbag being careful not to restrict breathing.

Vertebrae: Maintain the sternum and vertebrae in the same vertical plane.

Comments and Tips

- Ensure that the wings of the ilia are parallel to the table.
- A cleansing enema 1 to 2 hours prior to radiography should be considered to remove any feces in the colon that could obscure spinal lesions.

MEASURE: Wings of the ilia.

CENTRAL RAY: On the lumbosacral junction, caudal to the wings of the ilia, at an angle of 20 to 30 degrees in a caudocranial direction.

BORDERS: L6 to the most cranial caudal vertebra (from just cranial to the wings of the ilia to the femoral head).

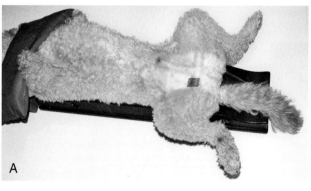

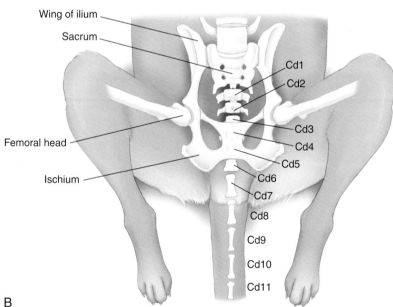

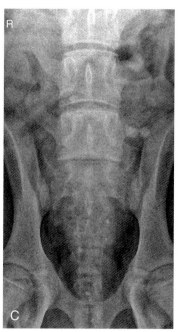

FIGURE 22-21 **A,** Positioning for the ventrodorsal view of the lumbosacral vertebrae. **B,** Radiographic anatomy of the ventrodorsal lumbosacral vertebrae. **C,** Ventrodorsal radiograph of the lumbosacral vertebrae.

Caudal Vertebrae

Lateral View

Positioning

Place In: Lateral recumbency.

Hind Limbs: Superimpose and pull the pelvic limbs in a neutral position; secure with a sandbag.

Forelimbs: Superimpose and cranially position the forelimbs slightly; secure with a sandbag if needed.

Head and Neck: Keep the head in a natural position; support with a sandbag if needed.

Vertebrae: Raise the cassette with a foam pad to keep at the same plane as the tail. Secure the tail to the cassette if needed.

Comments and Tips

- A grid is not used.
- Divide the plate so that both views are on one cassette.

MEASURE: Thickest part of the tail.

CENTRAL RAY: Area of interest.

BORDERS: Four or five vertebrae on either side of the area of interest, or the full tail.

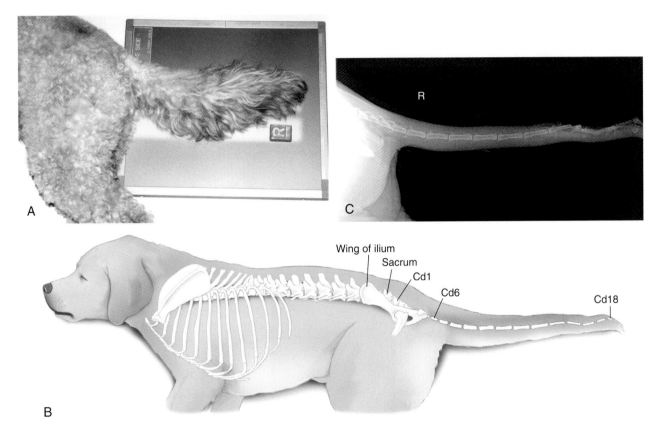

FIGURE 22-22 **A,** Positioning of the lateral caudal vertebrae. **B,** Radiographic anatomy of the lateral caudal vertebrae. **C,** Lateral radiograph of the caudal vertebrae that are fractured near the tip.

Ventrodorsal View of the Caudal Vertebrae

Positioning

Place In: Dorsal recumbency in a V-trough or supported by tape or sandbag if needed.

Hind Limbs: Extend the pelvic limbs; secure with sandbags if needed.

Forelimbs: Position the forelimbs cranially; secure with sandbags if needed.

Head/Neck/Sternum: The head can be in a natural position. Secure if needed.

Vertebrae: Secure the tail with tape if required, and keep it in a straight line with the body.

Comments and Tips

A grid is not needed.

MEASURE: Thickest part of the tail.

CENTRAL RAY: Area of interest.

BORDERS: Four or five vertebrae on either side of the area of interest, or the full tail.

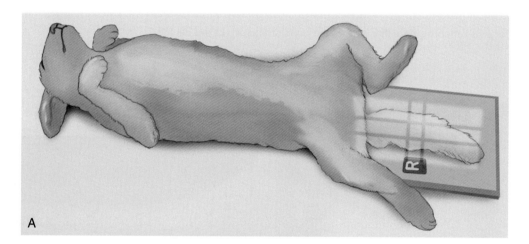

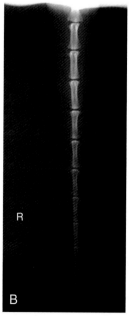

FIGURE 22-23 A, Positioning for the ventrodorsal view of the caudal vertebrae. B, Ventrodorsal radiograph of the coccygeal (caudal) vertebrae.

TABLE 22-2	Vertebral Number and Characteristics for Some Common Species		
		VERTEBRAL (NO.)- AND CHARATERISTICS	
ANATOMICAL LOCATION	**DOG**	**CAT**	**HORSE**
Cervical vertebrae (C)	7 Standard in most species.	7	7
Atlas (C1)	No spinous process. Reduced body. Two large lateral wings. Modified cranial and caudal processes (articular fovea) articulate via synovial joints allowing greater movement.	Similar to the dog.	Similar to the dog.
Axis (C2)	Large "blade-like" spinous process. Has peglike dens (odontoid process) at the cranial aspect to form the atlantoaxial joint. No intervertebral disc between C1 and C2; articulates caudally with C3 via an intervertebral disc.	Similar to the dog.	Similar to the dog.
C6	Large transverse processes (ventral lamina).	Similar to the dog.	Similar to the dog.
Thoracic vertebrae (T) (also varies within species)	13 +13 pairs of ribs. Same as cattle, sheep, and goats (Humans have 12.) Tall spinous processes. Large articular facets that form joints with the heads of the ribs.	13 +13 pairs of ribs. Rib heads are cranial to respective vertebral body.	18 +18 pairs of ribs.
T11(Anticlinal vertebrae)	Spinous processes project up straight, as opposed to the caudal reclining of the spinous processes of the cranial vertebrae and the cranial inclination of the vertebrae caudal to it. T10-T11 has narrowest intervertebral disc space.	T11	T16
Lumbar vertebrae (L)	7 (Humans have 5.) Large bulky bodies. Short spinous processes. Large, cranially angulated lateral processes. The diaphragmatic crura attach to L3 or L4 ventral margins, which may be ill defined. Straight or kyphotic curvature.	7 Same as goats. Pigs and sheep can have 6 or 7 Greater ratio of vertebral body length to height (longer). Lordotic curve.	6 Cattle also have 6.
Sacrum (S)	3 fused vertebrae. Pig and sheep have 4 fused vertebrae. Laterally forms sacroiliac joint with pelvis.	3 fused vertebrae.	5 fused vertebrae. Same for cattle, goats, and humans.
Caudal (Cd) or coccygeal(Cy) vertebrae	20–25. Humans have 4–5 fused as the coccyx. May have hemal arches ventral to craniocaudal vertebral bodies.	5–23 Hemal arches more commonly seen.	15–20 Hemal arches ventral to first few.

Optional Views

A ventrodorsal view of the spinal column with a vertical beam may not always be feasible because of patient injury or other concerns. Alternatives include a lateral decubitus view, an oblique view, and a dorsoventral view (Figure 22-24). Keep the principles of measuring, centering, and borders in mind for each of the positions described here. Center the beam on the area of interest.

Lateral Decubitus View (Ventrodorsal View with a Horizontal Beam)

The ventrodorsal view can also be achieved using a horizontal beam with the dog in lateral recumbency as described for the thoracic and abdominal views in Chapters 18 and 19 (Figure 22-24A).

Oblique View

To help localize a lesion identified on the lateral or VD views, an oblique view may be desired. Place the patient

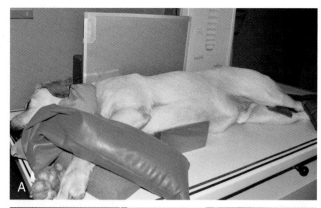

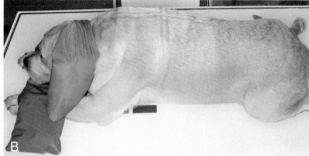

FIGURE 22-24 A, Positioning for ventrodorsal views of the vertebrae with a horizontal beam. Tightly collimate the beam on the area of interest. **B,** A dorsoventral view can be obtained if it is difficult to obtain a ventrodorsal view. Object film distance and magnification will be increased with the dorsoventral view, and the vertebrae are more difficult to keep parallel. Collimate the beam in tightly for spinal radiographs.

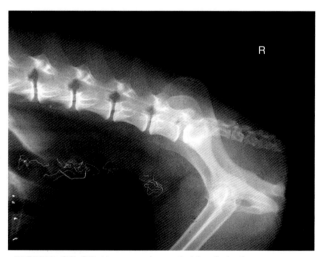

FIGURE 22-25 Mystery radiograph: Identify the foreign images.

in dorsal recumbency and rotate the body either to the right or to the left. Use padding under the mandible and cranial sternum to obtain a 30 to 45 degree oblique projection. Both the right and left oblique views should be compared.

Dorsoventral View

A dorsoventral view with the dog in sternal recumbency can also be completed, but it is more difficult to maintain the vertebrae parallel to the table. Also, object film distance (OFD) and thus magnification will be increased. For completion of this view, keep a pad under the head so that all the vertebrae are parallel to the table (Figure 22-24B).

KEY POINTS

1. General anesthesia or sedation should be considered for accurate positioning.
2. The common views are lateral and ventrodorsal views of each spinal area. Optional views may further assist diagnosis.
3. It is essential that each vertebra being imaged is parallel to the table/image receptor and perpendicular to the central ray. This minimizes distortion that could lead to misdiagnosis.
4. Measure at the thickest part of the area of interest.
5. Collimate tightly to the vertebrae, being conscious of the placement of the labels and markers.
6. Multiple views are recommended. Limit the number of vertebrae on an image.
7. If the patient has a spinal column injury, manipulation of the limbs and spine may be contraindicated.

References

1. Thrall DE: *Textbook of veterinary diagnostic radiology*, ed 5, St. Louis, 2007, Saunders.
2. Han C, Hurd C: *Practical diagnostic imaging for the veterinary technician*, ed 3, St. Louis, 2005, Mosby.
3. Sirois M, Anthony E, Mauragis D: *Handbook of radiographic positioning for veterinary technicians*, Clifton Park, NY, 2010, Delmar Cengage Learning.
4. Lavin L: *Radiography in veterinary technology*, ed 3, St. Louis, 2007, Saunders.
5. Morgan JP: *Techniques of veterinary radiography*, Ames, Iowa, 1993, Iowa State University Press.

Bibliography

Colville T, Bassert J: *Clinical anatomy and physiology for veterinary technicians*, St. Louis, 2008, Elsevier.
Done SH, Goody PC, Stickland NC, Evans SA: *Color atlas of veterinary anatomy, the dog and cat*, London, 2009, Mosby.
Dyce KM, Sack WO, Wensing CJG: *Textbook of veterinary anatomy*, ed 4, St. Louis, 2010, Saunders.
Evans H, de Lahunta A: *Guide to the dissection of the dog*, ed 7, St. Louis, 2010, Saunders.
Owens JM: *Radiographic interpretation for the small animal clinician*, St. Louis, 1982, Ralston Purina.
Ryan G: *Radiographic positioning of small animals*, Philadelphia, 1981, Lea & Febiger.
Tighe M, Brown M: *Mosby's comprehensive review for veterinary technicians*, ed 3, St. Louis, 2008, Mosby.

Small Animal Skull

We live in a world of possibilities ... when we believe it, we will see it.

—Dewitt Jones, Photographer and Inspirational Speaker

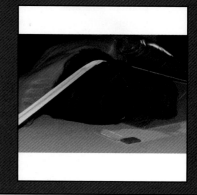

OUTLINE

LEARNING OBJECTIVES

When you have finished this chapter, you will be able to:

1. Know the common positions and principles used to radiograph the small animal skull.
2. Properly and safely position a dog or cat for the various common positions of the skull with an emphasis on where to measure and center the beam, where the borders are, and how to properly position, so that the body part is parallel to the film and both are perpendicular to the central ray.
3. Understand other views that may need to be completed as an alternative.
4. Identify normal skull anatomy found on a radiograph.

KEY TERMS

Mesaticephalic
Positional terminology
Rostrocaudal
Rostroventral-
  caudodorsal oblique
RV-CdD0 / RD-CdV0
Skyline

TECHNICAL NOTE

To preserve space, the radiographs presented in this chapter do not show collimation. For safety, always collimate so that the beam is limited to within the image receptor edges. You should see a clear border of collimation on every radiograph. In some jurisdictions, use of collimation is the law.

The skull along with the spine make up the axial skeleton. Proper imaging of the skull can be challenging because of complicated anatomy, superimposition of many of the structures, and the variation in size and shape of the various breeds. Images of the skull (Table 23-1) are often taken to evaluate trauma, congenital abnormalities, inflammatory lesions, tumors, or degenerative changes.

Radiographic Concerns and Anatomy

Heavy sedation or general anesthesia will be required for most patients for views other than the routine lateral and dorsoventral survey. Recognize that the endotracheal tube, tongue, and pinnae could all cause dense shadows that may interfere with the diagnosis, so they should be repositioned or removed from the field of view when possible.

Fortunately, the skull is relatively symmetrical and, in most small animals, approximately the same width in lateral and dorsoventral/ventrodorsal dimensions. Both positions are measured at the widest area of the cranium. If air-filled sinus cavities are to be radiographed, measure just rostral to the thickest part of the cranium to avoid overexposure.

High-contrast exposure is recommended. Use a grid for measurements over 11 cm. When possible, the radiograph should be tightly collimated to the primary area of interest, to reduce scatter radiation and to improve the image quality. Keep the thickest part of the skull toward the cathode. No special preparation is required other than cleaning the hair coat and removing any collar or halter.

Various-sized radiolucent wedges are required to properly and consistently position for extra-oral oblique radiographs of the mandible and maxilla. Place the appropriate marker toward the nose. Correctly identifying the film with right and left markers is essential, especially for any oblique views. Both markers should be placed on the film for oblique images so that there is no confusion as to which is the dependent jaw. The markers also help identify the different quadrants of the teeth. The oblique mandible and maxilla views are further discussed in Chapter 24.

For the lateral and dorsoventral (DV)/ventrodorsal (VD) views, symmetry of the skull is essential to help identify asymmetrical structures and opacities, because most disease processes of the skull are not bilateral.[1]

For a review of some of the terminology associated with the skull, see Figure 23-1. Figures 23-2, 23-3, and 23-4 show basic anatomy of the canine and feline skull.

TABLE 23-1	Protocol for Skull Radiography
ANATOMICAL LOCATION	**VIEW(S)**
Routine Views	
Skull—routine or survey	Lateral (affected side down) Dorsoventral (DV) or ventrodorsal (VD)
Optional Views	
Nasal cavity and frontal sinuses	Routine –DV/VD, Lateral Opposite lateral (L) Ventrodorsal open-mouth (rostroventral-caudodorsal oblique; —R20-30V-CdDO open-mouth) Frontal 90 Degree Rostrocaudal-Closed Mouth View Intraoral dorsoventral
Foramen magnum	Routine –DV/VD, Lateral Rostrocaudal (rostral 30 degree dorsal-caudoventral) (fronto-occipital) view
Tympanic bullae	Routine –DV/VD, Lateral Open-mouth rostrocaudal (rostral 10 degree ventral-caudodorsal) (R10-30V-CdD) Feline: closed-mouth rostral 10-degree ventral-caudodorsal (R10V-CdD) Lateral oblique views: LeD-RtVO/RtD-LeVO, affected side up Lateral oblique [LeV-RtDO/RtV-LeDO], affected side down
Temporomandibular joint	Routine –DV and Lateral Lateral oblique (LeV-RtDO/RtV-LeDO), affected side down Lateral oblique [LeD-RtVO/RtD-LeVO], affected side up
Zygomatic bone and orbit	Routine –DV/VD, Lateral
Maxilla and dental extraoral studies*	Right or left open-mouth lateral Intraoral dorsoventral Lateral oblique (LeV-RtDO/RtV-LeDO)
Mandible and dental extraoral studies*	Right or left open-mouth lateral Intraoral ventrodorsal Lateral oblique views (LeD-RtVO/RtD-LeVO)

*For the extraoral views, please see Chapter 24.

Strategically use positioning aids to give the patient the *illusion* that it is being held. A sandbag over the neck and limbs, and tape is essential if the patient is not properly sedated. Keep talking to it in a calm, low voice.

Remember the rules of nomenclature if the full term or its abbreviations are used. The first part of the term before the hyphen is where the central ray enters the body. This part of the body is closest to the tube head. The part after the hyphen is where the central ray exits. This is the body part closest to the table or image receptor.

Take, for example, a LeD-RtVO (Left dorsal-right ventral oblique) view:

LeD—the beam enters the head from the patient's left side at the dorsal aspect of the head

RtV—the part closest to the table is the right side, and the beam exits from the ventral part of the head

O—it is an oblique /view

Thus the patient is lying in right lateral recumbency in a dorsoventral oblique position; its nose is pointing to the table (Figure 23-1B).

A rostroventral-caudodorsal oblique view (RV-CdDO) means that the beam enters the front of the head from a ventral direction and exits at the back of the head on the dorsal side. The patient is lying on its back with the nose pointing towards the tube head. (See Figure 23-1D). The mouth can be open or closed. The descriptions are more accurate if the angle of either the beam or the position of the head away from the vertical plane is also included.

Thus an open mouth rostral 20 degree ventral-caudodorsal oblique (R20V-CdDO) means that the patient is lying on its back, with its mouth open and pointing to the tube head.

The head is positioned so that the central ray enters from the front of the head inside the mouth (RV) and exits toward the back of the mouth and head (CdD) at an angle (O) 20 degrees ventral from the plane of the hard palate.

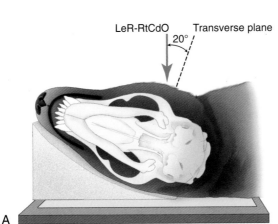

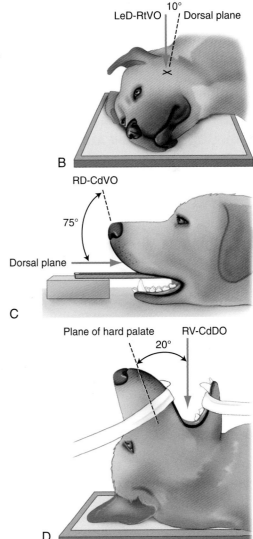

FIGURE 23-1 **A,** LeR-RtCdO: Left rostral–right caudal oblique view. The beam is entering rostrally (from the nose) on the left side of the skull (LeR). The beam exits on the caudal aspect (back) of the skull on the patient's right side (RtCd). Because the central ray is not on the transverse plane, it is an oblique view (O). The most accurate description, which includes the angle of the beam from perpendicular (20 degrees), is Le20R-RtCdO. **B,** LeD-RtVO: Left dorsal–right ventral oblique view. The central beam enters the skull dorsally (from the top of the head) on the patient's left side (LeD) and exits the skull ventrally (towards the chin) on the patient's right side (RtV). Because the skull is not in a true lateral position, it is an oblique (O). The most accurate description is Le10D-RtVO. This locates the entrance angle at 10 degrees dorsal to the dorsal plane through the area of interest such as for the left temporomandibular joint. **C,** RD-CdVO: Rostrodorsal-caudoventral oblique view of the maxillary incisor teeth. The center beam enters the maxilla directly from the front at the dorsal aspect of the skull (RD) and exits toward the back of the skull down toward the ventral side (CdV) at an angle (O). In this case the angle is 75 degrees dorsal to the dorsal plane. The most accurate description is R75D-CdVO (intraoral). The "R75D" indicates that the beam is angled at 75 degrees dorsal to the dorsal plane through the area of interest. The image receptor is inside the mouth. **D,** RV-CdDO: Rostroventral-caudodorsal oblique view. The central ray enters from inside the mouth or the front and ventral aspect of the head (RV) and exits toward the back and top of the head (CdD) at an angle (O) 20 degrees ventral from the plane of the hard palate. R20V-CdDO (open mouth) is a more accurate description. Another term for when the nose points up is rostrocaudal tangential.

Routine Views

Lateral View of the Skull

Place the affected side closer to the table.

Positioning

Place In: Right or left lateral recumbency with the affected side to the image receptor (see Figure 23-2).

Hind Limbs: Leave in a natural position; support with a sandbag or ties if needed.

Forelimbs: Pull caudally, and support with a sandbag or ties.

Head and Neck: Position the head so that the mandible is parallel to the long edge of the image receptor. Put padding under the cranioventral cervical region. Place a foam pad under the ramus of the mandible to superimpose the rami and to prevent rotation of the skull. Tape the head over the nose and neck area so that the tape is extended across the table. A sandbag may be placed over the neck and against a foam pad at the dorsal aspect of the head to keep the head in position.

Comments and Tips

- When viewing the skull in a rostrocaudal direction, an imaginary line drawn through the medial canthi of the eyes should be perpendicular to the tabletop.
- The rami of the mandible and the tympanic bullae should be superimposed on the image.
- The nasal septum should be parallel to the image receptor and tabletop.
- Ensure that the pinnae of the ears and tape are not superimposed over areas of interest.
- Pulling the pectoral limbs caudally may help keep the skull in a true lateral position.

MEASURE (ON THE AREA OF INTEREST): Survey: Highest point of the zygomatic arch at the center of the cranium.
Temporomandibular Joint: Highest point of the zygomatic arch over the joint.
Tympanic Bullae: Highest point of the zygomatic arch over the bullae.
Nares: Highest point of the zygomatic arch just rostral to the medial canthi.

CENTRAL RAY (ON THE AREA OF INTEREST): Survey: Lateral canthus of eye. Midway between the eye and ear, or on area of interest.
Temporomandibular Joint: Center just rostral to the ears.
Tympanic Bullae: Palpate and center on the base of the ear.
Teeth and Nares: Just rostral to the lateral canthus.

BORDERS (DEPENDS ON THE AREA OF INTEREST): Survey: Full skull—tip of the nose to the occipital protuberance.
Tympanic Bullae: Cranial and caudal to the ear.
Temporomandibular Joint: Cranial and caudal to the joint.
Teeth and Nares: Tip of the nose to the lateral canthi.

> **TECHNICIAN NOTES** Pads under the nose and neck will help keep the skull in a horizontal plane and minimize rotation.

> **TECHNICIAN NOTES** Quickly go through your mental checklist *before* pushing the exposure button: settings correct; image receptor/machine/grid in position; proper location of markers and identification (if using at this stage); correct body part and view; properly centered; borders correct and collimated; patient properly prepared, positioned, and restrained so the part will be parallel to the image receptor and both will be perpendicular to the central ray.

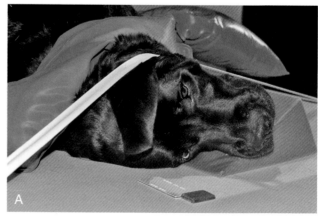

FIGURE 23-2 A, Positioning for the lateral skull view.

Lateral View of the Skull—*cont'd*

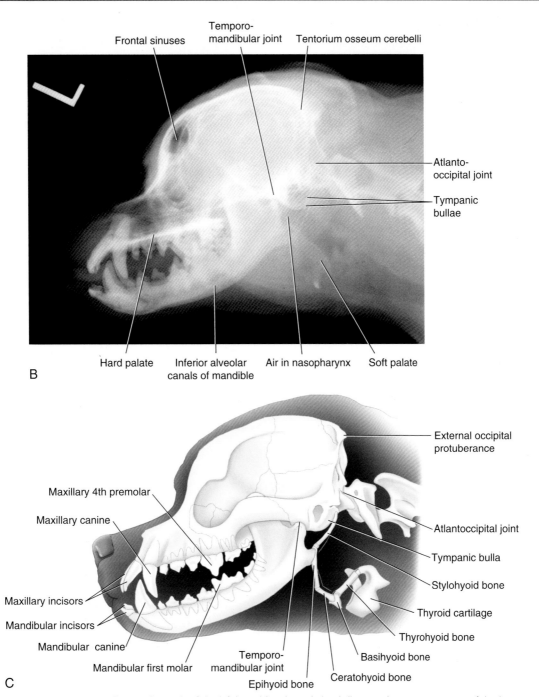

B

Frontal sinuses
Temporo-mandibular joint
Tentorium osseum cerebelli
Atlanto-occipital joint
Tympanic bullae
Hard palate
Inferior alveolar canals of mandible
Air in nasopharynx
Soft palate

C

Maxillary 4th premolar
Maxillary canine
Maxillary incisors
Mandibular incisors
Mandibular canine
Mandibular first molar
Temporo-mandibular joint
Epihyoid bone
Ceratohyoid bone
Basihyoid bone
Thyrohyoid bone
Thyroid cartilage
Stylohyoid bone
Tympanic bulla
Atlantoccipital joint
External occipital protuberance

FIGURE 23-2, cont'd B, Radiograph of the left lateral brachycephalic skull. Note the superimposition of the bones and teeth in a true lateral view. C, Lateral left-to-right radiographic anatomy of the skull.

Dorsoventral View of the Skull

Positioning

Place In: Sternal recumbency in a V-trough if required.

Hind Limbs: Place in a natural position and support them with a sandbag or ties.

Forelimbs: Pull caudally or leave them in a natural position alongside the head, out of the field of view; support them with a sandbag or ties.

Head and Neck: Extend the neck and head. Place a sandbag over the neck for support, being careful not to restrict breathing. Tape across the nasal septum and the cranium to keep the sagittal plane of the head perpendicular to the image receptor. Make sure the ears are positioned laterally, equidistant from the head.

Comments and Tips

- When viewing the skull in a rostrocaudal direction, an imaginary line drawn between the medial canthi should be parallel to the table.
- To prevent unwanted shadows, minimize the use of tape over the area of interest when lower exposure factors are used.
- Have the thickest part of the skull toward the cathode to help diminish changes in opacity.
- The endotracheal tube can be left in place, with the possibility of its causing a shadow kept in mind.

MEASURE (ON THE AREA OF INTEREST): Survey: Highest point of the cranium just caudal to the lateral canthi.

Temporomandibular Joint: Rostral to the ears on the dorsal midline of the skull.

Tympanic Bullae: Highest point of the cranium just caudal to the lateral canthi.

Nares: Rostral to the medial canthi.

CENTRAL RAY (ON THE AREA OF INTEREST): Survey: Between the two lateral canthi of the eyes on the sagittal crest or on the area of interest.

Temporomandibular Joint: Center just rostral to the ears on the dorsal midline of the skull.

Tympanic Bullae: Palpate the base of the ear and center on the dorsal midline between the ears.

Teeth and Nares: Center more rostral.

BORDERS (DEPENDS ON THE AREA OF INTEREST): Survey: Tip of the nose to the occipital protuberance.

Tympanic Bullae: Cranial and caudal to the ear.

Temporomandibular Joint: Cranial and caudal to the joint.

Teeth and Nares: Tip of the nose to lateral canthi.

TECHNICIAN NOTES To maintain symmetry for the DV view, ensure that an imaginary line drawn between the medial canthi is parallel to the table. Look from the rostrocaudal direction. Keep the hard palate parallel to the table and image receptor.

TECHNICIAN NOTES To be more efficient for any view, ensure that the body parts that are not in the beam are positioned and secured first. Position the area of interest last.

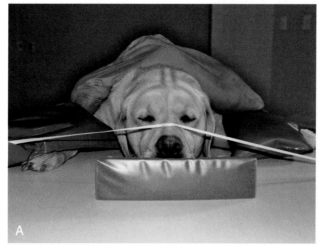

FIGURE 23-3 A, Positioning for the dorsoventral skull view.

Dorsoventral View of the Skull—*cont'd*

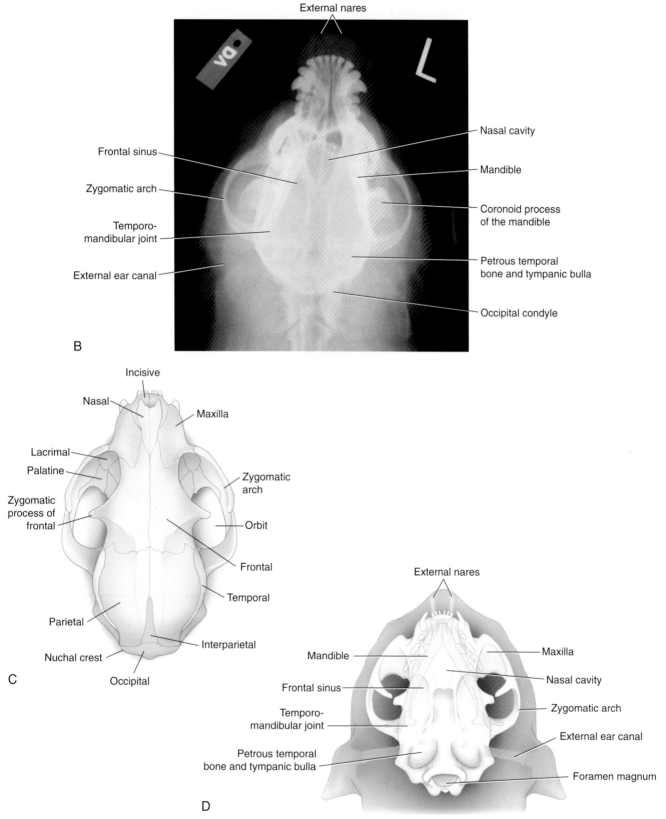

FIGURE 23-3, cont'd B, Labeled radiograph of the dorsoventral skull. C, Skull of the dog, dorsal view. D, Radiographic anatomy of the normal feline skull, projections.

Ventrodorsal View of the Skull

This view is used for a routine skull radiograph and for evaluation of the nasal sinus because the nasal passages are located dorsally.

Positioning

Place In: Dorsal recumbency in a V-trough if required, and support with sandbags.

Hind Limbs: Leave the hind limbs in a natural position, and support with sandbags or ties.

Forelimbs: Pull the front limbs caudally, lateral to the chest, and support with sandbags or ties.

Head and Neck: Position a foam pad or sandbag under the neck so that the hard palate is parallel with the image receptor. Place a small foam pad under the nose, and tape across the mandible to keep the head aligned with the table.

Comments and Tips

- Note the location of the tongue so that it does not create objectionable shadows on the area of interest.
- Ensure that there is symmetry of the head.
- The DV/VD view are compared in Figure 23-5.

> **TECHNICIAN NOTES**   For the VD view, extend the neck so that the nose/hard palate is parallel with the table.

> **TECHNICIAN NOTES**   True symmetry in a lateral view of a normal patient has been achieved if there appears to be only one structure on the image because the two sides are superimposed on each other.
>
> True symmetry in a DV/VD view of a normal patient has been achieved if the left and right sides are mirror images.

MEASURE (ON THE AREA OF INTEREST): Survey: Highest point of the cranium just caudal to the lateral canthi.

Temporomandibular Joint: Rostral to the ears on the ventral midline of the skull.

Tympanic Bullae: Highest point of the cranium just caudal to the lateral canthi.

Nares: Rostral to the medial canthi.

CENTRAL RAY (ON THE AREA OF INTEREST): Survey: Between the two lateral canthi of the eyes on the ventral midline, or on area of interest.

Temporomandibular Joint: Center just rostral to the ears on the ventral midline of the skull.

Tympanic Bullae: Palpate the bases of the ears, and center on the ventral midline between the ears.

Teeth and Nares: Center more rostral.

BORDERS (DEPENDS ON THE AREA OF INTEREST): Survey: Tip of the nose to the occipital protuberance.

Tympanic Bullae: Cranial and caudal to the ear.

Temporomandibular Joint: Cranial and caudal to the joint.

Teeth and Nares: Tip of the nose to the lateral canthi.

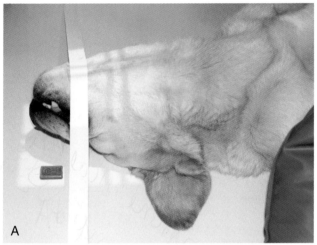

A

FIGURE 23-4 A, Positioning for the ventrodorsal skull view.

Ventrodorsal View of the Skull—*cont'd*

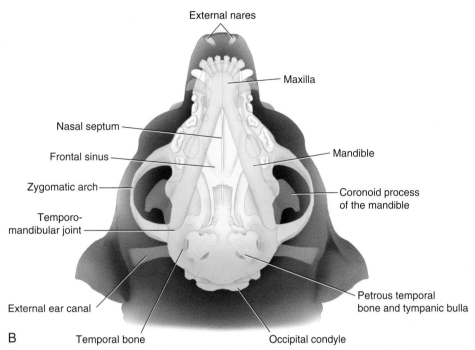

External nares

Maxilla

Nasal septum

Frontal sinus

Mandible

Zygomatic arch

Coronoid process
of the mandible

Temporo-
mandibular joint

External ear canal

Temporal bone

Occipital condyle

Petrous temporal
bone and tympanic bulla

B

FIGURE 23-4, cont'd B, Overlay and radiographic anatomy of the ventrodorsal skull.

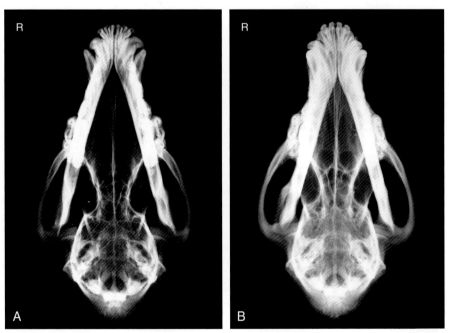

R

R

A

B

FIGURE 23-5 A, Ventrodorsal radiograph of the skull. B, Comparison of the same skull in a dorsoventral position. Different exposure factors have been used in each case.

Further Views

Ventrodorsal Open-Mouth (Rostroventral-Caudodorsal Oblique (R20-30V-CdDO) Open-Mouth) View[2]

The ventrodorsal open-mouth view images the nasal sinus and ethmoid regions without superimposition of the mandible. The position can be used only if the tube head is movable or can rotate.

> **TECHNICIAN NOTES**   "Rostroventral-caudodorsal oblique- (R20-30V-CdDO) (open-mouth)" means that the central ray enters the body from the nose rostro ventrally at an angle of 20 to 30 degrees and then exits obliquely toward the patient's back in a caudal direction. The patient is thus lying on its back.

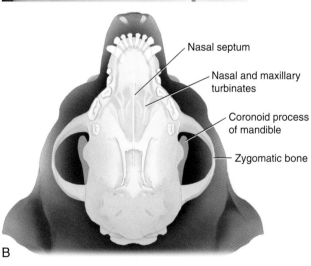

MEASURE: At the thickest area near the commissure of the lip (over the level of the third maxillary premolar).

CENTRAL RAY: On the nasal cavity—at the back of the palate about the level of the third premolar. Angle the tube head rostrocaudally 20 to 30 degrees.

BORDERS: Tip of the maxilla to the pharyngeal region (all of the upper palate).

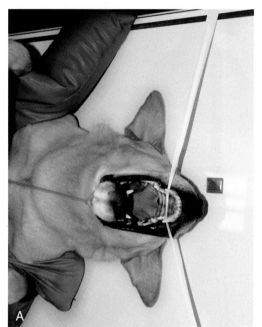

Nasal septum

Nasal and maxillary turbinates

Coronoid process of mandible

Zygomatic bone

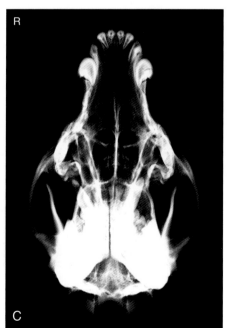

FIGURE 23-6 **A,** Positioning for the ventrodorsal open-mouth view (rostroventral-caudodorsal oblique; -(R20-30V-CdDO) open-mouth) for the nasal sinuses. **B,** Overlay and radiographic anatomy of the ventrodorsal open-mouth view. Tilt the tube head about 20 to 30 degrees in relation to the table in a rostrocaudal direction. **C,** Open-mouth ventrodorsal radiograph of the skull (rostroventral-caudodorsal oblique; (R20-30V-CdDO)open-mouth) view of the nasal sinuses.

Ventrodorsal Open-Mouth (Rostroventral-Caudodorsal Oblique (R20-30V-CdDO) Open-Mouth) View—cont'd

Positioning

Place In: Dorsal recumbency in a V-trough if required, and support with sandbags.

Hind Limbs: Leave in a natural position, and sandbag or secure them to the table with ties.

Forelimbs: Pull the front limbs caudally, lateral to the chest, and support them with sandbags or ties.

Head and Neck: Place a small foam pad under the nose, and have the hard palate parallel to the table. Position a strip of tape inside the mouth and securely adhere the ends to the table in a cranial direction so the maxilla is parallel to the table. Open the mouth wide by securing tape or gauze around the mandible and pulling caudally and ventrally. Depending on how wide the mouth is opened, the beam should be directed at 20 to 30 degrees from the vertical into the mouth and parallel to the mandible.[3]

Comments and Tips

• This position is similar to the ventrodorsal view except that the mouth is kept open and the tube head is angled.

• Decrease the kilovoltage peak (kVp) slightly from that on the skull chart to account for decreased density.

• The mouth can also be propped open with a tongue depressor, plastic speculum, or 1-mL syringe barrel placed between or over the canine teeth.

• The positioning device, tongue, and endotracheal tube may cause shadows. Keep the pinnae equally lateral to the head. Secure the endotracheal tube to the mandible to help prevent shadows on the area of interest.

• On a normal healthy patient, the nasal opacity and turbinate detail should be equal on both sides of the head.

Brachycephalic Breeds

• A better projection to image the nasal cavity of these breeds, is a closed-mouth caudoventral-to-rostrodorsal oblique (CdV-RDO) projection with the nose (hard palate) tipped down toward the film approximately 30 degrees and the vertical beam centered 2–3 cm rostral to the angular processes of the mandible (Figure 23-7).[3]

TECHNICIAN NOTES For the nasal sinuses, have the patient in a VD position and open the mouth. Keep the maxilla parallel to the table. Tilt the tube head. The collimator light should be on the hard palate back to the rear molars, and the image receptor must capture the primary beam.

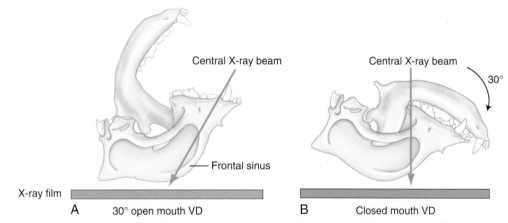

A   30° open mouth VD

B   Closed mouth VD

FIGURE 23-7 **A,** The ventrodorsal open-mouth view (rostroventral-caudodorsal oblique) is not as effective at imaging the nasal cavity in brachycephalic breeds. **B,** The closed-mouth caudoventral- rostrodorsal oblique (CdV-RDO) projection is more satisfactory. The nose (hard palate) is tipped down toward the film about 30 degrees with the central beam 2 to 3 cm rostral to the angular processes of the mandible.

Frontal 90-Degree-Rostrocaudal-Closed-Mouth View

This rostrocaudal view images the frontal sinuses.

Positioning

Place In: Dorsal recumbency in a V-trough if required; support with sandbags.

Hind Limbs: Leave in a natural position and secure with sandbag or ties.

Forelimbs: Pull the front limbs caudally, lateral to the chest, and support with a sandbag or ties.

Head and Neck: Position a foam pad or sandbag under the neck so that the hard palate is perpendicular with the image receptor. Point the nose up so it is perpendicular to the image receptor and to the long axis of the body. Keep it in position by placing tape, tubing or gauze around the nose. Secure caudally, keeping the nose pointed up.

Comments and Tips

- The hard palate should be perpendicular to the table. An imaginary line joining the medial canthi of the eyes should be parallel to the image receptor.
- Note the location of the tongue so it does not create objectionable shadows on the area of interest.
- Reduce the kVp because there is minimal tissue to penetrate.
- Another term for this view is *skyline view*.
- Mesaticephalic and dolichocephalic breeds usually have a well-developed frontal sinus. A rostrocaudal image of the frontal sinuses in a brachycephalic breed that does not have a recognizable frontal sinus on a lateral radiograph, will not be useful.[1]

> **TECHNICIAN NOTES** Keep the nose straight up and pointed at the tube head for the frontal sinuses in medium- (mesaticephalic) and long-nosed (dolicochephalic) dogs.

MEASURE: Over the site of the nasal sinuses (nasal stop).

CENTRAL RAY: Between the eyes (on the frontal sinuses).

BORDERS: Occipital crest to the dorsal aspect of the nasal planum (tip of nose).

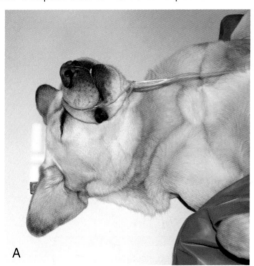

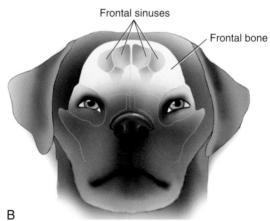

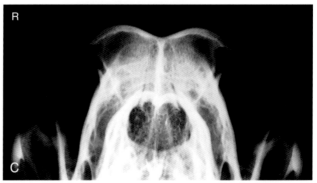

FIGURE 23-8 **A,** Positioning for the frontal 90-degree rostrocaudal closed-mouth view of the skull for the frontal sinuses. The nose is pointing straight up, and the beam is centered between the eyes. **B,** Overlay and radiographic anatomy of the frontal 90-degree rostrocaudal closed-mouth view of the skull. **C,** A frontal 90-degreee rostrocaudal closed-mouth radiograph to show the frontal sinus. The nose is pointing straight up.

Rostrocaudal Closed-Mouth (Rostral 30-Degree Dorsal-Caudoventral Oblique) View

The rostrocaudal closed-mouth or fronto-occipital view demonstrates the foramen magnum, cranial vault, calvarium, and sagittal crest.

Positioning

Place In: Dorsal recumbency in a V-trough if required, and support with sandbags.

Hind Limbs: Leave in a natural position; support with sandbags or tie if needed.

Forelimbs: Pull caudally, lateral to the chest; support with sandbags or ties.

Head and Neck: Point the nose upward and apply a long strip of tape or tubing to the nose. Angle the hard palate in a caudal direction toward the chest by pulling on the strip and securing it caudally.

Comments and Tips

- The central ray should intersect the bridge of the nose at an angle of 30 degrees to the dorsum of the nose or at an angle of 45 degrees to the hard palate.[3] The actual angle depends on the type of skull.
- This position is the same as the rostrocaudal frontal sinus view except that the nose is pulled more caudally.
- The tongue and endotracheal tube may cause shadows. Try to keep the pinnae equally lateral to the head.
- Some sources suggest that the nose should be positioned down for an occipitofrontal projection, and the beam centered at the junction of the right and left frontonasal sutures for dolicocephalic and mesaticephalic breeds and about the top of the nasal fold for brachycephalic breeds.[3]

MEASURE: At the site of the frontal sinuses.

CENTRAL RAY: Midway between the eyes so that the cranium is centered and the beam intersects the bridge of the nose.

BORDERS: Entire cranium.

> **TECHNICIAN NOTES** The eyes are looking up at the tube head for both the frontal sinuses and foramen magnum in the rostrocaudal views. The difference is that the nose is pointing caudally for a view of the foramen magnum.

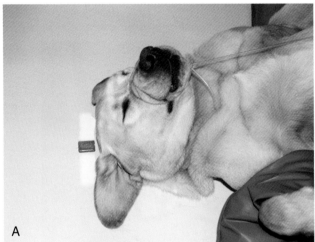

A

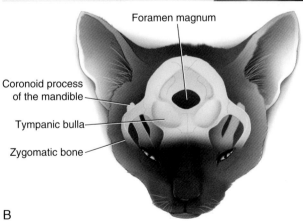

B

Foramen magnum

Coronoid process of the mandible

Tympanic bulla

Zygomatic bone

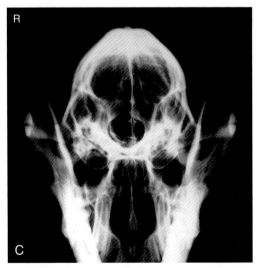

R

C

FIGURE 23-9 **A,** Positioning for the rostrocaudal or fronto-occipital (rostral 30-degree dorsal-caudoventral) view of the skull to image the foramen magnum, cranial vault, calvarium, and sagittal crest. The nose is pulled more caudally than for the frontal 90-degree view. **B,** Overlay and radiographic anatomy of the rostrocaudal view (R30D-CdV) or fronto-occipital of the skull to view the foramen magnum. **C,** A skull radiograph of the rostrocaudal (R30D-CdV) or fronto-occipital view.

Rostrocaudal Open-Mouth (Rostral 10 Degree Ventral-Caudodorsal Oblique) View

The rostrocaudal open-mouth view demonstrates the tympanic bullae, the base of the skull, and the odontoid process. There is minimal superimposition of the petrous temporal bone.[4]

Positioning

Place In: Dorsal recumbency in a V-trough if required, and support with sandbags.

Hind Limbs: Leave in a natural position; support with sandbags or ties if needed.

Forelimbs: Pull caudally, lateral to the chest, and support with sandbags or ties.

Head and Neck: A small amount of padding under the neck may help keep the head in position. Point the nose upward, and apply a long strip of tape just below the maxillary canines. Pull the nose about 10 degrees cranially, and secure. Apply tape or gauze to the mandibular canines, encompassing the endotracheal tube if used. Pull and secure the tape so that mandible is about 10 degrees caudal from the perpendicular.

Comments and Tips

- This position is similar to the frontal sinus view, except that the mouth is opened for dogs.
- The hard palate should be at about a 10-degree angle from the vertical for mesaticephalic breeds.[5]
- The mouth can also be propped open with a tongue depressor, plastic speculum, or 1-mL syringe barrel placed between or over the canine teeth.
- The tongue and positioning devices may cause shadows. Try to keep the pinnae equally lateral to the head.
- The beam should bisect the angle of the open mouth or at the junction of the hard palate and the horizontal rami of the mandible. The bullae should be projected freely.

MEASURE: At the commissure of the lips (level of maxillary third premolar).

CENTRAL RAY: At the commissure of the mouth just dorsal to the tongue from a rostroventral direction.

BORDERS: Entire nasopharyngeal region of the cranium.

> **TECHNICIAN NOTES** Point the nose to the tube head, open the mouth, and separate the mandible and maxilla, securing them slightly in each direction for evaluation of the tympanic bullae of dogs in the rostrocaudal open mouth view. Secure the tongue to the mandible.

> **TECHNICIAN NOTES** Collimate, ensuring that labels/markers are included and borders are visible for every image.

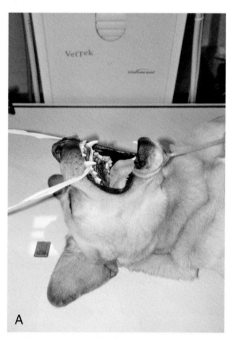

A

FIGURE 23-10 A, Positioning for the rostrocaudal open-mouth (rostral 10-30-degree ventral-caudodorsal oblique) view. This rostrocaudal view demonstrates the tympanic bullae, the base of the skull, and the odontoid process. Measure and center at the level of the commissure of the lips.

Rostrocaudal Open-Mouth (Rostral 10 Degree Ventral-Caudodorsal Oblique) View—cont'd

- The angle of the beam varies with the patient and with how wide the mouth can be opened. Brachycephalic breeds likely require a larger palatial angle (21 degrees), and dolichocephalic breeds a smaller angle (4 degrees).[3]
- It may also be better in brachycephalic breeds to keep the mouth closed and position as for a cat with the hard palate at a 10-degree angle from the perpendicular (Figure 23-11).[1]
- Slightly less kVp is required because there is less tissue density.

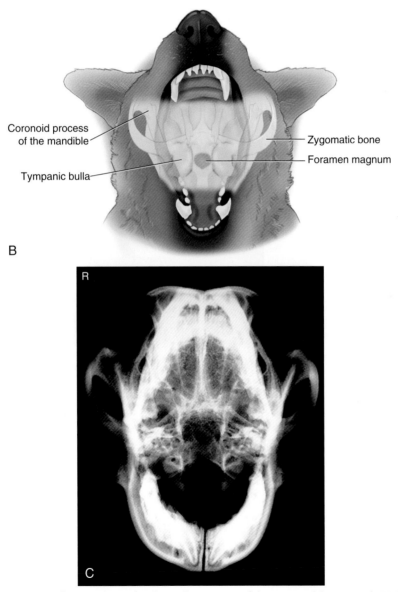

Coronoid process of the mandible

Tympanic bulla

Zygomatic bone

Foramen magnum

B

R

C

FIGURE 23-10, cont'd B, Overlay and radiographic anatomy of the rostrocaudal open-mouth (R10V-CdDO) view of the skull. C, An open mouth R10V-CdDO radiograph of the skull demonstrating the tympanic bullae.

Closed-Mouth Rostral 10 Degree Ventral-Caudodorsal Oblique View for Cat Tympanic Bullae

Comments and Tips

- Because the cat tympanic bullae are positioned anatomically more caudally than the dog bullae, keep the cat's mouth closed to view the tympanic bullae and odontoid process.
- Rest the dorsal aspect of the head on an angled foam wedge so that the hard palate is at an angle of 10 degrees from the vertical.
- Apply tape over the maxilla to secure.
- Center the beam at the level of the base of the mandibular body at the commissure of the mouth about 1 cm ventral to the external nares.[5]

TECHNICIAN NOTES Point the nose to the tube head, keep the mouth closed, and pull slightly cranially for evaluation of the tympanic bullae of feline patients and possibly for brachycephalic breeds.

TECHNICIAN NOTES Remember to apply the label appropriately in each image and to collimate the beam as tightly as possible.

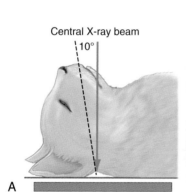

Central X-ray beam

10°

A

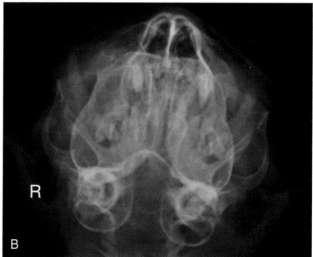

R

B

FIGURE 23-11 **A,** Positioning for the rostrocaudal closed-mouth (rostral 10-degree ventral-caudodorsal) view of the skull for the cat tympanic bullae. The mouth is closed, and both mandible and maxilla are displaced dorsally 10 degrees. **B,** A rostrocaudal close-mouth (R10V-CdDO) radiograph of the skull for the cat tympanic bullae.

Lateral Oblique View for the Tympanic Bullae (LeD-RtVO/RtD-LeVO)

The lateral oblique or LeD-RtVO (dorsoventral oblique) view with the head lying in a natural position isolates the tympanic bullae.

Positioning

Place In: Right or left lateral recumbency with the unaffected side to the image receptor.
- Right lateral—to view the left oblique tympanic bulla
- Left lateral—to view the right oblique tympanic bulla

Hind Limbs: Leave the hind limbs in a natural position; support with sandbags or ties if needed.

Forelimbs: Position caudally and support with sandbags or ties.

Head and Neck: Position the head so that the mandible is parallel to the long edge of the table. Allow the head to lie oblique naturally, with the nose pointing to the table. If needed, tape the head over the nose and neck area, extending the tape across the table.

Comments and Tips

- The degree of rotation from the true lateral depends on the species and type of skull. There should be enough rotation to allow isolation of each tympanic bulla.
- Use both labels, so that if the patient is positioned in right lateral recumbency, the right marker (unaffected bulla) will be dorsal and the left marker (affected bulla) ventral.
- This view can also be used for an oblique view of the temporomandibular joint (TMJ).

> **TECHNICIAN NOTES** Have the patient lie in a natural oblique lateral position with the nose and the unaffected tympanic bulla closest to the table. This could be considered a modified DV oblique view.

MEASURE: At the base of the ear over the tympanic bullae at the widest part of the cranium.

CENTRAL RAY: At the base of the ear over the tympanic bullae.

BORDERS: Cranial and caudal to the ear.

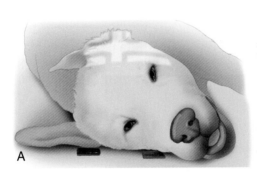
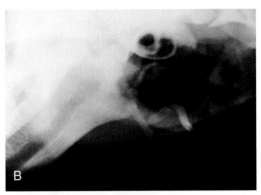

FIGURE 23-12 A, A left lateral oblique (LeD-RtVO) view with the head lying naturally, to show the tympanic bullae in isolation. The unaffected tympanic bullae is closer to the film. The dependent side marker is placed dorsally, and the marker for the affected side is placed ventrally. **B,** Radiograph of the lateral oblique view of the tympanic bullae. The affected bulla is magnified and positioned ventrally.

Lateral Oblique (Ventrodorsal Oblique; LeV-RtDO/RtV-LeDO)

This lateral oblique or ventrodorsal oblique (nose up) view can be used for the tympanic bullae and temporomandibular joints. This provides a different view of the mandibular condyle than is projected on the lateral and DV/VD views. This view can also be used to visualize the maxillary teeth. Another way to describe the view is laterorostral-laterocaudal oblique.

Positioning

Place In: Right or left lateral recumbency with the affected side to the image receptor.

Hind Limbs: Leave the hind limbs in a natural position; support with sandbags or ties if needed.

Forelimbs: Position caudally and support with sandbags or ties.

Head and Neck: Position the head so that the mandible is parallel to the long edge of the image receptor. Keep the skull in a straight lateral position. Place a foam pad under the mandible to raise the nose from 10 degrees to 30 degrees, depending on the breed of dog. The mouth can be partially opened. If needed, tape the head over the nose and neck area, extending the tape across the table. A sandbag may be placed over the neck and against a foam pad at the dorsal aspect of the head (Figure 23-13).

Comments and Tips

- This position displaces the nondependent bulla caudally and the dependent (down) bulla rostrally.
- The distance the mandible is raised depends on the breed. Dolichocephalic breeds require an angle of about 10 degrees, and mesaticephalic breeds about 15 degrees, whereas brachycephalic breeds generally require an angle of 25 to 30 degrees from the table.[3,6]
- Both right and left lateral oblique views should be taken for comparison.
- Ensure that the pinnae, tongue, and endotracheal tubes do not create objectionable shadows on the area of interest.
- The marker indicating the dependent side should be placed ventrally near the joint. The nondependent side marker should be placed dorsal to the nares to indicate that the raised joint is dorsal to the joint on the table.
- Use the skull technique chart, because more exposure is required to penetrate the cranium.

MEASURE: Just caudal to the lateral canthus over joint.

CENTRAL RAY: Between the caudal mandibular ramus and the base of the ear.

BORDERS: Cranial and caudal to the joint.

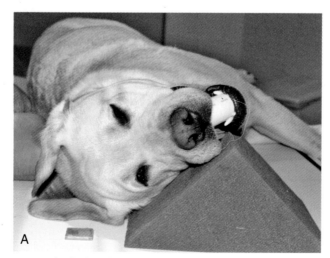

FIGURE 23-13 A, Positioning for the lateral oblique (LeV-RtDO) view of the skull for the maxillary teeth. The affected side is against the table. A smaller angle is used to visualize the tympanic bullae and temporomandibular joints. The left marker indicates that the left or nondependent side will be positioned more dorsally than the right maxilla. The R marker shows that the side closest to the film will be more ventral. It is under the foam pad nearer the right maxilla. The R and L marker in oblique cases do not show the side the animal is lying on. The markers only show the position of the jaws relative to each other.

Lateral Oblique (Ventrodorsal Oblique; LeV-RtDO/RtV-LeDO)—cont'd

Upper Dental Arcade

- This view can also be used to radiograph the upper dental arcade or bony lesions of the nondependent maxilla.
- A foam pad under the mandible, creating a 30- to 45-degree angle of the mandible with the table, is usually required (Figure 23-13A).
- The affected maxilla is closer to the table if imaging the teeth.
- The mouth should be widely opened, and the central ray is over the fourth premolar.
- The endotracheal tube should be tied to the mandible.
- The teeth should be marked with both positional markers—the dependent marker placed ventrally, and the upper side marker dorsally. (The dependent teeth will be grayer because there is minimal superimposition of the palate.)

TECHNICIAN NOTES For a lateral oblique view of the TMJ or maxillary teeth, position the nose up on a foam pad and have the affected joint or teeth closer to the table.

TECHNICIAN NOTES This view could also be called a ventrodorsal oblique view because the nose is tipped up at an angle and the beam enters the head more from the ventrodorsal aspect. The maxilla is closer to the table than the mandible (nose up).

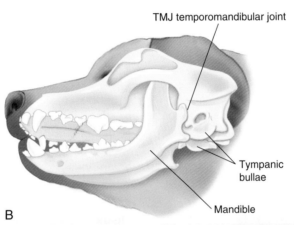

TMJ temporomandibular joint

Tympanic bullae

Mandible

B

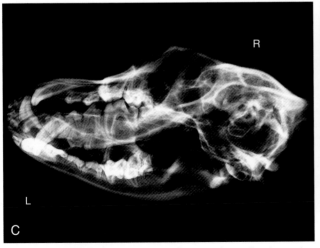

R

L

C

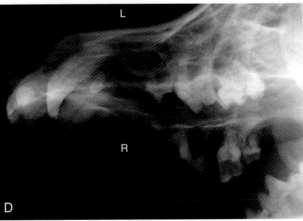

L

R

D

FIGURE 23-13, cont'd B, Overlay and radiographic anatomy of the lateral oblique or ventrodorsal oblique view to visualize the tympanic bullae, temporomandibular joints, and maxilla. C, Radiograph of the lateral oblique (ventrodorsal oblique or LeV-RtDO) view of a skull in right lateral D, Centering on the maxilla and opening the mouth wider in the open-mouth lateral oblique (LeV-RtDO open-mouth) radiograph provides this image of the maxillary dental arcade.

Lateral Oblique View for the Mandible (LeD-RtVO/RtD-LeVO)

The lateral oblique view for the mandible is used to radiograph the lower dental arcade or bony lesions of the nondependent mandible. It is similar to the ventrodorsal oblique except that the maxilla is raised (nose is down).

Comments and Tips

- The right side is down for visualizing the right mandibular teeth.
- A foam pad under the maxilla, creating a 20- to 45-degree angle of the mandible with the table, is required. (The affected mandible is closer to the table.)
- The actual angle depends on how wide the mouth is open and on the breed. There should be no superimposition of the affected mandibular premolars and molars by the other teeth.
- The mouth should be widely opened, and the beam centered over the fourth premolar.
- The endotracheal tube is tied to the maxilla.
- The teeth should be labeled with both positional markers, the dependent marker dorsally and the upper side marker ventrally. (The dependent teeth will be grayer because there is minimal superimposition of the rami of the mandibles.)
- This view is referred to as a left (20°- to 45-degree) dorsal, right ventral oblique view if the right side is down, and a right (20°- to 45-degree) dorsal, left ventral oblique view if the left side is down.

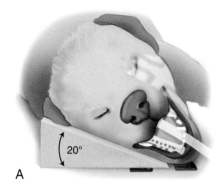

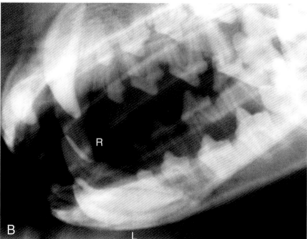

FIGURE 23-14 A, Lateral oblique or dorsoventral oblique (Le20D-RtVO) positioning for viewing the mandibular dental arcade. The maxilla is raised from 20 to 45 degrees, depending on how wide the mouth is open or the breed of the patient. **B,** Lateral oblique (LeD-RtVO) view for the mandibular arcade. Note that the teeth of the affected side appear grayer because there is no superimposition with the mandible. If the mouth is opened wider, there is less overlapping by the maxillary teeth.

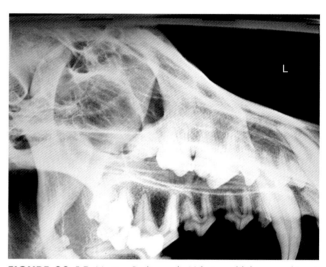

FIGURE 23-15 Mystery Radiograph: What would the correct terminology be for this view?

Lateral Oblique View for the Mandible (LeD-RtVO/RtD-LeVO)—cont'd

TECHNICIAN NOTES For the lateral oblique view of the mandibular teeth, raise the maxilla with a foam wedge. This could be considered a DV oblique view because the beam enters at the top of the head and exits ventrally. The nose is pointing down.

TECHNICIAN NOTES When placing the positional markers for an oblique view, consider the following:
- What quadrant are you attempting to image? When that quadrant is in the correct position, look at which part of the jaw is touching the table. Will it appear more ventral, or will it be displaced dorsally in relation to the opposite side of the jaw?
- For the right mandible, the patient is lying on its right side and the nose is down. With raising of the maxilla, the left or upper side of the mandible is tipped more ventral than the right mandible which, because of the sponge, is displaced dorsally. Thus, you would place the R marker near the tips of the right premolars and the L marker at the ramus of the left mandible. In these views, the markers do not indicate which side the patient is lying on but, rather, the specific quadrant.[1]

KEY POINTS
1. General anesthesia or sedation is required for accurate positioning for all skull views.
2. In order to achieve symmetry of the skull to minimize distortion and possibly misdiagnosis, the anatomical structures being examined must be parallel to the table/image receptor and perpendicular to the central ray:
   a. To help maintain symmetry for a lateral view, draw an imaginary line between the medial canthi. This line should be perpendicular to the table.
   b. To help maintain symmetry for a dorsoventral view, draw an imaginary line between the medial canthi. This imaginary line should be parallel to the table.
3. Collimate tightly to the area of interest, being conscious of the placement of the labels and markers.
4. Views other than the standard views depend on the area of interest and the reason for imaging the patient.
5. When labeling oblique views, think of which part of the jaw is against the film and how the opposite side is positioned.
6. In rostrocaudal projections, the angle of the central ray with the head varies, because of breed variations.

References

1. Thrall DE: *Textbook of veterinary diagnostic radiology*, ed 5, St. Louis, 2007, Saunders.
2. Smallwood JE, Shively MJ, Rendano VT, Habel RE: A standardized nomenclature for radiographic projections used in veterinary medicine, *Vet Radiol* 26:2-9, 1985.
3. Kus S, Morgan J: Radiography of the canine head: optimal positioning with respect to skull type, *Vet Radiol* 26:196-202, 1985.
4. Han C, Hurd C: *Practical diagnostic imaging for the veterinary technician*, ed 3, St. Louis, 2005, Mosby.
5. Hammond Gawain J, Sullivan M, Weinrauch S, King AM: A comparison of the rostrocaudal open mouth and rostro 10 degrees ventro-caudodorsal oblique radiographic views for imaging fluid in the feline tympanic bulla, *Vet Radiol Ultrasound* 46:205-209, 2005.
6. Morgan JP: Techniques of veterinary radiography, Ames, Iowa, 1993, Iowa State University Press.

Bibliography

Aspinall V, Cappello M: *Introduction to veterinary anatomy*, London, 2009, Butterman-Heineman.
Colville T, Bassert J: *Clinical anatomy and physiology for veterinary technicians*, St. Louis, 2008, Elsevier.
Done SH, Goody PC, Stickland NC, Evans SA: *Color atlas of veterinary anatomy, the dog and cat*, London, 2009, Mosby.
Douglas SW: *Principles of veterinary radiography*, London, 1980, Bailliere Tindall.

Dyce KM, Sack WO, Wensing CJG: *Textbook of veterinary anatomy*, ed 4, St. Louis, 2010, Saunders.
Evans H, de Lahunta A: *Guide to the dissection of the dog*, ed 7, St. Louis, 2010, Saunders.
Fauber TL: *Radiographic imaging and exposure*, ed 3, St. Louis, 2009, Mosby.
Lavin L: *Radiography in veterinary technology*, St. Louis, 2007, Saunders.
Owens JM: *Radiographic interpretation for the small animal clinician*, St. Louis, 1999, Ralston Purina.
Romich J: *An illustrated guide to veterinary medical terminology*, Clifton, NY, 2009, Delmar Cengage Learning.
Ryan G: *Radiographic positioning of small animals*, Philadelphia, 1981, Lea & Febiger.
Sirois M: *Principles and practice of veterinary technology*, ed 3, St. Louis, 2011, Mosby.
Sirois M, Anthony E, Mauragis D: *Handbook of radiographic positioning for veterinary technicians*, Clifton Park, NY, 2010, Delmar Cengage Learning.
Smallwood JE, Shively MJ, Rendano VT, Habel RE: A standardized nomenclature for radiographic projections used in veterinary medicine, *Vet Radiol* 26:2-9, 1985.
Thrall DE: *Textbook of veterinary diagnostic radiology*, ed 4, St. Louis, 2002, Saunders.
Ticer J: *Radiographic technique in small animal practice*, Philadelphia, 1984, WB Saunders.
Tighe M, Brown M: *Mosby's comprehensive review for veterinary technicians*, ed 3, St. Louis, 2008, Mosby.

Dental Radiography

Susan MacNeal, RVT, CVDT, BSc

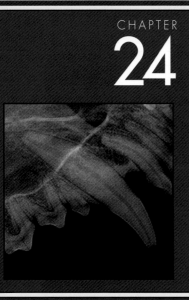

*A man begins cutting his wisdom teeth the first time
he bites off more than he can chew.*

—Herb Caen, San Francisco columnist, 1916–1997

KEY TERMS

Alveolar bone
Apical
Arch
Bisecting angle
Buccal
Carnassial tooth
Caudal
Cementoenamel
  junction (CEJ)
Concave
Contralateral
Convex
Coronal surface
Cusp
Distal
Distolateral oblique
Dorsal
Elongation
Enamel bulge
Extraoral
Facial
Foreshortening
Frenulum
Furcation
Incisal
Intraoral
Ipsilateral
Labial
Lamina dura
Lateral (side) lingual
Mental foramina
Mesaticephalic
Mesial
Mesiobuccal
Mesiolateral oblique
Mesiolingual
Occlusion

OUTLINE

LEARNING OBJECTIVES

When you have finished this chapter, you will be able to:

1. Produce diagnostic high-quality dental radiographs of the dog and cat with special
   emphasis on the following:
   • The proper dental terminology and the tooth surfaces.
   • The basic anatomy and formula of the teeth, including the number of roots for each
     tooth.

- Proper viewing of dental films.
- Use of parallel and bisecting angles.
- The normal views and protocol for extraoral and intraoral dental radiographs, keeping in mind where to measure, center, collimate, and properly position.
- Further concerns and idiosyncrasies, including the variations between dogs and cats.

Palatal surface
Parallel technique
Periapical
Position indicating
  device
Proximal surface
Radicular groove
Rostral
Rostrocaudal oblique
Sectorial occlusion
SLOB rule
Source image distance
Ventral

For true diagnostic radiographs of the canine and feline mouth, a dental x-ray machine should be used. The articulating arm on a dental x-ray machine enables one to obtain quality radiographs quickly and easily with minimal maneuvering of the patient. If there is no access to a dental x-ray unit, extraoral and intraoral radiographs can still be taken with a regular x-ray machine. The same techniques for intraoral radiographs can be performed with a conventional machine and nonscreen film. Extraoral radiographs can also be taken with regular screen/film cassettes, although the resulting extraoral images will not be as detailed as those obtained with the intraoral technique.

> **TECHNICIAN NOTES** In this chapter the term film is used with the understanding that in digital radiography, the digital sensor is substituted for the film.

Indications

In veterinary medicine it is essential to have dental radiographs as part of a comprehensive oral health examination. The visual inspection and tactile examination (probing) of the tooth is only a small part of the information required to make informed treatment decisions. Dental radiography is an essential component of a proper diagnosis, treatment planning, and monitoring.

Oral disease is very common in dogs and cats. A particular challenge with these patients is their inability to communicate pain and discomfort until oral disease is well advanced. Even then, isolating the exact origin and extent of the disease is difficult. Dental radiographs enable us to thoroughly evaluate the entire tooth and surrounding tissues, including bone.

Full-mouth radiographs should be taken as part of a complete oral examination. Specific indications for radiographs include, but are not limited to, periodontal disease, missing teeth, resorptive lesions, oral tumors and gingival inflammation, malformed teeth, discolored teeth, dental extractions, and dental trauma.

Positional Terminology

Some of the terms you should be familiar with are those associated with the direction of the beam and the intraoral terminology (Figure 24-1).

Tooth Anatomy and Dental Formula

Tooth Anatomy

In Figure 24-2, the crown is above the gums (supragingival) and the root below the gums (subgingival). The apex is the tip of the root. At the tip of the root there are small openings to allow the blood supply and nerves to enter the tooth; these openings are referred to as the apical delta. On a radiograph, the pulp chamber is the darker inner content of the tooth extending throughout the crown and the root. The root portion of the pulp chamber is generally referred to as the root canal. The dentin constitutes the bulk of the tooth and appears lighter than the pulp chamber on a radiograph. As a patient ages, secondary dentin is continuously produced.

Over time, the pulp chamber decreases in size because of the secondary dentin. Figure 24-3 illustrates how the size of the pulp chamber evident on a radiograph of the lower first molar can help with aging of an animal. The enamel is the outer covering of the crown, and the cementum is the outer covering of the root. The area that they meet is termed the cementoenamel junction (CEJ). The enamel and cementum are difficult to distinguish from the dentin. The periodontal ligament forms the attachment of the cementum to the alveolar bone. It appears as a thin gray line surrounding the roots. The lamina dura is the wall of the alveolar socket that surrounds the tooth. It appears as a dense white line adjacent to the periodontal ligament space.

The four basic tooth types in dogs and cats are as follows:
- Incisors (I or i) are used for grooming as well as grasping and cutting food. All incisor teeth are single rooted.
- Canine teeth (C or c) are single-rooted teeth that are used for grasping and holding prey. The structure of feline canine teeth supports that cats are true carnivores. There are shallow longitudinal groves on the buccal surfaces of

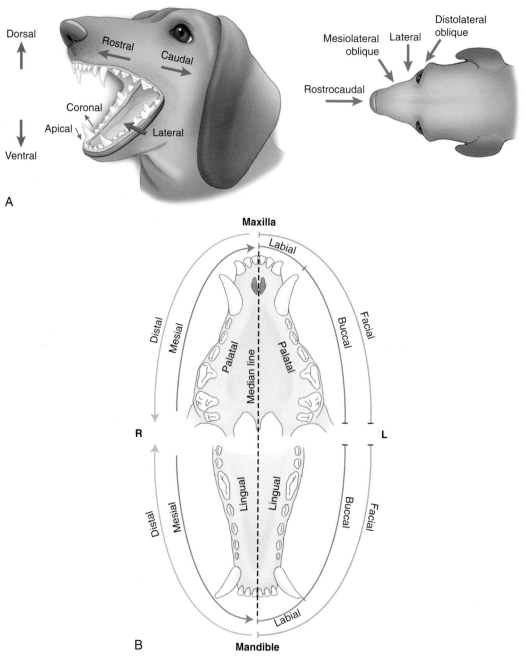

FIGURE 24-1 A, Anatomical directions. **B,** Positional terminology of the oral cavity.

the canine teeth. These grooves "wick" away blood from held prey.

- Premolar teeth (P or p) are designed for cutting and shearing meat. Premolar teeth have prominent sharp cusps and have one to three roots.
- Molar teeth (M or m) generally have flattened occlusal surfaces with the exception of the mandibular first molar tooth in dogs, which does have a cutting edge on the mesial cusp. The first mandibular molar tooth in cats has no flattened occlusal table; instead it has two cutting edges. Molar teeth have two or three roots, but some roots appear to be fused together to give the appearance of

being single rooted (feline maxillary first molar). Molar teeth in dogs are used for grinding food.

Dental Formula

The *dental formula* illustrates how many of each tooth type are present in half of a dog and cat's mouth. The short form for the type of tooth is followed by the number of that particular type there are. The formula is presented in a "fraction," with maxillary teeth shown above the teeth in the mandible, using the following conventions:

Tooth type: refer to description given in former discussion of tooth anatomy

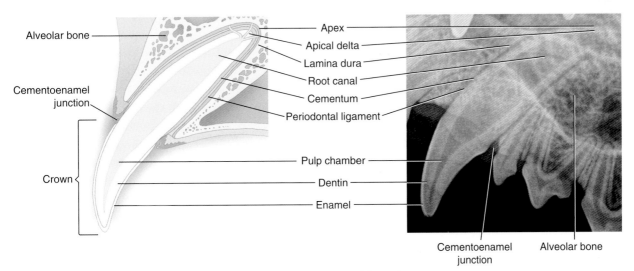

FIGURE 24-2 Anatomy of the tooth.

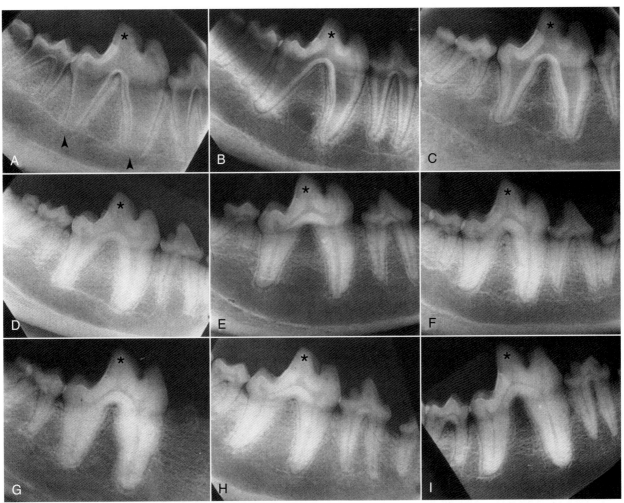

FIGURE 24-3 A to I, Radiographs show how the pulp chamber decreases in size as animals age (youngest, **A**; oldest, **I**). **A**, 6 months, open apex (arrowheads); **B**, 9 months, apical colsure; **C**, 16 months; **D**, 2 years; **E**, 3 years; **F**, 4 years; **G**, 6 years; **H**, 8 yeras; **I**, 12 years.

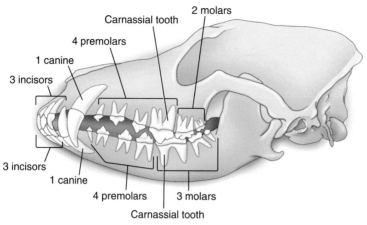

FIGURE 24-4 Canine dental formula.

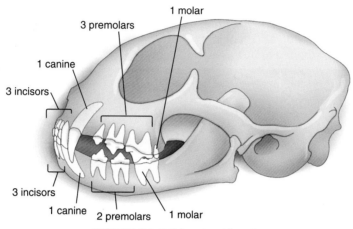

FIGURE 24-5 Feline dental formula.

Permanent: Upper case (I, C, P, M)
Deciduous: Lower case (i, c, p, m)

Canine Dental Formula

Figure 24-4 shows the canine dental formula, which is as follows:

$$\text{Deciduous teeth:} \; 2 \times \left(\frac{\text{i3c1p3m0}}{\text{i3c1p3m0}} \right) = 28 \text{ in total}$$

(shortened version to remember is 313/313

$$\text{Permanent teeth:} \; 2 \times \left(\frac{\text{I3C1P4M2}}{\text{I3C1P4M3}} \right) = 42 \text{ in total}$$

(a shortened version to remember is $\dfrac{3142}{3143}$)

> **TECHNICIAN NOTES** There are no deciduous precursors for the first premolar of the adult dog. Cat and dog molar teeth never have deciduous precursors.

Feline Dental Formula

Figure 24-5 shows the feline dental formula, which is as follows:

$$\text{Deciduous teeth:} \; 2 \times \left(\frac{\text{i3c1p3m0}}{\text{i3c1p2m0}} \right) = 24 \text{ in total}$$

A shortened version to remember is 313/312

$$\text{Permanent teeth:} \; 2 \times \left(\frac{\text{I3C1P3M1}}{\text{I3C1P2M1}} \right) = 30 \text{ in total}$$

A shortened version to remember is $\dfrac{3131}{3121}$

Nomenclature

Two types of numbering systems are used in veterinary medicine for identifying teeth. The anatomical system is an older system but still used in veterinary clinics. The modified Triadan system is the current numbering system of choice. It is easily integrated into paperless records and using it is much faster than using the anatomical system once it has been learned. Figure 24-6 illustrates the anatomical orientation and structure of the teeth with each system illustrated.

Anatomical System for Notation

The anatomical system uses a combination of short forms for tooth type (I, C, P, M for permanent teeth; or i, c, p, m

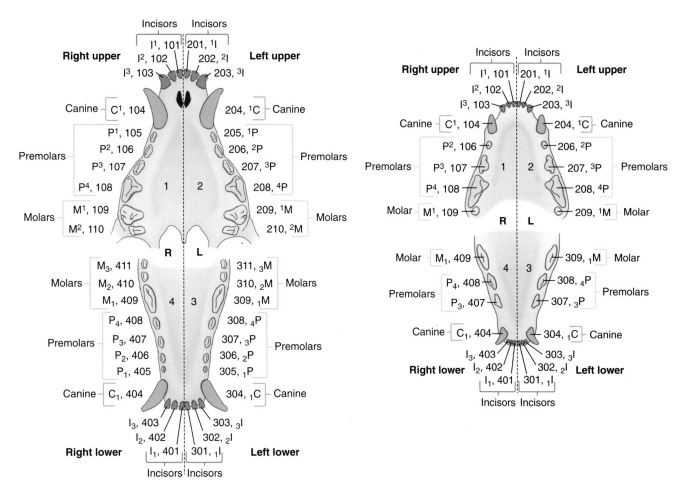

FIGURE 24-6 Anatomical and modified Triadan numbering systems in canine (*left*) and feline (*right*) teeth.

for deciduous teeth) and the numbers of those teeth in their group (i.e., premolars 1–4) to designate a specific tooth. The number of the tooth is placed on the left for a left-sided tooth and the right for a right-sided tooth; the number is superscript for a maxillary tooth and subscript for a mandibular tooth.; For example, I^2 designates the right maxillary second incisor (intermediate incisor).

Modified Triadan System

The modified Triadan system labels each tooth by a code of 3 numbers, starting at the midpoint of the arch in each quadrant. The first number designates the quadrant. The upper right quadrant uses the number 1 as the quadrant designation, the upper left quadrant uses 2, the lower left quadrant uses 3, and the lower right quadrant uses 4. Deciduous teeth use the series 5 through 8 for the quadrants.

The second two numbers are determined by the tooth position, counting back from the midline of the arch in each quadrant. Incisors are numbered 01, 02, and 03; the canine tooth is 04; premolars are 05, 06, 07, and 08; and the molars are 09, 10, 11. So for example, the Triadan number for ^3I is 203.

The Triadan system is adaptable to any species regardless of how many teeth are normally present for that species. However, in order to assign the Triadan numbers to species that are normally missing teeth in the dental formula, you need to know the anatomical number designations, especially for the premolars. Because the cat is missing the upper first premolar, there are no 105 or 205 teeth in a cat. Likewise, for the mandibular premolars, because the cat is missing the first and second premolars, the numbers 305, 306 or 405, and 406 are not used.

> *TECHNICIAN NOTES* The canine tooth always ends in a 4, and the first molar always ends in a 9. From there you can count forward or backward in the dental arch as needed.

Roots of the Various Teeth

It is very important to appreciate the structure and number of tooth roots (Figure 24-7). The appreciation of this anatomy is vital to determine tooth angle and to decide when

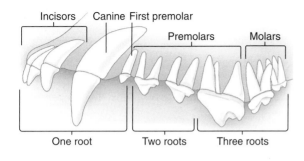

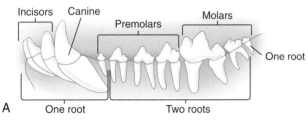

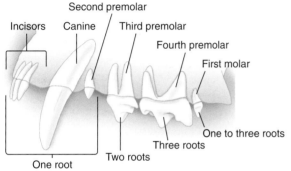

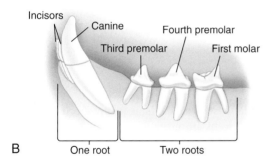

FIGURE 24-7 A, Roots of the permanent teeth of a canine. B, Roots of the permanent teeth of a feline.

to change the direction of the x-ray beam to isolate the roots. It is also important in the interpretation of radiographs to recognize extra or malformed roots.

Normal Radiographic Anatomy in Dogs and Cats

The following radiographs illustrate normal radiographic findings of the areas listed here. It is important to be able to distinguish between mandible and maxilla when viewing radiographs. It is also important to become familiar with the orientation of the teeth and the anatomical differences in root and crown structure. The more familiar you are with

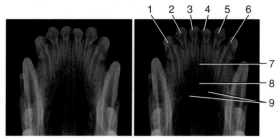

FIGURE 24-8 Normal radiographic anatomy of the canine adult maxillary incisors. 1, 203; 2, 202; 3, 201; 4, 101; 5, 102; 6, 103; 7, incisive canal; 8, interincisive suture; 9, palatine fissure.

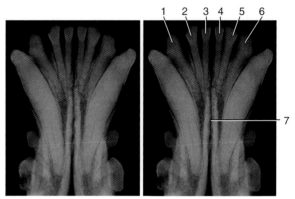

FIGURE 24-9 Normal radiograph anatomy canine adult mandibular incisors. 1, 403; 2, 402; 3, 401; 4, 301; 5, 302; 6, 303; 7, mandibular symphysis.

these areas, the easier it will be to distinguish between teeth on a radiograph.

- Normal adult maxillary incisors and teeth: look for white space distal to incisors, with two oval (dark) spaces, which are the palatine fissures (Figure 24-8).
- Normal adult mandibular incisors: look for a dark black line distal to incisors that separates mandibular rami (mandibular symphysis) (Figure 24-9).
- Normal adult maxillary premolars and molars: Look for the fine white line representing the maxillary recess apical to the roots (Figure 24-10).
- Normal adult mandibular premolars and molars: Look for dark black areas above and below the mandible (Figure 24-11).

Equipment and Supplies

Refer to Chapter 10 for information on the actual x-ray units used for the film, and the processing if applicable.

If choosing a digital system make sure to research the limitations and advantages of each type of system. The bulkier and less flexible sensor of some systems make some systems harder to work with. The size of the sensor may also be limited.

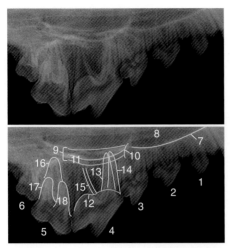

FIGURE 24-10 Normal radiograph anatomy canine maxillary premolars and molars. 1, 105; 2, 106; 3, 107; 4, 108; 5, 109; 6, 110; 7, nasal surface of the alveolar process of maxilla; 8, nasal cavity; 9, infraorbital canal; 10, infraorbital foramen; 11, palatine canal; 12, palatal marginal enamel; 13, mesiopalatal root; 14, mesiobuccal root; 15, radicular groove on distal root; 16, palatal root; 17, distobuccal root; 18, mesiobuccal root.

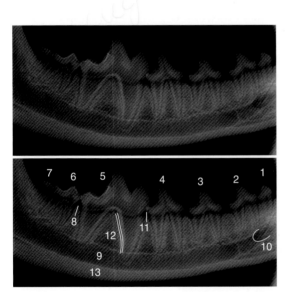

FIGURE 24-11 Normal radiograph anatomy canine mandibular premolars and molars. 1, 405; 2, 406; 3, 407; 4, 408; 5, 409; 6, 410; 7, 411; 8, alveolar margin; 9, mandibular canal; 10, middle mental foramen; 11, overlap of enamel; 12, radicular groove; 13, ventral mandibular cortex.

TECHNICIAN NOTES The same parallel and bisecting angle techniques are used for digital radiography as for the film system. The digital sensor replaces the film.

Viewing Dental Radiographs

Film is always exposed with the convex dot at the rostral end of the mouth; therefore, views on the right side have the dot in a different location from those on the left side. Figure 24-12 demonstrates with digital films how the locations of the dot ("a" on digital plates) differ. Once the film has been developed, hold it so the convex dot is raised toward you (as it was placed in the mouth). Determine whether you are looking at a maxilla or a mandible (see earlier discussions of tooth anatomy and normal anatomy radiographs). Orient the radiograph so the cusps of the maxillary teeth are pointing down toward the floor and the cusps of the mandibular teeth are pointing up toward the ceiling (Figure 24-13). Look at the film as if you were looking at the animal with the film positioned in its mouth. The anatomical structures and orientation of the teeth will allow you to determine if it is a maxilla or mandible and left or right (Figure 24-14).

TECHNICIAN NOTES With the convex dot facing you, visualize the film inside the patient's mouth to determine whether the film is showing the left or right side.

Mounting Dental Radiographs

If a full-mouth set of radiographs is taken, the practitioner may want them organized in a film mount (Figure 24-15). The film mount allows the films to be organized in a prearranged layout and filed for future reference. Digital systems also have templates built into the software to mount the digital radiographs.

A full-mouth set of dental radiographs should always be mounted as if you were looking at the animal. The animal's right side of the mouth should be on your left when viewing the full set of radiographs (Figure 24-16).

Projection Geometry

Parallel Technique

Parallel technique involves placing the dental film directly behind and parallel to the tooth and then directing the x-ray beam perpendicular to the film (Figure 24-17A). The anatomy of dog and cat mouths allows the parallel technique to be used in only one area. This area encompasses the teeth distal to and including the mandibular third premolars ($_3P_3$ or 307/407).

Bisecting Angle Technique

Because of the anatomical structure of the mouths of dogs and cats, film cannot be placed directly behind most teeth. The bisecting angle technique is used to image these teeth. This technique is used on all maxillary teeth, all incisors and canines, and mandibular premolars 1 and 2.

The bisecting angle is an angle formed by the intersection of the plane of the film and the long axis of the tooth. If the central ray is perpendicular to a line that bisects this angle, the resulting image is as accurate as possible (Figure 24-17B).

In order to accurately visualize the long axis of the tooth, you should stand at the patient's front (premolar teeth) or the patient's side (incisor and canine teeth) to find the bisecting angle (Figure 24-18).

Right maxilla   Left maxilla

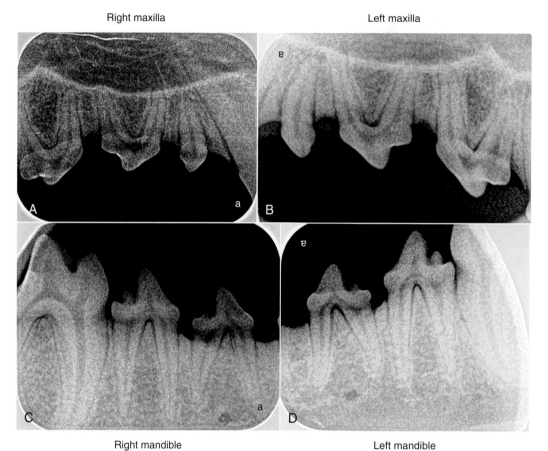

Right mandible   Left mandible

FIGURE 24-12 A to D, Digital films showing how placement of dot (a) differs.

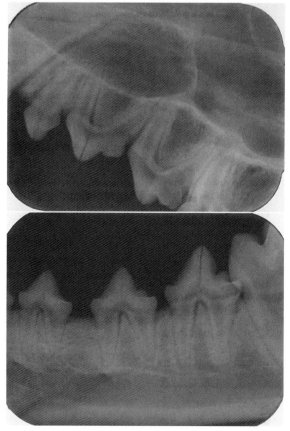

FIGURE 24-13 Proper viewing of a radiograph. Note that the maxillary cusps are pointing down and the mandibular cusps are pointing up.

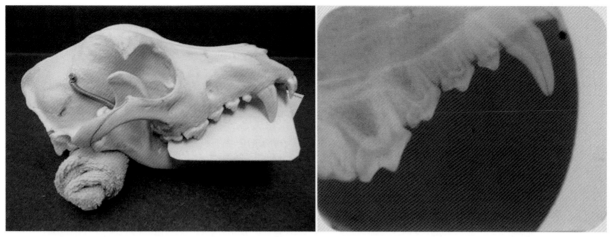

FIGURE 24-14 Proper film placement in mouth and accompanying radiograph (right maxilla), note: convex dot in upper right hand corner or film.

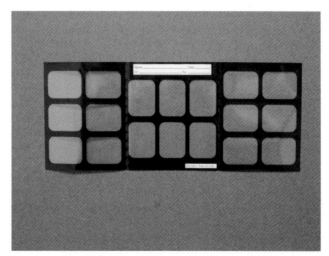

FIGURE 24-15 An example of a film mount.

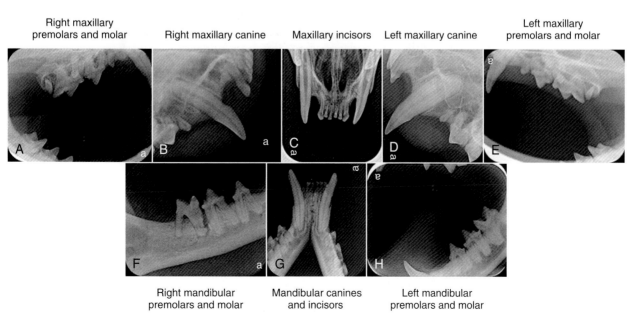

| Right maxillary premolars and molar | Right maxillary canine | Maxillary incisors | Left maxillary canine | Left maxillary premolars and molar |

Right mandibular premolars and molar   Mandibular canines and incisors   Left mandibular premolars and molar

FIGURE 24-16 A to H, An example of full-mouth feline radiographs.

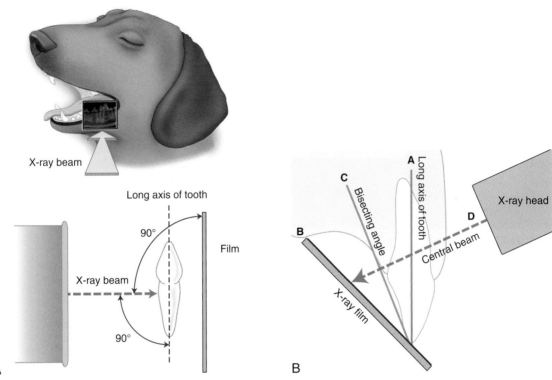

FIGURE 24-17 **A,** Parallel technique. **B,** Bisecting angle.

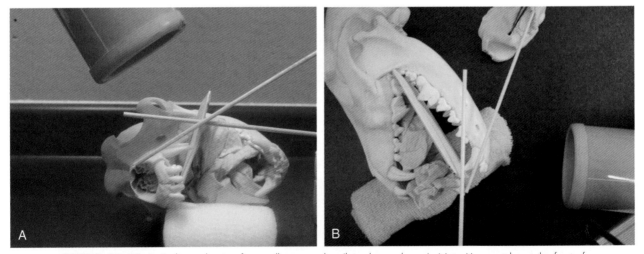

FIGURE 24-18 **A,** Radiograph setup for maxillary premolars (lateral recumbency). *Note:* You must be at the front of the patient to appreciate the angle that the tooth enters the skull. **B,** Radiograph setup for mandibular incisors (lateral recumbency). *Note:* You must be at the side of the patient to appreciate the angle that the tooth enters the skull.

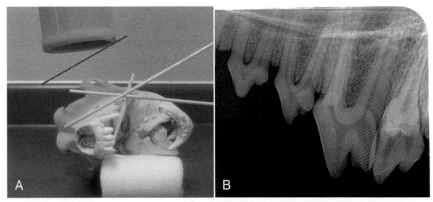

FIGURE 24-19 Radiograph setup (**A**) and resulting radiograph (**B**) demonstrating elongation. The red line is the bisecting angle that the x-ray beam should be perpendicular to. In this setup, the x-ray beam is focused too much on the tooth angle.

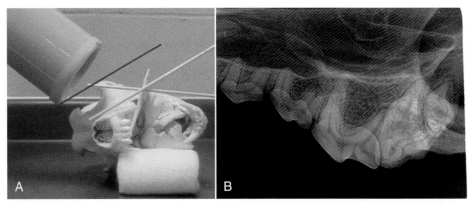

FIGURE 24-20 Radiograph setup (**A**) and resulting radiograph (**B**) demonstrating foreshortening. The *red line* is the bisecting angle that the x-ray beam should be perpendicular to. In this setup the x-ray beam is focused too much on the film angle.

> *TECHNICIAN NOTES* Another way to think of the bisecting angle is to split the difference between pointing the beam at the tooth angle and the film angle. This difference is the bisecting angle

Foreshortening and Elongation

If the x-ray beam is not aimed directly at the bisecting angle, the image will not be a true representation of the tooth. An artifact: elongation, or foreshortening will result.

The analogy of using the shadows created by the position of the sun overhead is one way to explain elongation and foreshortening. If you were standing in the middle of a field, the shadow created on the ground by the sun coming up on the horizon would create quite different shadows from those created by the sun directly overhead. When the sun is coming up on the horizon, a very long shadow is created; this effect

is elongation. At noon the sun is overhead, and your shadow is smaller than you are; this effect is foreshortening.

Elongation is the result of the central ray's being at a right angle to the long axis of the tooth instead of to the bisecting angle. Because the beam is directed at the angle of the tooth, the image will appear "stretched out," and the entire tooth may not have been captured on the film (Figure 24-19).

Foreshortening is the result of the central ray's being at a right angle to the film instead of to the bisecting angle. Because the beam is directed at the angle of the film, the tooth will appear to have the crown overlapping on the root (Figure 24-20).

> *TECHNICIAN NOTES* If the beam is perpendicular to the film, the image is foreshortened. If the beam is perpendicular to the tooth, the image is elongated. If you split the difference, the image is truer. The bisecting angle is splitting the difference.

Dental Radiography with Conventional Cassette: Common Views

- The use of conventional cassettes is not the ideal way to image teeth, but if there is no dental x-ray machine or nonscreen film, it is the only option.
- See the discussion of intraoral radiography with conventional machine later in this chapter.
- Screened cassettes and radiolucent positioning devices are required.
- Difficulties expected include: positioning of the cassettes in the mouth, because of the general characteristics of cassettes (size, thickness, weight).
- Teeth in the distal aspect of the mouth may be difficult to image owing to superimposition of the contralateral arch.

Maxillary Premolar and Molars: Ventrodorsal Oblique Extraoral Views

Positioning

Position the patient in lateral (side) recumbency, affected side down on the cassette; then rotate the patient so it is placed midway onto its back, between the lateral and ventral-dorsal (ventrodorsal [VD]) positions. Ensure patient is in true lateral by placing a foam wedge or roll under nose.

Place the mandible on a foam wedge, rotating the mandible at a 45-degree angle with the table surface.

The mouth should be wide open with a radiolucent mouth gag in place, see Figure 24-21A, B.

Comments and Tips

- Make sure the contralateral maxillary teeth and roots do not superimpose against interested maxilla premolars and molars.

MEASURE: Caudal hard palate at commissure of lips.

CENTRAL RAY: Maxillary third premolar.

INCLUDE: Maxillary premolars and molars.

> *TECHNICIAN NOTES*   The contralateral maxillary premolars and molars appear whiter because of bone superimposition. The affected side's premolars and molars appear magnified because of the angle of the head (causing elongation).

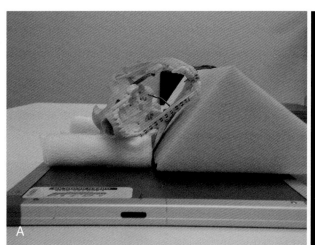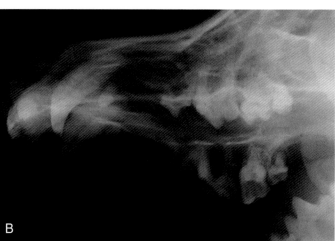

FIGURE 24-21 Extraoral technique setup (**A**) and radiograph (**B**) of maxillary premolars and molars.

Mandibular Premolar and Molars: Dorsoventral Oblique Extraoral Views

Positioning

Position the patient in lateral recumbency with the affected side down on the cassette.

Place the maxilla on a foam wedge, rotating the maxilla at a 20-degree angle with the table surface.

The mouth should be wide open with a radiolucent mouth gag, see Figure 24-22A, B.

Comments and Tips

- Make sure the contralateral mandibular teeth and roots do not superimpose over the areas of interest, which are the mandibular premolars and molars.
- The contralateral mandibular premolars and molars appear whiter because of the bone superimposition. The affected side's premolars and molars appear magnified because of the angle of the head (causing elongation).

MEASURE: Thickness of mandible at the commissure of lips.

CENTRAL RAY: Site of interest.

INCLUDE: Mandibular premolars and molars.

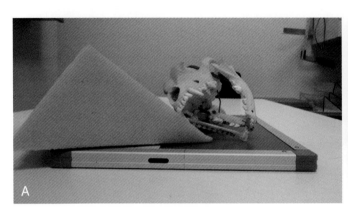 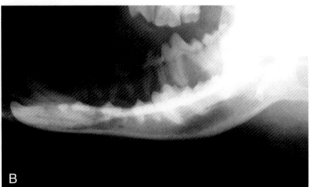

FIGURE 24-22 Extraoral technique setup (**A**) and radiograph (**B**) of mandibular premolars and molars.

Maxilla Incisors and Canine: Dorsoventral Intraoral/Occlusal View

Positioning

Position the patient in sternal recumbency.

A foam sponge should be placed under the mandible and cassette to keep it parallel to table top. Place one corner of the film cassette into the mouth as far as possible, see Figure 24-23A, B.

Comments and Tips

Source-image distance (SID) will have to be adjusted because of the raised cassette. The roots of the canine teeth will be superimposed over the premolars distal to the canine tooth The rostral nasal sinus cavity can be assessed with this view.

MEASURE: At the level of the commissure of the lips (maxilla thickness).

CENTRAL RAY: Site of interest.

INCLUDE: All incisors and canines, including roots.

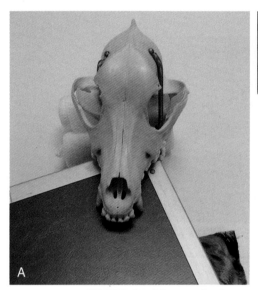
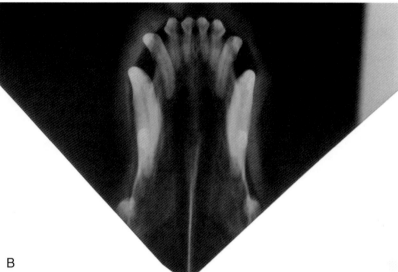

FIGURE 24-23 Intraoral technique with cassette setup (**A**) and radiograph (**B**) of maxillary incisors and canine.

Mandibular Incisors and Canine: Ventrodorsal Intraoral/Occlusal View

Positioning

The patient should be positioned in dorsal recumbency with a foam sponge placed under the nose and cervical spine to keep the mandible and cassette parallel to the tabletop.

Place one corner of the film cassette into the mouth as far as possible, see Figure 24-24A, B.

Comments and Tips

Raise the tube head, because the SID has decreased. The mandibular canine tooth will be slightly superimposed over the first premolar.

MEASURE: At the level of the commissure of the lips (mandible thickness, which is $_1M_1$ in dogs).

CENTRAL RAY: Site of interest.

INCLUDE: All incisors and canines, including roots.

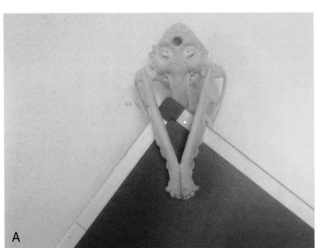 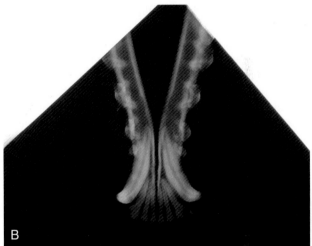

FIGURE 24-24 Intraoral technique with cassette setup (A) and radiograph (B) of mandibular incisors and canine.

Intraoral Dental Radiography with a Dental X-Ray Machine

The size of film chosen for each view depends on the size of the animal and the tooth to be radiographed. In general, size 4 film should be used for all x-rays of the canine teeth except for small dogs and cats. Most views in cats utilize size 2 films. The following views are demonstrated with the patient in lateral recumbency. This is the recommended patient position because it greatly reduces moving the patient during anesthesia.

The mandible and maxilla should be kept parallel with the tabletop. A small roll or foam wedge can be used to accomplish this goal. If maxillary views are taken, the endotracheal tube should be tied to the mandible, and vice versa. A paper towel should be used to position the film in the mouth.

The distance between the cone and the film depends on the size of film used. If small film (sizes 0, 1 or 2) is used, the cone can be against the patient's face with a source image distance (SID) of 1 to 2 inches. If size 4 film is used, the SID should be increased to at least 6 inches to allow for a wider area of x-rays (Figure 24-25).

The exposure will have to be increased if the SID is increased. Each machine varies, but generally, if the distance is approximately 6 inches from the film, the exposure will have to be increased by 1.5 times the normal exposure for that area. Remember the inverse square law from Chapter 6. Digital systems may not need an increase in exposure because of the greater sensitivity of digital plates.

Always center the cone on the tooth in question.

Dental x-ray machines have no collimator light; therefore the direction and width of the x-ray beam must be estimated with applicator sticks (Figure 24-26). Remember that once the beam leaves the collimator cone, it gets wider the farther it must travel.

Also remember that the "dot" should be rostrally placed with the convex side of the film (white side) facing the tube head ("a" on digital plates).

> **TECHNICIAN NOTES**   To find the bisecting angle: If the cone is coming from the side (premolars), you should be standing at the patient's front (kneel down at the nose level to visualize the tooth angle). If the cone is coming from the patient's front (incisors and canines), you should be standing at the patient's side.

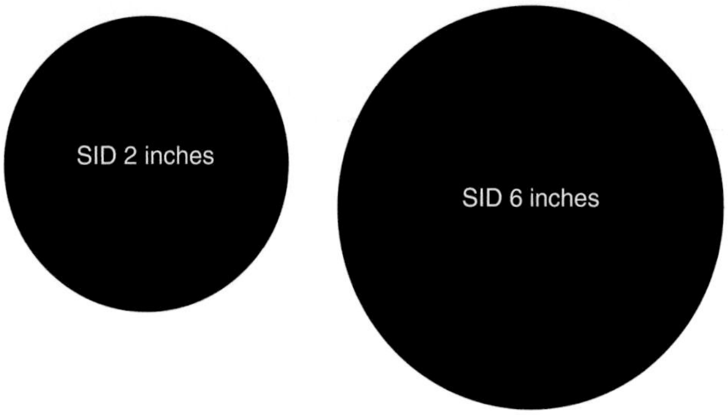

FIGURE 24-25 Comparison of focal size with a 2-inch and 6-inch source image distance (SID).

SID 2 inches

SID 6 inches

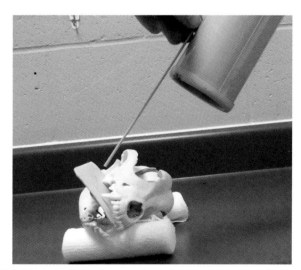

FIGURE 24-26 Applicator sticks used to estimate the size of the x-ray beam.

Canine Radiographs

Canine Maxillary Premolars

FILM: The opposite edge of the film should be touching the hard palate, resting against the palatal surface of the contralateral teeth. The tips of the premolar/molar should be at the edge of the film closest to the cone to allow ample space for the roots of the tooth to "fall onto" the film. A size 2 film is likely necessary to capture distal molars because of anatomical space constraints.

CENTRAL RAY: The cone is directed laterally and centered over the tooth in question. The SID depends on the size of film. For a size 4 film, the SID is 6 inches.

ANGLE: The bisecting angle is found by standing at the patient's front (Figure 24-27).

> **TECHNICIAN NOTES** Superimposition of multi-rooted teeth is always a concern. Multiple radiographs may be necessary to isolate specific roots if required (see later).

> **TECHNICIAN NOTES** When placing the film packet inside the mouth, remember, "the white side faces the white teeth" and the dot should be at the front of the mouth.

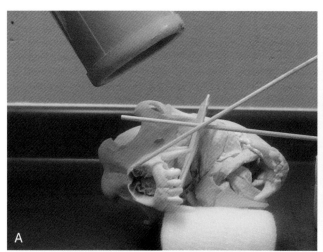 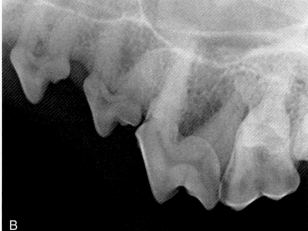

FIGURE 24-27 Intraoral technique radiograph setup (**A**) and radiograph (**B**) of maxillary premolars and molars (lateral recumbency).

Maxillary Premolars: SLOB Rule

The maxillary fourth premolar (108 [P^4] or 208 [^{4}P]) is a triple-rooted tooth that has one large distal root and two smaller mesial roots. The mesial roots superimpose over each other if the beam is directed from the lateral aspect. If a desired root needs to be isolated, the direction of the beam can be directed from the mesial or the distal aspect to "split" the roots on the film.

The SLOB rule stands for "same lingual opposite buccal." This term is used to help identify the particular root when the beam is directed from the mesial or distal aspect. "Same lingual" means that the lingual-mesial root (which is actually the palatal root-maxilla) appears to move in the same direction as where the x-ray beam is being directed from. "Opposite buccal" means that the buccal-mesial root appears to move in the opposite direction from where the x-ray beam is coming from.

The SLOB rule can be illustrated using your hands as shown in Figure 24-28. In this diagram the root structure of 208 or ^{4}P is depicted. In the first diagram, you can see the

Continued

Canine Maxillary Premolars—*cont'd*

thumb and one finger. In the second diagram, you can see an additional finger. If the direction the beam is coming from is changed, you will be able to see objects that were superimposed from the initial view. In the second diagram, you can see that if the beam (your eyes) is directed from the distal aspect, the palatal root appears to move in the same direction as where the beam is being directed from.

If the beam is directed from the distal aspect, the palatal root will appear as the middle of the three roots on the radiograph. If the beam is directed from the mesial aspect, the buccal root will appear as the middle of the three roots on the radiograph.

Technique

The same setup for the film, cone, and bisecting angle are used as described previously for maxillary premolars and molars is used as the starting point. Once the bisecting angle is found and the cone is aimed perpendicular to it from the lateral aspect, the cone can be directed from the mesial or distal aspect (Figure 24-29).

Mesiolateral Oblique View

For the mesiolateral oblique view, the cone is directed from the mesial aspect (mesial to distal), approximately 30 degrees from the initial position. Figure 24-30 shows the mesial roots

isolated on the radiograph. However the distal root will superimpose over the first maxillary molar tooth.

Distolateral Oblique View

For the distolateral oblique view, the cone is directed from the distal aspect (distal to mesial), approximately 30 degrees from the initial position. Figure 24-31 shows the mesial roots separated on the radiograph. However, the mesial roots may superimpose over the third maxillary premolar tooth.

Comments and Tips

Two radiographs are always necessary to evaluate all three of the roots of the maxillary fourth premolar tooth—the standard radiograph with the central ray directed at the bisecting angle from the lateral aspect and an oblique radiograph. The distolateral oblique view is preferred by the author to isolate the mesial roots.

> **TECHNICIAN NOTES** The SLOB rule states that if the beam is directed from the distal aspect, the palatal root will appear as the middle of the three roots on the radiograph. If the beam is directed from the mesial aspect, the buccal root will appear as the middle of the three roots on the radiograph.

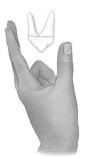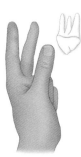

FIGURE 24-28 SLOB rule: Left hand used to demonstrate root isolation of 208 by changing x-ray beam direction.

Canine Maxillary Premolars—*cont'd*

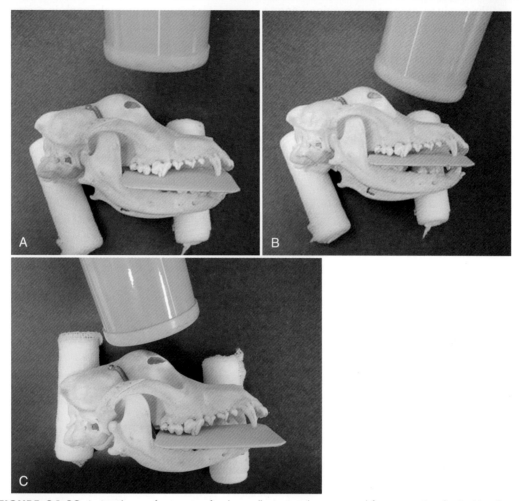

FIGURE 24-29 A, Initial setup for imaging fourth maxillary premolar as viewed from patient's side. B, Mesiolateral oblique radiograph setup of maxillary fourth premolar (lateral recumbency). showing final oblique x-ray cone. C, Distolateral oblique radiograph setup of maxillary fourth premolar (lateral recumbency) showing final oblique x-ray cone.

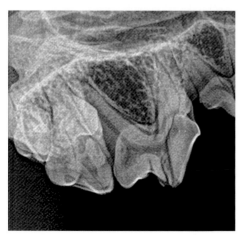

FIGURE 24-30 Mesiolateral oblique radiograph; the central root is the mesial-buccal root.

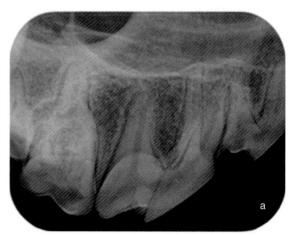

FIGURE 24-31 Distolateral oblique radiograph; the central root is the mesial-palatal root.

Maxillary Canine Tooth

The radiograph of the maxillary canine tooth is set up using the long axis of the tooth, which can be visualized from the side of the patient; *then* the x-ray cone is directed in an oblique angle toward the midline of the animal. This change in beam angle helps prevent superimposition of the canine tooth over the premolar teeth. The canine tooth curves distally, with its apex typically over the root of the second premolar; always use the root of the tooth to find the bisecting angle, not the crown. This view can also be used to visualize the ipsilateral incisors. When changing the beam angle it is helpful to utilize the angle meter on the tube head. With an animal in true lateral recumbency the angle should be on zero degrees.

> **TECHNICIAN NOTES** Remember that the same parallel and bisecting angle techniques are used for digital radiography as for the film system. The digital sensor replaces the film but some sensors are bulkier and less flexible than other sensors and the film.

FILM: Size 4 film is used for most dogs. Both canine teeth should be touching the film ("biting on it"). The tip of the canine tooth desired should be at the lateral edge of film to allow ample space for the root of the canine to "fall onto" the film.

CENTRAL RAY: The film to cone distance should be about 6 inches for a dog's canine tooth. The cone is directed in a rostrocaudal direction and centered over the tooth in question. The angle meter should read 0 on the tube head if the animal is in true lateral. The tube head is then moved up approximately 30 degrees vertically from the starting point so that the canine tooth does not superimpose over the premolars distal to it.

ANGLE: The bisecting angle of the tooth is found by standing at the patient's side using the long axis of the tooth. If root cutoff occurs and both canine teeth are "biting" on film, you need to foreshorten the angle slightly. To foreshorten the angle, focus more on the film.

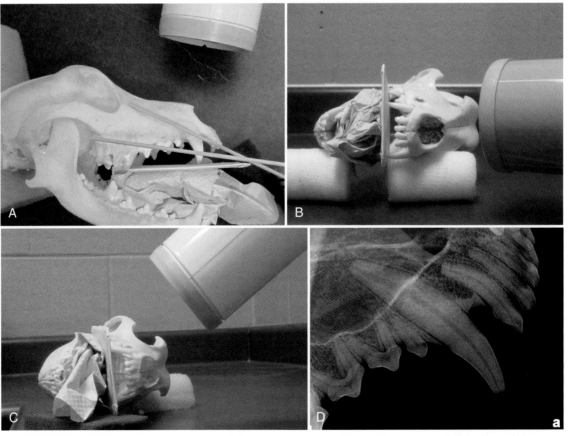

FIGURE 24-32 Three views of the intraoral technique radiograph setup of the maxillary canine tooth (lateral recumbency): (A) view from the patient's side to aim at bisecting angle; (B) and view from front while finding bisecting angle, (angle meter should be at 0 degrees); (C) view from the patient's front after final tilt (30 degrees) of x-ray cone; and (D) the radiograph (of the maxillary canine tooth. Note: ipsilateral incisors can be imaged as well.

Maxillary Incisors

The typical rostrocaudal view can capture all the incisors on one film. Because they converge at the midline, the roots cannot always be isolated because they may overlap slightly. In some instances, if a specific incisor needs to be isolated, the x-ray cone can be directed obliquely from the left or right side so its root is more isolated (similar to technique for maxillary canine tooth). Elongation is a common artifact for this view. Dog incisors have long roots that curve distally, like the root(s) of a canine tooth.

> **TECHNICIAN NOTES** When changing the beam angle it is helpful to utilize the angle meter on the tube head. With an animal in true lateral recumbency the angle should be on zero degrees.

FILM: The tips of the incisor teeth should be at the rostral edge of the film to allow ample space for the roots of the incisors to "fall onto" the film. The canine teeth will both be in contact with the film if a size 4 film is used.

CONE: The cone is directed in a rostrocaudal direction and centered over the nose.

ANGLE: The bisecting angle is found by standing at the patient's side. Remember that the incisor teeth in dogs curve distally, see Figure 24-33.

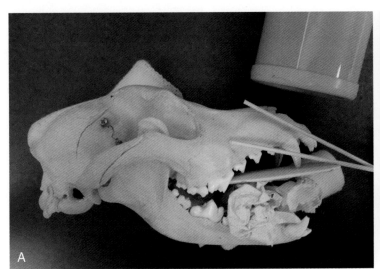
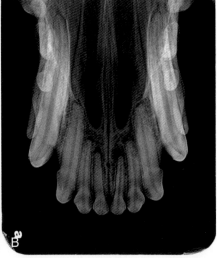

FIGURE 24-33 Setup for an intraoral technique radiograph (**A**) and the radiograph (**B**) of the maxillary incisors (lateral recumbency).

Mandibular Incisors

The typical rostrocaudal view can capture all the incisors on one film. Because they converge at the midline, the roots cannot always be isolated because they will overlap slightly. In some instances, if a specific incisor needs to be isolated, the x-ray cone can be directed obliquely from the left or right side so its root is more isolated (similar to mandibular canine tooth). Elongation is a common artifact for this view. Dog incisors have long roots that curve distally like the root(s) of a canine tooth.

FILM: The tips of the incisor teeth should be at the rostral edge of the film to allow ample space for the roots of the incisors to "fall onto" the film. Both canine teeth will be in contact with the film if a size 4 film is used.

CENTRAL RAY: The cone is directed in a rostrocaudal direction and centered over chin.

ANGLE: The bisecting angle is found by standing at the patient's side. Remember that the incisor teeth in dogs curve distally, see Figure 24-34.

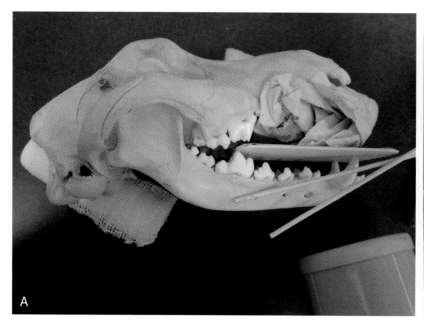
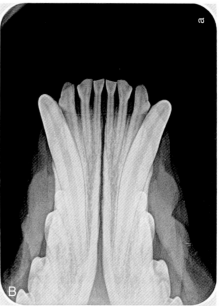

FIGURE 24-34 Setup for an intraoral technique radiograph (**A**) and the radiograph (**B**) of the mandibular incisors (lateral recumbency).

Mandibular Canine Tooth

The radiograph of the mandibular canine tooth is set up using the long axis of the tooth which can be visualized from the side of the patient; then the x-ray cone is slightly directed in an oblique angle toward the midline of the animal. This change in beam angle helps prevent superimposition of the canine tooth over the premolar teeth. When changing the beam angle it is helpful to utilize the angle meter on the tube head. With an animal in true lateral recumbency the angle should be on zero degrees. Mandibular canine teeth converge towards midline therefore the angulation toward midline is less than required for the maxillary canine tooth.

FILM: Size 4 film is used for most canine teeth. Both canine teeth should be touching the film ("biting on it"). The tongue is positioned on the opposite side of the film. The tip of the canine tooth desired should be at the lateral edge of the film to allow ample space for the root of the canine to "fall onto" the film.

CENTRAL RAY: The film-to-cone distance should be about 6 inches for a dog's canine tooth. The cone is directed in a rostrocaudal direction and centered over the tooth in question. The angle meter should read 0 on the tube head if the animal is in true lateral. The tube head is then moved up approximately 15 degrees vertically from the starting point so that the canine tooth does not superimpose over the premolars distal to it.

ANGLE: The bisecting angle of the tooth is found by standing at the patient's side using the long axis of the tooth. If root cutoff occurs and both canine teeth are "biting" on the film, you need to foreshorten the angle slightly. To foreshorten the angle, focus more on the film, see Figure 24-35 A-C.

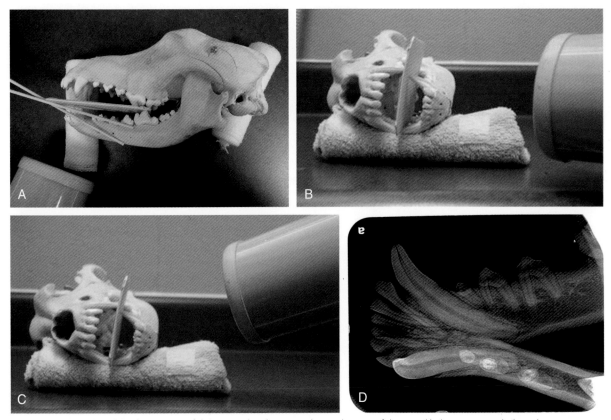

FIGURE 24-35 Three views of the intraoral technique radiograph setup of the mandibular canine tooth (lateral recumbency): (**A**) view from patient's side to aim at bisecting angle (**B**) view from patient's front while finding bisecting angle, (angle meter should be at 0 degrees) (**C**) view from the patient's front after final tilt (15 degrees) of x-ray cone (**D**) and the radiograph of the mandibular canine tooth.

Mandibular Premolars 1 and 2

FILM: The film (size 2) should be resting on both first and second premolars (left and right), behind the canine teeth, facing the floor of the mandible. The tips of the premolars to be radiographed should be at the edge of film closest to you (lateral) to allow ample space for the roots of the tooth to "fall onto" the film.

CENTRAL RAY: The cone is directed laterally and centered at the tooth to be radiographed.

ANGLE: The bisecting angle is found by standing at the patient's front. The x-ray beam will be angled through the floor of the mandible see Figure 24-36.

> **TECHNICIAN NOTES** Parallel technique cannot be used on mandibular premolars 1 and 2. Dogs have an elongated mandibular symphysis, which makes correct film placement impossible. Bisecting angle technique must be used on these teeth.

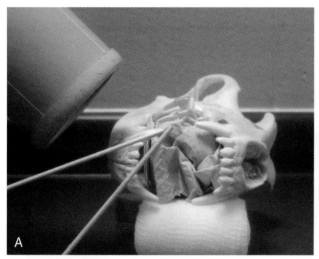
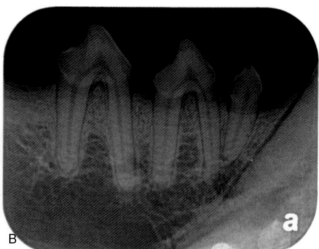

FIGURE 24-36 Setup for an intraoral technique radiograph (**A**) and the radiograph (**B**) of mandibular premolars 1 and 2 (lateral recumbency).

Mandibular Premolars 3 and 4 and Molars

FILM: The film is placed between the tongue and the mandible, parallel to the long axis of the teeth. It is necessary to *push the film* down until you can feel the film pop out under the ventral mandible. This maneuver ensures that the entire tooth is captured. A paper towel can be used to keep the film pushed down. The film can be gently bent to accommodate placement, and if a larger film is used, it can be placed behind the tooth diagonally so it fits.

CENTRAL RAY: The cone is directed laterally and centered on the tooth to be radiographed, perpendicular to film.

ANGLE: Parallel technique, see Figure 24-37.

> *TECHNICIAN NOTES* Parallel technique can be used for the mandibular premolars 3 and 4 and the mandibular molars because there is no hard palate to interfere with film placement behind the roots of these teeth.

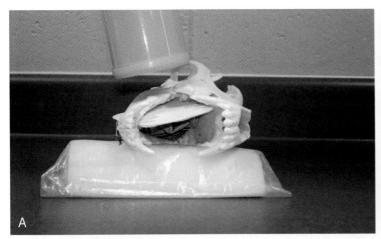
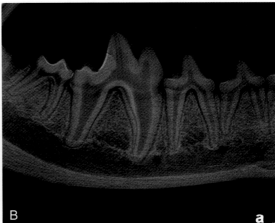

FIGURE 24-37 Setup for an intraoral technique radiograph (**A**) and the radiograph (**B**) of mandibular premolars 3 and 4, and molars (lateral recumbency).

Feline Radiographs

Maxillary Premolars: Intraoral Technique

FILM: The top edge of the film (size 2) is resting against the palatal aspect of the maxillary premolar teeth on the side of the mouth opposite to the teeth you are imaging. The bottom edge of the film rests against the lingual aspect of the mandibular canine tooth on the side of the mouth you are radiographing. The tongue should be behind the film on the mandible. The endotracheal tube will be on the tube side of the film. It may have to be untied and secured on one side only (with hemostats clamped to fur) for this view. The maxillary arcade should be parallel to the tabletop.

CENTRAL RAY: The x-ray cone is directed perpendicular to the film visualized from the front and ventral aspect of the patient.

ANGLE: The angle is referred to as a modified parallel technique. It is very important that the beam is perpendicular to the film from the front and side. NOTE: If root cutoff occurs, the beam must be centered more on the roots of the teeth, see Figure 24-38.

TECHNICIAN NOTES The standard bisecting angle that is traditionally used for maxillary premolars in a dog cannot be used for feline teeth because the zygomatic arch will be superimposed on these teeth. A "modified parallel technique" is used to minimize this superimposition.

TECHNICIAN NOTES It is very important that the beam is perpendicular to the film from the front and side when using the modified parallel technique for the feline intraoral maxillary premolars.

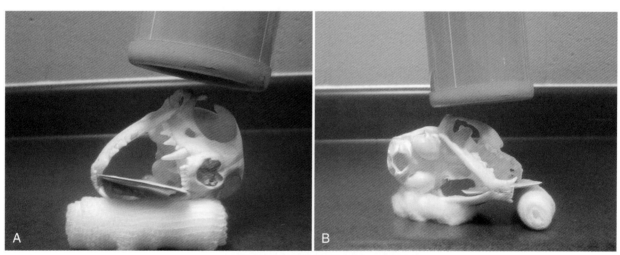

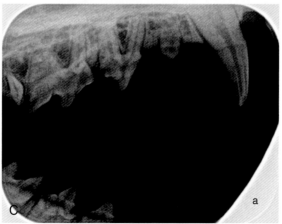

FIGURE 24-38 Setup for an intraoral technique radiograph of feline maxillary premolars and molar (lateral recumbency), (**A**) viewed from the front and (**B**) from the ventral aspect; (**C**) the radiograph of feline maxillary premolars and molar.

Maxillary Premolars: Extraoral Technique

Another option for imaging the maxillary premolars in cats is to use an extraoral technique. This is the preferred technique if a direct digital radiography (DDR) sensor is used, because film placement using the standard technique with the bulky sensors is problematic.

Comments and Tips

On the radiograph, you will see the premolars on the opposite side but they should not be superimposing on the maxillary premolars in question.

The film will have to be identified properly because the extraoral technique was used.

POSITION: The cat should be positioned in lateral recumbency with the mouth propped open. A 1-mL syringe (cut down) can be used to prop the mouth open. The endotracheal tube should be gently pulled ventrally so it is not superimposed over the premolars.

FILM: Size 2 film is positioned extraorally under the side to be radiographed. The cusps of the premolars should be at the edge of the film, allowing ample space for the roots of the teeth to be imaged (most of the maxilla should be on the film). The film must be parallel to the roots of the premolars; a small roll of tape or foam wedge under the film can be used to position it (Figure 24-39A).

CENTRAL RAY: As a starting point, with the patient in lateral recumbency, the cone is aimed at both maxillary arcades as if to superimpose them on the radiograph. Then the cone is directed toward the film, centering at the roots of the premolars near the film and bypassing the opposite arcade (Figure 24-40).

ANGLE: The beam is aimed at the film in a "near-parallel" technique.

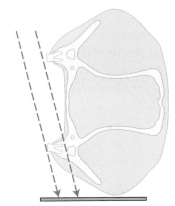

FIGURE 24-40 Labeled extraoral sketch.

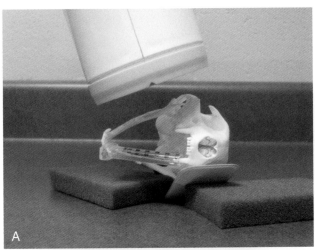

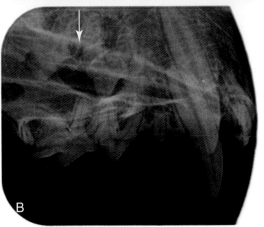

FIGURE 24-39 **A,** Setup for an extraoral technique radiograph of the feline maxillary premolars. **B,** The radiograph . Note the contralateral premolars at the top of the film edge (*arrow*).

Maxillary Canine Tooth

The radiograph of a maxillary canine tooth in a cat is set up using the long axis of the tooth, which can be visualized from the side of the patient; *then* the x-ray cone is directed in an oblique angle toward the midline of the animal. This change in beam angle helps prevent superimposition of the canine tooth over the premolar teeth. The canine tooth curves distally but not in as pronounced a way as the same tooth in a dog. When changing the beam angle it is helpful to utilize the angle meter on the tube head. With an animal in true lateral recumbency the angle should be on zero degrees.

Comments and Tips

The ipsilateral maxillary incisors cannot be captured in one image as those of dogs can because of anatomical differences between these species in tooth placement and the rostral maxilla.

FILM: Size 2 film is used. Both canine teeth should be touching the film ("biting on it"). The tip of the canine tooth desired should be at the lateral edge of film to allow ample space for the root of the canine to "fall onto" the film.

CENTRAL RAY: The cone is directed in a rostrocaudal direction and centered over the tooth in question.

The degree of angulation should read 0 on the tube head if the animal is in true lateral. The tube head is then moved up approximately 30 degrees vertically from the starting point so that the canine tooth does not superimpose over the premolars distal to it, see Figure 24-41.

ANGLE: The bisecting angle of the tooth is found by standing at the patient's side using the long axis of the tooth. If root cutoff occurs even though both canine teeth were "biting on" the film, you should ensure that the beam is centered on the film, and you may need to foreshorten the angle slightly. To foreshorten the angle, focus more on the film.

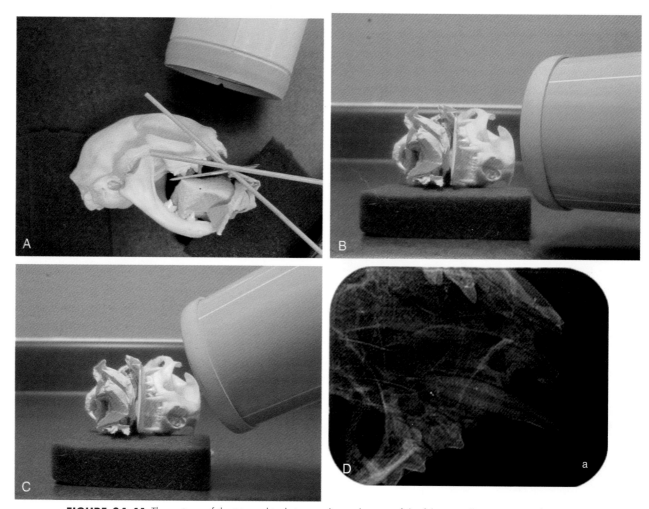

FIGURE 24-41 Three views of the intraoral technique radiograph setup of the feline maxillary canine tooth: (**A**) view from patient's side to aim at the bisecting angle and (**B**) view from patient's front while finding bisecting angle (angle meter should read 0); (**C**) view from the front after final tilt (30 degrees) of x-ray cone. (**D**) The radiograph of feline maxillary canine tooth.

Maxillary Incisors

FILM: Size 2 film is used for the maxillary incisors. The tips of the incisor teeth should be at the edge of the film closest to you (rostral) to allow ample space for the roots of the incisors to "fall onto" the film.

CENTRAL RAY: The cone is directed in a rostrocaudal direction and centered over the nose, see Figure 24-42.

ANGLE: The bisecting angle is found by standing at the patient's side.

> **TECHNICIAN NOTES** The typical rostrocaudal view can capture all the maxillary incisors on one film. Feline maxillary incisors are similar to little "pegs"; they curve slightly distally and do not converge in the middle like dog incisors.

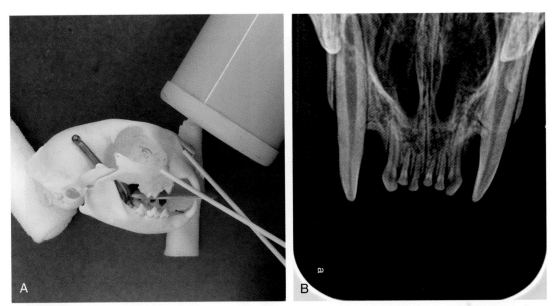

FIGURE 24-42 Setup for an intraoral technique radiograph (**A**) and the radiograph (**B**) of the feline maxillary incisors.

Mandibular Canines and Incisors

FILM: Size 2 film is used. Both canine teeth should be touching the film ("biting on it"). The tongue is positioned on the opposite side of the film.

CENTRAL RAY: The cone is directed in a rostrocaudal direction and centered over the patient's chin.

ANGLE: The bisecting angle is found by standing at the patient's side. The long axis of the canine tooth, not the incisors, should be used to find the bisecting angle. Remember that the canine tooth has a large root that curves in a caudal direction (Figure 24-43).

> **TECHNICIAN NOTES** Both mandibular canines and all incisors of the cat can be imaged in one view. The reason is that cats are missing premolar 1 and 2, thus allowing for a rostrocaudal beam without superimposition on other teeth.

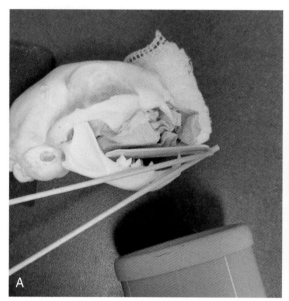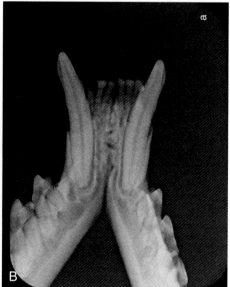

FIGURE 24-43 Setup for an intraoral technique radiograph (**A**) and the radiograph (**B**) of the feline mandibular incisors and canine teeth (lateral recumbency).

Mandibular Premolars and Molar: Standard Technique

Parallel technique can be used to image the mandibular premolars and molar of the cat because there is no hard palate to interfere with film placement behind the roots of these teeth. The mesial root of premolar 3 can be difficult to capture owing to interference with film placement and the mandibular symphysis. A bisecting angle technique can be used to image these teeth if this problem occurs.

FILM: The film (size 0 works best) is placed between the tongue and the mandible, parallel to the long axis of the teeth. It is necessary to *push the film down* until you can feel it pop out under the ventral mandible. This maneuver ensures that the entire tooth is captured. A paper towel can be used to keep the film pushed down. The film can be gently bent to accommodate placement, and if a larger film is used, it can be placed behind the tooth diagonally to fit behind it.

CENTRAL RAY: The cone is directed in a lateral direction and centered at the tooth to be radiographed, perpendicular to film (Figure 24-44).

ANGLE: Parallel technique.

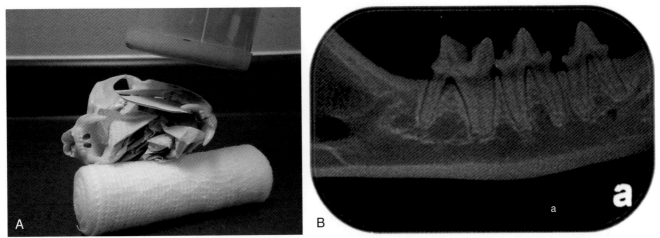

FIGURE 24-44 Setup for an intraoral technique radiograph (**A**) and the radiograph (**B**) of the feline mandibular premolars 3,4 and molars (lateral recumbency).

Mandibular Premolars and Molar: Bisecting Angle Technique

If the mesial root of the third premolar continues to be cut off and the film is placed as rostral as possible, then a bisecting angle technique can also be used to image these teeth. If a digital radiography sensor is used, this is the preferred technique because film placement using the standard technique with the bulky sensors is problematic.

FILM: The film (size 2) should be resting on the floor of the mandible, preferably with the tongue on the opposite side of the film. If this is not possible, the tongue can be left between the film and the teeth.

CENTRAL RAY: The cone is directed in a lateral direction at the tooth to be radiographed.

ANGLE: The bisecting angle is found by standing at the patient's front. The x-ray beam is angled through the floor of the mandible (Figure 24-45).

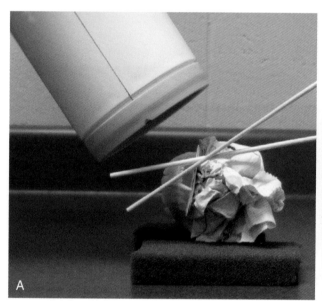
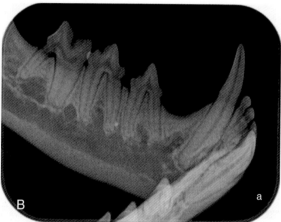

FIGURE 24-45 Setup for a radiograph of the feline mandibular premolars 3, 4 and the molar with the use of the bisecting-angle technique (**A**). The radiograph (**B**).

Canine and Feline Nasal Sinus Radiographs

Indications for radiographs of the nasal sinus cavity in either the dog or cat include evaluation of disease such as neoplasia as well as the detection of foreign bodies.

POSITION: The patient should be in sternal recumbency with the maxilla parallel to the tabletop.

FILM: For dogs, size 4 film is inserted as far as possible into the patient's mouth between the maxilla and the endotracheal tube. For cats, the film may need to be placed in on an angle or a size 2 film may be used.

CENTRAL RAY: The cone is 6 to 8 inches away from the film and centered on the nasal cavity. Use settings for a maxillary canine tooth, and adjust for the distance from the film.

ANGLE: The cone is directed perpendicular to the film (Figuer 24-46).

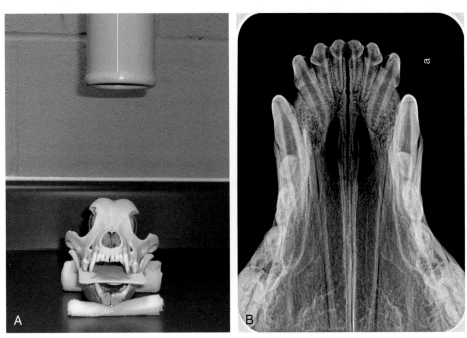

FIGURE 24-46 Setup for radiograph of nasal sinus (**A**) and radiograph (**B**).

Intraoral Dental Radiography with a Conventional Machine

If a dental radiography machine is not available, the intraoral radiographs previously described can be accomplished with a conventional machine. In the descriptions of the intraoral views, the x-ray cone was maneuvered to focus on the bisecting angle or film where indicated. With use of a conventional x-ray machine, the patient's body position and skull must be rotated so the previously described angles will line up with the x-ray beam, which is coming from overhead.

Procedure and Supplies
- Nonscreen film
- Foam wedges or rolls (assortment of sizes)
- SID should be 15 inches from the tabletop
- Settings: 60–70 kilovolts (kV), 100 milliamperage (mA), 1.6 milliamperes-seconds (mAs)
- If SID cannot be reduced, the following settings should be used: 40 inches SID, 60–70 kV, 100 mA, 3.2 mAs

Any of the previously described views can be accomplished with this technique, as illustrated by two examples. Figure 24-47 shows a radiographic setup for imaging the maxillary premolars with a conventional machine. The bisecting angle is found as previously described (as in Figure 24-27), but note that in the setup shown, the skull is rotated ventrally so that the stationary x-ray beam from overhead is aimed at the bisecting angle. In Figure 24-48, the mandibular incisors are imaged with a conventional machine. The patient is in dorsal recumbency with a small foam wedge placed under the nose. This positioning allows the beam to be directed at the bisecting angle.

Errors in Film Placement and Artifacts

Some common errors in film placement (not including previously described elongation and foreshortening) are as follows:

- Not pushing film in far enough (root cutoff) (Figure 24-49A)
- Cone not centered on tooth (cone cutoff) (Figure 24-49B)
- Light exposure in darkroom (Figure 24-49C)
- Processing errors (Figure 24-49D)
- Fingerprints on film (Figure 24-49E)
- Bent film (crescent line) (Figure 24-49F)
- Double exposure (Figure 24-49G)

Radiographs of Abnormal Dental Pathology

- Horizontal bone loss (Figure 24-50A)
- Vertical bone loss (Figure 24-50B)
- Periapical lucency (Figure 24-50C)
- Resorptive lesions (Figure 24-50D)
- Ankylosis (Figure 24-50E)
- Missing teeth (Figure 24-50F)
- Unerupted teeth (Figure 24-50G)
- Supernumerary teeth (Figure 24-50H)
- Retained root tip (Figure 24-50I)
- Complete extraction (Figure 24-50J)

> **KEY POINTS**
>
> 1. Dental radiography is essential for a proper assessment of the oral cavity in dog and cat mouths.
> 2. Dental radiographs can be accomplished in any veterinary hospital, even those without a dental x-ray unit.
> 3. Bisecting angle technique is used in most areas of dog and cat mouths.
> 4. Manual processing of films can be a source of many errors.
> 5. The SLOB rule helps identify specific roots when the x-ray cone is directed obliquely.

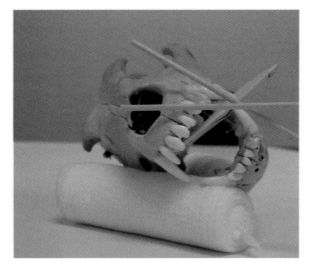

FIGURE 24-47 Setup for a radiograph of the canine maxillary premolars using a conventional x-ray machine. Note: beam comes from straight above.

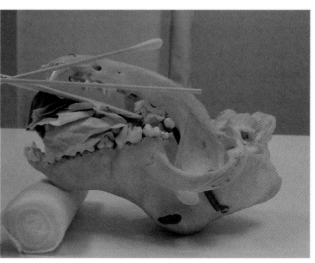

FIGURE 24-48 Setup for a radiograph of the canine mandibular incisors using a conventional x-ray machine. Note: beam comes from straight above.

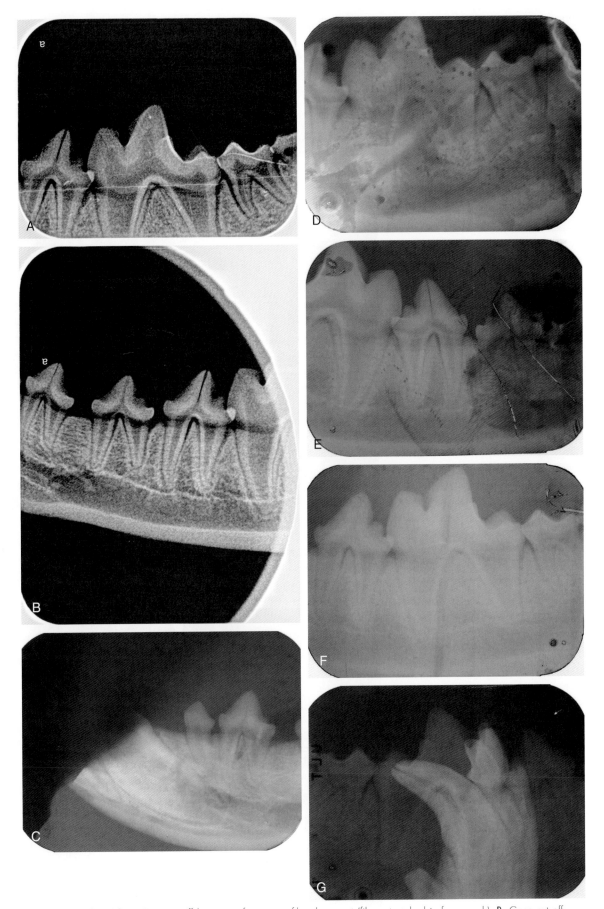

FIGURE 24-49 A, Root cut off because of improper film placement (film not pushed in far enough). B, Cone cut off. C, Light exposure in chairside darkroom. D, Film processing error: fixer not rinsed off film. E, Fingerprints and scratches on film. F, Bent film (crescent line). G, Double exposure.

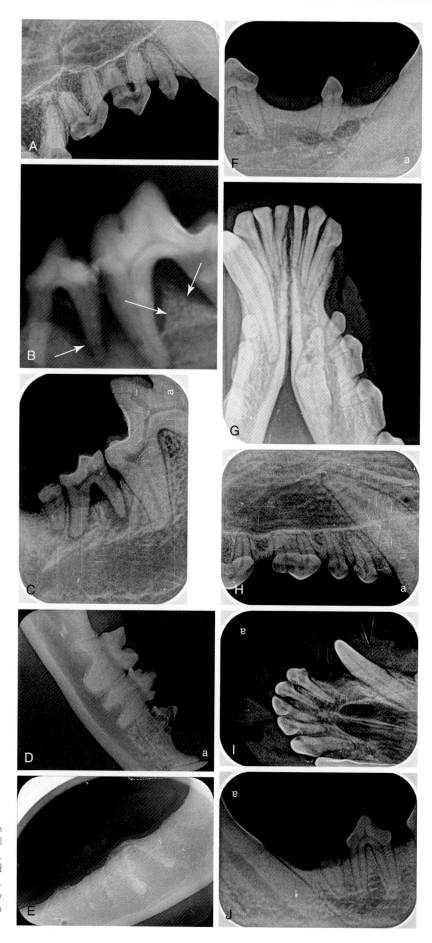

FIGURE 24-50 A, Horizontal bone loss evident on 106. **B,** Vertical bone loss (*arrows*). **C,** Periapical lucency on 410. **D,** Feline resorptive lesion 407. **E,** Ankylosis of canine mandibular premolar and molars. **F,** Congenitally missing tooth 406. **G,** Unerupted canine tooth 304. **H,** Supernumerary 105. **I,** Retained root tip 305. **J,** Complete extraction of 103.

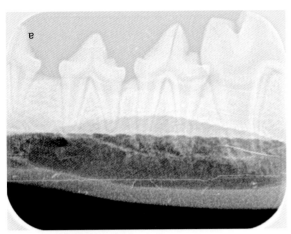

FIGURE 24-51 Mystery radiograph.

Bibliography

Bellows J: *Small animal dental equipment, materials and techniques: a primer*, Iowa, 2004, Blackwell Publishing.

Bellows J: *The practice of veterinary dentistry: a team effort*, Iowa, 1999, Iowa State Press.

Derbyshire G: *Veterinary dentistry for the nurse and technician*, St. Louis, 2005, Elsevier.

Emily PP: *Handbook of small animal dentistry*, New York, 1990, Pergamon Press.

Hale, F. Veterinary dentistry. Presented at 28th Ontario Association of Veterinary Technicians Conference, Toronto, 2006.

Han C, Hurd C: *Practical diagnostic imaging for the veterinary technician*, 3rd ed, St. Louis, 2005, Mosby.

Harvey CE: *Small animal dentistry*, St Louis, 1993, Mosby.

Holmstrom SE: *Veterinary dentistry for the technician and office staff*, St. Louis, 2000, Saunders.

Holmstrom SE, editor: *Veterinary clinics of North America*, vol 35, issue 4, St. Louis, 2005, Elsevier.

Iannucci J, Howerton, LJ: *Dental radiography: principles and techniques*, St. Louis, 2012, Saunders.

Mulligan TA: *Atlas of canine and dental radiography*, Yardley, PA, 1998, Veterinary Learning Systems.

Niemic BA: *A color handbook of small animal dental, oral and maxillofacial disease*, London, 2010, Manson Publishing.

Piasentin W: Techniques of veterinary dental radiography, *Vet Tech* 17:419-424, 1996.

Tutt D: *BSAVA manual of canine and feline dentistry*, 3rd ed, Gloucester, UK, 2007, British Small Animal Veterinary Association.

CHAPTER

25

Small Animal Special Procedures

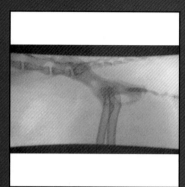

*Do not go where the path may lead, go instead
where there is no path and leave a trail.*

—Ralph Waldo Emerson, American Essayist and Poet, 1803–1882

KEY TERMS

Antegrade
Barium sulfate
Cathartic
Contrast medium
Cystography
Dimer
Double contrast
Dyschezia
Esophagography
Excretory urography
Filling defects
Functional study
Gastrography
Granuloma
Lower gastrointestinal
  (LGI) study
Morphological
Myelography
Negative-contrast agents
Nephrogram
Osmolality
Parasympatholytic agents
Pneumocystogram
Positive-contrast agents
Pyelogram
Radiolucent
Radiopaque
Retrograde
Tenesmus
Triiodinated compounds
Upper gastrointestinal
  (UGI) study
Urethrography
Viscosity
Vaginocystourethrography

OUTLINE

LEARNING OBJECTIVES

When you have finished this chapter, you will be able to:

1. Recognize the types of contrast media, including the differences between positive- and negative-contrast media, the physiological effects, the appearances on a radiograph, the indications, and the contraindications.
2. Comprehend the value of proper survey radiographs and patient preparation prior to the performance of contrast studies.
3. Summarize the procedures and protocols for common contrast studies.
4. Understand other radiographic contrast studies that may be utilized in practice.
5. Appreciate the other modalities used in addition to or in lieu of contrast studies.
6. Identify normal contrast study anatomy found on a radiograph.

TECHNICAL NOTE

To preserve space, the radiographs presented in this chapter do not show collimation. For safety, always collimate so that the beam is limited to within the image receptor edges. You should see a clear border of collimation on every radiograph. In some jurisdictions, use of collimation is the law.

Organs or soft tissue structures are often difficult or impossible to identify on plain or survey abdominal radiographs because the densities and atomic numbers of many organs are similar and thus have no natural contrast. A contrast medium attenuates the x-ray beam and therefore causes a difference in density between one tissue and another.

Contrast studies can use either a positive or a negative medium that can be administered to increase the radiographic contrast within an organ or system. In normal radiographic imaging, positive-contrast agents appear white or radiopaque on the completed radiograph, whereas negative-contrast agents appear black or radiolucent. The agents are administered so that they will either demonstrate the anatomy, by outlining or filling a cavity or organ such as the stomach or urinary bladder; or demonstrate the physiology, by being excreted through an organ such as the kidney.

Contrast medium introduced into the body, changes the density or atomic number within an organ, to make the tissue or organ visible upon imaging. The introduction of radiolucent or radiopaque media, differentiates these structures from the surrounding tissues. They can be useful in determining the anatomy such as size, shape, location, position, contour; defects in mucosal surface of an organ; the luminal contents; or the presence of extramural lesions. Functional assessment of the organ can be obtained through transit time after giving a contrast meal or by injecting a water-soluble organic iodide (functional study); however, this is more time-consuming and detailed.

These special contrast studies are used to provide information that might not otherwise be available to make a diagnosis, further evaluate the character of a suspected lesion, or determine appropriate treatment. However, endoscopy, ultrasound, and other imaging modalities, when available, have replaced contrast radiography for many evaluations.

The desired effect of any contrast substance injected into the body is to cause a difference in density and organ visibility yet still be harmless to the patient. However, with any procedure there are contraindications. These are discussed in the descriptions of the particular studies. To minimize risks, certain questions must to be asked prior to administration of a contrast agent. Depending on the procedure, the veterinarian needs to determine whether the contrast study will be useful, whether it is the best diagnostic tool, and whether it will furnish enough information. Risks may be involved, and it has to be determined whether the procedure could harm the patient. The patient may not tolerate fasting, which is usually required, or may not be a good anesthetic risk if anesthesia is recommended. Also, because of the time and costs involved, other diagnostic procedures may be more useful.

Patient preparation, equipment, and technique vary depending on the special procedure. A contrast study should never replace a routine survey radiograph. Survey radiographs performed prior to the contrast study help determine proper exposure and patient preparation for the contrast study. The need for contrast media may also be eliminated if a diagnosis can be achieved with a survey radiograph. Ultrasound and other imaging modalities, when available, have replaced contrast radiography for many evaluations; however, some modalities use similar agents.

Contrast Media Used for Radiographic Imaging

Positive-Contrast Media

Barium sulfate and water-soluble organic iodides—both ionic and nonionic—are the agents used to produce a positive-contrast image (Figure 25-1; Table 25-1). The atomic numbers of barium (56), and iodine (53) are higher than that of tissues and bones. As a comparison, 20 is the atomic number of calcium, an element of the bone.

Barium sulfate is used exclusively for radiographic examination of the gastrointestinal tract and can be administered orally or rectally. It is an insoluble white crystalline powder that is chemically inert. It does not alter normal physiological function and is available commercially as a powder, colloid suspension, or paste. Proper viscosity is required for the specific area being studied. Esophageal studies require a paste, whereas a thin mixture is needed for a single-contrast enema. If there is a suspected bowel perforation, the contrast agent of choice is a water-soluble organic iodide. When first manufactured, barium separated easily, like chalk in water. Barium is currently refined so that each molecule is covered with a wetting agent to keep the barium in suspension.[1]

> ### TECHNICIAN NOTES
>
> - Osmosis is the movement of water through a semipermeable membrane from a liquid of low concentration to one of a higher concentration until the two concentrations are equal.
> - Osmotic pressure is the pressure of a solution against a semipermeable membrane to prevent water from flowing inward across that membrane. It is determined solely by the concentration of dissolved particles.
> - An osmole is the unit of measurement that refers to the number of moles of a compound that contributes to this osmotic pressure of a solution.
> - Osmolality is the number of osmoles of solute per kilogram of solvent and is usually expressed as mOsmol/kg (milliosmoles/kg). (Osmalarity is the concentration of the osmotic solution and is expressed as mOsm/L).
> - Tonicity is the measure of this osmotic pressure.
> - A solution can be described as having an osmotic pressure or equilibrium that does not cause osmosis between the blood vessels and the surrounding fluids. This is an isosmolar fluid and it has the same osmolality as the plasma, so there will be no water exchange.
> - A hyperosmolar or hypertonic fluid will have a higher osmolality than the plasma, and thus liquid will be pulled into the plasma.
> - A hypotonic or hyposmolar fluid will have a lower osmotic pressure than plasma, so water will leave the plasma.

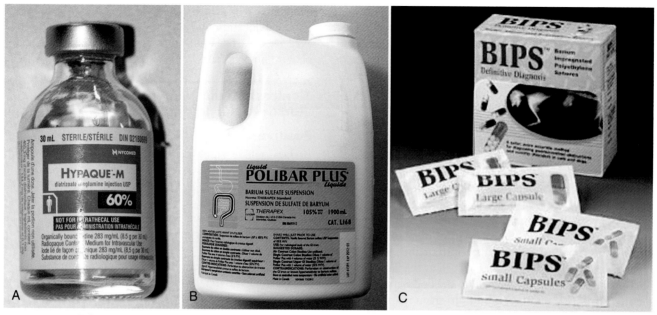

FIGURE 25-1 Positive contrast media. **A,** Iodine. **B,** Barium. **C,** Barium-impregnated polyurethane spheres (BIPS).

Water-soluble organic iodides are generally used in intravascular studies or injected into other body cavities. Iodides mix readily with blood or other body fluids and are excreted through the kidneys. The iodine atoms in the contrast medium molecule, are the primary attenuators of the x-ray beam, so the concentration of the iodine in the contrast agent is important. A higher iodine concentration shows more contrast on an image. The two major types of iodinated contrast media are ionic and non ionic.

Water-soluble organic ionic iodides are triiodinated compounds derived from the benzoic acid ring structure. These compounds are called ionic because an anion (negative) and cation (positive) make up each compound. The cation is a salt, usually sodium (Hypaque) or meglumine (Conray), or a combination of the two. Sodium is slightly more toxic than either the meglumine or the combination. The salts increase the solubility of the compound. The cation is combined with a negatively charged component called an anion. The benzene ring with three iodine atoms attached, plus other chemical components (side chains) make up the anion. Diatrizoate and iothalamate are common anions.

In an ionic contrast medium, there are three iodine atoms to two particles in the solution, which will give a 3:2 ratio (3 components of the iodine: 1 positive cation + 1 negative ion) resulting in higher osmolality. These are referred to as high-osmolar contrast agents (HOCA). The higher the osmolality, the greater the risk of anaphylactic reactions. The media whose molecules dissociate in this way and cause changes in osmolality are termed ionic and the media whose molecules remain whole in solution are termed nonionic.[1]

In the water-soluble organic nonionic iodide contrast agent, the ionizing carboxyl group is replaced with a group such as amide or glucose that does not dissociate into ions. When dissolved in water, a nonionic compound forms with each molecule containing three iodine atoms, for a ratio of 3:1 (3 iodine: 1 non dissociating molecule). Owing to their nonionizing nature, these contrast media are referred to as low-osmolality contrast agents (LOCAs) and therefore they do not increase the osmolality of the blood plasma. The nonionic contrast agent is closer to being isotonic and is therefore better tolerated by the body, causing fewer anaphylactic reactions, although it is more viscous and more expensive to purchase.

Along with describing intravascular contrast media molecules as ionic versus nonionic, they are also classified according to a second characteristic—monomer versus dimer. Both ionic and nonionic contrast agents come in a monomer form (one benzene ring) and a dimer form (two benzene rings, which means there are more iodine molecules, which lowers the osmolality). The ionic monomer has the highest osmolality and the nonionic dimer has the lowest osmolality. When low osmolar agents are administered intravenously (IV), they cannot cross an intact blood-brain

TABLE 25-1 Positive Contrast Agents for Gastrointestinal (GI) Studies in Animals

CONTRAST AGENT	USES	ADVANTAGES	DISADVANTAGES	CHARACTERISTICS CONCERNS OR COMMENTS	COMMON TRADE NAME(S)
Barium sulfate suspensions	Routine GI contrast studies—use only rectally or orally. Do not use if a GI perforation is suspected.	Low cost. Palatable. Delineates the mucosal walls well. Excellent opacity. Remains in suspension. Does not become diluted with secretions. Not absorbed through the intestines—no fear of absorption. Good density.	Slow to be transmitted. Insoluble—cannot use with perforation. Aspiration in lung can be fatal. Very irritating to the peritoneum.	Radiodense. Physiologically inert. Resists dilution. Completely insoluble. If leaked into peritoneal cavity, may induce granulomas or adhesions. Hygroscopic nature absorbs water from the bowel so may cause a bowel obstruction from barium impaction in debilitated patients.	Liquid Polibar Plus Esobar esophageal cream (60% w/w)
Barium sulfate USP	Not recommended.	Inexpensive.	Flocculates, poor mucosal detail.		
Oral organic iodine—ionic solution	Suspected intestinal perforation or obstructions.	Rapid transit time. Nonirritating to serosal surfaces and peritoneum. Readily absorbed from peritoneal cavity if leakage. Can be absorbed across the mucosa and excreted by the urinary tract.	Has a bitter taste. Expensive in comparison with barium suspension. Hypertonicity can cause: • fluid movement into the lumen • dilution of the contrast medium • electrolyte imbalance • dehydration • nausea, vomiting • decreased blood pressure	Common oral forms are meglumine diatrizoate and sodium diatrizoate.	Oral: Gastrografin

Continued

TABLE 25-1	Positive Contrast Agents for Gastrointestinal (GI) Studies in Animals—cont'd			
CONTRAST AGENT	USES	ADVANTAGES	DISADVANTAGES	CHARACTERISTICS CONCERNS OR COMMENTS	COMMON TRADE NAME(S)
Organic iodine—ionic solution—injectable	Intravenous (IV) injections for urinary radiography, infusion in hollow organs.	Less viscous.	The hypertonicity effects listed above are more likely to occur after rapid IV bolus. Irritating to the brain and spinal cord. Can cause toxicity and tissue irritability (e.g., in kidney, bladder).	Sodium diatrizoate provides better opacification for excretory urography. Because they are water soluble and absorbed into the bloodstream, hypertonicity is a real concern. Common IV solutions are meglumine and sodium diatrizoate, and sodium diatrizoate alone. Cannot be used for myelography.	IV: Sodium diatrizoate (Hypaque M)
Organic iodine—nonionic solution	Myelography. Can be used IV especially for young or debilitated patient.	Fewer side effects than with ionic form—rapid transit time. Nonirritating. Resorbed after extraluminal leakage. Does not become increasingly dilute. Endoscopy and ultrasonography will not be impaired if a contrast study is first completed.	Expensive.	Low osmolarity and chemical nature. Nonionic dimer contrast media is virtually isotonic with blood and cerebrospinal fluid.	Iohexol (Omnipaque), iopamidol (Isovue), ioversol (Optiray), iopromide (Ultravist), iotrolan, ioxilan (Oxilan), nonionic dimer iodixanol (Visipaque)
Radiopaque markers	Determine orocolic transit rate. Note obstructive disease.	Easy to administer. Not likely to be aspirated or to cause peritonitis. Can be given with food. Time frame for radiographs not as important. Do not obscure abdominal detail. More likely to detect motility disorders.	Cannot visualize mucosal detail or luminal margins. Expensive in comparison with barium suspension. Studies can take longer.	If delayed emptying occurs, the cause will not be known. Do not use barium-impregnated spheres (BIPS) for 24–48 hours after barium suspension.	BIPS

barrier and are excreted via glomerular filtration through the kidneys.[2]

> **TECHNICIAN NOTES** The most isotonic iodine contrast media currently on the market are the water-soluble organic nonionic dimers.

Because of the number of agents and concentrations available, trade names constantly vary.

See Table 25-2 for further comparisons among positive contrast media used for radiographic imaging.

> **TECHNICIAN NOTES** The normal osmolalities of the sera of humans and dogs are relatively equivalent.

Physiological Effects of Intravenous Contrast Media

If the contrast medium has a high osmolality, water will move into the vessels both from the extravascular tissues and from the red blood cells. The red blood cells begin to shrink or crenate. With crenation, circulating blood volume and peripheral blood flow increase; systemic vascular resistance and blood pressure decrease. All of this happens because of the introduction of a solution such as organic ionic iodine that has a higher concentration (hyperosmolar) than blood.

Many of the side effects of using ionic and nonionic contrast media have been alleviated with the introduction of the ionic and nonionic dimers, which have lowered the osmolality of contrast media to an almost isosmolar level.

Vasodilation, produced by the injection of a contrast medium, is thought to be the primary cause of the accompanying pain, discomfort, and flushing. When an isotonic contrast agent is used, the discomfort and flushing are reduced. Isotonic means that the osmolalities or concentrations of the two fluids (contrast media and blood) are the same relative to each other. Many of the adverse physiological effects of contrast media can be related to osmolality, but there are other factors to consider as well.

Viscosity refers to the resistance of fluid to flow. This influences the injectability or delivery of the contrast agent. Nonionic dimers such as iodixanol (Visipaque) have the lowest osmolality but the highest viscosity of the water-soluble organic iodides. This means that the solution will pass slowly through the syringe. Warming of the solution decreases the viscosity. A centipoise (cPs) is the unit used to describe the viscosity of a solution. It is one hundredth of a poise and is the amount of force needed to move one layer of liquid in relation to another liquid. The thinner the liquid the lower the viscosity and the cPs (water at 21°C [70°F] is about 1cPs). See Table 25-2.

The clearance or elimination of the molecules of injectable contrast media, occurs primarily by glomerular filtration and renal clearance. None of the molecules is reabsorbed or secreted by the renal tubules. The speed of elimination depends on the glomerular filtration rate, but virtually 100% of the contrast agent will be out of the body in 24 hours.

In the case of complete cessation of renal function, elimination takes place through the liver and gut at a much slower rate. The thyroid and liver retain about 1.5%, which can result in elevation of blood values after a procedure. Nuclear medicine scans of the thyroid should not be attempted after a contrast medium injection because the results will be inaccurate.

Negative- and Double-Contrast Media

Negative-Contrast Media

Negative-contrast media are the low–atomic number or low-density agents such as air, nitrous oxide, oxygen, and carbon dioxide. These substances absorb fewer x-rays than soft tissue and appear dark or radiolucent on the radiograph. This effect enhances the contrast between the soft tissues.

	CHEMICAL			OSMOLALITY	VISCOSITY	VISCOSITY
TABLE 25-2	**Chemical Structure and Physiochemical Properties of Iodine-Based Contrast Agents**					
IONICITY	STRUCTURE	OSMOTIC CLASS	REPRESENTATIVE COMPOUNDS	(MOSM/KG)	(CPS AT 20° C)	(CPS AT 37° C)
Ionic	Monomer	High osmolality	Diatrizoate, meglumine (Renografin, Conray, Hypaque)	1400–1800	6	4
	Dimer	Low osmolality	Ioxaglate (Hexabrix)	600	15	8
Nonionic	Monomer	Low osmolality	Iohexol (Omnipaque), iopamidol (Isovue), ioversol (Optiray), iopromide (Ultravist)	600–850	9–21	5–10
	Dimer	Iso-osmolality	Iodixanol (Visipaque)	280	27	12

cPS, centipoise is a unit to describe the viscosity of a solution.

There is less mucosal detail with the use of negative-contrast than with positive-contrast media. Oxygen and carbon dioxide are more soluble than water. Be careful not to over-inflate organs such as the bladder, especially if using room air, because air embolism can result if an organ ruptures or if there are ulcerative lesions. Embolism can lead to cardiac arrest.[3]

Double-Contrast Procedures

Double-contrast procedures utilize both positive-contrast and negative-contrast agents to image an organ, commonly the urinary bladder, stomach, or colon. To avoid air bubbles, which can be misinterpreted as lesions, the negative-contrast medium is generally administered first, followed by the positive-contrast agent.

Gastrointestinal Tract Studies

Patient and Other Preparation

Patient preparation is essential. Actual preparation does vary slightly according to the procedure, but generally the area that is being radiographed should not have any radiodense artifacts, such as food, bowel contents, and gas, that could be misdiagnosed as lesions or abnormalities.

The animal should be fasted so that the gastrointestinal tract is emptied. A cathartic or enema should be administered in a timely manner to minimize gas production. Make sure the hair coat is clean and dry with no mats. Any sedation or anesthetics given need to be taken into account if transit time for the contrast agent through the gastrointestinal tract, is of concern. Anticholinergics such as atropine, decrease gastrointestinal time. It is essential to take a survey radiograph prior to giving contrast media, to ensure that the procedure is still necessary and that the proper radiation techniques are utilized.

Along with proper preparation of the patient, it is important to give the correct amount of contrast medium to properly coat or distend the organ as required (Figure 25-2).

Another error is not taking enough radiographs in the proper sequence. Imagine judging a book by reading the front and back covers and perhaps a few pages in the middle. One would not appreciate the information that is in the book. Make sure that the required number of radiographs is taken. For accurate diagnosis of the stomach, all four views (ventrodorsal [VD], dorsoventral [DV], and right and left lateral views) should be imaged. Depending on the study, oblique views or abdominal compression may be required. The views must be properly positioned and centered and must include the appropriate landmarks. See Chapter 18 to review the positions of the abdomen and common anatomy.

Indications

Special studies of the gastrointestinal (GI) tract are usually completed when there are concerns about vomiting, diarrhea, constipation, hematochezia, melena, abdominal mass, abdominal pain, foreign bodies, or post-abdominal trauma.

In the study, the barium is administered and the GI tract is generally evaluated for morphological changes, blockages, and functional changes such as the rate of gastric emptying or small bowel transit time.

Contraindications

Special studies should not be completed if the animal has a fluid-filled distended esophagus or stomach or if the bowel is atonic. Patients with ileus due to torsion (Figure 25-3) or other conditions are not good candidates.

Contrast Agents

The suspension form of barium is the positive-contrast agent generally used, because its particles do not flocculate or separate. The barium sulfate does settle upon standing, so the suspension should be shaken prior to use. Barium is found in containers from 280 mL to 1900 mL. Barium sulfate is not hypertonic and does not increase the intraluminal fluid. A disadvantage is the slow transit time through the small bowel. Chilling the barium sulfate for an upper gastrointestinal (UGI) study does speed up the transit time; however, for a lower gastrointestinal (LGI) study, barium temperature between room and body temperature, is more comfortable for the patient.

> **TECHNICIAN NOTES** To decrease the viscosity of organic nonionic dimer solutions such as iodixanol, warm the solution prior to use. If you chill the barium, the transit time is quicker in UGI studies. For LGI studies, have the solution at room to body temperature for patient comfort.

Barium is not sterilely produced and once the container is open, there is a possibility for contamination to occur. Any equipment that is reused, such as a reservoir-type container, enema tube, or syringes, must be thoroughly cleaned and sterilized prior to use.

If there is a perforation of the bowel, a combination of diatrizoate meglumine and diatrizoate sodium (Gastrografin) iodinated water-soluble organic iodine can be used. The nonionic compounds are safer than the ionic agents because they are more isosmolar, so they draw less fluid into the bowel with minimal dilution of the contrast agents. The hyperosmolality of the solution and the resulting complications that could arise with use in dehydrated patients or those with severe electrolyte imbalance, need to be considered. The high cost limits their use to mostly small patients.

> **TECHNICIAN NOTES** To minimize artifacts, always make sure that the patient has a clean dry hair coat, with no traces of contrast medium. Remove the collar if cranial body radiographic views are to be taken.

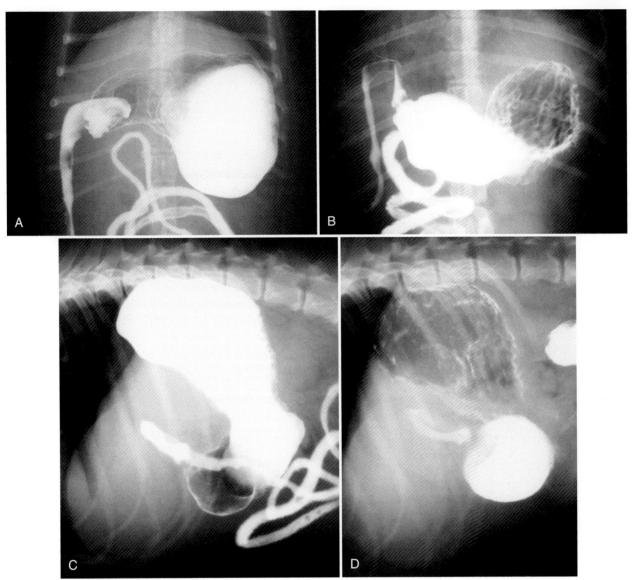

FIGURE 25-2 Normal variations in barium (fluid) and gas distribution within the stomach with different patient positions. **A,** Ventrodorsal view, in dorsal recumbency. Gas is located in the body and pyloric antrum. Fluid settles dependently to fill the fundus, body, and pyloric portions. **B,** Dorsoventral view, in ventral recumbency. Gas rises to the cardia and fundus, and fluid settles dependently to fill pyloric portions and part of the body. **C,** Left recumbent lateral view. Gas rises to the pyloric portion, and fluid settles dependently to fill the fundus and body. **D,** Right recumbent lateral view. Gas rises to the fundus and dorsal body, which are coated with barium. Fluid settles dependently to fill the pyloric portion and part of the body.

Esophagography

Contrast radiography of the esophagus, or esophagography, is often needed to accurately identify lesions or further characterize survey radiographic findings. It is best used to evaluate morphological or structural alterations of the esophagus. Nonstatic imaging such as fluoroscopy is recommended for specific evaluation of functional abnormalities (see Figure 25-5).

Indications

Dysphagia, regurgitation of undigested food, acute gagging or retching, excessive salivation, megaesophagus (Figure 25-4), abnormal swallowing, esophageal dysfunction, and foreign body are all indications for esophagography. The double-contrast study evaluates morphological abnormalities such as mucosal abnormalities, intraluminal foreign bodies, and partial strictures or stenosis.

Precautions

Patients with dysphagia may aspirate the contrast agent. It may not be necessary to add contrast media to a dilated, fluid-filled, or food-filled esophagus because there may be enough contrast present for visualization of lesions or abnormalities. If asphyxiation is a concern, barium sulfate paste should not be used. Consider the use of organic iodine preparation in cases of perforation.

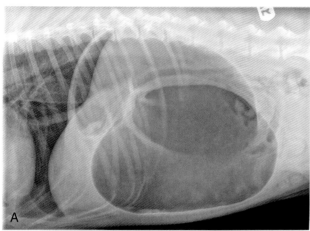

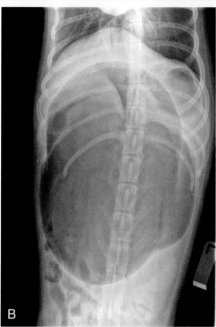

FIGURE 25-3 Gastric torsion. Note the characteristic double bubble. **A,** Right lateral abdomen. **B,** Ventrodorsal abdomen.

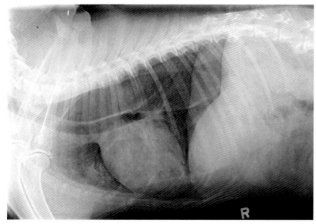

FIGURE 25-4 Lateral thorax showing megaesophagus.

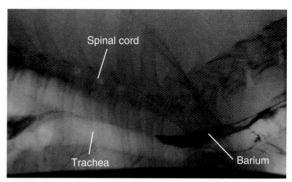

FIGURE 25-5 A barium swallow during an esophageal study utilizing fluoroscopy. Note the reversal of the densities. The barium is darkest, and the bones are also black. The trachea is white, as is the spinal cord.

Contrast Media and Dosage

- Barium sulfate paste, 60%–100%
- Barium sulfate liquid, 45%–85%
- Barium sulfate liquid (30%) mixed with canned food or kibble
- Oral aqueous iodine solutions
  The dosage is 5 to 20 mL to induce several swallows.[4]

Equipment/Supplies

- Large dose syringe.
- Optional—canned food or kibble.

Patient Preparation

- Remove collar, clean hair coat.
- If megaesophagus is to be evaluated, the esophagus should be emptied prior to administration of a contrast agent.
- If further gastrointestinal studies are being completed, the animal should be fasted.
- Fractious animals can be given a low dose of a phenothiazine, but because the esophagus is affected by most central nervous system depressant drugs, motility will be affected.

> **TECHNICIAN NOTES**   To minimize opacity of the brachium musculature over the thoracic inlet, keep one limb cranial and the other caudal. Usually the limb of the side the animal is lying on is pulled cranially.

Positions

Lateral: Generally a right lateral.
Optional: Ventrodorsal or oblique views (VLe-DRt/VRt DLeO).
Dorsoventral: See "Dorsoventral Thoracic Inlet View" in Chapter 19.

Borders

Full length of esophagus: Cervical and thoracic areas to expose atlanto-occipital junction (oropharynx) to T12 (cranial portion of stomach) (Figure 25-5).

Procedure for Barium Esophagogram

1. Expose survey radiographs—lateral and VD.
2. Position the animal in lateral recumbency on the x-ray table.
3. Place paper towels on tabletop or towels around the patient's mouth and neck.
4. Slowly infuse the barium into the buccal pouch. Close the mouth and wait for the animal to swallow.
5. Take serial radiographs of the animal in lateral recumbency—the right is usually easier for the positioner.
6. Administer additional barium or barium-soaked kibble in the buccal pouch. Close the mouth and wait for the animal to swallow.
7. Obtain further lateral radiographs if required, or place the patient in ventral recumbency for VD or oblique views as required. The oblique projections avoid superimposition of the esophagus over the spine (see Chapter 18 for technique).
8. If a lesion has been noted by esophagoscope or with the passage of a tube, a partial esophagram can be made: pass the tube till the point of the abnormality, and administer barium sulfate at the site.

Double-Contrast Study

1. Obtain survey radiographs and perform an esophageal study using liquid barium suspension as described previously.
2. Pass a stomach tube through an oral speculum if required. Avoid forcing the tube through partial obstructions.
3. Perform a lateral radiograph to confirm the placement of tube in case the tip of the tube needs to be readjusted for study of a specific portion of the esophagus.
4. Attach a syringe and inject barium sulfate, 3–5 mL for a small dog or cat and 8–10 mL for a large dog.
5. Keeping the patient in lateral recumbency, attach an air syringe and inject 20–30 mL of air for a small dog or cat and 40–50 mL of air for a large dog.
6. Immediately radiograph the dorsal thorax.
7. Reposition the patient in sternal recumbency. Repeat the air injection and radiograph immediately.

Comments and Tips

- Avoid getting contrast medium on the patient, image receptor and table, as the artifacts may interfere with the diagnosis.
- The patient is usually sedated or anesthetized for the double-contrast study. This is usually completed following gastrography after the stomach tube is retracted to the esophagus. If there is gastroesophageal reflux, further barium sulfate suspension is not needed. Administer only the air.
- A very small amount of aspirated barium sulfate is generally well tolerated in healthy lungs and cleared from the airways within 24 hours.[5]

- Oropharyngeal issues are best evaluated in the midst of a swallow and during a pause after completion of the swallow.
- Oblique views may eliminate superimposition of the spine and sternum for better visualization of the esophagus.

> **TECHNICIAN NOTES** Quick overview of the esophagus contrast study:
> 1. Prepare the animal including survey radiographs.
> 2. Administer the barium, and immediately expose radiographs with the patient in lateral position.
> 3. Administer more barium, and take further positions as required.

> **TECHNICIAN NOTES** For dilution of contrast medium, saline is best, especially for barium studies. To calculate the dilution, it is easiest to use either a ratio and proportion method or a fraction method.
> For example: You need to use 120 mL of a final dilution of 20% barium. The initial barium sulfate comes as a 60% concentrated solution. How much of the concentrated barium will you use, and how much diluent will you need?
> Ratio and proportion method:
>
> Final diluted percentage : Initial concentration
> = Volume needed : Final volume administered
>
> $$20\% : 60\% = X : 120 \text{ mL}$$
>
> Fraction method:
>
> $$\frac{\text{Final diluted percentage}}{\text{Initial concentration}} = \frac{\text{Volume needed}}{\text{Final volume administered}}$$
>
> $$\frac{20\%}{60\%} = \frac{X}{120}$$
>
> In both cases, now continue as:
>
> $$(20)(120) = X(60)$$
>
> $$60X = 2400$$
>
> $$X = 40$$
>
> 40 mL of the concentrated barium is needed.
> Since you will use 120 mL total volume with 40 mL of concentrated solution, you need 80 mL of diluent (120 − 40 = 80).

Upper Gastrointestinal Study

The patient is given the contrast medium orally, and images are taken during the transit of the contrast medium through the stomach and small bowel, and into the colon as required. The full procedure will be described, although actual timing and centering depend on the patient's condition.

Morphological studies of the stomach and intestines are made to examine (1) the size, shape, and position of the organs, (2) the character of the stomach wall and the stomach contents, or (3) extramural, mural, or intramural lesions of the gastrointestinal tract. Gastric motility and pyloric and intestinal function can be determined by noting gastric and intestinal emptying, keeping in mind that the times vary, depending on the size and nature of the test meal. Functional studies are performed slightly differently from morphological ones. Sedation or anesthesia affects transit time in functional studies.

Barium food mixture studies have also been completed to further evaluate gastric function. There appears to be evidence that there is a wide range of normal gastric emptying time. Unless there are gross abnormalities, a barium solid food meal is not useful. Barium-impregnated polyethylene spheres (BIPS, Chemstock Animal Health Ltd., Christchurch, New Zealand) have been used as an alternative to evaluate the emptying of solids in dogs and cats (Figure 25-1C).

Endoscopy is an alternative modality that can be used, although it is difficult to adequately access the mesenteric small intestine with the endoscope. Ultrasonography can often provide diagnostic information about the small bowel, negating the need for a contrast radiographic study.

TECHNICIAN NOTES Make sure to give the complete volume for proper distention of the lumen in order to complete a diagnostic barium study.

Indications

Recurrent unresponsive vomiting, diarrhea, hematemesis, anorexia, melena, mass lesions, suspected foreign body or obstruction, wall distortions, wall lesions, abdominal organ displacement, chronic weight loss, persistent abdominal pain, and inconclusive results of a survey radiograph are all indications for an upper gastrointestinal study.

TECHNICIAN NOTES Remember that when radiographing the abdomen, you are generally:
* Measuring at the thickest part (liver), at the thoracolumbar (TL) junction.
* Centering caudal to the 13th rib in the dog or 2–3 fingerbreadths caudal to 13th rib in the cat.
* Including cranially from T9 (for VD views) and T7 (for lateral views) and caudally to the acetabulum.
For the cranial abdomen for gastrography:
* Measure and center at the TL junction.
* Include cranially from T9 (for VD views) and T7 (for lateral views) to L5-L6.

Precautions
* If rupture or perforation is suspected, use water-soluble organic iodides, but in dehydrated patients, avoid the use of such agents. Ultrasonography would be an overall safer means for diagnosis in compromised patients.
* Delay the study if the stomach is filled with ingesta.
* The use of barium in gastric dilatation/volvulus, chronic obstructive bowel disease, and paralytic ileus cases is complicating.
* Gastric distention is not recommended immediately after gastric surgery or deep biopsy. Prior use of tranquilizing or other drugs affects the transit time. If tranquilization

is required in morphological studies, consider acetylpromazine for dogs and ketamine for cats. Avoid parasympatholytic agents and drugs used for treatment in gastrointestinal disorders, which may cause gaseous distention or decrease motility prior to the contrast study. Use of anticholinergics should be suspended at least 24 hours, though preferably 48 to 72 hours, prior to the administration of contrast media.[4]

TECHNICIAN NOTES Slightly higher kilovolt peak (kVp) values up to 6 to 8 kVp, are generally needed for positive-contrast studies.

Contrast Media and Dosage
Barium sulfate suspension, 60%:[5]
* 8–10 mL/kg for dogs lighter than 10 kg and cats
* 5–8 mL/kg for medium-sized dogs, 10–40 kg
* 3–5 mL/kg for dogs heavier than 40 kg
For double-contrast or negative-contrast study:
* Air: 50–100 mL for dogs lighter than 10 kg and cats
* 100–200 mL for medium-sized dogs, 10–40 kg
* 200–300 mL for dogs heavier than 40 kg
Effervescent granules (Baros, E-Z-Gas II).

Equipment/Supplies
Gastric tube, oral speculum, 50-mL syringe, towels.

Survey
Take lateral and ventrodorsal radiographs prior to the administration of an enema (Figure 25-6).

Patient Preparation
* The gastrointestinal tract should be empty so that it does not interfere with interpretation of transit time. Foreign bodies or small gastric and intestinal lesions may be obscured by ingesta. If the animal is not anorectic or vomiting, fast at least 12 hours prior to administration of the contrast meal. Twenty-four hours is best if mucosal disease of the small intestine is being evaluated.
* If an enema is required, as indicated by the survey radiograph, administer at least 2 to 4 hours prior to the procedure to minimize gas artifacts.
* If the patient has severe abdominal stress, neither fasting nor an enema or laxative is suggested.

TECHNICIAN NOTES Prior to administering the barium, have everything ready, such as the image receptors in position, technique set, protective gear, animal near the table, etc. If administering the barium with the animal on the table, keep in mind that barium spillage will create artifacts on the image.

TECHNICIAN NOTES If using the orogastric tube, make sure its placement in the esophagus and not in the trachea, has been verified. Before removing the tube, clear it with a small amount of air, and kink the tube to minimize aspiration.

TABLE 25-3	Upper Gastrointestinal Tract Positive-Contrast Film Sequence		
SPECIES	BARIUM	IONIC AND NONIONIC ORGANIC IODINE	STRUCTURES TYPICALLY OPACIFIED IN NORMAL ANIMALS*
Dog	Immediate	Immediate	Stomach
	15 minutes		Stomach, duodenum fills
	30 minutes	15 minutes	Stomach, duodenum, jejunum
	1 hour		Stomach, duodenum, jejunum
	2 hours	30 minutes	Stomach, complete small intestine, cecum reached
	4 hours	1 hour	Small and large intestine
Cat	Immediate	Immediate	Stomach
	5 minutes	5 minutes	Stomach, duodenum fills
	30 minutes	30 minutes	Complete small intestine, cecum fills
	1 hour	1 hour	Small and large intestine

*These are only approximations of the components of the gastrointestinal tract visible at these times, as individual transit times vary greatly.

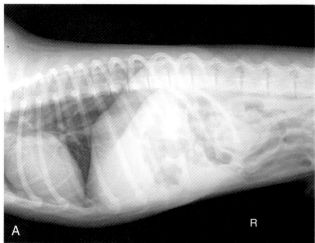

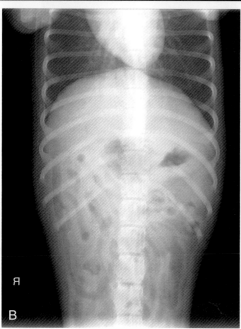

FIGURE 25-6 A, Right lateral survey. B, Ventrodorsal survey radiograph.

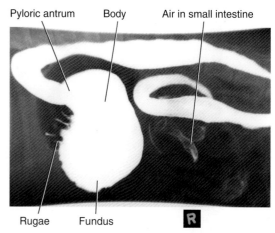

FIGURE 25-7 An upper gastrointestinal radiograph taken within minutes of the administration of barium. This is an inverted fluoroscopic image.

Procedure for Positive-Contrast Upper Gastrointestinal Study

The image sequence for positive-contrast UGI study is shown in Table 25-3.

1. Using either the buccal pouch and syringe, or a gastric tube, administer barium sulfate.
2. If completing a gastrogram, immediately take four radiographs centering over the cranial abdomen: ventrodorsal, right and left lateral, and dorsoventral views (Figure 25-7).
3. At 15 minutes post administration: take ventrodorsal and right lateral views (Figure 25-8).
4. At 30 minutes post administration: take ventrodorsal and right lateral views (Figure 25-9).
5. At 60 minutes post administration: take ventrodorsal and right lateral views (Figure 25-10).
6. Hourly post administration: take ventrodorsal and right lateral views until the study is completed (Figures 25-11). See Figure 25-12 for feline image.

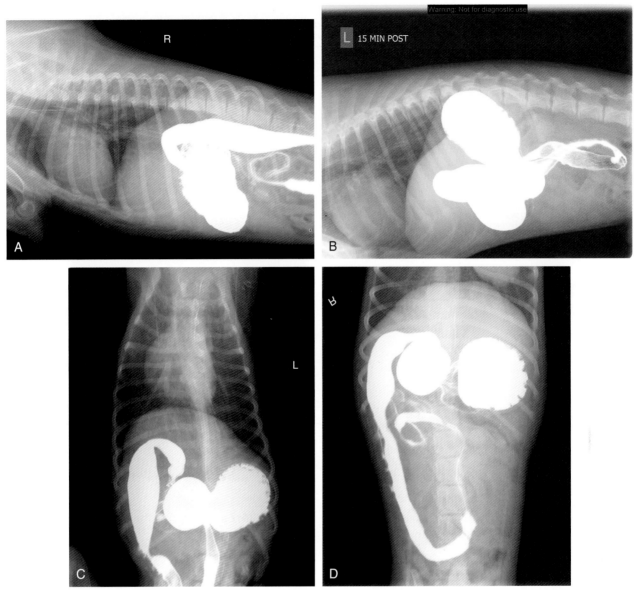

FIGURE 25-8 Fifteen minutes post administration of barium in a dog. **A,** Right lateral abdomen. Note that there is gas in the fundus and barium in part of the body and the duodenum. **B,** Left lateral abdomen. There is more gas in the pyloric portion and duodenum in comparison with the right lateral 15-minute exposure. The heart is also more slightly rounded than in the right lateral. **C,** Ventrodorsal abdomen. The gas is in part of the body and pyloric antrum. **D,** Dorsoventral abdomen. The gas rises to the cardia and fundus. The diaphragm has a slightly more "bumpy" appearance than in the ventrodorsal view because the trilobed crura are lateral to the central cupula.

> **TECHNICIAN NOTES** The 15-minute radiographs may be eliminated in dogs, depending on the nature of the study, but are highly recommended in cats because of the rapid GI transit time. An extra radiograph at 90 minutes may also reveal further information for the cat.

Comments and Tips

- If gastric and intestinal emptying time is of concern, perform the study early enough in the day to be able to properly complete the procedure.
- If an orogastric tube is not used, barium may leave the stomach before all the agent is administered, meaning that the stomach will not have optimal distention.
- It is important to give sufficient volume of barium sulfate suspension.
- The gastrogram is finished when the majority of the barium is not visible in the stomach; the small bowel study ends when there is little evidence of barium in the small intestine.
- If the pylorus is of interest, oblique views may be required.
- The rugal folds are best seen on gastric emptying.

> **TECHNICIAN NOTES** Strategically used positioning aids give the patient the *illusion* that it is being held. A sandbag over the neck and limbs, and/or the use of tape is essential if the patient is not sedated. Keep talking to it while taking the images.

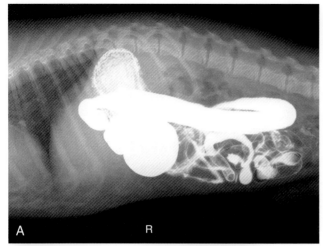
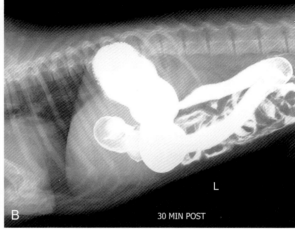
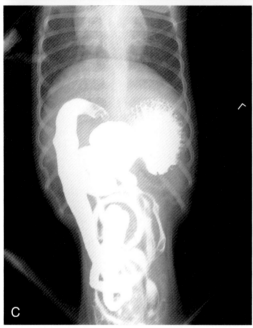

FIGURE 25-9 Thirty minutes after the administration of barium. **A,** Right lateral abdomen. The gas is more evident in the fundus than in the left lateral. **B,** Left lateral abdomen. Gas is more evident in the pyloric antrum. **C,** Ventrodorsal abdomen. Gas is more evident in the pyloric antrum and part of the body.

> **TECHNICIAN NOTES** The UGI is complete when the barium is in the colon.

> **TECHNICIAN NOTES** To convert kg to pound multiply by 2.2. Thus 10 kg is basically 22 lb. 40 kg is 88 llb.

Procedure for Double-Contrast Upper Gastrointestinal Study

Double-contrast imaging may provide further information primarily for the stomach wall and by allowing further visualization of the gastric location or extramural gastric lesion. Evaluation of mural and intraluminal gastric lesions may also benefit by the ability to "see through" the stomach. A double-contrast study does not evaluate motility or emptying. It should not be performed if the animal is not fasted.
1. The patient is best chemically restrained.
2. Complete a routine noncontrast survey.
3. Using a gastric tube, administer barium sulfate.
4. Attach an air-filled syringe, and administer air until the stomach is distended.
5. Withdraw the tip of the tube into the caudal esophagus or remove completely.
6. Gently rotate the patient to coat the gastric mucosa.
7. Immediately take the four views of the stomach—right and left laterals, ventrodorsal, and dorsoventral (Figure 25-13). Center the beam over the cranial abdomen.
8. Administer more negative-contrast medium if air has been lost by regurgitation or has passed into the small bowel, and repeat the radiographs.

Comments and Tips
- It is difficult to determine the exact dosage. Judge the amount required by noting the resistance to injection of air as well as by palpating for the distended stomach.

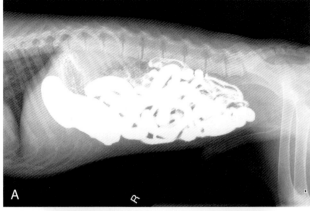

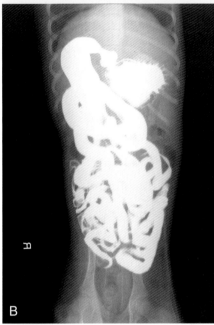

FIGURE 25-10 Sixty minutes after the administration of barium. A, Right lateral abdomen. B, Ventrodorsal abdomen.

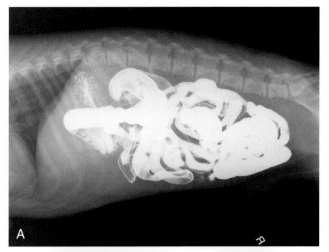

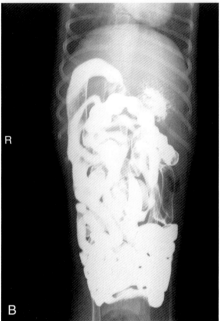

FIGURE 25-11 Two hours after the administration of barium. A, Right lateral abdomen. B, Ventrodorsal abdomen.

- Make sure stomach is distended so that the gastric wall will appear thin and uniform.
- Negative-contrast gastrography or a pneumogastrogram can be substituted for a positive-contrast study or a double-contrast study. Follow the same procedure as for the double-contrast study, omitting the barium sulfate.
- If required, the study can be continued as a double-contrast or negative-contrast morphological study of the small intestine:
  - Take lateral and ventrodorsal radiographs at 15 minutes, 30 minutes, 60, minutes and hourly as required.
  - The distended small bowel can be easily evaluated.
- If inserting a gastric tube is not practical, carbon dioxide–producing granules or spansules that cause effervescence, such as Baros, or E-Z-Gas II, can be substituted for the air in both the double-contrast and negative-contrast studies. Place the granules/spansules in the patient's buccal pouch and close the mouth to prevent foam

from dissipating before it reaches the stomach. Radiograph immediately because the gas produced may be belched.[5]
- The procedure in the cat is the same for a double-contrast or negative-contrast morphological study.

> **TECHNICIAN NOTES**   Quickly go through your mental checklist *before* pushing the exposure button: settings correct; image receptor/machine/grid in position; proper location of markers and identification (if using at this stage); survey radiographs taken, proper fasting, enema, etc., agent administered; correct body part and view; properly centered; borders correct and collimated; thickest part to the cathode; patient properly positioned, and restrained so the body part will be parallel to the image receptor and both are perpendicular to the central ray; correct timing, full expiration for abdomen views.

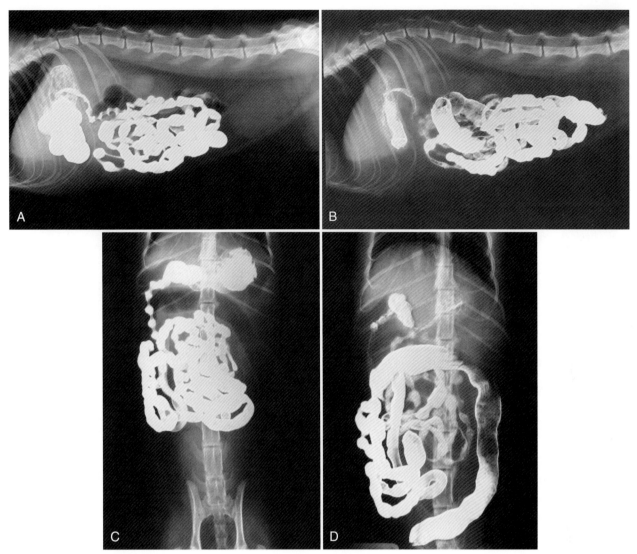

FIGURE 25-12 Normal feline upper gastrointestinal series. **A** and **B**, Lateral and venteodorsal views made 15 minutes after barium administration. **C** and **D**, Lateral and venteodorsal views made 3 hours after barium administration. Note the "string of pearls" appearance of the duodenum, which is not uncommon in cats.

> **TECHNICIAN NOTES**   Quick review of UGI study:
> - Prepare the patient, including fasting, an enema, survey radiographs.
> - Make sure everything is ready so the exposure can be made immediately.
> - Administer the barium antegrade.
> - Place the animal in position, and follow the required sequence for times and positioning for proper completion of positive-contrast UGI study.
> - Follow up with a negative-contrast study if required.

Lower Gastrointestinal Study

The radiographic examination of the cecum, colon, and rectum through retrograde administration of contrast medium generally evaluates extramural masses, mural or larger mucosal lesions, and intraluminal lesions. Smaller mucosal lesions are better determined endoscopically.

Disease in the area of ileocolic valves and the ascending and transverse processes is better examined with contrast studies. For visualization of the entire large bowel and small lesions such as mucosal irregularities, full distention with removal of feces is required. Oral administration of a positive-contrast medium does not fully distend the large bowel, so rectal administration is required for certain procedures. Chemical restraint is usually needed because many patients will not tolerate rectal infusion without sedation or general anesthesia.

Indications

Abnormal defecation especially in combination with excessive mucus or bright red stool, stricture, tenesmus, colonic obstruction, dyschezia, colonic or rectal neoplasia, colitis, and ileocolic intussusception are all indications to complete a barium enema study (Figure 25-14). The barium enema is most indicated when narrowing of the lumen prevents

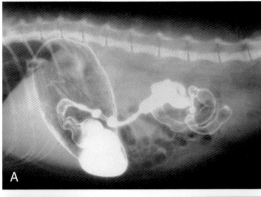

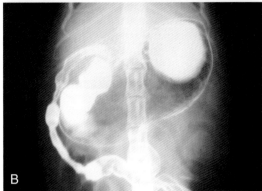

FIGURE 25-13 Double-contrast gastrogram. A, Lateral view. B, Ventrodorsal view.

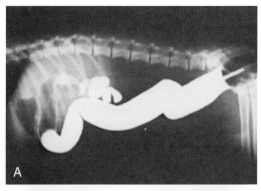

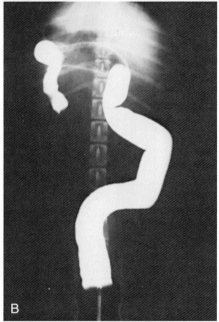

FIGURE 25-14 Barium enema. A, Lateral view. B, Ventrodorsal view.

passage of an endoscope, a mural or extramural lesion is suspected, or the mucus is found to be normal endoscopically.

Precautions

- Do not complete a retrograde administration or barium enema if perforation is suspected.
- Barium enemas are not recommended if the patient has had proctoscopy within 12 hours because the wall may be weakened.
- Reflux into the distal small bowel may occur without over-distention.
- Transient spasm may occur if the agent is cold, the wall is irritated by the tube, or narcotic premedication is used.[5]

Contrast Media and Dosage

Barium sulfate brought between room and body temperature, 20%.

Dosage to fill the large intestine:[5]
- 10–20 mL total in a small dog or cat.
- 30 mL in medium-sized dogs, 10–40 kg.
- 60 mL for dogs heavier than 40 kg.

Use half the dosage to evaluate the rectum or to partially fill the colon.

Dosage for double-contrast technique:
- In the dog: 5–10 mL of barium sulfate and 50–200 mL of air.
- In the cat: 2–3 mL of barium sulfate suspension and 25–50 mL of air.

Dosage for negative-contrast technique:
- In the dog: 60 to 100 mL of air.
- In the cat: 20 to 30 mL of air.

Equipment/Supplies

- Bardex or Foley catheter for the inflatable cuff.
- Syringe/enema bag/can/commercial enema set.
- Three-way stopcock valve.
- Lubricant.
- Compression paddle.

Survey

Ventrodorsal and lateral radiographs.

Patient Preparation

- The colon should be absent of fecal material if mucosal disease is being studied. Endoscopy will likely be more diagnostic than radiographic contrast for this study. No food is allowed for 24 to 36 hours. Water is allowed up to 4 hours prior to the procedure.
- Administer both cathartic and warm-water enemas the previous evening if the disease process has not emptied

the gastrointestinal tract. Consider using a low non-soap enema to stimulate defecation if stool is present. Just prior to the study, confirm with a warm-water enema that the effluent is clear.

- Sedate or anesthetize the patient.
- Take survey lateral and VD radiographs of the abdomen if not done so previously. This preparation is best completed 2–4 hours before the procedure. Unlike for endoscopy, the colon does not need to be washed clean, but any feces or ingesta in the colon could create confusing artifacts.
- For patients with acute abdominal pain, acute persistent vomiting, or palpable, enlarged fluid- or gas-filled bowels, no preparation is needed. The gas or fluid may be helpful in diagnosis.

Procedure for Positive Contrast Barium Enema for Both Dogs and Cats

1. Have the chemically restrained patient on the table.
2. Insert the catheter rectally and inflate the cuff to prevent leakage.
3. Keep the reservoir slightly above tabletop to maximize gravity or use minimum pressure on the syringe. Stop the infusion if there is resistance to the flow of the contrast agent. Close off the three-way stopcock.
4. Take ventrodorsal and both right and left lateral radiographs. Oblique views may be required, especially in males (see Chapter 18 for technique).
5. Process the films, and if no additional contrast agent or radiographs are required, remove as much of the contrast medium as possible prior to removal of the catheter.
6. Further radiographs may be obtained if desired once the barium is removed.

> **TECHNICIAN NOTES** Collimate, ensuring that labels /markers are included and borders are visible for every image.

Comments and Tips

- The catheter should be removed from the rectum away from the x-ray table, preferably above a container near a floor drain.
- Compression of the large bowel may further show the presence of a lesion.
- It is best to give small increments of the barium until the desired effect is seen on the radiographs.
- Soapy water enemas could irritate the large bowel mucosa, leading to spasms or gas accumulations that could cause radiographic artifacts during a barium enema.

Procedure for Double-Contrast Large Intestinal Study for Both Dogs and Cats

1. Have the chemically restrained patient on the table.
2. Insert the catheter rectally and inflate the cuff to prevent leakage. Place a three-way stopcock valve at the end of the catheter.

3. Infuse the barium sulfate suspension (2–10 mL; see dosages listed previously) through the three-way stopcock valve and close the valve.
4. Open the valve, infuse the air, and close the valve.
5. Take ventrodorsal and right and left lateral radiographs.
6. View the images and determine whether additional contrast agents or radiographs are required.
7. Release the stopcock valve. Gently remove as much air and barium as possible prior to removing the catheter.
8. Further images may be obtained if desired, once the barium is removed.

Comments and Tips

- Move the patient to an appropriate location for defecation.
- The amount of air infused can be decreased if distention is not required.

Pneumocolon

- This large intestine contrast study can be used if the colon is not emptied.
  - The same procedure is followed as for the double-contrast large intestinal study without barium sulfate.
  - Infuse 20–100 mL of air according to the weight of the animal as previously outlined.

Double-contrast technique

- This proceduse can also be used in conjunction with upper gastrointestinal study.
  - Indicated if the patient is unable to tolerate a conventional barium enema study or if a view of the ileocecal region is required.
  - When the swallowed barium reaches the right ileocolic junction, insufflate the calculated amount of air through a small catheter inserted into the rectum. Inflate the cuff and use a three-way stopcock valve to infuse the air and keep it in the colon.
  - Open the stopcock valve and remove the catheter. Continue the study if required.

> **TECHNICIAN NOTES** Exposure factors may need to be increased for a barium study.

> **TECHNICIAN NOTES** Quick review of LGI contrast study:
> 1. Prepare the patient, including fasting, enema, sedation, and survey radiographs.
> 2. Make sure everything is ready.
> 3. Administer the barium retrograde, and take required radiographs.
> 4. Place the patient in position and follow the required sequence for times and positioning for proper completion of a positive-contrast LGI.
> 5. Follow up with a negative-contrast study if required.

Use of Barium-Impregnated Polyethylene Spheres

Barium-impregnated polyethylene spheres are designed for evaluation of gastric dysmotility and intestinal transit time in dogs and cats. Note some of their advantages and disadvantages in comparison with barium suspension, mentioned in Table 25-1. The spheres are a mixture of plastic and barium sulfate and come in two diameters: 5-mm spheres to evaluate partial and complete obstruction and 1.5-mm spheres meant to mimic food passage. The number and size of the spheres, fasting period, and type and amount of food will affect the gastric emptying time and orocolic transit. Strict adherence to the manufacturer's suggestions should be followed for a proper functional study.

Dosage and Considerations

The inert spheres are available in capsules of two sizes that can be purchased as 5 or 10 dose packs. Regardless of the species or size, each dog or cat will have ingested 10 large spheres and 30 small spheres, which can be administered by giving either 1 large orange capsule or 4 small blue capsules (See Figure 25-1C). If gastrointestinal obstruction is suspected or there are acute gastrointestinal concerns, food is not generally given. For chronic gastric emptying or orocolic transit problems, feed with an intestinal diet following the BIPS package insert. As with liquid barium studies, sedatives and drugs influence gastrointestinal motility. The manufacturer of the spheres does provide a separate reference interval for gastric transit if acetylpromazine is administered.

Two views perpendicular to each other are concurrently required. These views are generally a right lateral and a ventrodorsal. Standard abdominal protocol should be followed to include the complete abdomen. The actual time that the radiographs are taken is not crucial, but the time elapsed between the administration of the spheres and when the images are taken is important to note and should be marked on the radiographs.

Generally, lateral and VD radiographs are simultaneously taken anywhere from 6 to 24 hours after administration, if the capsules are given on an empty stomach, to rule out pyloric and small intestinal blockage (Figure 25-15). For chronic vomiting or diarrhea, radiographs are taken 8 hours after food and the capsules are administered, to detect delayed gastric emptying. If none of the BIPS are in the colon, further images need to be taken later in the evening or early the next morning. If gastric dumping is suspected, one set of radiographs should be taken within 1 to 2 hours of BIPS administration.[6]

The study can also be used to assess large bowel transit. An enema or cathartic should be given to remove the retained feces. Give the BIPS with recommended diet, and radiograph at 24, 48, and 72 hours. Check the reference intervals to make sure to follow the time suggestions.[6]

The gastric emptying rate and orocolic transit rate are determined by applying a formula separately to the large and small spheres. Generally small BIPS are used to determine

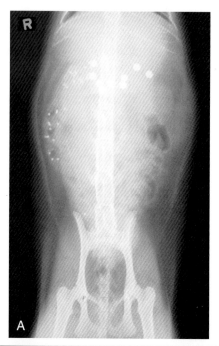

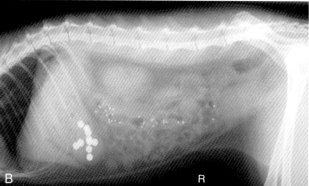

FIGURE 25-15 **A,** Ventrodorsal abdomen 4 hours after administration of BIPS. All of the small BIPS have left the stomach, but the majority of large BIPS are still present. None of the BIPS are in the colon, so the orocolic rate is 0% for both the small and large BIPS. **B,** Right lateral abdomen BIPS study 4 hours after administration. Both views are required to determine the actual location of the BIPS.

the gastric emptying for motility disorders, because they more closely mimic food, whereas the gastric emptying rate of the large BIPS is best considered for partial obstructions of the pylorus or intestine.[6] The results are then compared with a standardized chart, based on the size of the sphere, whether food is given, or the type of food given. Once the correct chart is used, the calculation is compared with the average and mean emptying rate/transit times that are probable at that point after administration. Times are quicker if the capsules are given without food.

If obstruction is noted, it is not necessary to calculate the formula. In an animal with obstruction, the large spheres are designed to become trapped at the orad aspect of an obstructing lesion, giving the appearance of dumping. If gravelling or the accumulation of indigestible material or a dilated bowel is not noted, a second set of radiographs should be

Formula for gastric emptying with use of BIPS:
1. Count the number of BIPS that have *left* the stomach.
2. Calculate as follows:

$$\frac{\text{Number of BIPS that have left stomach}}{\text{Total number of BIPS seen on image}} \times 100 = \frac{\text{\% BIPS that have}}{\text{left the stomach}}$$

Formula for orocolic transit rate:
1. Count the number of BIPS that are in the colon and calculate as follows:

$$\frac{\text{Number of BIPS in colon}}{\text{Total number of BIPS seen on radiograph}} \times 100 = \frac{\text{\% of BIPS in}}{\text{the colon}}$$

Remember to calculate the small and large spheres separately. The total number seen on the image will be a maximum of 10 large or 30 small spheres. Apply this percentage to the appropriate chart.

taken in 1 to 2 hours. Strong contractions of the stomach may have expelled the markers in small groups, or there may be bunching at the ileocolic valve. This transient bunching at the ileocolic valve is most often evident in healthy cats, animals with weak peristalsis, or toy dogs. On a VD view, the ileocolic valve will be at about the level of L3-L4. Two views are required to prevent misdiagnosis.

As the spheres are barium based, they appear white on the radiographs. Both views are required to determine exactly where the spheres are, because parts of the large intestine are superimposed over the cardia of stomach and over the stomach just caudal to left crus of the diaphragm in some animals in the lateral view (See Chapter 18). Also, on a VD, BIPS in the transverse colon can be mistaken for BIPS bunched in the small intestine if only a lateral abdominal view is taken. If the location of a sphere cannot be accurately determined, it is not included in the formula calculation.

Quick review of the use of BIPS:
1. Prepare the patient, including fasting or feeding as required and survey radiographs.
2. Administer the capsules.
3. Expose lateral and VD views at the suggested time, depending on the condition. Repeat radiographs if required.
4. Follow up with barium study or negative-contrast study if required.

Normal Radiographic Anatomy of the Gastrointestinal Tract

Normal Radiographic Appearance of the Esophagus with Contrast Media

The normal oropharyngeal region shows coating of the mucosa with no significant retention of the contrast agent. A small amount of medium may sometimes stay in the esophageal lumen immediately caudal to the cranial esophageal sphincter.

The normal canine esophageal mucosa appears as a series of longitudinal folds with its lines close together throughout, except at the thoracic inlet, where the esophagus passes along the left lateral side of the trachea. The normal feline esophagus also has parallel lines at the level of the heart base, with the caudal third of the esophagus being described as having a herringbone pattern. It consists of obliquely directed folds that correspond to the smooth muscle segment.[4] The esophagus is best evaluated on a lateral radiograph of the neck and on lateral and DV views of the thorax.

Normal Radiographic Stomach and Small Bowel Anatomy

Please review the anatomy in Chapter 18 to view what is generally visualized on a survey radiograph. Table 18-1 gives an overview of the anatomy in the various positions and Figure 25-2 shows the images.

Table 25-3 indicates image sequence for the positive-contrast upper gastrointestinal tract study. The gastric emptying time of normal animals varies greatly. Factors such as the effect of medication and the type or volume of meal given, also alters times. Low dosages of barium may delay emptying and transit time because the stomach empties slower when there is less volume in the stomach. Delay may also occur in nervous animals or in a stressful environment.

On an upper GI barium sulfate study without any food, delayed gastric emptying is diagnosed when gastric emptying is not completed after 3 hours in dogs and 1 hour in cats. Gastric emptying time longer than 8 hours for barium mixed with solid food is considered abnormal.[7]

Abnormal gastric emptying may be seen with incomplete pyloric obstruction. This can be associated with a pyloric tumor, congenital or acquired pyloric stenosis, or a gastric or duodenal foreign body. Delayed gastric or intestinal emptying can be evaluated by means of a simple or double contrast radiographic study, BIPS, scintigraphy, ultrasonography, or endoscopy. In some cases, gastric outflow obstruction may be documented only with food or with BIPS. Scintigraphy, using a radioactive meal, is the ideal modality to study gastric emptying because the study is very close to natural conditions and gives a quantitative index.[4,7] Scintigraphic evaluation of gastric emptying can be completed in 4 to 5 hours and is more consistent than gastric emptying times as measured by BIPS.[4,8,9] Magnetic resonance imaging (MRI) has not yet been applied for assessment of gastric emptying in small animals. Ultrasonography for determining gastric emptying can be subjective. Further methods are not practical outside the laboratory.[10]

The rugal folds are best seen at the periphery as the stomach begins to empty (see Figure 25-2). They are also more evident with negative contrast, but if the stomach is too distended in a double-contrast study, the folds may disappear. The rugae should be uniform, linear, or slightly tortuous and parallel.

In about a third of cats, the duodenum has a "string-of-pearls" appearance during a positive-contrast study (see Figure 25-12). This is due to the peristaltic contractions. In dogs, transient peristaltic contractions may be noted in the body of the stomach, pyloric canal, and antrum. Pseudoulcers or square outpockets may also be noted on the nonmesenteric descending duodenum of the dog.[4] They are not found in the cat.

The cecum in a cat appears pointed, whereas in a dog it has a corkscrew appearance. On VD or DV views, the cecum appears just to the right of midline in both species.

Variations do exist in the appearance of the normal stomach, when the patient changes position and as the amount and percentage of fluid and gas change. See the table in the Technician Notes box for a simplified version of where gas and fluid can be found as the position of the patient changes. A vertical beam is used.

TECHNICIAN NOTES   The following box capsulates how positioning affects the distribution of gas and liquid[4]:

View	Location of Gas	Location of Fluid
Dorsoventral	Fundus	Body/pylorus
Ventrodorsal	Body (± pylorus)	Fundus
Left lateral	Pylorus (± body)	Fundus
Right lateral	Fundus dorsal body	Pylorus

In the normal dog and cat, the rest of the small intestine should appear smooth. In dogs, barium between the intestinal villi may show up as a fine brush pattern.[4] Short lengths of the bowel may reveal peristalsis.

The colon wall is generally smooth, and the lumen uniform in width. Barium adhering to mucus or feces may create artifacts. Lymph follicles that are present in the mucosa of both the dog and the cat colon, and in the cecum of the dog, may appear as spicules on a barium enema study or as pinpoint radiopacities if viewed head-on in a double-contrast study.[4]

Upon removal of the positive-contrast medium, longitudinal folds are visible that are made more detailed with the infusion of air.

The VD or DV view of the colon shows a question-mark configuration.

Contrast Studies of the Urinary System

Contrast studies of the urinary system evaluate the kidneys, urinary bladder, ureters, prostate gland, and urethra. Survey radiographs of the kidneys may provide external anatomical information such as size, shape, and radiographic opacity if existing radiographic contrast is adequate. However, when kidneys cannot be assessed by survey radiographs or when qualitative functional urography is needed, excretory urography or ultrasonography may provide better information than survey radiographs.[4] There are different ways of evaluating the urinary system, and the method chosen is dictated by the clinical signs of the patient. Studies performed through contrast radiography have limitations, and with the advent of ultrasonography, a safer and more accurate method for evaluating the kidneys and prostate is available. The combination of the two methods may provide the greatest information.

Excretory Urography[4,5,7]

Indications

Excretory urography is primarily used to determine the size, shape, location, and integrity of the kidneys as well as the size, shape, and appearance of the collecting systems. Although excretory urography is not a quantitative measurement of renal function, it can be used to assess the relative function of the kidneys and, indirectly, the pathophysical mechanism of renal failure.[4] Ultrasound shows the anatomy. Specific indications include hematuria, dysuria, pyuria, straining at urination, and frequency of urination.

The principle of the study is that sterile, water-soluble, iodinated contrast medium is injected intravascularly, where it circulates; then the kidney concentrates and excretes the iodine, contrasting the kidneys, ureters, and urinary bladder. The study was formerly called an intravenous pyelogram (IVP) or an intravenous urogram (IVU).

Precautions

- Excretory urography can be used in both azotemic and nonazotemic patients provided there is adequate hydration.
- A temporary decrease in renal function may occur after excretory urography.
- Dehydration can result in kidney damage, so a dehydrated animal should be rehydrated prior to the procedure.
- Abdominal compression may have to be modified because of precluded conditions.
- Although they are rare, systemic reactions have occurred. Kidney function parameters such as blood urea nitrogen (BUN) and serum creatinine levels should be checked prior to the start of the procedure. It is important that the patient's hydration status be determined and corrected prior to administration of the agent.
- Even though the incidence of reaction to contrast media is low, especially with the use of low-osmolar, nonionic contrast media, it is imperative to be prepared and not to become complacent. Reactions can occur quickly and without warning. Most severe acute reactions occur within the first 1 to 5 minutes after administration. Signs can range from mild to fatal. The most common signs tend to be vomiting, defecation, urination, urticaria, tachycardia, and hypotension with or without collapse. Most reactions can be reversed with immediate and proper intervention. Vital signs should be monitored before, during, and after the procedure to observe for adverse reactions. An emergency resuscitation kit should be on hand prior to injection.
- Proper technique should be used to minimize iatrogenesis that may be caused by placement of the catheter.

> *TECHNICIAN NOTES* Some suggestions for minimizing reactions to contrast media injections are as follows[1]:
> * Prior to injection, check that the solution is clear and colorless.
> * Check the expiration date, and discard outdated contrast material.
> * Keep the media out of direct light for storage.
> * There are no preservatives, so immediately use the bottle once it is opened, and discard the remainder.
> * Keep the agent close to body temperature. The warmed solution decreases the viscosity for easier injection and reduces the potential for cardiovascular collapse.
> * To prevent incompatibility, do not administer other medications in the same syringe or IV administration set
> * Ensure patency of the catheter prior to the injection.
> * If a contrast medium needs to be injected into a line, use normal saline (NS), dextrose and water (D/W), or lactated Ringer's solution (R/L). Potassium chloride (KCl) added to the IV is the *only* compatible medication. However, fluids dilute the concentration, lessening the contrast noted on an image.
> * Stop injecting immediately if a reaction appears, and leave the catheter in the vein.
> * Monitor carefully throughout.

Contrast Media and Dosage

Water-soluble organic iodide, 850 mg/kg body weight.

Note: A concentration of 300–400 mg iodine per mL is the suggested dilution.

Ionic: Diatrizoate (Sodium Hypaque).

Nonionic: Iopamidol (Isovue), iohexol (Omnipaque), or iodixanol (Visipaque).

Equipment/Supplies

* Indwelling intravenous catheter, syringe, and system for abdominal compression.
* Urethral catheter if continuing the study.
* Emergency resuscitation kit.
* Markers to identify exposure time.

Survey

Right lateral (Figure 25-16) and ventrodorsal views.

Patient Preparation

* No food for 24 hours before the study; water ad libitum.
* Perform a cleansing enema the previous evening if possible or at least 2 hours before (best if 4 hours to minimize gas artifacts).
* If urine samples are required for examination, they should be collected prior to infusion of the medium. Contrast agents increase specific gravity, cause a false-positive increase in urinary protein as detected by sulfosalicylic acid, and may inhibit bacterial growth.
* Assess patient hydration, and proceed only if normal.
* Remove the urine so the contrast medium will not be diluted.

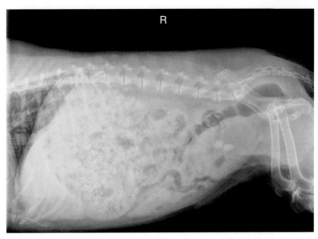

FIGURE 25-16 Lateral survey of the abdomen of a diabetic patient. Positive contrast studies would obliterate the bladder stones.

* Have image receptors, settings, markers, timers, protective gear, etc. ready, so that upon administration of the contrast agent, the image can be taken immediately.
* Position an indwelling catheter.

> *TECHNICIAN NOTES* Remember that for the full abdomen you are generally:
> * Measuring at the thickest part (liver), at the TL junction.
> * Centering the beam caudal to 13th rib in the dog, 2–3 fingerbreadths caudal to 13th rib in the cat.
> * Including cranially from T9 (for VD views) and T7 (for lateral views) and caudally to the acetabulum.
> For cystography only if a full abdominal view is not required:
> * Measure and center just cranial to the crest of the ilium.
> * Cranially include from the caudal aspect of the ribs (about L2) to caudal to the ischium.

> *TECHNICIAN NOTES* The cranial pole of the right kidney of a dog is generally found at T13.

Procedure

1. The patient is best sedated or anesthetized to minimize discomfort.
2. Obtain survey radiographs.
3. Place the animal in ventrodorsal recumbency with a patent indwelling catheter.
4. Inject the calculated warmed solution quickly as a bolus—within 2 minutes.
5. Flush the catheter with heparinized saline after the solution is administered.
6. Sequence the radiographs as follows after injection (Figures 25-17):
   a. Immediately—within 5 to 20 seconds: ventrodorsal.
   b. 5 minutes: ventrodorsal and right lateral.
   c. If there is evidence of contrast agent within both kidneys, compression may be applied.

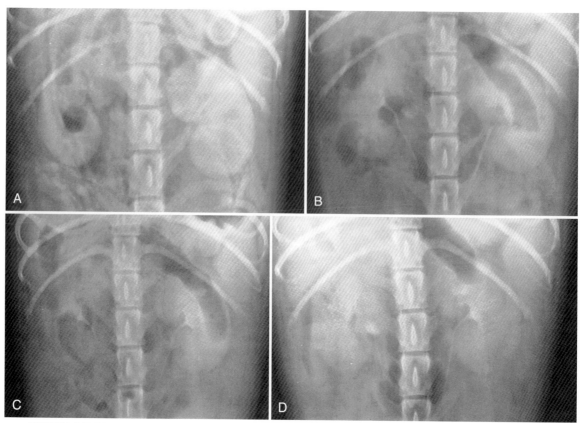

FIGURE 25-17 Ventrodorsal abdomen views of a normal dog after intravenous administration of 400 mg iodine per pound of body weight in the form of sodium iothalamate. **A,** 10 seconds after injection; **B,** 5 minutes; **C,** 20 minutes; **D,** 40 minutes.

d. 20 minutes: ventrodorsal (both collecting systems should be filled with contrast medium).

e. If compression has been applied, remove the compression band.

f. 30–40 minutes: right lateral and ventrodorsal obliques (optional if retrograde cystography is contraindicated).

g. Further contrast study of the bladder can be completed:

- Positive-contrast retrograde cystography: Infuse positive-contrast medium solution retrogradely via the urethral catheter. The amount would be determined by pressure and what is noted on the previous radiographic image.

- Double-contrast retrograde cystography: Infuse negative-contrast medium via the urethral catheter.

> **TECHNICIAN NOTES**   Make sure to properly use time markers for each view. Follow the recommended placement by placing at the cranial aspect for VD views and at the ventral cranial abdomen for lateral views.

Comments and Tips

- For diagnostic reasons it is best if the bolus is administered fairly quickly, but the patient may be nauseous and may vomit if it is given too quickly.

- Right lateral positioning is suggested as there is greater longitudinal separation of the right and left kidneys.

- Compression over the bladder can be applied for better visualization of the renal collecting system by delaying the drainage of the contrast media. If the urinary bladder is compressed, the intraluminal pressure increases and prevents drainage through the ureters.

- Compression can be applied by placing a flat radiolucent sponge on the central abdomen and securing it with elastic bandages. Commercially available compression devices can also be used.

- The agent can be administered more slowly and the sequence delayed for ureter examination.

- IV fluids should be stopped during the sequence because fluids reduce the concentration of the iodine and subsequent image on the radiograph.

- If the kidneys are highly compromised, contrast media may occur in the liver.

- Many sequences of images are available, but the one described here probably provides the most diagnostic information.[4]

- The excretory urogram consists of the nephrogram and the pyelogram:

  - Opacification of the functional renal parenchyma (nephrons) occurs immediately and is known as the nephrographic phase. The vascular supply and perfusion of the kidney are noted, helping differentiate the cortex from the medulla.

- The pyelographic phase shows the renal pelvis, pelvic recesses, and ureters. The renal collecting channels extend into the medulla from the pelvis of the kidneys. A compression band slows the drainage from the pyelogram.
- The drainage phase occurs when the agent is in the bladder.
- Proper distention of the urinary bladder cannot be achieved solely with an excretory urogram study. Retrograde cystography is required. However, in traumatized female cats, it may be difficult to position a urethral catheter.
- The status of patient hydration, dosage rate, and renal function all affect the concentration, excretion, and opacification of the positive-contrast medium.
- Opaque material in the intestinal lumen, intestinal gas over the urinary bladder or urethra, and nipples can be mistaken for uroliths or filling defects. Gas bubbles in the bladder or urethra introduced by urinary catheterization may appear as mineralized lesions in the tissues of the bladder wall.
- A maximum of 90 mL of contrast medium in dogs, and 15 mL in cats, is suggested.
- Additional views can be decided on the basis of individual findings.

TECHNICIAN NOTES Proper patient preparation is essential to ensure quality images.

TECHNICIAN NOTES Quick review of excretory urography:
1. Prepare the patient, including fasting, enema, emptying of the bladder, insertion of IV line and urinary catheters, survey radiographs, and sedation/anesthesia. Follow proper aseptic technique.
2. Have everything ready so exposures can be made immediately after administration of contrast medium.
3. Administer the warmed contrast water-soluble organic iodide IV as a quick bolus.
4. Expose the required radiographs in the correct time sequence.
5. Apply compression if required, and continue the sequence of exposure.
6. Follow up with a positive or negative retrograde contrast medium if required for the bladder or urethra.
7. Remove the contrast medium; insert an antibiotic if required; remove the catheter; and recover the animal.

Retrograde Cystography[4,5,7]

Cystography is the study of the bladder via the retrograde infusion of contrast media through a urinary catheter. Positive-, negative-, or double-contrast studies can be performed with or without an excretory urogram. The actual study used is dictated by clinical history, clinical signs, radiographic signs, and character of the urine obtained with bladder catheterization.

Indications

Clinical indications for retrograde cystography include unresponsive clinical signs due to abnormal urine (hematuria, crystalluria, and bacteriuria), abnormal urination (dysuria, pollakiuria), trauma, and abnormalities noted on survey radiographs such as abdominal masses, a change in bladder opacity or wall, or a change in location.

Precautions

Iatrogenesis due to catheterization and cystographic procedures—trauma, bacterial infections, kinked or knotted urethral catheters—can occur. Intramural or subserosal accumulation of contrast media occurs more frequently in cats and usually does not cause a clinical problem. Mucosal ulceration, inflammation, and granulomata reactions are usually transitory with no serious clinical problems.

Fatal, though rare complications can occur with the introduction of a gas embolism after administration of negative-contrast media. Nitrous oxide or carbon dioxide should be used, especially in patients with hematuria, because blood in the urine shows evidence of communication between the bladder lumen and vascular system. Nitrous oxide or carbon dioxide is 20 times more soluble in serum than air or oxygen. Left lateral recumbency may decrease the chance for any emboli to reach the lungs.[5]

TECHNICIAN NOTES Never use barium for any urinary studies including cystography.

Contrast Media and Dosage

Positive-contrast media: Water-soluble organic iodide diluted to 150–200 mg of iodine/mL, 3–12 mL /kg.
Negative-contrast media: Nitrous oxide, carbon dioxide, air 3–12 mL/kg.
Double-contrast media: Water soluble organic iodide diluted to 150–200 mg of iodine/mL:
- Cat: 0.5 mL–1 mL.
- Dog less than 10 kg: 1–3 mL.
- Dog greater than 10 kg: 3–6 mL.

Equipment/Supplies

- Sterile male or female urinary catheter.
- Vaginal speculum or adapted otoscope for female dogs.
- Sterile lubricating jelly.
- Light source.
- 20- to 50-mL syringe.
- 2% lidocaine jelly.
- Three-way valve.
- Source to deposit urine.
- 2–5 mL total of 2% lidocaine without epinephrine (optional).
- Broad-spectrum antibiotics (optional).

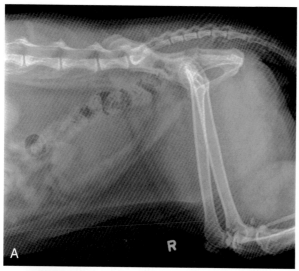

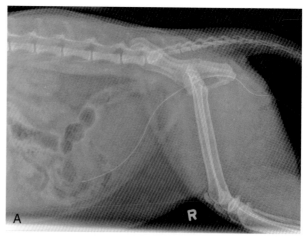

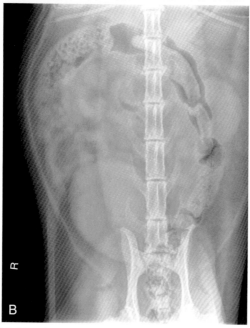

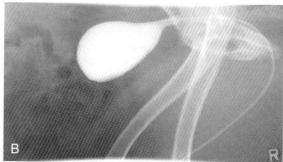

FIGURE 25-19 A, Catheter injected with iodine prior to a cystogram. B, Lateral positive-contrast cystogram.

FIGURE 25-18 A, Right lateral survey prior to a cystogram. Note the presence of stool, which could mask lesions. B, Ventrodorsal abdomen survey prior to a cystogram.

Survey Radiographs

Ventrodorsal and right lateral (Figure 25-18) views.

Patient Preparation

- Sedation is suggested because urinary bladder distention can be uncomfortable especially in patients with cystitis.
- Withhold food for 24 hours if possible, and administer an enema 4 hours before the study to avoid superimposition of fecal matter and to minimize gas artifacts.
- Proper sterile technique is required. If a catheter was inserted to collect urine for an excretory urogram, leave it aseptically inserted.
- If urine samples are required for examination, they should be collected prior to infusion of the agent because contrast agents increase specific gravity, cause a false-positive

increase in protein as detected by sulfosalicylic acid, and may inhibit bacterial growth.

> **TECHNICIAN NOTES**   While inserting the contrast medium, stop the infusion when external palpation of the bladder shows that it is moderately distended, if reflux occurs around the catheter, or if you feel back-pressure on the syringe.

Procedure for Negative-Contrast Study (Pneumocystogram) or Positive-Contrast Cystography

Retrograde negative-contrast cystography is used to identify the integrity of the bladder wall following trauma or to locate the bladder. Retrograde positive-contrast cystography is used to evaluate the bladder wall character in a trauma patient or to locate the bladder after trauma or herniation (Figure 25-19). In the absence of ultrasound, both studies can help determine caudal abdominal masses; a pneumocystogram is best for cystic calculi.

1. Take ventrodorsal and lateral survey radiographs of the full urinary tract.
2. Apply sterile 2% lidocaine jelly on the tip of a premeasured urethral catheter, and aseptically and atraumatically insert until the catheter tip is within the urinary bladder.
3. Gently empty the bladder, and note the volume of urine removed.

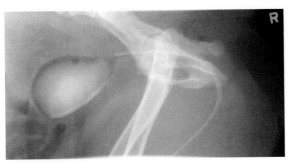

FIGURE 25-20 Double-contrast cystogram. Note the bubble of air at the tip of the urinary catheter.

4. Apply a syringe and three-way stopcock, and infuse with 2–5 mL total of 2% lidocaine without epinephrine to reduce bladder pain and spasm.
5. Carefully infuse the medium, noting appropriate distention. Close the stopcock valve when adequate distention is reached.
6. Take radiographs: right and left lateral and ventrodorsal views, centering over the bladder. An oblique view is optional but is suggested for evaluation of prostate or urethral problems in a male.
7. If further distention of the bladder is required, inject additional contrast agent and repeat the radiographs.
8. Carefully remove the contrast medium. Flush with a broad-spectrum antibiotic if the patient is not receiving systemic antibiotics as per the veterinarian. Remove the catheter.

Procedure for Double-Contrast Retrograde Cystography

Double-contrast cystography is best for assessing bladder wall lesions and intraluminal filling defects (Figure 25-20).
1. Take ventrodorsal and lateral survey radiographs of the full urinary tract.
2. Apply sterile 2% lidocaine jelly on the tip of a premeasured urethral catheter, and aseptically and atraumatically insert until the catheter tip is within the urinary bladder.
3. Gently empty the bladder, and note the volume of urine removed.
4. Apply a syringe and three-way valve (stopcock), and infuse with 2–5 mL total of 2% lidocaine without epinephrine, to reduce bladder pain and spasm (optional).
5. Carefully infuse the negative-contrast medium, noting appropriate distention. Close the stopcock valve when adequate distention is reached.
6. Take right lateral, left lateral, and ventrodorsal radiographs (oblique view for evaluation of prostate or urethral problems in a male). Center over the bladder (cranial to the crest of the ilium).
7. Slowly infuse the organic water-soluble iodine into the bladder.
8. Gently rotate the animal from side to side to coat the bladder wall with iodine.
9. Take right and left lateral and ventrodorsal radiographs (oblique view for evaluation of prostrate or urethral problems in a male). Center over the bladder.

10. If further distention of the bladder is required, inject additional contrast agent, and repeat the radiographs.
11. Remove the contrast medium when appropriate. Flush with a broad-spectrum antibiotic if required. Remove the catheter.

Comments and Tips
- Both lateral views are suggested because a change in position may define a lesion more accurately.
- Ensure that the catheter has been premeasured and is in the correct location just within the urinary bladder.
- If urine is removed from a relatively full bladder, the same amount of contrast medium can be infused.
- It is best if the small bowel is empty and the colon is void of fecal material.
- Using lidocaine without epinephrine, helps decrease the possibility of spasm and helps obtain complete bladder distention.
- A neurogenic bladder may hold two to three times, but a diseased bladder, only a fraction of the anticipated volume of air or positive-contrast medium. Palpate carefully, noting resistance in the syringe and watching for leakage.
- If the catheter has an inflatable cuff, deflate after the radiographs have been taken.
- Any urine leakage with positive-contrast medium should be cleaned from the table, image receptor, or patient to minimize artifacts on the image.
- Reduce the kVp by 4 to 6 in cats and small dogs and by up to 10 to 15 for medium and large dogs, if completing a pneumocystogram, because of inherent contrast.
- Compression through the use of a paddle will help move the contrast pool for better evaluation of the integrity of the bladder wall.
- After taking the positive-contrast cystography radiographs, the catheter tip can be repositioned into the urethra to perform an urethrogram. This will better evaluate the bladder neck.
- Urethral reflux of positive-contrast agent may be a normal finding.
- If a ruptured bladder is suspected, contrast agent can be used without dilution to better visualize the agent in the peritoneal cavity.
- Extravasation of the positive-contrast agent in the extraperitoneal soft tissues or peritoneal cavity is well tolerated.[5]

Cystography via Cystocentesis in the Dog and Cat

Cystography via cystocentesis is not common but can be performed if necessary, especially if urethral obstruction prevents catheterization. It is more useful in cats than in dogs. Either negative- or positive-contrast media can be administered in this way.

Procedure
1. Manually palpate the urinary bladder, immobilizing it with your fingers against the ventral or lateral abdomen.

> **📋 TECHNICIAN NOTES**   To calculate the concentration of contrast medium needed, use the following formula:
>
> $$\frac{\text{Final diluted percentage}}{\text{Initial concentration}} = \frac{\text{Volume needed}}{\text{Final volume administered}}$$
>
> A 15-kg dog requires 60 mL of a 10% iodinated contrast medium for a urinary study. If the stock bottle is 50%, what is the amount in mL taken from the bottle?
>
> $$\frac{10\%}{50\%} = \frac{X}{60 \text{ mL}}$$
>
> $$\left(\frac{1}{5}\right)(60 \text{ mL}) = X \text{ mL}$$
>
> 12 mL should be taken from the bottle.
> *Note:* The sterile diluent required will be 60 mL – 12 mL = 48 mL.

2. Aseptically introduce a 1-inch, 22-gauge needle in a cat or a 2-inch 22-gauge needle in the dog through the midline abdominal wall.
3. Extract the urine, noting the volume.
4. Infuse positive-contrast media or air so that there is minimal bladder distention.
5. Remove the needle.
6. Take lateral and ventrodorsal or oblique radiographs.

Comments and Tips

- There will likely be minimal leakage into the peritoneal cavity.
- To minimize possible leakage, do not apply any bladder compression following injection.

> **📋 TECHNICIAN NOTES**   Quick review of retrograde cystography:
>
> 1. Prepare the patient, including fasting, enema, emptying of the bladder, insertion of the urinary catheter, survey radiographs, and sedation/anesthesia. Follow proper aseptic technique.
> 2. Have everything ready before administering the contrast media.
> 3. Administer the required solution—warmed positive-contrast water-soluble organic iodide and/or negative-contrast medium.
> 4. Obtain the required radiographs shortly after administration.
> 5. If required, follow up with the opposite-contrast media for the bladder or urethra.
> 6. Remove contrast medium; insert antibiotic if required; remove the catheter, and recover the animal.

Urethrography[4,5,7]

Urethrography consists of filling the urethra with contrast medium to evaluate it (Figure 25-21). This can be accomplished in either a retrograde manner with a positive-, negative-, or double-contrast medium or by applying compression on a positive-contrast–filled bladder to cause a voiding urethrogram. The actual technique varies with the sex and species of the patient. Often this study is

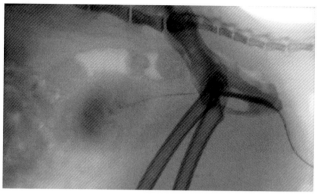

FIGURE 25-21 Urethrogram with fluoroscopy of a dog positioned in right lateral recumbency. Iodine has been injected retrograde via a catheter. Some of the iodine has dispersed in the bladder.

performed after completion of a retrograde cystogram merely by repositioning the catheter tip more caudally.

Indications

Urethrography is indicated to determine the abnormal passage of urine due to urethral trauma, stricture, obstruction, or other pathological disturbances.

Precautions

If injury results upon catheterization, injected air may enter the venous system, leading to fatal venous air embolism. Compression for a voiding urethrogram is contraindicated if the bladder is diseased because of the greater possibility of rupture.

Contrast Media and Dosage

Positive-contrast organic ionic or nonionic agent (diluted to 150–200 mg of iodine/mL):
- Dogs: 10–15 mL volume
- Cats: 5–10 mL volume

Equipment/Supplies

- Sterile catheter with inflatable bulb if possible.
- Sterile lubricating jelly.
- Catheter adapter.
- Large syringe.
- Sterile saline solution.
- 2% lidocaine jelly and lidocaine solution.

Survey Radiographs

Ventrodorsal and right lateral.

Patient Preparation

- Sedation is suggested, as the procedure may cause discomfort.
- Give a cleansing enema to remove fecal matter from the descending colon and rectum.
- Proper sterile technique is required. If the catheter was used for cystography, leave it aseptically inserted.
- If urine samples are required for examination, they should be collected prior to infusion of contrast media.

Procedure for Retrograde Positive-Contrast Urethrography

This procedure is most often performed in male dogs for evaluation of the urethra and suspected prostatic disease. Only indirect evidence of prostatic disease is provided, however.

1. If not previously done, take ventrodorsal and lateral survey radiographs of the full urinary tract.
2. If the catheter is not yet inserted, fill the lumen of the catheter with contrast medium.
3. Insert the lubricated tip about 1 to 3 cm into the urethral orifice, and inflate the balloon.
4. Depending on the size of the patient, inject the contrast medium until you feel back pressure.
5. Take lateral radiographs toward the end of the infusion, repeating the administration if needed. A ventrodorsal oblique radiograph may be helpful.
6. Remove the catheter.

Procedure for Antegrade or Voiding Urethrogram

Because it is harder to catheterize female dogs and cats the antegrade or voiding urethrogram is easier to complete than the retrograde study.

1. Apply gentle pressure on the positive-contrast–filled, distended bladder with a paddle or wooden spoon. Place a towel under the patient to absorb any leakage.
2. Take a lateral radiograph when urine is noted at the urethral orifice.

Procedure for Vaginocystourethrography[4]

Vaginocystourethrography is another method of evaluating the urethra in female dogs (Figure 25-22).

1. If not previously done, take ventrodorsal and lateral survey radiographs of the full urinary tract.
2. Patients should be given general anesthesia for vaginocystourethrography.
3. If the catheter is not yet inserted, fill the lumen of the catheter with contrast medium.
4. Insert the lubricated tip into the vestibule and inflate the balloon to occlude outflow. The tip of the catheter distal to the balloon should be as short as possible to prevent it from entering the vagina.
5. It may be necessary to clamp the vulvar lips tightly to prevent reflux.
6. Inject amount of positive-contrast media for the size of the patient. The vagina will fill preferentially.
7. Infuse so the contrast medium will reflux into the urethra and bladder. Overdistention may result in expulsion of the contrast medium.[4]
8. Take lateral radiographs at the end of the infusion. The catheter can be pulled out at the same time.

Comments and Tips

- Make sure the pelvic limbs are pulled cranially to prevent superimposition of the femurs over the urethra (modified lateral view; see Chapter 18).
- If the catheter does not have a cuff, use a larger catheter to limit leakage of the contrast medium. Place a towel to absorb leaking contrast agent. Avoid using a stiff catheter to minimize iatrogenesis.
- Avoid the use of sterile lubricating jelly with a positive-contrast agent to prevent filling defects and false-positive diagnosis.
- Minimize the length of time the catheter balloon is inflated to avoid mild reversible inflammatory reaction.
- If the urinary bladder is fully distended with urine, contrast medium, or sterile saline during urethrography, there may be better distention of the urethra, especially the prostatic urethra.
- Vesicoureteral reflux and urethroprostatic reflux occur frequently in mature healthy dogs undergoing maximum distention urethrocystography.
- Left lateral recumbency is suggested when gas is being put in the bladder because the position will help the animal recover if an air embolus develops. Some radiographers prefer the typical right lateral position because it helps decrease renal overlap on images. If you suspect that an air embolus has developed during the procedure, immediately deflate the bladder and place the patient in left lateral recumbency.

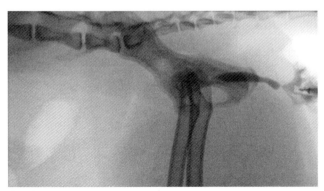

FIGURE 25-22 Fluoroscopy of a vaginogram iodine study with the patient positioned in lateral recumbency.

> **TECHNICIAN NOTES**   Quick review of retrograde urethrography and vaginocystourethrography:
> 1. Prepare the patient, including fasting, enema, emptying of the bladder, insertion of the urinary catheter, survey radiographs, and sedation/anesthesia. Follow proper aseptic technique.
> 2. Have everything ready before administering the contrast medium.
> 3. Administer the warmed positive-contrast water-soluble organic iodide via the catheter.
> 4. Obtain the required radiographs shortly after administration.
> 5. Remove the contrast medium; insert antibiotic if required; remove the catheter; and recover the animal.

TABLE 25-4	Summary of Complete Urinary Tract Examination
Preparation	• No food for 12–24 hours with water given ad libitum.
	• Withhold water at least 1–2 hours or as required prior to sedation or anesthesia.
	• Give an enema at least 4 hours prior to lessen the chance of gas artifacts.
	• Assess patient hydration and proceed only if normal.
	• Have plates, settings, markers, protective apparel, etc., ready.
	• Sedate animal and obtain survey radiograph—right lateral and ventrodorsal (VD)
	• Aseptically place intravenous (IV) catheter in vein, and urethral catheter in bladder.
	• Place a 3-way stopcock valve on the urethral catheter.
	• Remove any urine from the bladder.
	• Place the patient in dorsal recumbency.
Excretory urography	• Inject iodinated contrast medium at 880 mg/kg as a bolus within 2 minutes. Note maximum limits.
	• Flush catheter with heparinized saline after the solution is administered.
	• Take VD radiograph within 20–40 seconds of completing injection (nephrogram).
Double-contrast cystogram	• Distend bladder with negative contrast media at about 1–2 mL/kg to keep iodine in kidney.
	• Take VD and right lateral radiographs of the kidneys 5 minutes after IV injection (pyelogram).
	• Gently palpate the bladder and determine whether more negative-contrast agent should be administered.
	• At 20 minutes after IV injection, obtain VD, lateral, and oblique radiographs (optional) of kidneys, ureters, bladder (drainage and cystogram).
Urethrogram	• Inject iodinated medium (5–15 mL) into the urethra as you withdraw the catheter.
	• Take lateral radiograph as soon as you see contrast agent leaking from the external orifice of the urethra.

Complete Urinary Tract Examination

Table 25-4 gives a summary of a complete urinary tract examination. Combining the procedures just described allows one to perform a complete urinary tract examination at one time.

> **TECHNICIAN NOTES**
> • Properly prepare patient.
> • Obtain survey radiographs.
> • Give correct dose.
> • Follow proper procedure.
> • Monitor, monitor, monitor.

Normal Radiographic Anatomy of the Urinary Tract

Review the anatomy of the kidneys, bladder, urethra, and prostate found in Chapter 18.

Excretory urograms allow further quantitative measurements of the kidney and proximal ureters. The cortex is more radiopaque than the medulla in the early nephrogram phase. Generally the pyelogram is more radiopaque than the nephrogram. The normal nephrogram is most radiopaque within 10 to 30 seconds after administration of a bolus injection of contrast medium.[4] The pyelogram should be consistently opaque. The ureter width varies because of peristalsis. The normal bladder wall is about 1 mm thick regardless of the amount of distention.[4]

Prostate enlargement can be viewed on a survey radiograph as a soft tissue mass in the caudal abdomen. The displacement of the bladder due to prostatomegaly is more obvious with positive-contrast media.

Additional Techniques

Myelography[4,5]

Myelography (Figure 25-23) is the placement of an injection of radiopaque contrast agent into the subarachnoid space in either the cerebellomedullary cistern or the lumbar region for evaluation of the spinal cord. Computerized tomography (CT) and MRI are replacing the use of myelography for spinal evaluation in many practices because they are quicker and noninvasive.

Indications

Myelography helps localize and identify the cause of suspected transverse spinal myelopathy, such as the size of the lesion or the extent of cord compression. The location helps determine prognosis and course of treatment. Specific indications for myelography include paresis, paralysis, proprioceptive or sensory deficit, and spinal pain thought to be due to a transverse myelopathy.

Precautions

General anesthesia is required; any contraindications need to be evaluated. The cerebrospinal fluid (CSF) should be examined to check that there is no systemic or local infection such as myelitis or meningitis. The needle must be placed through an aseptic site. The anesthetic regimen should not

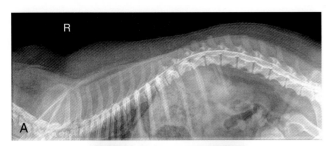

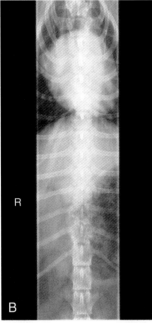

FIGURE 25-23 A, Lateral projection during myelography study. B, Ventrodorsal view during a myelography study.

include a phenothiazine derivative, which might lower the seizure threshold. Corticosteroids should not be administered intrathecally with the contrast agent. The animal should be adequately hydrated to help minimize side effects and complications due to delayed elimination of contrast medium from the subarachnoid space. Incorrect procedure can cause trauma and have fatal consequences. Myelography may also cause intensification of pre-existing neurological signs.

Contrast Media and Dosage
Organic nonionic positive-contrast iodine: iopamidol (Isovue®), 200 mg/mL, or iohexol (Omnipaque), 240 mg/mL.

Dosage for the dog:[5]
- 0.45 mL/kg to outline the entire spine; does depend on patient and nutritional status
- 0.30 mL/kg to study the cervical spine; does depend on patient and status

Dosage for the cat:
- 0.30 mL/kg for cervical study
- 0. 45 mL/kg for cervicothoracic study
- 0. 60 mL/kg for complete spinal study

Equipment/Supplies
- Clippers, scrub solutions, drape, sterile gloves.
- Dog: 20-gauge spinal needle with a flat bevel, 2–4 inches in length; two 10-mL syringes.
- Cat: 22-gauge spinal needle with a flat bevel, 1½ inches in length; two 5-mL syringes.
- Two 10 mL syringes for the dog and two 5 mL syringes for the cat. 18-gauge 1-inch needle, 3-mL syringe to collect cerebrospinal fluid.
- CSF collection tube, extension set, 0.22-μ nucleopore (Millipore) filter.

Survey
Lateral and ventrodorsal noncontrast studies of the entire spine collimated sharply over the area of interest—cervical, thoracic, thoracolumbar, or lumbar vertebrae (see Chapter 22 for positioning guidelines).

Patient Preparation
- Use general anesthetic without a phenothiazine derivative.
- Shave the hair caudal to the skull (for cisternal) or over the lumbar spine (lumbar), and complete three scrubs.

> **TECHNICIAN NOTES** Keep in mind the suggestions for minimizing reactions to contrast media injections as described in the Technician Notes box for excretory urography.

Procedure
For actual positioning of the needle, please consult more complete references. The veterinarian will usually perform the injection and administration of the agent.

1. After obtaining the survey radiographs and anesthetizing the patient, aseptically prepare the region by shaving a 4-inch (10-cm) square; complete a surgical scrub and drape as follows:
   a. For cervical myelography: caudal to external occipital protuberance
   b. For lumbar myelography: L5-L6.
2. Position the patient in perfect lateral recumbency with the aid of sandbags or foam sponges.
3. For cervical myelography:
   a. The head should be positioned in maximum ventral flexion (chin touching the sternum) with the aid of sandbags or foam pads, so that the midline of the head and neck are parallel to the table. The table can be tilted at 10 degrees with the patient's head at the raised end.
   b. With the stylet in place, insert the needle into the cerebellomedullary cistern through the atlantooccipital space.
4. For lumbar myelography:
   a. Flex the pelvic limbs forward so the feet are along the abdomen. Sandbag in place.
   b. With the stylet in place, insert the needle into the subarachnoid space.

5. Withdraw CSF, in a volume that is at least equal to the volume of contrast agent to be injected.
6. Slowly inject the contrast medium as follows:
   a. For cervical myelography: over 3 to 4 minutes, and remove the needle.
   b. For lumbar myelography: over 5 minutes. Keep the capped needle in place.
7. Rotate the patient to ensure equal mixing of contrast agent and CSF.
8. For cervical myelography:
   a. Keep the head elevated for a few minutes to allow contrast medium to flow caudally. The head may also need to be massaged.
   b. A lateral radiograph can confirm the location of the contrast volumes. Take lateral views beginning at the site of injection and move caudally.
   c. When contrast medium has reached the main area of interest, complete further lateral ventrodorsal and oblique radiographs for accurate identification and location of the lesion.
9. For lumbar myelography:
   a. Once the CSF has been collected and the contrast medium injected, the capped needle should remain in place while the lateral view is made. This prevents the contrast from leaking into the needle tract and the epidural space.
   b. Upon completion of the lateral view, remove the needle and immediately take the ventrodorsal view.[3]
10. Keeping the patient under general anesthesia for about an hour after injection lessens the frequency of post-myelography convulsions. Keep the head raised during recovery to prevent contrast medium from flowing into the ventricles of the brain, increasing the pressure and the risk of convulsions.

Comments and Tips

- The patient can remain in sternal recumbency for either injection. This position makes it more difficult to determine the depth of the needle, which is better evaluated and radiographed in the lateral position.
- Cautions for positioning of the needle for the cerebello-medullary cistern through the atlanto-occipital space:
  - Incorrect lateral positioning would puncture the vertebral sinus and cause bleeding.
  - Incorrect cranial positioning may put the tip in the hind brain, causing respiratory collapse and death.
  - Any movement during positioning may lacerate the spinal cord or medulla.
- If the needle position is accurate for the cervical injection, the most common problem is that the contrast medium does not flow caudally to fully visualize the lesion:
  - The contrast medium flows rostrally into the ventricular system when resistance to caudal flow is met, so only the cranial margin of a compressive lesion may be identified.
  - Positioning the head up during the injection or after removal of the spinal needle and massaging the neck may assist in the flow.

- Cervical myelography is not likely diagnostic if there is severe thoracolumbar cord swelling.
- There is less danger in incorrect positioning of the needle for lumbar myelography:
  - Lateral placement punctures the venous sinuses, creating a bloody tap and compromising the interpretation of the CSF.
  - The most common problem with lumbar punctures is the injection of the contrast agent into the epidural space and/or into the venous sinuses.
  - Extradural passage of contrast agent decreases the amount available in the subarachnoid space.
- If there is a bloody tap, do not inject the contrast agent, because the mixture of blood and contrast agent is highly irritative in the subarachnoid space.
- If post-myelography convulsions occur, intravenous diazepam in therapeutic doses is recommended. If this is not effective, intravenous barbiturates are suggested.

> **TECHNICIAN NOTES**   Quick review of myelography:
> 1. Prepare the patient, including fasting, enema (if required), survey radiographs, general anesthesia, and shaving and scrubbing of the site. Follow proper aseptic technique.
> 2. Have everything ready.
> 3. Place the needle; remove CSF, and slowly inject warmed organic nonionic positive-contrast iodine.
> 4. Obtain the required lateral, VD, and oblique radiographs.
> 5. Recover the animal when appropriate.

Further Contrast Studies

Table 25-5 gives a brief overview of additional contrast radiography techniques, many of which have been replaced by ultrasound or other modalities. See other sources for more complete information.

Contrast Agents Used for Other Modalities

Ultrasound

Many substances may act as contrast agents in ultrasonography. Orally ingested fluid may expel gas from the stomach and create an acoustic window to the pancreas. Echo-free fluids such as water and saline may distend body cavities to improve visualization of the luminal walls. Contrast media for intravenous use have been limited to encapsulated microbubbles, which may produce up to a 25-dB increase in echo strength. They are generally used in Doppler ultrasonography of the heart.

Computed Tomography

Generally, the nonionic contrast agents used in radiographic contrast studies are used in CT.

TABLE 25-5	Additional Contrast Radiography Techniques		
STUDY	AGENT(S) USED	INDICATION/PROCEDURE	COMMENTS
Angiocardiography (nonselective) (selective study is direct injection into the right ventricle)	Water-soluble organic iodide.	Inject into the cephalic or jugular vein to obtain information on cardiac abnormalities such as occlusion of a particular blood vessel, to demonstrate pathological lesions of the vascular system, or to provide evidence of a tumor noted on the survey.	Sedation or anesthesia usually required. Fluoroscopy or a method of rapidly exposing multiple images is recommended because a series of radiographs is to be taken every second.
Arthrography	Water-soluble organic iodide—nonionic low-osmolar agent. Pneumoarthrogram can be completed with carbon dioxide or nitrous oxide, which is preferred to air which could cause an air embolism. CO_2 is resorbed much more quickly than other gases.	Injection into the synovial fluid to contrast the articular surfaces and joint capsule. An arthrogram can be used to evaluate a ruptured joint capsule, the presence of a cartilaginous flap, meniscal injuries, or the necessity for surgery.	Dilute with sterile saline to a concentration of 20%-40%. General anesthesia and a surgically prepared 8 × 8-cm area is required. Contraindicated if there is infection of surrounding soft tissues.
Bronchography	Nonionic water-soluble iodine.	Tracheobronchial lesions that cause coughing or dyspnea.	CT and MRI have displaced this procedure.
Celiography—positive-contrast	Water-soluble organic iodide.	Evaluates the abdominal cavity and the integrity of the diaphragm often to determine a diaphragmatic hernia.	Surgical preparation of the site just caudal to the umbilicus.
Fistulography	Water-soluble organic iodide (preferred) or negative contrast media.	Evaluates the extent of fistulous tracts. Will detect radiolucent foreign bodies. Infuse into the fistulous tract with a syringe and flexible catheter, preferably one with a balloon tip.	Infection in the area may disseminate into the site. Often the site of the wound is distant from the site of drainage.
Pneumoperitoneography, peritoneography, herniography (generally replaced by computerized tomography [CT], magnetic resonance imaging [MRI], or ultrasound.)	Negative contrast media with carbon dioxide and nitrous oxide are preferred gases because of their more rapid absorption in the body. Room air also has an increased incidence of air embolism.	Evaluates the abdominal cavity and integrity of the diaphragm. Often used to determine a diaphragmatic hernia. A horizontal beam should be used. The gas does not need to be removed.	Sedation is usually required. Surgical preparation caudal to the umbilicus is required. Use a stylet and syringe. Fasting and a full bladder are suggested.

Magnetic Resonance Imaging

In cases in which it is difficult to differentiate between two types of tissue on MRI, the solution is to add a contrast agent to one of them. An MRI contrast agent works by affecting the time it takes for the hydrogen atoms to return to their original energy state. This increases the difference in the signal intensity from the two types of tissue, thus increasing the degree of contrast on the image. The contrast medium becomes evenly distributed in the blood and is then washed out by the kidneys. Most MRI contrast media contain the heavy metal gadolinium encapsulated in a chelate that makes it less toxic. Sometimes the gadolinium is given midway through the MRI session by injection into a vein to highlight areas of tumor or inflammation.

All gadolinium chelates are administered intravenously. Each injection of gadolinium is followed by a saline flush. The rate of injection should be slower than 10 mL per minute.

Some gadolinium products in common use today are as follows:

- Gadopentetate dimeglumine (Magnevist)
- Gadoteridol injection (ProHance)
- Gadodiamide injection (Omniscan)
- Gadobutrol (Gadovist)

Positron Emission Tomography and Nuclear Medicine Imaging Agents

Nuclear imaging (or scintigraphy) requires use of radioactive contrast agents (called radiopharmaceuticals) to obtain images. Some agents used for positron emission tomography (PET) provide information about tissue metabolism or some other specific molecular activity. The most commonly used agent in veterinary medicine is technetium 99mTc, which is used to radiolabel many different common radiopharmaceuticals. It is used most often in bone and heart scans. See Chapter 15 for further information.

KEY POINTS

1. Contrast medium changes the density or atomic number of a tissue or organ, making it more visible on imaging.
2. Positive-contrast medium has a greater atomic number than the elements of soft tissue and bone, and it is denser. Thus, agents such as barium, atomic number 56, attenuate the x-rays to a greater degree, absorb more x-rays, and create a whiter image on the radiograph.
3. Negative-contrast media have lower atomic numbers and are less dense than soft tissue, so the x-rays will not be attenuated. X-rays pass through more easily, causing a black image to appear on the radiograph. Carbon dioxide and nitrous are the negative-contrast agents of choice, because according to literature room air can create air emboli.
4. Double-contrast studies utilize both positive- and negative-contrast agents. Depending on the study, the negative-contrast medium is often administered first and the positive-contrast agent second.
5. A contrast study is generally more effective for determining the change in morphology than for determining the function of an organ.
6. There is a risk involved in any contrast study. The benefits of and contraindications to the patient, need to be weighed by the veterinarian.
7. Various dilutions of barium sulfate suspension are the most commonly used positive-contrast agent for gastrointestinal studies.
8. Barium should not be used if there is a suspected perforation, because barium is physiologically inert. It resists dilution in the peritoneal cavity and is completely insoluble. If it were leaked into the peritoneal cavity, a granuloma or adhesions may occur. Barium should never be injected intravenously.
9. Water-soluble organic iodides can be used if there is suspected intestinal perforation. They have a rapid transit time, are readily absorbed from the peritoneal cavity across the mucosa, and are excreted by the kidney.
10. Water-soluble organic ionic iodine is hypertonic and can cause electrolyte imbalance, dehydration, nausea, vomiting, decreased blood pressure, and other physiological problems.
11. Water-soluble organic nonionic iodine with a dimer chemical structure is almost isotonic to blood and cerebral fluid and has fewer side effects than ionic iodine.
12. Patient and other preparation is essential for the full benefit of the contrast study to be obtained. Depending on the study, this could include fasting, enema administration, and/or sedation. Make sure that the correct concentration in sufficient amount is given and that enough radiographs are made at the appropriate times. Have image receptors, markers, timers, protective apparel, etc. ready prior to the administration of the contrast agent.
13. Survey radiographs before the administration of the contrast agent are essential for ensuring that the correct exposure is made, that patient preparation is adequate, and that the contrast study still needs to be completed.
14. Keep in mind that with the addition of positive-contrast medium, kVp may have to be raised slightly. With the administration of negative-contrast medium, kVp may have to be lowered slightly.
15. The actual procedure and radiographs taken are dictated by the clinical signs in the patient and by the veterinarian's assessment. Only one area may need to be evaluated or a full-system contrast study may be required.
16. Ultrasound and other imaging modalities, when available, have replaced contrast radiography for many evaluations.
17. The nonionic contrast agents used for radiography are generally used for computerized tomography. Gadolinium can be used for magnetic resonance imaging, and radiopharmaceuticals are used for positron emission tomography or nuclear medicine imaging.

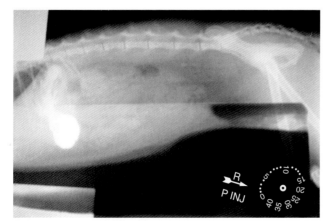

FIGURE 25-24 Mystery radiograph: Why is there a difference in density on the lower portion of the radiograph?

Acknowledgements

Special thanks to Evelyn Kelly, RN, AC(R), MRT(R) BSc, MA, for her assistance with the chapter.

References

1. Kelly EA: Ontario Association of Medical Radiation Technologists (OAMRT): Intravenous contrast injection for medical radiation technologists & related allied health professionals, revised November 2010. File No: 4010-4036. Ontario Association of Medical Radiation Technologists
2. American Society of Health-System Pharmacists: Quick guide to contrast media, 2010. http://www.ashp.org/Import/PRACTICEANDPOLICY/PracticeResourceCenters/ContrastMedia/QuickGuidetoContrastMedia.aspx.
3. Han C, Hurd C: *Practical diagnostic imaging for the veterinary technician*, ed 3, St. Louis, 2005, Mosby.
4. Thrall DE: *Textbook of veterinary diagnostic radiology*, ed 5, St. Louis, 2007, Saunders.

5. Morgan JP: *Techniques of veterinary radiography*, Ames, Iowa, 1993, Iowa State University Press.
6. Medical ID Systems, Inc: BIPS Manual. Published 2008. http://www.medid.com/manual_bipers.pdf.
7. Randano V: UGI-stomach-ohiostate.htm/Veterinary Radiography. In Proceedings of the Ontario Association of Veterinary Technician Conference, Toronto, February 2005.
8. Lester NV, Roberts GD, Newell SM, et al: Assessment of barium impregnated polyethylene spheres (BIPS) as a measure of solid-phase gastric emptying in normal dogs—comparison to scintigraphy, *Vet Radiol Ultrasound* 40:465-471, 1999.
9. Goggin JM, Hoskinson JJ, Kirk CA, et al: Comparison of gastric emptying times in healthy cats simultaneously evaluated with radiopaque markers and nuclear scintigraphy, *Vet Radiol Ultrasound* 40:89-95, 1999.
10. Wyse CA, McLellan J, Dickie AM, et al: A review of methods for assessment of the rate of gastric emptying in the dog and cat: 1898-2002, *J Vet Intern Med* 17:609-621, 2003.

Bibliography

Kelly EA: Ontario Association of Medical Radiation Technologists (OAMRT): Intravenous contrast injection for medical radiation technologists & related allied health professionals, revised November 2010. File No: 4010-4036. Ontario Association of Medical Radiation Technologists.

American College of Radiology Imaging Network: About imaging exams and agents. Published 2011. http://www.acrin.org/PATIENTS/ABOUTIMAGINGEXAMSANDAGENTS/ABOUTIMAGINGAGENTSORTRACERS.aspx.

Carrig CB: The use of compression in abdominal radiography of the dog and cat, *Vet Radiol* 17:178-181, 1976.

Colville T, Bassert J: *Clinical anatomy and physiology for veterinary technicians*, St. Louis, 2008, Elsevier.

Done SH, Goody PC, Stickland NC, Evans SA: *Color atlas of veterinary anatomy, the dog and cat*, London, 2009, Mosby.

Douglas SW: *Principles of veterinary radiography*, London, 1980, Bailliere Tindall.

Dyce KM, Sack WO, Wensing CJG: *Textbook of veterinary anatomy*, ed 4, St. Louis, 2010, Saunders.

Evans H, de Lahunta A: *Guide to the dissection of the dog*, ed 7, St. Louis, 2010, Saunders.

Lavin L: *Radiography in veterinary technology*, ed 3, St. Louis, 2007, Saunders.

Lester NV, Roberts GD, Newell SM, et al: Assessment of barium impregnated spheres (BIPS) as a measure of solid-phase gastric emptying in normal dogs-comparison to scintigraphy, *Vet Radiol Ultrasound* 40:465-471, 1999.

Owens JM, Biery DN: *Radiographic interpretation for the small animal clinician*, ed 2, Baltimore, 1999, Williams & Wilkins.

Sirois M, Anthony, Mauragis D: *Handbook of radiographic positioning for veterinary technicians*, Clifton Park, NY, 2010, Delmar Cengage Learning.

Solomon R: Role of osmolality in the incidence of contrast induced nephropathy: A systemic review of angiographic contrast media in high risk patients, *Kidney Int* 68:2257, 2005.

Tighe M, Brown M: Mosby's comprehensive review for veterinary technicians, ed 3, St. Louis, 2008, Mosby.

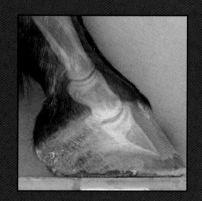

Equine and Large Animal Radiography

Marg Brown, RVT, BEd Ad Ed, and Shannon Brownrigg, RVT

*A horse is the projection of peoples' dreams about themselves—
strong, powerful, and beautiful—and it has the capability of giving us
escape from our mundane existence.*

—Pam Brown, Australian Poet, 1948—

LEARNING OBJECTIVES

When you have finished this chapter, you will be able to:

1. Have an understanding of the terminology used in equine and large animal radiography.
2. Identify skeletal anatomy.
3. Produce a diagnostic radiograph for common radiographic procedures of the equine/large animal patient, using proper safety and positioning techniques.
4. Be familiar with the less common views.
5. Identify normal equine and large animal anatomy found on a radiograph.

Imaging large animals requires good planning prior to taking the radiograph(s), good teamwork, and lots of patience. Be prepared to expect the unexpected. The common principles of radiography that apply to small animals also apply to large animals with the major differences being size and posture, which necessitate special consideration for areas of patient restraint, equipment, preparation, radiation safety and positioning devices. Safety of personnel and patient is critical.

Compare the large animal anatomy with human and small animal anatomy to familiarize yourself (Figure 26-1). The technical terms are similar but common terms differ.

Special Considerations

Restraint and Patient Preparation

Proper patient preparation is essential to obtain high-quality radiographs and to minimize radiation exposure. Large animals can easily become startled when confronted with unfamiliar objects, so it is important to minimize sudden movements and loud noises. Movement artifacts, poor positioning of the patient or the x-ray beam, and inadequate exposure are the most common reasons that radiographs must be repeated. Among other inconveniences, any repetition means further radiation dose for the restrainer or the patient.

Large animals in the standing position, are minimally restrained, which is cause for concern for human and machine safety. Sedation can help calm the animal and curtail startling it to help diminish movement blur. Keep the behavior of the particular patient in mind, and modify your restraint to take advantage of that behavior. Depending on the patient, consider raising the opposite limb, using a twitch, offering food, or using stocks, among other strategies. To help minimize repeat radiographs, take the time to make sure that the patient is properly positioned, the image receptor is properly placed, and the central ray is properly directed.

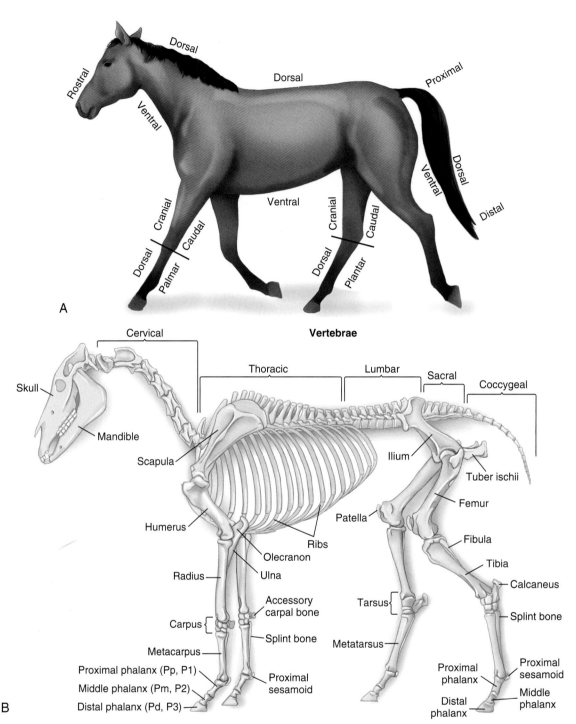

A

B

FIGURE 26-1 A, Key terms used in radiography. B, Equine skeleton.

> **TECHNICIAN NOTES** Debris such as shavings, mud, sand, small stones, and manure may cause radiographic artifacts. Visually inspect and clean the legs and hooves well before performing radiographs of the area.

The hair coat should be dry, brushed, and cleared of dirt or other debris. If the foot is being radiographed, it is important to prevent overlying shadows superimposed on the field of view. This is especially true of dorsopalmar/dorsoplantar and oblique views. Remove the shoe and trim back any overgrown portions of the foot. Pick and thoroughly clean the sole and clefts, and then pack the sulci adjacent to and in the center of the frog with a substance of similar radiographic opacity, such as Play-Doh, methylcellulose, or softened soap, to eliminate gas shadows caused by the grooves of the frog (Figure 26-2).

> **TECHNICIAN NOTES** A piece of paper, plastic wrap, paper towel, or dry gauze is suitable to keep the packing material from picking up particles. Try brown paper bags, craft paper, or sandwich bags, depending on the size of the foot.

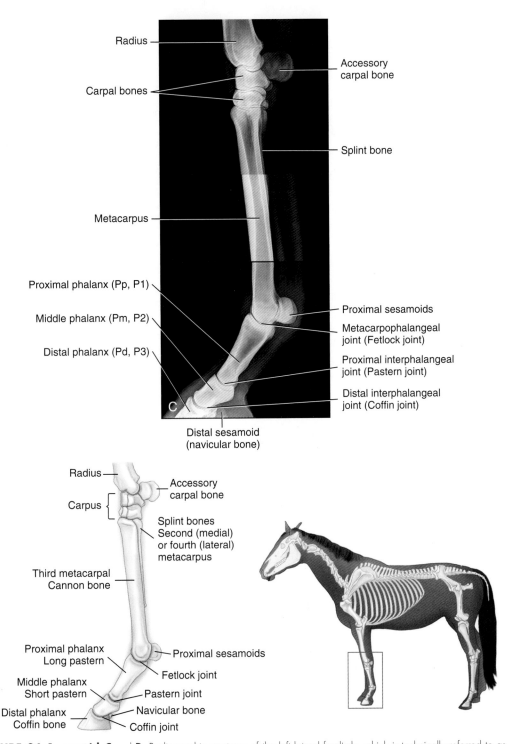

FIGURE 26-1, cont'd C and D, Radiographic anatomy of the left lateral forelimb, which is technically referred to as a lateromedial view.

If film cassettes are used and radiographs are being taken off site, make sure to take enough cassettes and film to the farm to allow for "repeats" and unexpected views. For digital radiography make sure that all required equipment is included.

Radiation Safety and Positioning Devices

All of the radiation safety principles applied to small animals also apply to large animals. When working with large animals, concern for physical safety often supersedes radiation concerns. It is essential to keep the three tenets of radiation safety in mind (shielding, distance, and time) at all times.

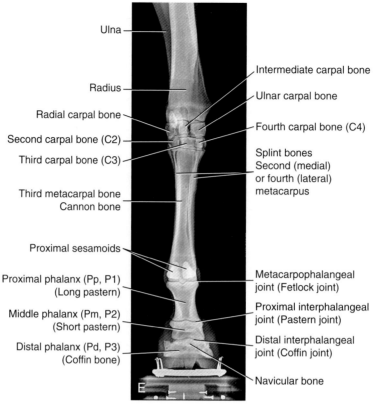

Ulna

Intermediate carpal bone

Radius

Ulnar carpal bone

Radial carpal bone

Fourth carpal bone (C4)

Second carpal bone (C2)

Third carpal bone (C3)

Splint bones
Second (medial)
or fourth (lateral)
metacarpus

Third metacarpal bone
Cannon bone

Proximal sesamoids

Metacarpophalangeal
joint (Fetlock joint)

Proximal phalanx (Pp, P1)
(Long pastern)

Proximal interphalangeal
joint (Pastern joint)

Middle phalanx (Pm, P2)
(Short pastern)

Distal phalanx (Pd, P3)
(Coffin bone)

Distal interphalangeal
joint (Coffin joint)

Navicular bone

E

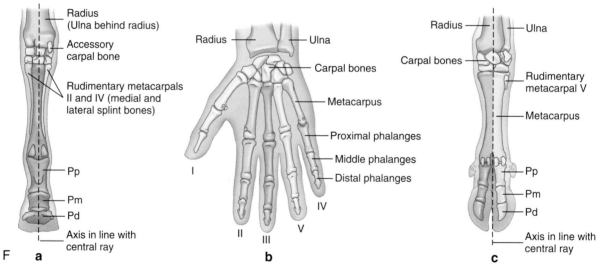

Radius
(Ulna behind radius)

Accessory
carpal bone

Rudimentary metacarpals
II and IV (medial and
lateral splint bones)

Pp

Pm

Pd

Axis in line with
central ray

F   a

Radius

Ulna

Carpal bones

Metacarpus

Proximal phalanges

Middle phalanges

Distal phalanges

I

II

III

IV

V

b

Radius

Ulna

Carpal bones

Rudimentary
metacarpal V

Metacarpus

Pp

Pm

Pd

Axis in line with
central ray

c

FIGURE 26-1, cont'd E, Radiographic anatomy of the DP or dorsopalmar (dorsoproximal-palmarodistal) of left fore-limb. F, Comparison of the palmar views of the (a) horse's limb, (b) human hand, and (c) ruminant's limb.

The extensive use of portable machines, such as those used in large animals, can be particularly dangerous with regards to radiation exposure. These machines can be aimed in any direction, and because of their limited power, they must use longer exposure times to produce diagnostic images. Caution must be taken to ensure no one is in the path of the primary beam. It is critical to wear a lead apron and gloves when holding the portable radiograph machine.[1]

Any assistants who will be near or in the path of the beam must have appropriate protective lead attire and a radiation dosimeter. The human positioning during radiographs can cause protective wear to shift. Thus a conscious effort to ensure proper fitting and positioning of protective gear must be made at all times during large animal radiographs. The most significant safety action is to increase one's distance from the primary beam through the use of a cassette holder (Figure 26-3). Avoid holding image receptors directly in your gloved hand.

Because the construction of x-ray machines does not allow the primary beam to be centered less than about 10 cm from the ground, a positioning block may need to be used to raise the affected foot (Figure 26-4). This is especially true

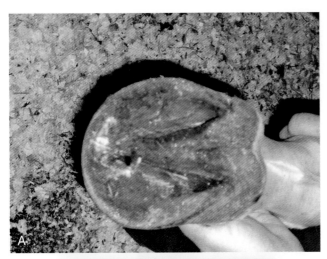

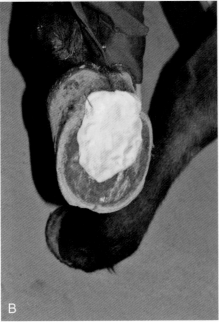

FIGURE 26-2 For diagnostic radiographs of the distal foot the shoe should be removed, and the sole cleaned (**A**) then packed with a radiolucent material (**B**).

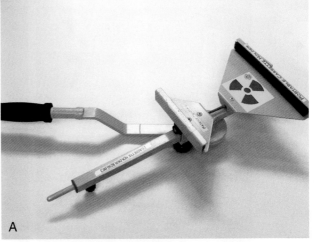

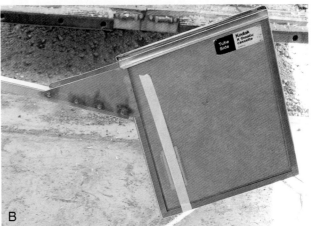

FIGURE 26-3 **A** and **B**, Commercial cassette holders used for equine positioning.

for the lateromedial view of the foot. A cassette tunnel is also useful for digit radiographs to protect the image receptors for dorsopalmar or dorsoplantar and oblique views of the foot. A cassette tunnel can be purchased or can be manufactured out of radiolucent wood (avoid use of nails) or hard plastic durable enough to withstand the weight of the horse.

Make sure that the primary beam is collimated to include only the area of interest. All margins of the primary beam should be visible on the processed film. Because a horizontal beam is standard for many radiographic positions, always be conscious of where the beam is directed.

To help decrease exposure time, use a fast combination of film and screen. The source-image distance (SID) is generally less for large animals, with the common SID being 26 to 30 inches, compared with 40 inches in radiography of small animals. Shorter SID also helps decrease the exposure time.

All personal protective equipment (PPE) must undergo a routine maintenance schedule to evaluate weaknesses and breakage. Proper storage of PPE is important; avoid folding gowns and gloves.

> **TECHNICIAN NOTES** *ALWAYS* keep the three principles of radiation safety in mind—time, distance and shielding when imaging large animals.

Equipment

Of the three types of x-ray machines available—portable, mobile, and ceiling-mounted—the portable unit is the most practical for those in ambulatory practices. Portable units are small and can be set up wherever there is a power supply. Depending on the type of unit, the kilovoltage peak (kVp) and milliampere (mA) are generally preset, giving power anywhere from 40 to 120 kVp and 15 to 100 mA. Time is usually the variable control, providing milliampere-seconds (mAs) values of 0.3 to 100. Newer units have variable kV and mAs. The digital displays

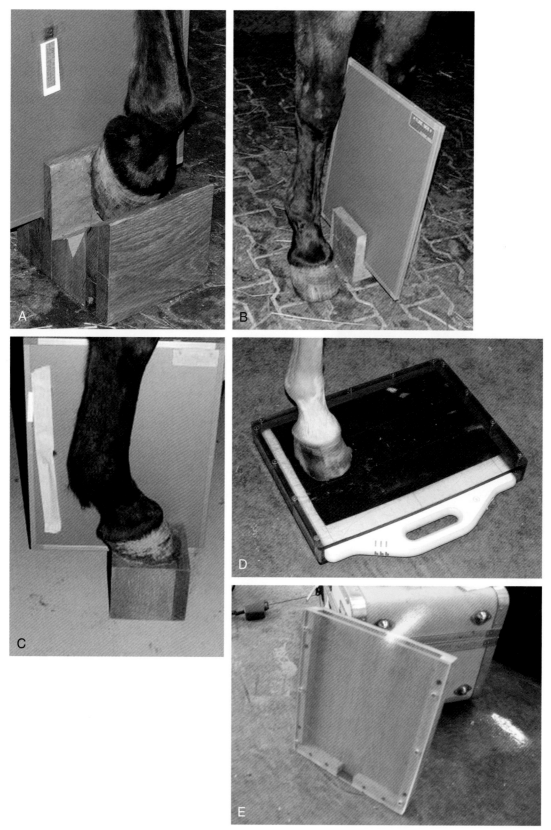

FIGURE 26-4 An example of positioning devices used to hold the cassette. **A,** Used for the upright pedal route DP positions. **B,** Ideal for lateral views of the metacarpus. **C,** Use for the lateral phalanx and sesamoids. The block can be rotated for a DP weight-bearing view so the beam is parallel to the ground. **D,** Use of a radiolucent cassette tunnel for the digital plate. **E,** Homemade cassette tunnel for film cassette.

allow adjustments of 1 kV to 5 kV increments. These units are generally adequate for radiography of the equine distal limbs, skull, and cranial cervical vertebrae. Disadvantages of these units are the relatively low mA capacity, making movement more of a concern. Line voltage may also vary, causing inconsistency in the exposures. It may be difficult to see the field of collimation in well-lit areas leading to increased radiation to personnel.

Although the portable equipment is built to withstand a certain amount of rough handling, transportation and frequent movement of radiographic equipment increase the opportunity for damage to x-ray equipment. The unit should never be left in the vehicle overnight during below freezing temperatures unless a sufficient warm up time is taken into consideration prior to the first exposure.

Mobile units can be wheeled from room to room in the same premises, but are generally too cumbersome to be easily moved and transported. The kVp and mA capacity is higher, allowing for shorter exposure times and less chance of blurring than with the portable units.

Veterinary specialty referral practices commonly use large permanently mounted ceiling units on a set of ceiling rails, to allow horizontal and vertical movement. It may be difficult to obtain parallel views of the feet because the unit may not reach the ground close enough to prevent obliquity. A supplementary portable unit is often used in these situations. These high capacity units have the greatest output range (between 800 to 1000 mA), capable of obtaining good quality radiographs of regions such as the chest, pelvis, and thoracolumbar vertebrae.

Regular maintenance and calibration of all x-ray units are essential to the production of quality radiographs and maintenance of a safe working environment. Inspections should be implemented as per local regulations.

See Chapter 9 for further information on digital equipment.

> **TECHNICIAN NOTES** Electrical power may vary in different barn settings. Power may not have the consistency (brown-outs) to produce quality radiographs. Have suitable and safety-approved extension cord(s) for exterior use as part of your equipment list. Cords with optimum length are best (the shorter the better).

Equine Radiography

Radiographic Interpretation and Diagnosis

Keep the same principles in mind as when viewing radiographs of small animals:

- The proximal end of the extremity is at the top of the viewer for DP/PD/CrCd/CdCr views. For the lateral or oblique radiographs, it points up and the cranial or dorsal aspect of the limb is to your left.
- You should have an understanding of the normal anatomy.

- Use a systematic approach making sure to view the whole film.
- Review the radiography check list found in Chapter 17.

The purpose of most radiographs taken in equine practice is to evaluate the bones of the skeleton; thus, any response of the bone to insult or disease is relevant. Any changes such as sclerosis (causing more of a radiopaque image) or demineralization (radiolucent appearance) may not be visible on the radiograph because a change of at least 30% in the bone mineral matrix is required before radiographic changes are evident.[2]

Consideration may need to be given to additional imaging for accurate diagnosis and prognosis. This would include ultrasonography as well as cross-sectional imaging modalities such as computerized tomography (CT), magnetic resource imaging (MRI), scintigraphy, and further diagnostic testing. Modalities such as nuclear scintigraphy and thermography not only show subtle changes to the bone but also demonstrate soft tissue, such as ligaments, tendons, and articular cartilage, that are poorly imaged on radiographs (Figure 26-60).

Pre-Purchase Examinations

Equine clients often request a pre-purchase examination of a horse prior to buying a competitive or breeding prospect. This examination is to reduce the buyer's risk and assess the current health and athletic soundness of the horse. The examination is not a guarantee of the health or soundness of the horse, but an interpretation of the ability of the horse to meet the intended purpose of the procurer.

Depending on the level of expected performance or value of the purchase, this examination may include extensive radiographs. It is critical for all parties to identify any potential conflict of interest that may exist. The veterinarian requested to perform such an examination must clearly identify his or her relationship with or prior knowledge of the horse, and its owners or trainers, to be purchased. It is recommended to have a legal agreement prepared and signed, that clearly identifies any relationship or knowledge, to protect the interest of the performing veterinarian.

> **TECHNICIAN NOTES** Unless otherwise indicated, when the limb is described the forelimb terminology is used, but it is understood that the same principles apply to the hind limb.

Labeling and Terminology

For proper diagnosis and legal requirements, correct labeling is mandatory. As with radiography of small animals, permanent identification of the patient and owner (or purchaser for a pre-purchase examination) is required. The specific limb being radiographed should also be identified, as well as the actual position. This includes indicating forelimbs and hind limbs, especially distal to the carpus/tarsus.

Conventionally, limb markers should be placed dorsally or laterally. If there is a swelling on the limb, a marker such as a BB pellet taped on the skin might be useful.

Because equine skeletal structures are large and complex, multiple views are required. Refer to Chapter 17 for a review of some of the basic terminology. In small animals, generally two views perpendicular to each other are taken. Horses generally require a minimum of four views for most positions, and six for many joints.

> **TECHNICIAN NOTES**   Here is a short review of the terms you should be familiar with especially in reference to equines (Figure 26-1):
> - Dorsal, palmar and plantar, cranial, and caudal: Remember these terms take precedence when combined with other terms.
> - From point of entrance of the beam to point of exit is how radiographic projections should be described.
> - Terminology of the limbs proximal to the tarsus and carpus is cranial (the part of the body facing the head) or caudal (the part of the body facing the tail).
> - Distal to and including the carpus and tarsus, the terms are dorsal (the part of the body facing the head) and palmar (front limb facing the tail) or plantar (hind limb facing the tail).
> - Oblique: Not parallel to one of the two major directional axes (Figure 26-5, Figure 17-3).
> - Tangenital or skyline. Refers to the central ray entering and exiting the same side of the limb so that the bone is in profile.
> - In those views requiring a combination of directional terms, a hyphen should be inserted to separate the point of entry and point of exit. Example: palmaroproximal-palmarodistal (PaPr-PaDi).

> **TECHNICIAN NOTES**   The lateromedial and dorso-palmar (plantar) views evaluate only 50% of the limb. Further views are required for proper diagnosis. These views are known as oblique views and are obtained with the radiographic beam at an angle to the midsagittal plane of the limb (between dorsal and lateral/medial).

Dorsolateral-Palmaromedial Oblique (DLPMO)

For the dorsolateral-palmaromedial oblique (DLPMO) or medial oblique view (Figure 26-6B), the central ray faces the dorsal part of the limb aimed 45 degrees laterally from the midline. The image receptor is on the palmaromedial aspect of the limb so that it is perpendicular to the beam. Remember "point of entry to point of exit"; the beam travels from dorsolateral to palmaromedial. The film marker is placed along the lateral aspect of the image receptor and appears to be along the palmar aspect of the limb in the radiograph. So that there is no confusion as to what angle should be used, the proper description for this 45-degree DLPMO view is dorsoproximal 45-degree lateral palmarodistomedial oblique (DPrL45-PaMO).

What is actually being highlighted on this medial oblique projection is the opposite bone that is being radiographed, specifically the lateral portion. To be more technical, specifically, it is the dorsomedial and palmarolateral surfaces of the limb (*red lines* on Figure 26-6B). This might seem confusing because it is the surface opposite to the name of the view. But keep in mind that the side that is closer to the film will be hidden behind the bone, allowing the projection farther from the film to be in profile. The radiograph is like a shadow–the way the beam is directed, the part on the film is superimposed, but the opposite edges are highlighted.

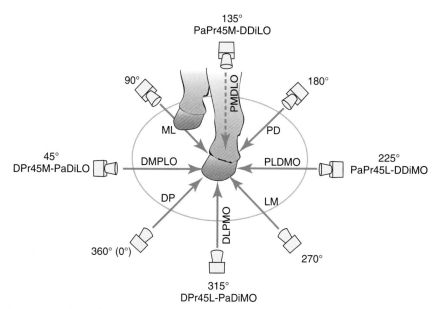

FIGURE 26-5 Terminology of the equine proximal limb views. Inner circle: Common terminology and angles. Outer circle: proper directional terms for the oblique views taken at the level of the metacarpus. P and Pa, palmar; D, dorsal; Pr, proximal; Di, distal; M, medial; L, lateral; O, oblique.

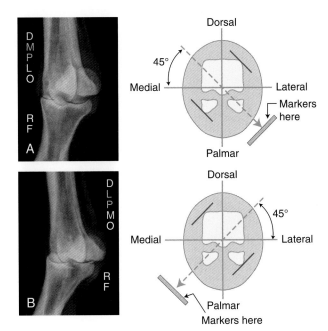

FIGURE 26-6 Description of the terminology of the oblique views on a fetlock radiograph. The dotted lines are the direction of the beam and the red lines are the surfaces of the limbs being imaged. **A,** Lateral oblique or dorsoproximal 45-degree medial–palmarodistolateral oblique (DPr45M-PaDiLO). Following the rule and taking the middle two and outer two letters, you are looking at the dorsolateral and palmaromedial surfaces of the limb/medial sesamoid. **B,** Medial oblique or dorsoproximal 45-degree lateral–palmarodistomedial oblique (DPr45L-PaDiMO). Following the rule and taking the middle two and outer two letters, you are looking at the dorsomedial and palmarolateral surfaces of the limb/lateral sesamoid.

TECHNICIAN NOTES To help remember which views are highlighted in the oblique views, look at the abbreviation for the view and ignore the "O." Take the middle two letters and then the outer two letters. In the case of DLPMO, the middle two letters are (LP) and the outer two letters are (DM). So you are looking at the dorsomedial and palmarolateral surfaces of the limb. The lateral portion, not the medial bone, is more in profile. The medial portion is against the image receptor.

Dorsomedial-Palmarolateral Oblique (DMPLO)

For the dorsomedial-palmarolateral oblique (DMPLO) or lateral oblique view (Figure 26-6A), the central ray is aimed at the dorsal part of the limb 45 degrees medially to the midline. The image receptor is on the palmarolateral aspect of the limb and is perpendicular to the beam. The beam is traveling from dorsomedial (point of entry) to palmarolateral (point of exit). The film marker is placed along the lateral aspect of the image receptor, appearing to be on the dorsal part of the limb in the radiograph. So that there is no confusion as to what angle should be used, the proper description for this 45-degree DMPLO is dorsoproximal medial 45-degree–palmarodistolateral oblique (DPrM45-PaLO).

Taking the two middle and two outer letters once the "O" is removed tells us that the dorsolateral and palmaromedial surfaces (*red lines* on Figure 26-6) will be highlighted. The medial part of the bone is in profile.

TECHNICIAN NOTES To demonstrate that the opposite projections will be in profile, tape two different objects, such as a pen and pencil, to an empty paper towel roll. Label four sides as dorsal, palmar, lateral, and medial, and place a piece of paper behind your "limb." Use your finger as the x-ray beam and try the oblique views. Notice that the opposite protrusion is in profile. Using a flashlight may also help you visualize the projections better. The radiograph is like a shadow with the way the beam is directed, the part on the film is superimposed, but the opposite edges are highlighted.

In practice, you may hear common terms that are used in lieu of the correct anatomical terms (Table 26-1). Keep in mind that these terms are for the purpose of further understanding and not necessarily the proper nomenclature. Anterior posterior, a human term, (AP) is used in practice; however, the correct nomenclature is dorsopalmar or dorsoplantar (DP).

TECHNICIAN NOTES A human middle finger is equivalent to the front foot of the horse, whereas the hind foot is basically a human's middle toe (Figure 26-7). It is no wonder the foot is the most frequently imaged for lameness issues.

Equine Radiographic Positions

Comments:
- If using a cassette tunnel, make sure it is strong enough to support the weight of the horse and is translucent to minimize artifacts on the film.
- If using a wooden block, have it high enough so that the beam can be directed in a horizontal plane on the area of interest. Ideally, the block should have a slot to support the cassette close to the limb to minimize distortion.
- For the foot, if only the lateromedial view of the digit is needed, then shoe removal, sole cleaning, and foot trimming are not required.
- For equal weight-bearing, ideally both front feet should be on a wooden block. If only the affected foot is placed on the block, the distal limb joints are extended.
- The opposite limb may need to be lifted to ensure full weight-bearing and to prevent motion if equal weight bearing is not required.
- Keep the image receptor as close and parallel to the limb as possible to minimize object-film distance (OFD) and distortion.
- Always ensure that the assistant is not standing behind the image receptor in the beam direction; a cassette holder should be used when possible.
- Collimate the beam inside the film edges.

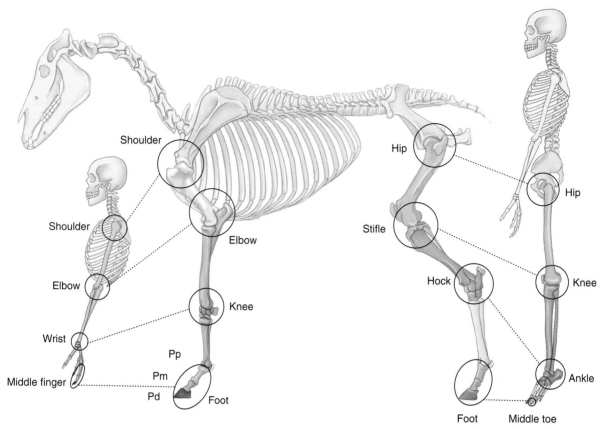

FIGURE 26-7 Comparison of human and equine skeletal structures.

TABLE 26-1	Comparative Terminology of the Human and Equine Limbs		
ANATOMICAL TERM	**FURTHER TERM/ABBREVIATION**	**COMMON LAY TERM**	**HUMAN EQUIVALENT (MIDDLE FINGER/MIDDLE TOE)**
Distal phalanx (Pd)	Third phalanx (P3)	Coffin or pedal bone	Distal phalanx (finger tip)
Distal interphalangeal joint		Coffin joint	Distal interphalangeal joint
Distal sesamoid		Navicular bone	
Middle phalanx (Pm)	Second phalanx (P2)	Short pastern	Middle phalanx
Middle interphalangeal joint		Pastern joint	Middle interphalangeal joint
Proximal phalanx (Pp)	First phalanx (P1)	Long pastern	Proximal phalanx
Proximal sesamoid bones		Fetlock	
Metacarpal interphalangeal joint		Fetlock joint	Metacarpal interphalangeal joint—knuckle
Metacarpus/metatarsus	3rd metacarpal/ metatarsal bone (M3)	Cannon bone	Metacarpus /Metatarsus
	2nd metacarpal bone/ metatarsal bone (M2)	Short splint bone	
	4th metacarpal bone/ metatarsal bone (M4)	Long splint bone	
Carpometacarpal/carpometatarsal joint		Knee joint /hock joint	Wrist joint/ankle joint
Carpus /tarsus		Knee /hock	Wrist /ankle
	Elbow/stifle		Elbow/knee
		Shoulder/hip	Shoulder/hip

TABLE 26-2 | Views of the Equine Limb Examination

STRUCTURES EVALUATED/ COMMENTS	VIEWS/COMMENTS*	COMMON TERMINOLOGY
P3	Dorsal 65-degree proximal–palmarodistal oblique (D65Pr-PaDiO); beam angled to ground, high coronary or upright pedal routes.	Dorsopalmar (DP)
	Dorsoproximal-palmarodistal (DPr-PaDi) with horizontal beam	
	Lateromedial (LM) with foot on block (optional).	Lateral (L)
	Oblique views especially if a P3 fracture is suspected:	
	(1) Dorsal 65-degree proximal, 45-degree lateral–palmarodistomedial oblique (D65Pr-45L–PaDiMO)	(1) Medial oblique or DLPMO
	(2) Dorsal 65-degree proximal, 45-degree medial–palmarodistolateral oblique (D65Pr-45M-PaDiLO)	(2) Lateral oblique or DMPLO
Distal interphalangeal joint	Dorsal 65-degree proximal–palmarodistal (D65Pr-PaDiO) high coronary route with beam angled to ground	Dorsopalmar (DP)
	Lateromedial (LM) with foot on block to include solar margin of P3 and soft tissues of sole on the radiograph	Lateral (L)
Optional	Oblique views	
	(1) Dorsal 65-degree proximal, 45-degree lateral–palmarodistomedial oblique (D65Pr-45L–PaDiMO)	(1) Medial oblique or DLPMO
	(2) Dorsal 65-degree proximal, 45-degree medial–palmarodistolateral oblique (D65Pr-45M-PaDiLO)	(2) Lateral oblique or DMPLO
Navicular	Lateromedial (LM)	Lateral (L)
	Dorsoproximal-palmarodistal oblique (DPr-PaDiO):	Dorsopalmar (DP)
	(1) High Coronary stand-on route:	
	45°: projects proximal border and extremities (D65Pr-PaDiO)	
	65°: projects both borders and extremities (D65Pr-PaDiO)	
	or	
	(2) Upright pedal route (on a block):	Dorsopalmar (DP)
	D90Pr-PaDiO Projects proximal border and extremities	
	D80Pr-PaDiO: Projects both borders and extremities	
	Palmaroproximal-palmarodistal oblique view (PaPr-PaDiO):	Flexor or skyline
	D65Pr45L-PaDiMO	Medial oblique (DLPMO)
	D65Pr45M-PaDiLO	Lateral oblique (DMPLO)
Pastern P1, proximal interphalangeal joint, P2	Lateromedial (LM)	Lateral (L)
	Dorsoproximal-palmarodistal oblique (D30-45Pr-PaDiO)	Dorsopalmar (DP)
	Dorsal 35-degree proximal, 35-degree lateral–palmarodistomedial oblique (D35Pr-35L-PaDiMO)	Medial oblique (DLPMO)
	Dorsal 35-degree proximal, 35-degree medial–palmarodistolateral oblique (D35Pr-35M-PaDiLO)	Lateral oblique (DMPLO)
Metacarpophalangeal/ Metatarsophalangeal Joint/Proximal Sesamoid Bones (Fetlock)	Dorsal 10-degree proximal–palmarodistal oblique (D10Pr-PaDiO)	Dorsopalmar (DP)
	Lateromedial (LM) extended	Lateral (L)
	Lateromedial (LM) flexed	Flexed lateral (L)
	Dorsoproximal 45-degree lateral–palmarodistomedial oblique (DPr45L-PaDiMO)	Medial oblique (DLPMO)
	Dorsoproximal 45-degree medial–palmarodistolateral oblique (DPr45M-PaDiLO)	Lateral oblique (DMPLO)
Optional views	Palmaroproximal-palmarodistal oblique view (PaPr-PaDiO)	Flexor/skyline/caudal tangential
	Dorsoproximal-dorsodistal oblique (DPr-DDiO)	Extensor surface/skyline
Metacarpal/metatarsal canon bone (M3)	Dorsoproximal-palmarodistal (DPr-PaDi)	Dorsopalmar (DP)
	Lateromedial (LM)	Lateral (L)
Lateral splint bone (M4)	Dorsoproximal 45-degree lateral–palmarodistomedial oblique (DPr45L-PaDiMO)	Medial oblique (DLPMO)
Medial splint bone (M2)	Dorsoproximal 45-degree medial–palmarodistolateral oblique (DPr45M-PaDiLO)	Lateral oblique (DMPLO)

Continued

TABLE 26-2	Views of the Equine Limb Examination—cont'd	
STRUCTURES EVALUATED/ COMMENTS	**VIEWS/COMMENTS***	**COMMON TERMINOLOGY**
Carpus	Dorsoproximal-palmarodistal (Dorsopalmar) (DPr-PaDi)	Dorsopalmar (DP)
	Lateromedial extended (LM)	Lateral (L)
	Lateromedial flexed (LM)	Flexed Lateral (L)
	Dorsoproximal 45-degree lateral–palmarodistomedial oblique (DPr45L-PaDiMO)	Medial oblique (DLPMO)
	Dorsoproximal 45-degree medial–palmarodistolateral oblique (DPr45M-PaDiLO)	Lateral oblique (DMPLO)
Optional views	Dorsoproximal-dorsodistal oblique flexed (DPr-DDiO)	Skyline
Tarsus	Dorsoproximal-plantarodistal (DPr-PlDi)	Dorsoplantar (DP)
	Lateromedial (LM) extended	Lateral (L)
	Lateromedial flexed (LM)	Flexed lateral (L)
	Dorsoproximal 45-degree lateral–plantarodistomedial oblique (DPr45L-PlDiMO)	Medial oblique (DLPMO)
	Dorsoproximal 45-degree medial–plantarodistolateral oblique (DPr45M-PlDiLO)	Lateral oblique (DMPLO)
Tuber calcaneus	Flexed plantaroproximal-plantarodistal (PlPr-PlDi)	Skyline
Radius	Cranioproximal-caudodistal (CrPr-CdDi)	Craniocaudal (CrCd)
	Lateromedial (LM)	Lateral (L)
Optional	Caudoproximal-craniodistal (CdPr-CrDi)	Caudocranial (CdCr)
	Cranioproximolateral-caudodistomedial oblique (CrPrL-CdDiMO)	Medial oblique (CrLCdMO)
	Cranioproximomedial-caudodistolateral oblique (CrPrM-CdDiLO)	Lateral oblique (CrMCdLO)
Elbow joint	Cranioproximal-caudodistal (CrPr-CdDi)—standing	Craniocaudal (CrCd)
	Mediolateral standing (ML)	Lateral (L)
Optional views	Proximodistal (skyline or flexor) of olecranon	
	Lateromedial (LM)	Lateral (L)
	Mediolateral through the thoracic cavity	
	Cranioproximal-caudodistal (CrPr-CdDi)—recumbent	Craniocaudal (CrCd)
	Mediolateral (recumbent) (ML)	Lateral (L)
	Craniomedial-caudolateral oblique	Lateral oblique (CrMCdLO)
Shoulder	Mediolateral (ML)	Lateral (L)
Optional view	Cranioproximal 45-degree medial–caudodistolateral oblique (CrPr45M-CaDiLO)	Lateral oblique (CrMCdLO)
Optional	Cranioproximal 45-degree lateral–caudodistomedial oblique (CrPr45L-CaDiMO)	Medial oblique (CrLCdMO)
Stifle	Lateromedial (LM)	Lateral (L)
	Caudoproximal-craniodistal (CdPr-CrDi)	Caudocranial (CdCr)
Lateral trochlear ridge and medial femoral condyle (stifle)	Caudoproximal 60-degree lateral–craniodistomedial oblique (Cd60L-CrMO)	Medial oblique (CdLCrMO)
Optional Stifle	Cranioproximal-caudodistal (CrPr-CdDi)	Craniocaudal (CrCd)
	Cranioproximal-craniodistal oblique (CrPr-CrDiO)	Skyline patella
	Lateromedial flexed (LM)	Flexed lateral (L)

Palmar is used in this chart and chapter with the understanding that *plantar* can be substituted when referring to the hind limb.

- The central ray should always be perpendicular to the axis being radiographed. The suggested angle with the ground may change depending on the limb confirmation of the patient.
- Place directional markers (right/left, front/rear) on the lateral aspect of the limb for DP(CrCd) and oblique views and at the dorsal/cranial aspect for lateromedial views.

Table 26-2 lists the views that are used in equine limb examination.

TECHNICIAN NOTES Remember to keep the principles of good radiography in mind with every view. The body part should be close to and parallel to the image receptor, and the central ray is perpendicular to both.

TECHNICIAN NOTES Keep the principles of radiation safety in mind for each exposure.

The Digit (Foot)

The distal phalanx and the navicular bone are considered as the digit or foot. Common indications for imaging of the equine foot include lameness localized to the foot by clinical examination (pain on pressure from foot testers, increased digital pulses, etc.) or by diagnostic analgesia, laminitis, penetrating wounds, or a pre-purchase examination.[2]

Dorsopalmar DP (Dorsoproximal-Palmarodistal) View

The three following views can be taken for the dorsoproximal-palmarodistal (DPr-PaDi) (DP) view:

High coronary view: Dorsal 65-degree proximal–palmarodistal oblique (D65Pr-PaDiO). The beam is angled to the ground 65 degrees dorsoproximal (stand-on route) (see Figure 26-8). The foot is on top of the cassette tunnel, which is placed on the ground. The foot is placed near the center, and the toe close to the front edge of the tunnel.

Upright pedal route: Dorsoproximal-palmarodistal oblique (DPr-PaDiO). The beam is horizontal and parallel to the ground with the toe pointed down (Figure 26-9). Point toe of foot downward so it is resting on a block or use a navicular block. The sole is perpendicular to the ground, and the dorsal hoof wall is 45 degrees to the horizontal for the coffin bone.

Position 3: True Dorsopalmar view: Figure 26-10. The beam is horizontal and parallel to the ground, but the foot is weight-bearing. The foot is placed on the wooden block to raise it to the level of the x-ray tube. The image receptor is positioned vertically and directly caudal to the foot on the floor or in the cassette groove.

Central Ray and Collimation

Center on the *midsagittal plane* of the pedal bone (dorsal foot wall) just distal to the coronary band. Include the full digit—foot wall, pedal bone, superimposed navicular bone,

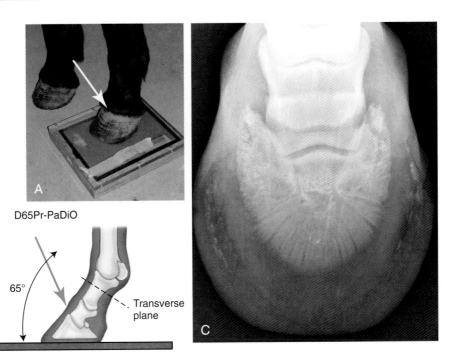

D65Pr-PaDiO

65°

Transverse plane

Supporting
B   surface

C

FIGURE 26-8 A, Positioning for the dorsoproximal (DP) view of the digit using a tunnel cassette for the high coronary stand-on view angled 65 degrees to the ground (65-degree proximal–palmarodistomedial oblique). The foot is best placed closer to the front of the cassette so that none of the foot shadow and thus relevant structures is missed. **B,** Dorsoproximal-palmarodistal oblique (DPr-PaDiO) view of the equine distal phalanx and distal sesamoid bone (navicular) made at 65 degrees proximal to the supporting surface. The accurate description is D65Pr-PaDiO but is often referred to as a DP, high coronary view. **C,** Radiograph of the dorsoproximal distal phalanx with the high coronary view route.

Continued

Dorsopalmar DP (Dorsoproximal-Palmarodistal) View—*cont'd*

middle phalanx (P2), and the distal part of the proximal phalanx (P1). Collimate, ensuring that labels are included and borders are visible.

Comments

- Aim the central ray at right angles to the correctly trimmed foot wall.
- Lift the opposite limb for restraint for the high coronary view.
- Proper full preparation of the sole is essential.
- Wings of the coffin bone and distal sesamoids should be equidistant.
- The purpose of the high coronary study is to note the number, size, and character of the vascular channels. The

crena, which is the large notch in the solar border, the palmar processes or wings formed by the solar border, and the *ungular or collateral cartilages* are all noted.[3] This is the preferred view for the interphalangeal joint.

- The upright pedal route better shows the extensor process, conformation, quality of hoof care, and relationship of foot to the surface, and is preferred for the bones.[3]
- The study with the foot weight-bearing on a block and the beam parallel to the ground is slightly more limited than the high coronary view, but does assess lateromedial foot imbalance, some distal phalanx fractures, and ossification of the collateral cartilages of P3.[2]
- This view also applies to the hind limb.

TECHNICIAN NOTES The high coronary stand-on route literally means stand on the casette tunnel. The upright pedal route has the pedal bone (digit) pointing downward, sole flat on plate and both perpendicular to the ground.

TECHNICIAN NOTES A common cause of non-diagnostic radiographs of the foot is lack of preparation. Artifacts need to be eliminated—remove the shoe, remove dirt, debris and excess horny tissue, and pack the sulcus to eliminate air artifacts.

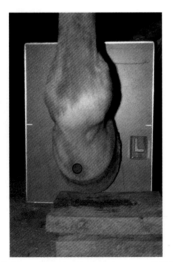

FIGURE 26-9 Positioning for the dorsoproximal (DP) digit and the navicular bone using the upright pedal route. The beam is horizontal and parallel to the ground. Referred to as the dorsal 65-degree proximal–palmarodistal oblique (D65Pr-PaDiO).

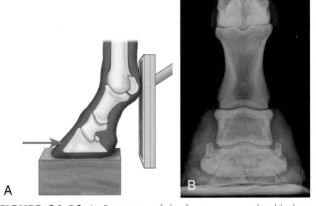

A

FIGURE 26-10 A, Positioning of the foot on a wooden block to obtain a weight-bearing DP view of the digit. **B,** Radiograph of the true dorsopalmar view with the foot on a block.

Lateromedial View

The lateromedial view of the distal phalanx is used for all of the bones and joints of the foot.

Positioning

Place the foot on a wood block and the image receptor on the medial side of the leg in the positional slot of the wood block (Figure 26-11).

Central Ray and Collimation

Aim the central ray 90 degrees to the midsagittal plane of the foot wall, just below the coronary band. The beam should be parallel to the ground, midway between the dorsal foot wall and the bulbs of the heel. The view should include the entire foot—whole foot wall, distal phalanx (P3), middle phalanx (P2), distal portion of P1, navicular bone, and distal interphalangeal and proximal interphalangeal joints. Collimate, ensuring that labels are included in front of the foot and borders are visible.

Comments

- The bulbs of the heel should be superimposed and in a straight line with the central ray.
- Care must be taken when assessing the foot pastern axis, which may be altered if the horse is not fully weight-bearing on a level surface.[4]

- Position the foot forward on the tunnel cassette, especially for the pelvic limb.
- Wings of the coffin bone and distal sesamoids should be superimposed when viewing the radiograph.
- Consider taping radiodense wire to the dorsal hoof wall to help evaluate the hoof wall thickness, especially if there is overexposure.
- This view also applies to the hind limb.
- For this view of the distal phalanx, the purpose is to see the relationship between the dorsal foot wall and the dorsal border of the distal phalanx. The palmar processes may appear to be irregular with separate bony fragments. They are normally separated from the distal phalanx cartilages by a prominent parietal *sulcus*.[3]

> **TECHNICIAN NOTES**   Obliquity is a concern so it is important to make sure that the central ray is lined up so that the bulbs of the heel are superimposed.

> **TECHNICIAN NOTES**   The same principles apply to the hind limb. Substitute the term *plantar* for *palmar*.

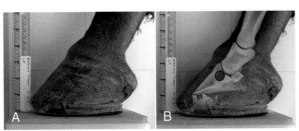

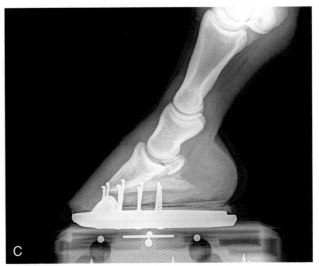

FIGURE 26-11 **A,** Positioning for the lateromedial view of the distal phalanx. **B,** Radiographic anatomy of the lateromedial left equine distal phalanx. **C,** Radiograph of the lateromedial left equine distal phalanx of the above patient with the shoe in place. The shoe needs to be removed for other views of the digit.

Oblique Views

Oblique views of the distal phalanx and navicular bone are as follows:

Medial oblique–DLPMO: Dorsal 65-degree proximal, 45-degree lateral–palmarodistomedial oblique (D65Pr45L-PaDiMO) (See Figure 26-12)

Lateral oblique–DMPLO: Dorsal 65-degree proximal, 45-degree medial–palmarodistolateral oblique (D65Pr45M-PaDiLO) (See Figure 26-13)

The medial oblique–DLPMO view allows visualization of the lateral wing of the coffin bone (see Figure 26-12).

Positioning

Place the foot on the tunnel cassette with the foot off-center, slightly toward the side to be studied. The angle to be projected is closer to the edge of the image receptor.

Central Ray and Collimation

Angle the beam 65 degrees downward to the supporting surface on the DP line just below the coronary band and 45 degrees either lateral or medial to the midsagittal plane. Center the beam just distal to the coronary band, half the distance between the dorsal wall and the heels. Collimate, ensuring that labels are included and borders are visible.

Comments

- Keep the beam perpendicular to the foot axis; this is normally about 65 degrees to the ground.
- Ensure that the foot is clean and shoes have been removed.
- The oblique views help detect nondisplaced fractures in the quarters of the solar border and in the plantar or palmar processes of the distal phalanx.

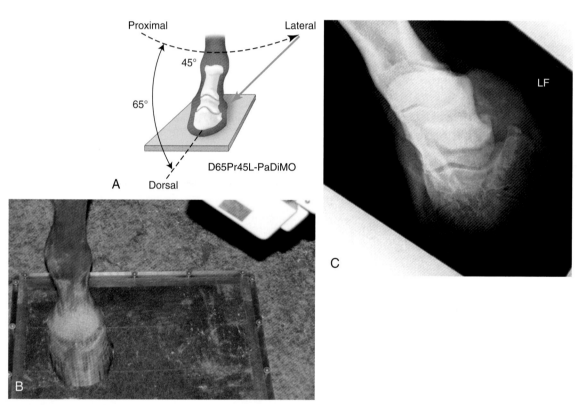

FIGURE 26-12 **A,** A DLPMO or medial oblique view of the equine distal phalanx made at 65 degrees proximal to the supporting surface and 45 degrees lateral to the dorsopalmar line or the midsagittal plane. The blue arrow indicates the side the beam is directed from. Specifically, this projection would be termed D65Pr45L-PaDiMO. **B,** Positioning for the medial oblique–DLPMO radiograph of the left front distal phalanx to view the lateral wing of the coffin bone. The beam is 65 degrees to the ground and 45 degrees lateral to the midsagittal plane. The foot is best placed closer to the side of the cassette facing the tube head to allow the full foot shadow to appear on the image. **C,** Radiograph of the medial oblique–DLPMO position of the digit as described in A and B.

Oblique Views—cont'd

- In the medial oblique view, which is used to visualize the lateral wing of the coffin bone, this wing appears larger due to increased OFD. Because there is no superimposition, the lateral wing of the coffin bone appears grayer.
- In the lateral oblique view, which is used to visualize the medial wing of the coffin bone, this wing appears larger due to increased OFD. Because there is no superimposition, the medial wing of the coffin bone appears grayer.
- This positioning also applies to the hind limb.

> **TECHNICIAN NOTES** As with small animal imaging, be prepared prior to making the exposure to minimize retakes. Your mental check list includes but is not limited to: machine ready and settings correct, PPE donned, use of a cassette holder or positioning device if possible, proper location of markers, patient properly prepared and restrained, correct body part and view, properly centered and borders included, correct angle of the central ray so it is perpendicular to the body part and the image receptor.

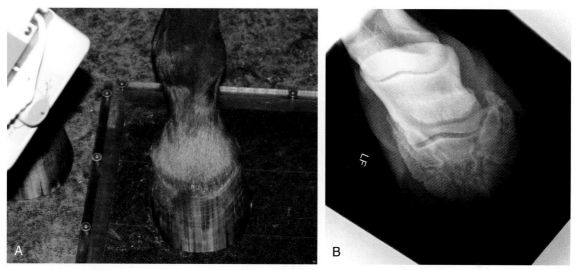

FIGURE 26-13 A, Positioning for the lateral oblique-DMPLO [D65Pr45M-PaDiLO] view of the left front distal phalanx. The beam is 65 degrees to the ground and 45 degrees medial to the midsagittal plane. Note placement of foot to ensure the full image will be shown. **B,** Lateral oblique—DMPLO radiograph of the distal phalanx to view the medial wing of the coffin bone.

Navicular Bone (Distal Sesamoid)

Lateromedial View

Positioning, Central Ray, and Collimation

Positioning, central ray, and collimation instructions are the same as those for the lateromedial view of the distal phalanx (Figure 26-14).

Comments

- This view assists in evaluating the changes in the shape of the bone that are often associated with chronic degenerative changes of navicular disease.[3]
- If only a lateral view is required, the shoe does not have to be removed; only cleaning and brushing of the wall are required.

- This view gives a foreshortened projection along the axis of the bone. Both borders and both surfaces will be projected in profile.

> **TECHNICIAN NOTES**   If a radiodense wire is taped or barium is applied on the midsagittal plane of the dorsal hoof wall, it is easier to see the hoof wall axis on an image.

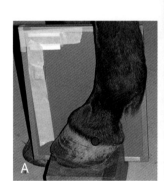
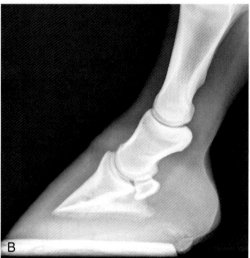

FIGURE 26-14 A, Positioning for the lateromedial view of the navicular bone standing on a block. B, Lateromedial radiograph of the navicular bone.

Dorsopalmar (DP): Dorsoproximal-Palmarodistal Oblique Views

High Coronary Stand-on Routes

Dorsal 65-Degree Proximal–Palmarodistal Oblique (D65Pr-PaDiO)

The D65Pr-PaDiO view projects both borders and extremities, and the distal border can be seen through the distal and palmar (plantar) portions of the middle phalanx (Figure 26-15).

Positioning

Place the foot on the cassette tunnel, which is flat on the ground. Position the foot near the center and the toe close to the front edge of the tunnel.

> **TECHNICIAN NOTES** The 45-degree high coronary stand-on and the 90-degree upright pedal routes show the undistorted proximal navicular border.
>
> The 65-degree high coronary stand-on and the 80-degree upright pedal routes show both the distal and proximal borders.

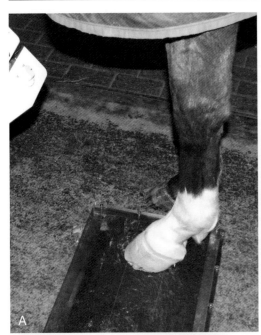
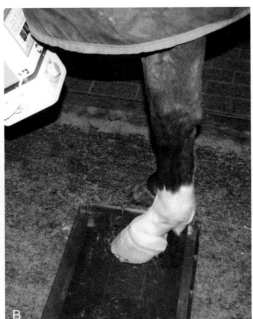
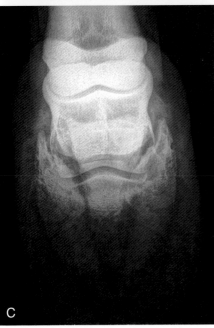

FIGURE 26-15 A, Positioning for the dorsoproximal (DP) view of the navicular with the high coronary view angled 45 degrees to the ground (dorsal 45-degree proximal–palmarodistomedial oblique). B, Positioning for the dorsoproximal (DP) view of the navicular with the high coronary view angled 65 degrees to the ground. C, Radiograph of the DP (D60-65Pr-PaDiO)-high coronary navicular position.

Continued

Dorsopalmar (DP): Dorsoproximal-Palmarodistal Oblique Views—cont'd

Central Ray and Collimation

The beam is 65 degrees with the ground and at 110 degrees with the hoof wall. The central ray is on the midsagittal plane just distal to the coronary band centered between the bulbs of the heel. All of P3, the navicular, and P2 are included. Collimate, ensuring that labels are included and borders are visible.

Dorsal 45-Degree Proximal–Palmarodistal Oblique (D45Pr-PaDiO)

The D45Pr-PaDiO view projects the proximal border and extremities.

Positioning

Place the foot on the cassette tunnel, which is flat on the ground. Position the foot near the center and the toe close to the front edge of the tunnel.

Central Ray and Collimation

The beam is 45 degrees with the ground and 90 degrees with the foot wall. The central ray is on the midsagittal plane above the coronary band, centered between the bulbs of the heel. All of P3, navicular, and P2 are included. Collimate, ensuring that labels are included and borders are visible.

Upright Pedal Route[4]

Place the foot with the toe tipped so that the dorsal wall is positioned 80 or 90 degrees from the horizontal. The central ray is directed horizontally (Figure 26-16).

Dorsal 90-Degree Proximal-Palmarodistal Oblique (D90Pr-PaDiO)

The D90Pr-PaDiO view projects the proximal border and extremities (equivalent to 45-degree high coronary view).

Positioning

Place the foot on a block with the toe pointing downwards, the sole perpendicular to the ground, and the dorsal foot wall about 90 degrees to the horizontal. If the special navicular block is used, place the foot in the slot closest to the front of the block or the 45 degree slot.

Central Ray and Collimation

The beam is horizontal to the ground. The central ray is on the midsagittal plane just distal to the coronary band, centered between the bulbs of the heel. All of P3, navicular, and P2 are included. Collimate, ensuring that labels are included and borders are visible.

Dorsal 80-Degree Proximal–Palmarodistal (D80Pr-PaDiO)

The D80Pr-PaDiO view projects both the proximal and distal borders and the extremities (equivalent to 65-degree high coronary view).

> **TECHNICIAN NOTES** Be consistent with laterality when viewing a series of radiographs from the same patient. In other words the lateral and medal aspect of all views (except the LM) must be in the same orientation.

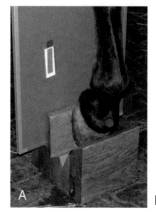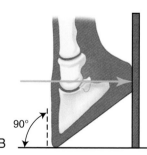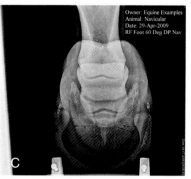

FIGURE 26-16 A, An alternate upright pedal route for navicular positioning. The hoof is placed in one of two slots that change the angle at which the central ray strikes the navicular, giving both 80-degree and 90-degree DP views. This was made but commercial 45 and 65 degree navicular blocks can be purchased. **B,** Positioning for the upright pedal route of the navicular with the foot tipped so that the dorsal wall is positioned 90 degrees from the horizontal to show the proximal border of the distal sesamoid. The arrow indicates the horizontally directed central ray. **C,** Radiograph of the DP equine upright pedal route for the navicular with the dorsal wall positioned 80 degrees.

Dorsopalmar (DP): Dorsoproximal-Palmarodistal Oblique Views—*cont'd*

Positioning

Place the foot on a block with the toe pointing downwards, the sole perpendicular to the ground, and the dorsal foot wall perpendicular or about 80 degrees with the ground. If using the special navicular block, place the toe in the position closest to the image receptor or the 65 degree slot (Figure 26-16).

Central Ray and Collimation

The beam is horizontal and parallel to the ground. The central ray is on the midsagittal plane 2 cm proximal to coronary band between the bulbs of the heel. All of P3, the navicular, and P2 are included. Collimate, ensuring that labels are included and borders are visible.

Comments

- Important: The foot needs to be properly trimmed and the sole cleaned for the DP views.
- Proper angulation of the central ray is important for the high coronary views.

- The high coronary view requires less restraint but involves more geometric distortion because the beam is not perpendicular to the image receptor.
- Collimate the beam for better image quality by decreasing scatter radiation.
- A lead shield (navicular mask) can be cut so that only the area of interest is exposed. This shield, along with placement of a lead sheet under the cassette tunnel for the high coronary stand-on route or behind the image receptor for the upright pedal route, limits scatter radiation and fogging.
- These views also apply to the hind limb.

TECHNICIAN NOTES When using the cassette tunnel, keep in mind how the "shadow" or image will project onto the receptor. If the affected limb is not properly positioned on the image receptor for the oblique or DP views, you may miss the area of interest.

Flexor/Caudal Tangential/Skyline (Palmaroproximal-Palmarodistal Oblique) View

Positioning

Place the image receptor directly under the foot in the center of the cassette tunnel. Position the affected navicular bone more caudally than the contralateral foot. Extend the fetlock, causing the middle phalanx to be vertical and isolating the navicular bone (Figure 26-17).

Central Ray and Collimation

Center on the midpoint between the bulbs of the heel at the distal-palmar (or distal-plantar) fetlock. Position the central ray along the palmar or plantar surface on the midsagittal plane. The angle is about 65 degrees with the ground but the central ray must be angled tangentially in the same plane as the flexor cortex. Collimate, ensuring that labels are included and borders are visible.

Comments

- This view shows the flexor surface, palmar cortex, and medulla of the navicular bones.[4]

- Decrease the SID to 20 inches and adjust the exposure factors accordingly.
- Full patient preparation is required.
- Take advantage of any nerve blocks, and perform the study before the anesthetic wears off, if possible.
- Keep a small field of exposure to minimize scatter radiation.
- This view also applies to the hind limb. For radiographing the rear feet, it is physically safer for the machine and restrainer if the hind limbs are kept in a normal position.

> **TECHNICIAN NOTES** Common problems for imaging the skyline of the navicular bone of the front limb include: not extending the foot far enough forward, improper foot preparation (cleaning and packing) and not angling the central ray proximally enough.

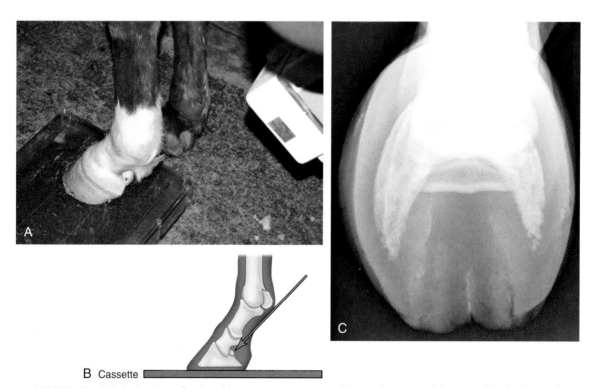

FIGURE 26-17 **A,** Positioning for the palmaroproximal-palmarodistal oblique (flexor/caudal tangential/skyline) view of the navicular bone. **B,** Anatomy of the skyline view of the navicular bone. This view highlights the flexor surface of the navicular bone and allows the distinction between the cortex and medulla to be visualized. **C,** Radiograph of the palmaroproximal skyline of the navicular bone.

Oblique Views

Oblique views of the navicular bone are as follows:

Medial oblique–DLPMO: Dorsal 65-degree proximal, 45-degree lateral–palmarodistomedial oblique (D65Pr45L-PaDiMO)

Lateral oblique–DMPLO: Dorsal 65-degree proximal, 45-degree medial–palmarodistolateral oblique (D65Pr45M-PaDiLO)

The oblique views do not superimpose the wings, so fractures are more easily diagnosed.

Positioning, Central Ray, and Collimation

Positioning, central ray, and collimation instructions are the same as those for the oblique views of the distal phalanx (see Figure 26-12).

The Pastern

Middle and Proximal Phalanx, Proximal Interphalangeal Joint (Pastern)

The main indications for radiography of the middle and proximal phalanx and proximal interphalangeal joint are lameness localized with clinical examination or diagnostic analgesia, and penetrating wounds. Specific views of this area are best obtained with the horse bearing weight on the limb.[4]

Lateromedial View of the Pastern

The lateromedial view of the pastern provides information on the character of the foot axis and the bones and joints in the digit.

Positioning

Place the foot on the wood block, and position the image receptor on medial side of leg, perpendicular to the ground (Figure 26-18).

Central Ray and Collimation

Center on the proximal pastern joint (interphalangeal joint) or the joint of interest. Include P2, the proximal interphalangeal joint, P1, and the interphalangeal-metacarpal joint. The beam is parallel to the ground and lateral or 90 degrees to the midsagittal plane. Collimate, ensuring that labels are included and borders are visible.

Comments

- Look at the foot from the front to see whether there is angulation of the digit.
- If there is a conformational problem, the angle of the beam may need to be adjusted.
- This view also applies to the hind limb.

> **TECHNICIAN NOTES** The technique is similar for imaging the lateromedial views of the lower limbs. What differs is the centering and collimation.

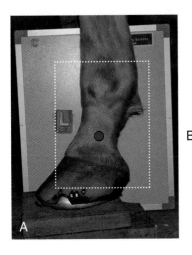
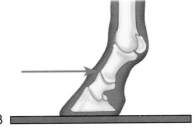
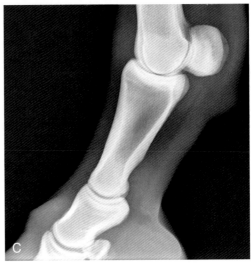

FIGURE 26-18 A, Positioning for the lateromedial view of the middle and proximal phalanx and proximal interphalangeal joint (pastern). B, Radiographic anatomy of the middle and proximal phalanx and proximal interphalangeal joint (pastern). C, Radiograph of lateromedial middle and proximal phalanx and proximal interphalangeal joint (pastern).

Dorsopalmar (DP): Dorsoproximal-Palmarodistal Oblique (D30-45Pr-PaDiO) View

The D30-45Pr-PaDiO view of the pastern is a standard view to evaluate the causes of forelimb and hind limb lameness. Additional views of the opposite limb are indicated in patients less than 9 months of age. Comparison studies permit evaluation of physeal closure.[3]

Positioning

Clean the hair coat. Position the image receptor caudal to the limb (palmar or plantar position), keeping it parallel to the phalanges (Figure 26-19).

Central Ray and Collimation

Center the beam on the midsagittal plane. Include P2, the proximal interphalangeal joint, P1, and the interphalangeal-metacarpal joint. The beam must be perpendicular to the foot axis. The central ray is at about a 30- to 45-degree angle with the ground but always perpendicular to the foot axis. Collimate, ensuring that labels are included and borders are visible.

Comments

- The joint space appears narrowed on one side if the horse is not standing straight. Elevate the opposite forefoot to ensure that the horse is bearing full weight.
- This view also applies to the hind limb.

> **TECHNICIAN NOTES** Because of the foot conformation, the central ray is angled to the ground but perpendicular to the hoof wall. Thus the DP views of the foot taken with an angled beam with the ground are, referred to as dorsoproximal-palmarodistal oblique views. There is no lateral or medial designation.

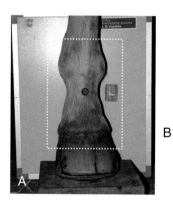
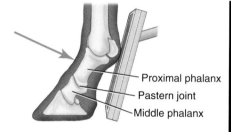
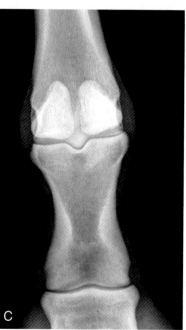

Proximal phalanx
Pastern joint
Middle phalanx

FIGURE 26-19 A, Positioning for the dorsopalmar/dorsoplantar view of the middle and proximal phalanx and proximal interphalangeal joint (pastern). B, Radiographic anatomy of the dorsal aspect of the middle and proximal phalanx and proximal interphalangeal joint (pastern). C, Radiograph of the dorsopalmar/dorsoplantar view of the middle and proximal phalanx and proximal interphalangeal joint (pastern).

Oblique Views

Oblique views of the pastern are as follows (Figure 26-20):

Medial oblique–DLPMO: Dorsal 35-degree proximal, 35-degree lateral–palmarodistomedial oblique (D35Pr35L-PaDiMO).

Lateral oblique–DMPLO: Dorsal 35-degree proximal, 35-degree medial–palmarodistolateral oblique (D35Pr35M-PaDiLO).

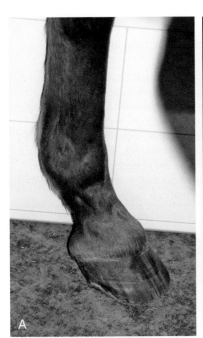

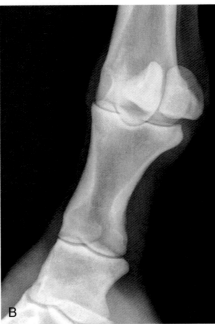

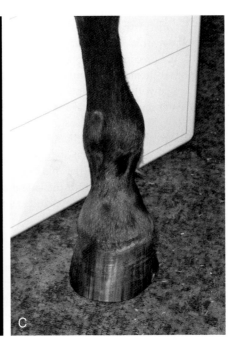

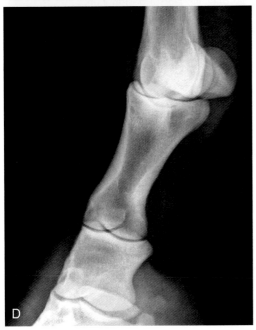

FIGURE 26-20 **A,** Positioning for the medial oblique view of the right front pastern. Ideally the limb should be placed on a wooden block to ensure the full area of interest is in the field of view. **B,** Radiograph of the medial oblique view of the pastern. **C,** Positioning of the lateral oblique view of the right front pastern. **D,** Radiograph of the lateral oblique view of the pastern.

Continued

Oblique Views—cont'd

Positioning

Place the foot on a wood block. Position the image receptor against the lateral side of the limb, for the lateral oblique view and against the medial side for the medial oblique. The limb can be positioned as for a DP view, with the image receptor directly caudal to the limb, if a cassette slot is used but there will be distortion of the limb.

Central Ray and Collimation

Include P2, the proximal interphalangeal joint, P1, and the interphalangeal-metacarpal joint. The central ray is at a 35-degree angle with the ground and perpendicular to the foot axis. Center on the proximal interphalangeal joint or the area of interest. Rotate the tube as follows:

- To a 35-degreee angle from the midsagittal plane toward the lateral side for the medial oblique view
- To a 35-degree angle from the midsagittal plane toward the medial part of the limb for the lateral oblique view.

Collimate, ensuring that labels are included and borders are visible.

Comments

- These oblique views detect areas of new bone production that are located medially and laterally from the palmar/plantar and dorsal borders of the phalanges, as well as indicating new bone formation around the joints.[4]
- Chip fractures of the phalanges are best visualized on oblique views.[4]

- Dorsoproximal-palmarodistal oblique views made by aligning the beam at right angles to the dorsal surface of the pastern and the parallel image receptor, result in less distortion, specifically for assessment of middle phalanx or proximal interphalangeal joint.[4]
- Using a wood block with a 35-degree groove (to hold the image receptor) alleviates the need for a person to hold the plate.
- These views also apply to the hind limb.

> **TECHNICIAN NOTES**   Remember that the last letter before the O (oblique) tells us which side is against the film, so the beam has to come from the opposite side. To tell which bones will be in profile, after the "O" is dropped take the middle two and outer two letters. Thus, for a DLPMO view, you can see the lateral sesamoid (which is grayer and more magnified), so it is the dorsomedial and palmarolateral surfaces that are highlighted.

> **TECHNICIAN NOTES**   Do not get confused with the oblique designation for the dorsoproximal-palmarodistal view for the lower limb in which the central ray focused on the mid sagittal plane is angled to the ground because of hoof confirmation. There is no lateral or medial designation in these DP views and the angle degree to the ground is placed right after the Dorsal designation.

Metacarpophalangeal/Metatarsophalangeal Joint/Proximal Sesamoid Bones (Fetlock)

Dorsopalmar (DP): Dorsal 10-Degree Proximal–Palmarodistal Oblique (D10Pr-PaDiO) View of the Fetlock

Positioning

This is a full weight-bearing view. Ensure that hair is free of all debris. Place the foot on the ground. Position the image receptor caudal to the limb (palmar or plantar position) (Figure 26-21).

Central Ray and Collimation

Center on the midsagittal plane of the fetlock joint. Include P1, the fetlock, and one third of the cannon bone. The central ray is at a 10- to 15-degree angle with the ground and perpendicular to the foot axis. Collimate, ensuring that labels are included and borders are visible.

Comments

- Superimposition of the proximal sesamoid bones over the joint space can be avoided by angling the central ray with the ground proximodistally 10 degrees for the dorsopalmar view and 15 degrees for the dorsoplantar view.[4]
- This view provides visibility of the fetlock joint and the proximal sesamoid bones.
- Additional views of the opposite limb are indicated in patients less than 12 months of age.[3]
- This view also applies to the hind limb.

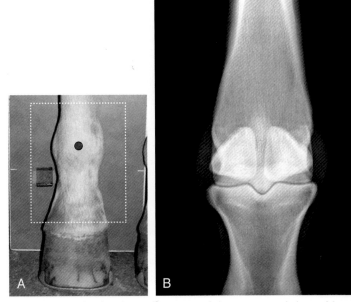

FIGURE 26-21 A, Positioning for the dorsopalmar view of the metacarpophalangeal/metatarsophalangeal joint/ proximal sesamoid bones (fetlock). B, Radiograph of dorsopalmar view of the metacarpophalangeal joint/proximal sesamoid bones (fetlock).

Lateromedial (LM) Extended View

Positioning

The lateromedial extended view of the fetlock is a fully weight-bearing view with the foot placed on the ground or a block. Clean the hair coat and place the image receptor against the medial side of leg (Figure 26-22).

Central Ray and Collimation

Center at the medial aspect of the fetlock, and include P1, the fetlock, and a third of the cannon bone. Keep the beam parallel to the ground and directed 90 degrees from the midsagittal plane. Collimate, ensuring that labels are included and borders are visible.

Comments

- Aligning the beam parallel to a line tangential to the bulbs of the heel results in a true lateromedial view. Palpation of the medial and lateral epicondyles of the third metacarpal bone may be helpful.[4]
- This view contains the fetlock joint and a portion of the bones proximal and distal to it. A true lateromedial view displays the metacarpal condyles and superimposed sesamoids, with a visible joint space.[5]
- This view also applies to the hind limb.

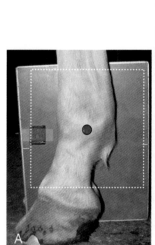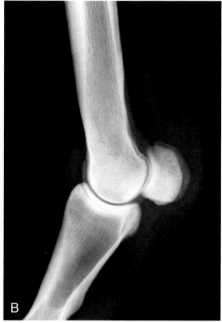

FIGURE 26-22 A, Positioning for the lateromedial view of the metacarpophalangeal/metatarsophalangeal joint/proximal sesamoid bones (fetlock). **B,** Radiograph of the lateromedial view of the metacarpophalangeal proximal sesamoid bones (fetlock).

Lateromedial Flexed (LM) View

Positioning

Support the foot off the ground, and completely flex the fetlock (Figure 26-23). Do not abduct the foot laterally.

Central Ray and Collimation

Center at the medial aspect of the fetlock joint, and include P1, the fetlock, and the proximal cannon bone. Keep the beam parallel to the ground and directed 90 degrees from the midsagittal plane. Collimate, ensuring that labels are included and borders are visible.

Comments

- The flexed lateromedial view allows for greater visualization of the spatial area of the metacarpophalangeal joint. The distal articular surface of metacarpal/tarsal bone is shown.
- This view also applies to the hind limb.

TECHNICIAN NOTES Ensure that the restrainer is not within the beam direction and is wearing the proper PPE.

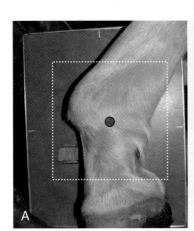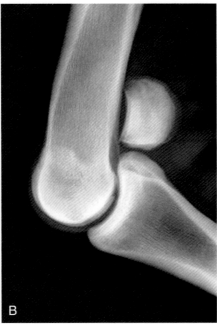

FIGURE 26-23 A, Positioning for the lateromedial flexion view of the metacarpophalangeal joint/proximal sesamoid bones or fetlock. **B,** Radiograph of the lateral flexion view of the fetlock.

Oblique Views

Oblique views of the fetlock are as follows:

Medial oblique–DLPMO: Dorsoproximal 45-degree lateral–palmarodistomedial oblique (DPr45L-PaDiMO) (Figure 26-24 A and B)

Lateral oblique–DMPLO: Dorsoproximal 45-degree medial–palmarodistolateral oblique (DPr45M-PaDiLO)

The medial oblique view is used to view the lateral sesamoid (see Figure 26-24A and B), and the lateral oblique to view the medial sesamoid (see Figure 26-24C and D).

Positioning

The foot is placed in a normal weight-bearing position under the body.

Central Ray and Collimation

The beam is parallel to the ground at the middle of the joint and angled 30 to 45 degrees from the midsagittal plane in the medial or lateral direction. Collimate, ensuring that labels are included and borders are visible.

Comments

* The oblique views of the fetlock allow visualization of the medial and lateral sesamoid bones on the palmar/plantar aspect of the limb.
* This view also applies to the hind limb.

> **TECHNICIAN NOTES** The precise position of the central ray may vary depending on the patient conformation. It is important to be perpendicular to the area of interest and the image receptor.

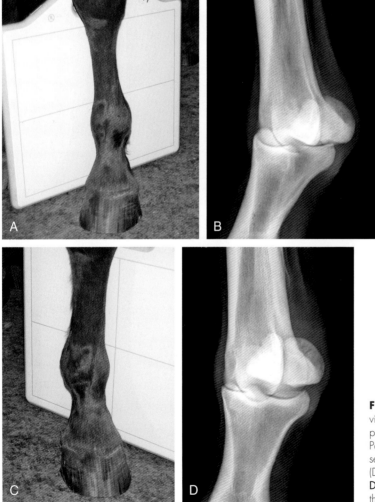

FIGURE 26-24 A, Positioning for the medial oblique (DLPMO) view of the left fetlock. Proper description of the view is dorsoproximal 45-degree lateral–palmarodistomedial oblique (DPr45L-PaDiMO). **B,** Medial oblique (DLPMO) view of the proximal sesamoids or fetlock joint. **C,** Positioning for the lateral oblique (DMPLO) view of the left front proximal sesamoids or fetlock joint. **D,** Radiograph of the lateral oblique (DPr45M-PaDiLO) view of the proximal sesamoids or fetlock joint.

Optional Views

Flexor/Skyline/Caudal Tangential (Palmaroproximal-Palmarodistal Oblique [PaPr-PaDiO]) View

Positioning

Place the foot as far back under (or behind for the hind foot) the horse as possible while maintaining weight-bearing on it. Position the image receptor in the tunnel with the foot centered on the tunnel.

Central Ray and Collimation

Center the ray in between the proximal sesamoid bones.[3] The central ray should be perpendicular to the ground caudal to the front limb. Collimate, ensuring that labels are included and borders are visible.

Comment

- SID is decreased because there is minimal space caudal to the front limb, when the x-ray tube is placed under the horse.
- This view allows visualization of the axial surface and abaxial recess of the proximal sesamoid bone.[2]
- This study can also be made using an oblique view with the tube shifted either medially or laterally.[3]
- This view also applies to the hind limb.

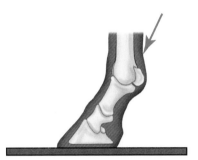

FIGURE 26-25 Flexor (skyline/caudal tangential) view of the fetlock. The proper term is palmaroproximal-palmarodistal oblique (PaPr-PaDiO).

Extensor Surface/Skyline (Dorsoproximal-Dorsodistal [DPr-DDi]) View of the Fetlock

Positioning

Fully flex the fetlock joint and position the leg forward. The image receptor is positioned against the dorsal surface of the proximal phalanx[3] and parallel to the ground (Figure 26-25).

Central Ray and Collimation

Center the beam on the dorsodistal end of the third metacarpal (tarsal) bone. Position the x-ray tube directly above the distal end of the third metacarpal (tarsal) bone. The central ray is almost perpendicular to the ground. Collimate, ensuring that labels are included and borders are visible.

Comments

- The SID is decreased to 50 cm.
- This study evaluates lesions dorsal to the distal end of the third metacarpal bone as well as soft tissue mineralization. It also detects the character of intra-articular fracture lines of the distal metacarpal bone.[3]
- This study can be performed on the hind limb, but positioning is more difficult.[3]

Metacarpus/Metatarsus (Cannon Bone, M2, and M4)

Dorsopalmar (DP): Dorsoproximal-Palmarodistal (DPr-PaDi) View

Positioning
The patient is standing in a natural weight-bearing position. The image receptor is caudal to the palmar or plantar aspect of the limb and perpendicular to the ground (Figure 26-26).

Central Ray and Collimation
Center on the midsagittal plane of the third metacarpus/third metatarsus (cannon bone). Include the cannon bone, fetlock, and carpal/tarsal joints. The beam is parallel to the ground and perpendicular to the limb and image receptor. Collimate, ensuring that labels are included and borders are visible.

Comments
- Larger image receptors are recommended for this area.
- This view may include both joints (distal and proximal to metacarpus). If the image receptor is not large enough, include one joint to provide orientation. Distortion is possible because of the length of the area.
- This view also applies to the hind limb.

> **TECHNICIAN NOTES** When taking radiographs, mark the center of the area to be examined with a radiolucent indicator such as tape. This maneuver may minimize repeat radiographs due to inaccurate centering and also gives a reference point if the position is to be repeated.

> **TECHNICIAN NOTES** Because the central ray is parallel to the ground and not angled, there is no oblique (O) distinction to the DP views proximal to and including the metacarpus/metatarsus.

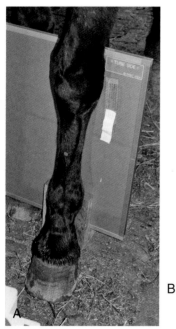

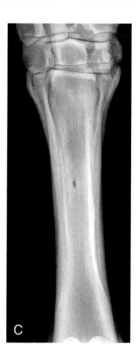

Radius
Radial carpal bone
Third carpal bone
Lateral splint bone
Intermediate carpal bone
Ulnar carpal bone
Fourth carpal bone
Medial splint bone
Metacarpus
Proximal sesamoid
Proximal phalanx (Pp, P1)
Middle phalanx (Pm, P2)
Distal phalanx (Pd, P3)

FIGURE 26-26 **A,** Positioning of the dorsopalmar or DP of the third metacarpals (canon bone), M2, and M4 (splint bones). Proper description of the view is dorsoproximal-palmarodistal (DPr-PDi). **B,** Anatomy of the third metacarpus (canon bone), M2, and M4 (splint bones). **C,** Radiograph of the dorsopalmar view of the third metacarpus (cannon bone), M2, and M4 (splint bones).

Lateromedial (LM) View

Positioning
The patient is standing in a natural weight-bearing position. The image receptor is against the medial aspect of the cannon bone (Figure 26-27).

Central Ray and Collimation
Center on the midshaft of the cannon bone (M3). Include from the carpus/tarsus to the fetlock. The beam is parallel to the ground and angled 90 degrees from the midsagittal plane. Collimate, ensuring that labels are included and borders are visible.

Comments
- The image receptor must be large enough to include at least one joint to provide orientation.
- This is a standard weight-bearing view.
- This view also applies to the hind limb.

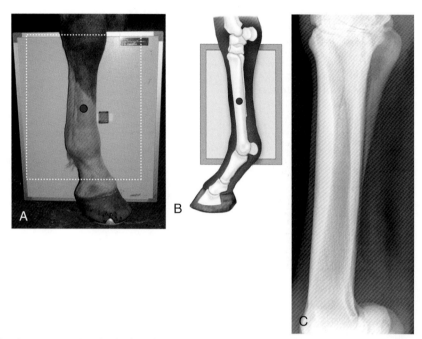

FIGURE 26-27 **A,** Positioning for the lateral extended (lateromedial) view of the third metacarpus (cannon bone), M2, and M4 (splint bones). **B,** Anatomy of the lateral extended (lateromedial) view of the third metacarpus (cannon bone), M2, and M4 (splint bones). **C,** Radiograph of the lateral extended (lateromedial) of the third metacarpus (cannon bone), M2, and M4 (splint bones).

Oblique Views to View the Splint Bones

Oblique views of the metacarpus/metatarsus to view the splint bones are as follows:

Medial Oblique–DLPMO: Dorsoproximal 45-degree lateral–palmarodistomedial oblique (DPr45L-PaDiMO)

Lateral oblique–DMPLO: Dorsoproximal 45-degree medial–palmarodistolateral oblique DPr45M-PaDiLO

The medial oblique view is used to evaluate the lateral splint bone (M4), and the lateral oblique to evaluate the medial splint bone (M2).

Positioning

The image receptor is placed on the lateral or medial aspect of the limbs, against the plantar or palmar surface (Figure 26-28).

Central Ray and Collimation

The beam is centered on the midshaft of the cannon bone parallel to the ground as follows:

- For the medial oblique view: The central ray is directed 35 to 45 degrees laterally from the midsagittal plane. The image receptor is against the medial plane of the metacarpus.
- For the lateral oblique view: The central ray is directed 35 to 45 degrees medially from the midsagittal plane. The image receptor is against the lateral plane of the metacarpus.

Collimate, ensuring that labels are included and borders are visible.

Comments

- The oblique views also apply to the hind limb.
- The oblique views provide an unobstructed view of the splint bones (second and fourth metacarpus/metatarsus).

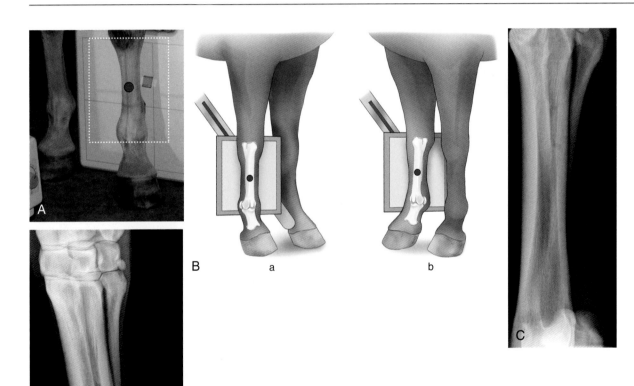

FIGURE 26-28 **A,** Positioning for the lateral oblique (DMPLO) view of the third metacarpus (cannon bone), M2, and M4 (splint bones). The proper description is dorsoproximal 45-degree medial–palmarodistolateral oblique (DPr45M-PaDiLO). **B,** Anatomy of the medial oblique (a) and lateral oblique (b) radiographic views of the third metacarpus (cannon bone), M2, and M4 (splint bones). **C,** Radiograph of the DLPMO view of the third metacarpus (cannon bone), M2, and M4 (splint bones), to show the lateral splint bone or M4. **D,** DMPLO radiograph to show the medial splint bone or M2.

Carpus

The carpus consists of three principal joints with articulation between adjacent bones in each row of carpal bones. This causes overlying images, which may confuse interpretation. Consequently, it is recommended to obtain a minimum of five standard views.[4]

Dorsopalmar (DP): Dorsoproximal-Palmarodistal (DPr-PaDi) View

Positioning
The image receptor is placed vertically on the palmar aspect of the limb and perpendicular to the beam. Full weight-bearing is used. The opposite limb may have to be elevated (Figure 26-29).

Central Ray and Collimation
Direct the ray to the middle of the carpus at a true DP plane, centering on an imaginary line from the middle of the foot wall to the radius. Include the entire carpus and a portion of each of the metacarpal bones and radius/ulna. The beam is parallel to the ground and perpendicular to the carpus and image receptor. Collimate, ensuring that labels are included and borders are visible.

Comments
- To see whether there is closure of the distal radial physis in young horses, the other limb may be required for comparison.
- The orientation of the central ray is to be relative and perpendicular to the limb in question, not to the body of the horse.
- On the radiograph, the intercarpal space between the radial and intermediate carpal bones should be visible with no superimposition.

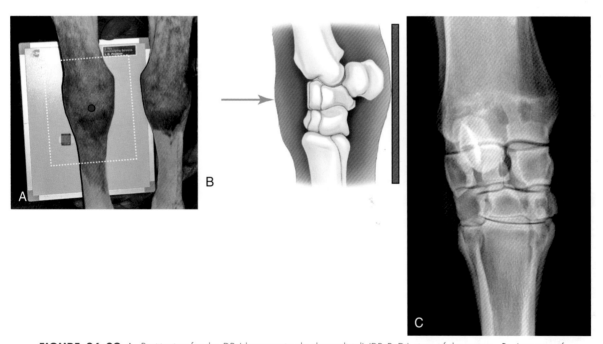

FIGURE 26-29 A, Positioning for the DP (dorsoproximal-palmarodistal) (DPr-PaDi) view of the carpus. B, Anatomy of the DP (dorsoproximal-palmarodistal) (DPr-PaDi) view of the carpus. C, Radiograph of the DP (dorsoproximal-palmarodistal) (DPr-PaDi) view of the carpus.

Lateromedial (LM) Extended View

Positioning

The image receptor is placed vertically at the medial aspect of the limb (Figure 26-30).

Central Ray and Collimation

The beam is parallel to the ground and perpendicular to the carpus and image receptor. The central ray is angled 90 degrees from the dorsal midline. Collimate, ensuring that labels are included and borders are visible.

Comments

- A true LM view displays all carpal bones superimposed over one another, allowing for a clear view of the dorsal surfaces. A small portion of the distal and proximal bones along with a full view of the carpus should be visible.
- The carpus is a very complex joint. Multiple views may be required.
- Consideration must be given to mature versus immature development.

Lateromedial (LM) Flexed View

Positioning

Place the image receptor vertically against the medial aspect of the carpus. Elevate the limb of interest, and flex the carpus to approximately three quarters of full flexion. Support the foot at the level of the carpus of the opposite limb so the carpus is slightly dorsal to the limb. Keep the carpus under the body, and prevent abduction (Figure 26-31).

Central Ray and Collimation

The central ray is over the lateral aspect of the limb in the middle of the carpus. Include the entire carpus. The central ray is parallel to the ground, 90 degrees from the midsagittal plane, and perpendicular to the image receptor. Collimate, ensuring that labels are included and borders are visible.

Comments

The lateromedial view of the carpus is used to see the articular and proximal surfaces of the three rows of carpal bones.

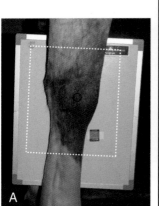
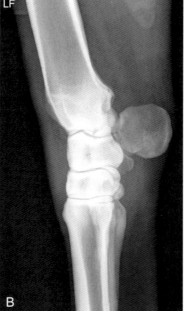

FIGURE 26-30 A, Positioning for the lateromedial view of the carpus. B, Radiograph of the lateromedial view of the carpus.

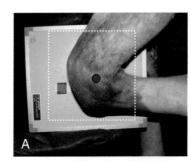
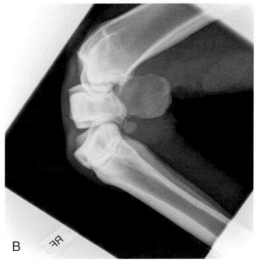

FIGURE 26-31 A, Positioning for lateromedial flexed view of the carpus. B, Radiograph of the lateromedial flexed view of the carpus.

Oblique Views

Oblique views of the carpus are as follows:

Medial oblique–DLPMO: Dorsoproximal 45-degree lateral–palmarodistomedial oblique (DPr45L-PaDiMO).

Lateral oblique–DMPLO: Dorsoproximal 45-degree medial–palmarodistolateral oblique (DPr45M-PaDiLO).

Positioning

The image receptor is placed vertically against the palmarolateral or the palmaromedial side, depending on the projection (Figure 26-32).

Central Ray and Collimation

The x-ray tube is in front of the limb and perpendicular to the image receptor. The beam is centered on the middle of the carpus. Include the entire carpus and a portion of the metacarpal bones and radius. The beam is parallel to the ground and perpendicular to the image receptor.

- For the lateral oblique view: Position the central ray medially 45 to 60 degrees from the dorsal midline (with the image receptor against the palmarolateral aspect).
- For the medial oblique view: Position the central ray laterally 45° to 60 degrees from the dorsal midline (with the image receptor against the palmaromedial aspect).

Collimate, ensuring that labels are included and borders are visible.

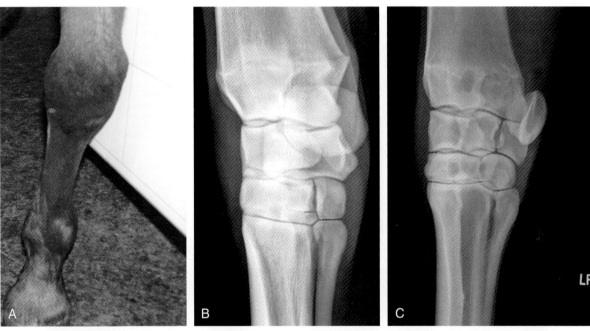

FIGURE 26-32 **A**, Positioning for the DMPLO (lateral oblique) view of the carpus. The proper description is the dorsoproximal 45-degee medial–palmarodistolateral oblique (DPr45M-PaDiLO). Place the limb as close as possible to the image receptor. **B**, Radiograph of the lateral oblique or DMPLO view of the carpus. **C**, Radiograph of the medial oblique or DLPMO view of the carpus.

Skyline: Flexed Dorsoproximal–Dorsodistal Oblique (DPr-DDiO) Views of the Distal Radius, Proximal Row of Carpal Bone, and the Distal Carpal Row[2]

Positioning

Elevate the limb and flex the carpus, so the metacarpals are horizontal, and parallel to the ground, for all the views. Place the image receptor firmly against the dorsal surface of proximal metacarpus, parallel to the ground (Figure 26-33).

Central Ray and Collimation

Include the dome of the carpus. Aim the central ray toward the midsagittal plane of the dorsal surface of the carpus.

The exact location and angle of the beam to the image receptor vary, depending on the row of carpal bones being imaged, as follows:

- For the flexed D65Pr-DDi for a skyline view of the dorsodistal radius:
  - The radius is vertical to ground at the level of the opposite carpus.
  - The central ray is angled to 65 degrees with the image receptor.
- For the flexed D45Pr-DDi for a skyline view of the dorsal aspect of the proximal row of carpal bones:

- The radius is angled at 45 degrees with the ground and slightly cranially so the flexed carpus is slightly in front of the opposite carpus.
- The central ray is angled to 45 degrees from vertical or to the plate.
- For the flexed D30Pr-DDi for a skyline view of the dorsal aspect of the distal carpal row:
  - The carpus is maximally flexed so that the radius is angled to 60 degrees with the ground.
  - The flexed carpus is positioned cranial and proximal to the opposite carpus.
  - The central ray is angled 30 degrees with the image receptor.

Collimate, ensuring that labels are included and borders are visible.

Comments

- There will be distortion if the image receptor is not perpendicular to the carpal bones.
- Avoid the tendency to abduct the flexed carpus.

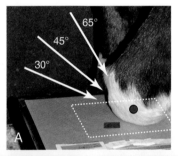

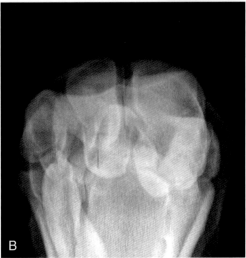
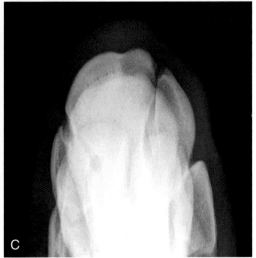

FIGURE 26-33 **A,** Positioning for the skyline view of the carpus or the dorsoproximal–dorsodistal oblique flexed views (DPr-DDiO). **B,** Radiograph of a 60-degree, dorsoproximal-dorsodistal oblique flexed (skyline) view (D60Pr-DDiO) of the distal row of carpal bones. **C,** Radiograph of the distal row of carpal bones with a 30-degree angle.

Tarsus

Dorsoplantar (DP): Dorsoproximal-Plantarodistal (DPr-PlDi) View

Positioning
The limb being evaluated is bearing full weight. The opposite limb may have to be elevated. The vertical image receptor is caudal to the limb on the plantar aspect (Figure 26-34).

Central Ray and Collimation
From the middle of the tarsal joint at true DP plane, center on the imaginary line from the middle of the foot wall to the tibia. Include the entire tarsus, a portion of each of the metatarsal bones, and the medial and lateral malleoli of the tibia. The beam is parallel to the ground and perpendicular to the carpus and image receptor. Collimate, ensuring that labels are included and borders are visible.

Comments
- This view demonstrates the tarsal joint and a portion of the bones proximal and distal to it.
- The primary beam is usually directed horizontally, but in some horses, it is best to direct the beam 5 to 10 degrees proximodistally to visualize the joint more clearly.

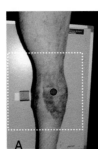
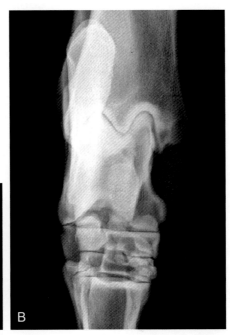

FIGURE 26-34 A, Positioning for the DP (dorsoproximal-plantarodistal) (DPr-PlDi) view of the tarsus. **B,** Radiograph of the DP view of the tarsus.

Lateromedial (LM) Extended View

Positioning

The patient is standing in a natural weight-bearing position. Place the image receptor perpendicular to the ground against the medial aspect of the tarsus. Keep the tarsus under the body, and prevent abduction (Figure 26-35).

Central Ray and Collimation

Center over the lateral aspect of the limb in the middle of the tarsal joint. Include the entire tarsal joint. The beam is parallel to the ground and 90 degrees from the midsagittal plane. Collimate, ensuring that labels are included and borders are visible.

Lateromedial Flexed (LM) View

Positioning

Place the vertical image receptor against the medial aspect of the tarsus. Elevate the limb of interest, and flex the tarsus as the horse will allow. Support the foot at the level of the tarsus of the opposite limb with the affected tarsus slightly dorsal to the limb. Keep the tarsus under the body, and prevent abduction (Figure 26-36).

Central Ray and Collimation

Center over the lateral aspect of limb at the talus. Include the point of the hock, distal tibia, and proximal metatarsal bones. The beam is parallel to the ground and angled 90 degrees from the midsagittal plane.

The central ray is perpendicular to the image receptor. Collimate, ensuring that labels are included and borders are visible.

Comments

- Care must be taken when flexing the tarsus to monitor the comfort level of the patient.
- Wear protective PPE.

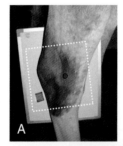

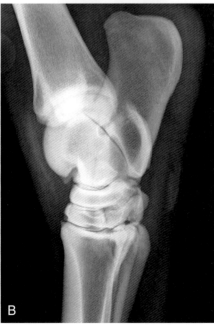

FIGURE 26-35 A, Positioning for the lateromedial (LM) view of the tarsus. B, Radiograph of lateromedial (LM) view of the tarsus.

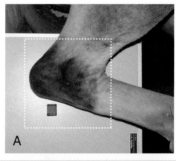

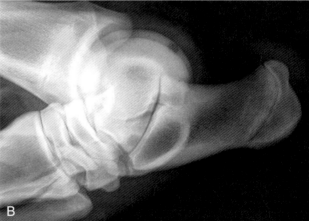

FIGURE 26-36 A, Positioning for the lateromedial flexed view of the tarsus. B, Radiograph of the lateromedial flexed view of the tarsus.

Oblique Views

Oblique views of the tarsus are as follows:

Medial oblique–DLPMO: Dorsoproximal 45-degree lateral–plantarodistomedial oblique (DPr45L-PlDiMO).

Lateral oblique–DMPLO: Dorsoproximal 45-degree medial–plantarodistolateral oblique (DPr45M-PlDiLO).

Positioning

The patient is standing in a normal weight-bearing position. The image receptor is placed vertically against the plantaromedial or plantarolateral aspect of the tarsus (Figure 26-37).

Central Ray and Collimation

The x-ray tube is in front of the limb and perpendicular to the image receptor. The central ray is directed horizontally to center on the central tarsal bone. The beam is parallel to the ground.

• For the medial oblique view: Position the central ray laterally 45 to 60 degrees from the dorsal midline (with the image receptor against the plantaromedial aspect) (see Figure 26-37A and B).

• For the lateral oblique view: Position the central ray medially 45 to 60 degrees from the dorsal midline (with the image receptor against the plantarolateral aspect) (see Figure 26-37C).

Collimate, ensuring that labels are included and borders are visible.

Comments

• The actual position of the central ray in relation to the dorsal midline may vary depending on the confirmation.

• There will be greater magnification with the medial oblique view owing to increased OFD, which is caused by the angulation of the distal tibia.

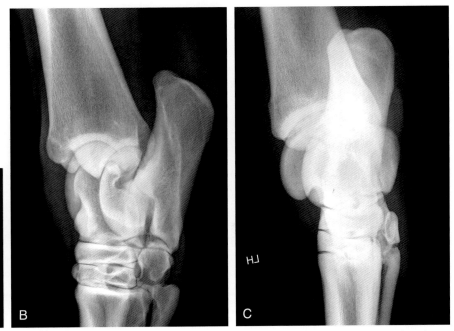

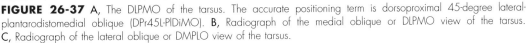

FIGURE 26-37 A, The DLPMO of the tarsus. The accurate positioning term is dorsoproximal 45-degree lateral-plantarodistomedial oblique (DPr45L-PlDiMO). **B,** Radiograph of the medial oblique or DLPMO view of the tarsus. **C,** Radiograph of the lateral oblique or DMPLO view of the tarsus.

Skyline: Flexed Plantaroproximal-Plantarodistal (PlPr-PlDi) View of the Tuber Calcaneus and Sustentaculum Tali

Positioning

Elevate the limb and flex the tarsus joint so that the metatarsal bones are parallel with the ground and horizontal for all views. Place the image receptor horizontally and firmly against the plantar surface of the calcaneus, parallel to the ground (Figure 26-38).

Central Ray and Collimation

Position the x-ray tube directly above the tarsus, perpendicular to the ground with the central ray on the tuber calcaneus. Ensure that the beam is straight down, as perpendicular to the image receptor as possible, with a slight cranial angulation, to avoid the thigh musculature. Include only the calcaneus and sustentaculum tali. Collimate, ensuring that labels are included and borders are visible.

Comments

- This skyline flexed view provides evaluation of the calcaneus and the sustentaculum tali from a proximal-to-distal direction without overlying bony shadows.[3]
- The use of a ceiling-mounted x-ray unit is preferred, because of the height of the positioning of the tube head required.

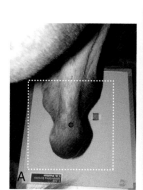
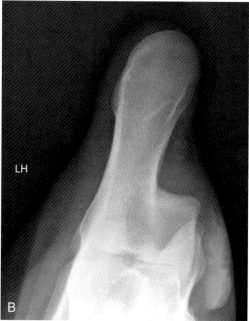

FIGURE 26-38 A, Positioning of the tuber calcaneus for the skyline flexed or plantaroproximal-plantarodistal (PlPr-PlDi) view. **B,** Radiograph of the tuber calcaneus for the skyline flexed or plantaroproximal-plantarodistal (PlPr-PlDi) view.

Radius/Ulna

Craniocaudal (CrCd): Cranioproximal-Caudodistal (CrPr-CdDi) View

Positioning

The patient is standing in a natural weight-bearing position. The image receptor is caudal to the palmar aspect of the limb and perpendicular to the ground (Figure 26-39).

Central Ray and Collimation

Center on the midsagittal plane of the radius/ulna. Include at least one joint. Ensure that the beam is parallel to the ground and perpendicular to the limb and image receptor. Collimate, ensuring that labels are included and borders are visible.

Comments

- The positioning is easier in a young horse or a recumbent patient.
- Include at least one joint to provide orientation if more than one view is required.
- The central ray is usually directed at the point of injury or the location of pain or swelling.

Lateromedial (LM) View

Positioning

The patient is standing in a natural weight-bearing position. The image receptor is against the medial aspect of the cannon bone (Figure 26-40).

Central Ray and Collimation

Position the beam parallel to the ground and angled 90 degrees from the midsagittal plane. Center on the radius/ulna at the point of injury or pain. Collimate, ensuring that labels are included and borders are visible.

Comments

- Include at least one joint to provide orientation.
- If the affected limb can be pulled forward to position the plate laterally, the beam can be directed in a medial-to-lateral direction.

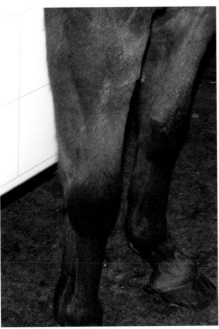

FIGURE 26-39 Positioning for the craniocaudal (CrCd) or cranioproximal-caudodistal view of the radius and ulna.

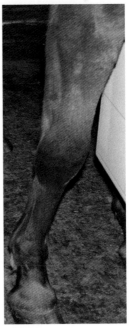

FIGURE 26-40 Positioning for the lateral view of the radius and ulna.

Elbow (Brachioantebrachial Joint)

The elbow joint is difficult to radiograph while the animal is in a standing position because of its proximity to the ventral body wall. The use of general anesthesia is preferred if possible. Because of the increased thickness of the limb, higher-capacity x-ray equipment is required.

Craniocaudal (CrCd): Cranioproximal-Caudodistal (CrPr-CdDi) View

Positioning

With the patient anesthetized and in lateral recumbency, abduct the limb and extend it away from the body wall. With the patient in standing position, extend the limb as far cranial as possible. The foot is elevated off the ground. Place the image receptor against the radius/ulna, pushing medially against the ventrolateral thorax caudal to the olecranon (Figure 26-41).

Central Ray and Collimation

Direct the central ray in a cranioproximal-caudodistal direction through the cranial aspect of the joint. The beam should be perpendicular to the image receptor and the limb. Include the olecranon and a portion of the radius and ulna. Collimate, ensuring that labels are included and borders are visible.

Comments

* Because of its proximity to the ventral body wall, this joint is difficult to radiograph; anesthesia is preferred.
* This view shows the humeroradial joint space and medial and lateral aspects of the humerus and radius.
* Lifting the foot off the ground partially separates the elbow from the chest wall.
* If the patient is weight-bearing, the central ray will be more horizontal to the ground. Place the image receptor with the long edge pressed firmly against the ventrolateral thorax at the caudal aspect of the elbow. Extend the lower inner corner ventral to the thorax to include the distal humerus.

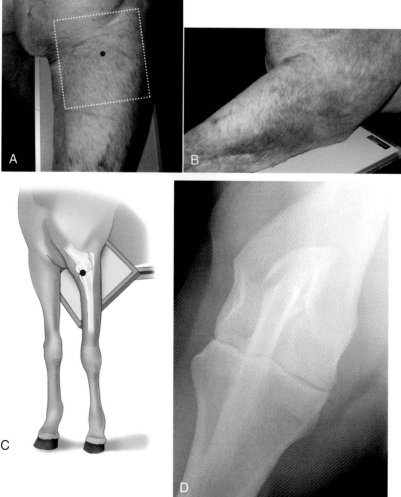

FIGURE 26-41 A and B, Positioning for the craniocaudal view of the elbow. C, Anatomy of the craniocaudal view of the elbow. D, Radiograph of the craniocaudal view of the elbow.

Mediolateral (ML) View

With the patient standing, the mediolateral view is the easiest positioning for the elbow and is often suitable for a portable x-ray unit.

Positioning

Extend the affected limb cranially as far as possible. Elevate the limb, and manually pull it forward so the radius is parallel to the ground. Place the image receptor firmly against the lateral aspect of the limb, with the elbow joint centered to the image receptor. The image receptor must remain perpendicular to ground (Figure 26-42).

Central Ray and Collimation

Center on the elbow joint. Include the entire joint in collimation. Direct the beam parallel to the ground, toward the medial side of the elbow joint just cranial to the opposite forelimb. Collimate, ensuring that labels are included and borders are visible.

Comments

- Forward extension is required for an adequate projection.
- If the limb cannot be extended, the patient may need to be bearing weight on the limb and a lateromedial view obtained with the image receptor positioned against the medial aspect. The distal humerus or olecranon is not as well visualized with this position.
- A recumbent study is best with the patient in lateral recumbency.

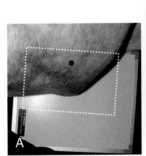
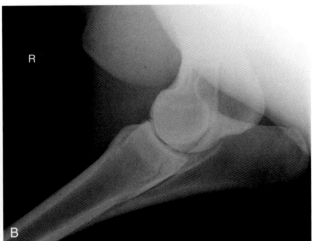

FIGURE 26-42 A, Positioning for the lateromedial view of the elbow. B, Radiograph of the lateromedial view of the elbow.

Shoulder

To attain quality projections of the shoulder joint, the use of general anesthesia and placement of the patient in lateral recumbency are recommended. The standing position may be possible if the patient tolerates manipulation. The easiest and maybe only view of the shoulder that can be obtained is the mediolateral.

Mediolateral (ML) View

Positioning

Elevate the affected limb and pull cranially with the radius parallel to the ground. Superimpose the humeral head over the soft tissue of the neck. Firmly place the image receptor against the lateral aspect of the shoulder joint (Figure 26-43).

Central Ray and Collimation

The x-ray tube is on the opposite side of the patient. Direct the beam parallel to the ground and perpendicular to the image receptor, centered on the joint. Include the proximal humerus and distal spine of the scapula. To center on the scapulohumeral joint, palpate the distal aspect of the spine of the scapula of the opposite limb. Direct the central ray 10 cm cranial and proximal to this.[2] Collimate, ensuring that labels are included and borders are visible.

Comments

· If injury to the supraglenoid process is suspected, direct the central ray more dorsocaudally.
· If there is injury to the tubercles, direct the central ray more ventrocaudally.[3]

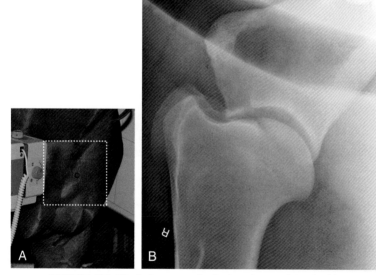
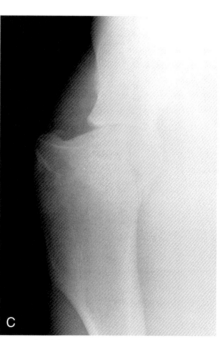

FIGURE 26-43 A, Positioning for the lateral view of the shoulder joint. B, Radiograph of the mediolateral view of the equine shoulder joint. C, Radiograph of the craniocaudal view of the shoulder joint.

Oblique Views[3]

Oblique views of the shoulder are as follows:

Lateral oblique (CrMCdLO): Cranioproximal 45-degree medial–caudodistolateral oblique (CrPr45M-CaDiLO).

Medial oblique (CrLCdMO): Cranioproximal 45-degree lateral–caudodistomedial oblique (CrPr45L-CaDiMO).

Positioning

The patient is standing with the affected limb in a normal position slightly cranial to the opposite limb. Place the image receptor cranial and medial to the affected shoulder joint, against the pectoral muscle mass, for the medial oblique view, and lateral to the affected shoulder for the lateral oblique view.

Central Ray and Collimation

The ray is centered at the craniolateral aspect of the proximal humerus. The beam is parallel to the ground or directed downward.

- For the medial oblique: Position the x-ray tube caudally and lateral to the thorax.
- For the lateral oblique: Position the x-ray tube cranial and medial to the opposite limb.

Collimate, ensuring that labels are included and borders are visible.

Comments

- Because the central ray hits the image receptor at an angle, there is distortion of the underlying bones.
- It is difficult to adequately evaluate the shoulder joint space with this view.
- These views are used to evaluate an area of suspected injury at the point of the shoulder.

Stifle (Femorotibial Joint)

Radiography of the femorotibial joint (stifle) is difficult because of the thickness of the surrounding tissue and the sensitive nature of this region. Because of the depth of the muscle in the femoral region, the caudocranial projection demonstrates little above the joint space. Radiographs of this region should be attempted only if the patient is cooperative. Safety is paramount in radiography of the hind region of the horse. Sedation or a twitch may be used; general anesthesia is also to be considered.

Lateromedial (LM) View

Positioning

The patient remains in a natural standing, fully weight-bearing position; angle and cautiously place the image receptor against the medial side of the stifle joint. Use gentle force to push the flat edge of the image receptor as far into the medial aspect of the stifle (flank) as possible. Most patients object to this image receptor placement.

Central Ray and Collimation

Center the ray over the femorotibial joint; approximately 10 cm distal to the patella and perpendicular to the image receptor. Collimate to the size of a large image receptor, ensuring that labels are included and borders are visible.

Comments

- It may also be helpful to visualize directing the central ray approximately 5 to 7 cm proximal to the tibial plateau, between the cranial and middle thirds of the stifle.[6]

- Great care must be taken because of the sensitivity of the patient in this region of the body. All personnel involved must be prepared to respond to the patient at any moment.
- Touching the medial stifle region and the flank prior to inserting the image receptor may help with patient compliance.
- It is helpful to elevate the opposite limb to minimize motion and the risk of being kicked.
- Sedation is highly recommended.
- This view visualizes the articular surfaces of the femorotibial joints.
- To obtain a **flexed** view: Either lift the limb or rest the toe on the ground, creating a "dropped" stifle position. The horse may prefer to rest the toe over a full weight-bearing position of the opposite limb.

Caudocranial (CdCr): Caudoproximal-Craniodistal (CdPr-CrDi) View

Positioning

With the patient in a natural standing position, position the x-ray tube caudally to the stifle joint. To increase the ease of image receptor placement, extend the hind limb caudally and angle the central ray 10 to 20 degrees proximodistally.[4] Place the image receptor cranially to the stifle and tilt it so that the long edge is snug against the body wall (Figure 26-44).

Central Ray and Collimation

Center the ray over the stifle joint approximately 10 cm distal to the patella with the beam almost perpendicular to the image receptor. Aim to angle the central ray 10 to 15 degrees proximodistally so that it exits at the proximal cranial tibia level.[2]

Collimate, ensuring that labels are included and borders are visible.

Comments

- This view is indicated to identify secondary bone growth within the joint space. Consider that the distal growth center of the femur closes at age 20 to 30 months. The apophyseal center of the tibial tuberosity joins the proximal tibial growth center at 9-12 months, and the combined growth centers join the tibial shaft at 20–30 months.[3]
- This view helps detect changes indicative of secondary joint disease and evaluate the joint width.

> **TECHNICIAN NOTES**   A firm touch is less irritating than a light touch for the patient. Introduce a gloved hand prior to the introduction of the image receptor. Be sure not to come in contact with the sheath of a male horse. Keep alert to any signs of agitation displayed by the patient.

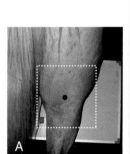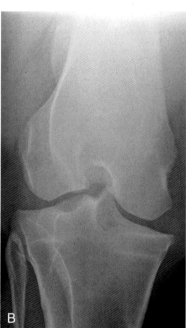

FIGURE 26-44 A, Positioning for the caudocranial view of the stifle. B, Radiograph of the caudocranial view of the stifle.

Medial Oblique (CdLCrMO): Caudoproximal 60-Degree Lateral–Craniodistomedial Oblique (CdPr60L-CrDiMO) View

Positioning

The horse is standing in a natural, weight-bearing position (Figure 26-45).

Central Ray and Collimation

Center the ray approximately 10 cm on the caudal aspect of the limb at the level of the femorotibial joint[4] at a downward angle of 10 degrees.[2] Direct the x-ray tube horizontally and position it caudally and laterally. Push the image receptor as far into the flank as possible, resting it against the medial ridge of the trochlea.[3]

Collimate, ensuring that labels are included and borders are visible.

Comments

The flexed lateromedial view displaces the patella distally to better visualize the proximal femoral trochlear ridges, proximal tibia, and apex of the patella.

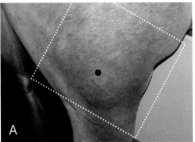

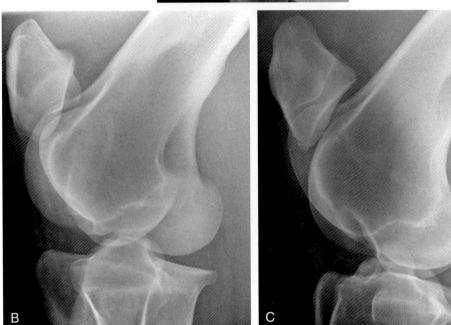

FIGURE 26-45 A, Positioning of the medial oblique (caudolateral-craniomedial oblique) view of the stifle. B, Radiograph of the medial oblique (caudolateral-craniomedial oblique) view of the stifle. C, Compare the oblique view in B to this lateral view of the stifle, and note the superimposition of the bones in the lateral view.

Skyline: Cranioproximal-Craniodistal Oblique (CrPr-CrDiO) View

Positioning

With the patient in a natural standing position, lift the distal hind limb, flex and retract it caudally to place the tibia horizontally. Position the image receptor horizontal to the ground facing the stifle, so the caudal part of the plate touches the tibial crest. Position the x-ray tube dorsally and angled down to the stifle (Figure 26-46).

Central Ray and Collimation

Direct the central ray distally (downwards) distally and 10 degrees lateral to medial. Tightly collimate to the cranial patella. Ensure that labels are included and borders are visible.

Comments

This view is used to access fractures of the patella. The medial and lateral trochlear ridges as well as the intertrochlear groove of the femur are visualized.[2]

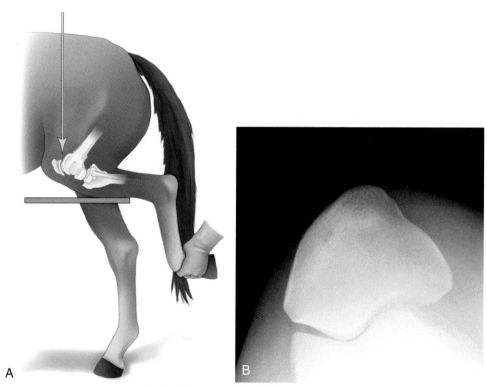

FIGURE 26-46 A, Positioning for the skyline view of the stifle joint. B, Skyline radiographic view of the patella.

Pelvis and Hip Joints

General anesthesia is required for the pelvic radiographic study of a large animal patient. Young foals or calves can be successfully radiographed in the field, whereas larger patients (horses or cows) must be radiographed in the hospital setting because of the specific high-powered radiographic equipment required, such as a mobile or ceiling-mounted unit, to provide proper output (high kV exposure). Views may be segmented to obtain a complete pelvic view (multiple images used for a single view). If using film, the use of a table with an embedded cassette tunnel is preferred to increase ease of positioning and cassette exchange. Owing to the thickness of this region, the use of a grid is suggested.

Before administration of a general anesthetic, special consideration must be given to the anesthesia recovery process for patients with pelvic fractures or luxation. As a result, a pelvic radiographic study may be contraindicated.

Ventral Dorsal (VD) View

Positioning

Place the patient in dorsal recumbency with the hind limbs flexed in a "frog-leg" position (Figure 26-47). Angle the limbs about 20 to 30 degrees above the surface, not touching the ground or table. Evacuation of the rectum may be required to minimize artifacts for an evaluation of the pelvic symphysis.

Central Ray and Collimation

Position the tube directly vertical to the pelvis with the beam centered over the image receptor. Multiple views may be required, depending on the size of the patient. Center the beam over specific areas of interest and perpendicular to the image receptor to minimize distortion. Collimate, ensuring that labels are included and borders are visible.

Comments

- It is important for the two legs to be positioned at the same angle and flexion to maintain symmetry of the pelvic joints.
- If more than one projection is necessary, each centering point should be marked with a marker or tape. Marking the centering points allow adjustments to be made from the previously exposed site.
- For a thorough assessment, five to seven overlapping radiographs may be required.

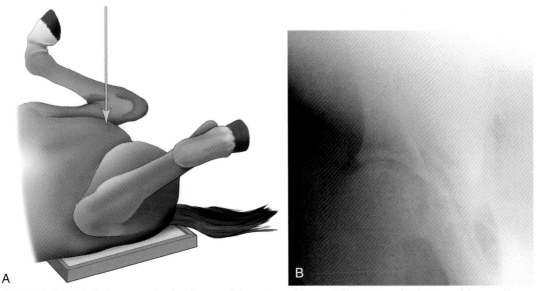

FIGURE 26-47 A, Positioning for the VD view of the pelvis and hip joint. The arrow is the direction of the central ray. **B,** Radiograph of the acetabulum of an anesthetized patient in a ventrodorsal view.

Ventrodorsal Oblique View (for Each Hip)

Positioning

Place the patient in a ventrodorsal position, with the hind limbs flexed (frog-leg), and pelvis then shifted 10 to 20 degrees to elevate the unaffected side away from the tabletop. Rectal evacuation is not required for this position. Image receptor is positioned under the patient.

Central Ray and Collimation

Position the beam directly vertical to the hip joint and center laterally from the midline over the hip joint of interest.[3] Angle the beam perpendicular to the image receptor. Collimate, ensuring that labels are included and borders are visible.

Comments

- The oblique views are to isolate and evaluate the individual hip joint. Comparative radiographs are recommended.

- A specific angle is not critical, provided it is possible to repeat the same angle on the opposite side.
- X-ray positioning devices may be helpful to maintain and repeat the angle of the pelvis. Ensure that both the hind and front ends of horse are rotated.
- Secure the patient to prevent injury and unexpected movement. The use of ropes is critical to secure the patient on the tabletop.
- Protective padding is recommended with the use of ropes to prevent tendon and ligament injuries.
- The use of a cassette tunnel is preferred for ease of changing image receptors.
- The proximal femur can also be radiographed if the beam is centered more laterally.

Head, Neck, Thorax, and Abdomen

- The image receptor is placed against the side of the skull (Figure 26-48) closest to the area of interest (i.e., lesion).
- The x-ray tube is positioned on the opposite lateral side. Note that for all positions:
- Position the patient in a natural standing posture.

- Direct the central ray on the area of interest and perpendicular to the image receptor.

Collimate, ensuring that labels are included and borders are visible.

See Table 26-3 for further specifics.

Skull Comments

- The area of interest must be isolated because of the density of the skull and multiple areas of interest.
- For best results, multiple views are recommended, including oblique views.
- Removal of the halter is required to avoid artifacts. A rope halter or a halter fashioned from a rope may be used. Inspect the rope for small metal clips, which are often present in manufactured rope products.
- It is difficult to minimize movement of the skull. Sedation may or may not be beneficial. Placing a cover over the patients' eyes may be helpful. Maintaining constant contact will keep the horse at ease and prevent reaction to changes in positioning.
- The head is held without rotation.
- Lowering the level of the head by extension or mild pressure allows for easier positioning of the unit and the image receptor.
- Because of the weight of the x-ray unit, it may be difficult and awkward to hold it motionless at the level of the skull. The use of a stand or ceiling-mounted unit may prove more successful.
- Flushing of the oral cavity is required to remove any foodstuffs to prevent artifacts.
- If the patient is sedated, an oral gag may be used to improve the isolation of the selected arcade for oblique views.

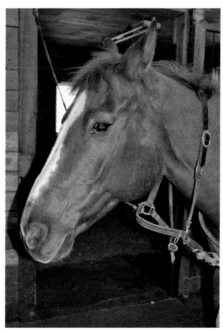

FIGURE 26-48 Use of halter or lead shank to prevent artifacts for skull imaging.

TABLE 26-3	Imaging of the Equine Head, Neck, Thorax, and Abdomen			
BODY PART	**PROJECTION**	**IMAGE RECEPTOR PLACEMENT**	**X- RAY TUBE**	**FURTHER COMMENTS (+SEE BELOW)**
Skull	Lateral (Figure 26-49)	Against the affected side.	Opposite lateral side.	From the opposite side on area of interest.	
Skull	Dorsoventral (DV) (Figure 26-50)	Horizontal ramus against the ventral aspect of the mandible.	At the dorsal aspect.	Along the midline of dorsal skull on area of interest, perpendicular to the horizontal ramus of mandible.	Easier to note asymmetry. Will need increased exposure.
Maxillary sinuses, nasal passage	Oblique views: Dorso 45-degree lateral–ventrolateral oblique (D45L-VLO) (Figure 26-51)	Ventral, against affected side. Plate is angled 45 degrees.	Dorsolateral above the head on the opposite unaffected side.	On 3rd and 4th cheek teeth and 45 degrees from parallel plane directed downward.	Avoids superimposition of cheek teeth. Best views for maxillary sinuses, frontal sinuses, and both dental arcades. Bilateral recommended.
Incisor	D45L-VLO	Below affected jaw and laterally.	Above affected jaw and opposite lateral.	45-degree angle directed downward on area of interest.	
Upper dental arcade	D45L-VLO	Against affected side laterally.	Position laterally against unaffected side on the dorsal head.	Downward 45 degrees from horizontal on area of interest.	Can reverse so image receptor against unaffected side and beam aimed upward 45 degrees (V45L-DLO).
Lower dental arcade	D45L-VLO	Unaffected side ventrally.	Laterally to affected side of head dorsally.	Downward 45 degrees from horizontal on area of interest.	
Frontal region	D30L-VLO	Affected side slightly ventrally.	Opposite unaffected side slightly above head.	30 degrees centered on midline behind eye on the affected side.	Avoid inadvertent rostrocaudal angulation. Will need less exposure than if imaging teeth.
Teeth	V45L-DLO (Figure 26-52)	Above affected jaw (dorsally) and laterally.	Below affected jaw (ventrally) and from opposite lateral.	45-degree angle directed upward.	Alternative view for oblique teeth. For upper dental arcade, the image receptor is placed against the unaffected side.
Teeth	Occlusal (Figure 26-53)	In the mouth as far caudal as the patient will allow.	Maxillary: dorsal to head Mandibular: ventral to head.	Maxillary: direct beam downward Mandibular: direct beam upward at 60–80 degrees from vertical, depending on the conformation of incisors.	Difficult as patient not likely to cooperate without chemical restraint. Need lower exposure than for cheek teeth.

Continued

TABLE 26-3	Imaging of the Equine Head, Neck, Thorax, and Abdomen—cont'd			
BODY PART	**PROJECTION**	**IMAGE RECEPTOR PLACEMENT**	**X- RAY TUBE**	**CENTRAL RAY**	**FURTHER COMMENTS (+SEE BELOW)**
Guttural pouch/ larynx/ pharynx/ hyoid bones	Lateral (Figure 26-54)	Lateral side of the caudal skull.	Horizontal beam opposite lateral side of the skull.	Caudal to vertical ramus of mandible (over guttural pouch region). At caudoventral angle of the mandible for the nasopharynx, larynx, and proximal trachea.	Portable unit may be used because it is soft tissue density. Position as for routine skull views. Oblique views can be taken with 10- to 20-degree caudorostral angle.[2] Endoscopy is preferred for nasopharynx, larynx, and proximal trachea.
	Dorsoventral (DV)	Ventral: under the mandible.	Dorsal to the head.	Midline of the skull over the area of interest.	Sedation is highly recommended.
Cervical spine	Lateral (Figure 26-55)	Side of the cervical region.	Opposite side of neck.	Centered on region of choice: C-2 C-4 C-6	Because of the size of the patient, the cervical spine must be exposed in three views. The patient can be standing or recumbent.
Thoracic spine	Lateral (Figure 26-56)	Side of the patient on area of interest.	Opposite side.	Area of interest perpendicular to the image receptor.	Often completed for the dorsal spinous processes (withers).
Thorax	Lateral (Figure 26-57)	Affected side	Horizontal beam on opposite side.	See comments below for specifics: (1) midcraniodorsal (2) midcaudodorsal (3) midcranioventral (4) midcaudoventral	Patient standing. Portable unit not powerful enough.
Abdomen	Lateral (Figure 26-58)	On side (most lesions on midline).	Opposite side.	Last rib for small horses: (1) midcranioventral (2) midabdominal (3) midcaudodorsal (4) midcaudoventral	Multiple laterals required for larger patients.

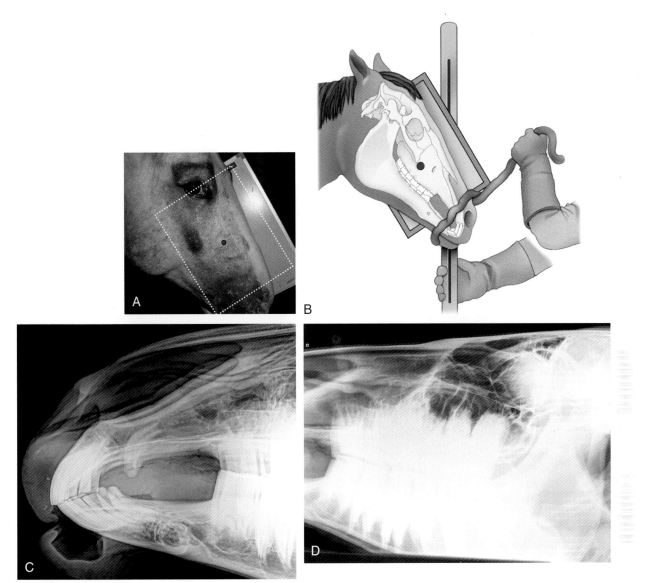

FIGURE 26-49 A, Positioning for the lateral view of the skull. B, Anatomy of the view of the lateral skull. Radiographs of the lateral skull, cranial aspect (C) and caudal aspect (D).

> **TECHNICIAN NOTES** The dental formula (see chapter 24 for further explanation) of the horse is:
> * Deciduous: 2(di3/3, dc 0/0, dp 3/3) = 24
> * Permanent: 2(I3/3, *C1/1, *P3-4/3, M3/3) = 36–42

*Mares often do not have canine teeth; the first premolars, called wolf teeth, are often not present in either species.

Cervical Spine Comments

* Remember that the cervical spine is located in the ventral portion of the neck.
* If the patient is in lateral recumbency, positioning devices are required to position the spine parallel to the table.
* An increase in exposure factors is needed.

* Flexed lateral, ventrodorsal, and oblique views are optional.
* Consider placing radiopaque markers dorsal to the vertebrae for identification and repeat radiographs.
* Collimate to the bones.

Thoracic Spine Comments

* A lower-powered unit can be used to visualize the dorsal spinous processes (withers) of the thoracic spine (Figure 26-56).
* For ventral portion of the thoracic vertebrae, a high-powered x-ray apparatus and a grid are needed.
* Patient positioning is similar to that for radiographs of the thorax, except that the central ray is over the thoracic spine.
* Mobile equipment may be used with smaller patients (i.e., foals).

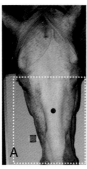

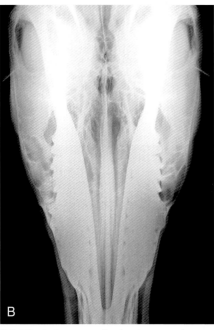

FIGURE 26-50 A, Positioning for the dorsoventral view of the skull. B, Radiograph of the dorsoventral view of the skull.

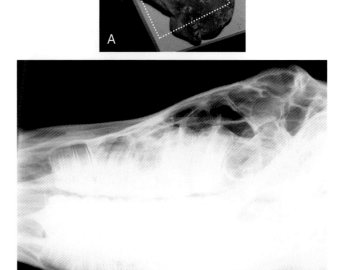

FIGURE 26-52 A, Positioning for the oblique view of the teeth. Also referred to as a latero 30 degree dorsal-lateroventral oblique. B, Radiograph of the oblique projection of the skull.

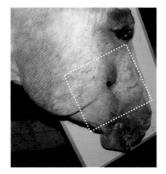

FIGURE 26-51 Positioning for the oblique view of the skull.

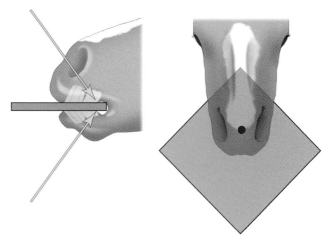

FIGURE 26-53 The position for an intraoral, rostrocaudal oblique radiograph to evaluate the rostral aspect of the incisive bone and the incisors. The downward arrow is the direction of the central ray for radiography of the maxilla and the upward arrow indicates the direction of the central ray for the mandibular structures.

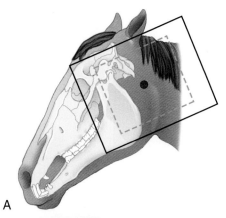

A

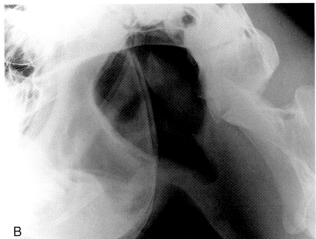

B

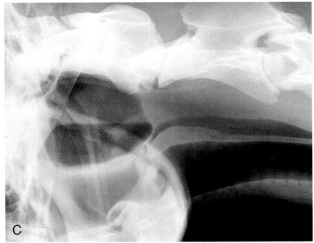

C

FIGURE 26-54 A, Positioning for the lateral view of the guttural pouch. Radiographs of the lateral (B) Guttural pouch (C). Larynx/pharynx.

Thorax Comments

- High kVp with a grid is used.
- The SID is usually increased to 80 inches.
- The caudodorsal region could be imaged with low-output equipment, short SID, and fast intensifying screens.
- Radiographs are generally taken at full inspiration.
- In a natural standing position, the elbows of a horse are superimposed over the cranial region of the thorax. Extend the forelimbs to prevent superimposition.
- Center for the following regions in an average size horse. Use a large image receptor and collimate to within the margins[2] (Figure 26-57):
  - Craniodorsal: 10–15 cm ventral to the most caudal point of scapula.
  - Caudodorsal: 20 cm caudal to and 15 cm ventral to the most caudal part of the scapula.
  - Cranioventral: 15 cm caudal to the shoulder joint.
  - Caudoventral: 20 cm ventral to and 10 cm caudal to most caudal point of the scapula.

Abdomen Comments

- Equipment and preparation are as for the thorax, high-powered equipment being needed to penetrate the thick tissue.

- The abdomen of the horse can be radiographed in standing or recumbent position.
- Diagnostic ultrasound is generally used in lieu of abdominal radiographs.

Other Large Animal Radiography

Bovine

Even if they are frequently handled, bovine patients have little to no experience of handling of their lower extremities. This fact poses a challenge to perform radiographs of any extremity. Maintaining image receptor placement close to the limb without proper restraint devices is almost impossible in most conditions. The use of stocks, ropes, and pulley, or ideally, a lift table, will aid in the production of quality radiographs of cattle. It is these challenges plus economic concerns, that radiographs are generally only completed in high-quality or high-producing livestock.

The use of stocks provides reduced mobility of the patient; however, they do not limit the mobility of the limbs. Securing the affected limb or, if weight-bearing, rigging an

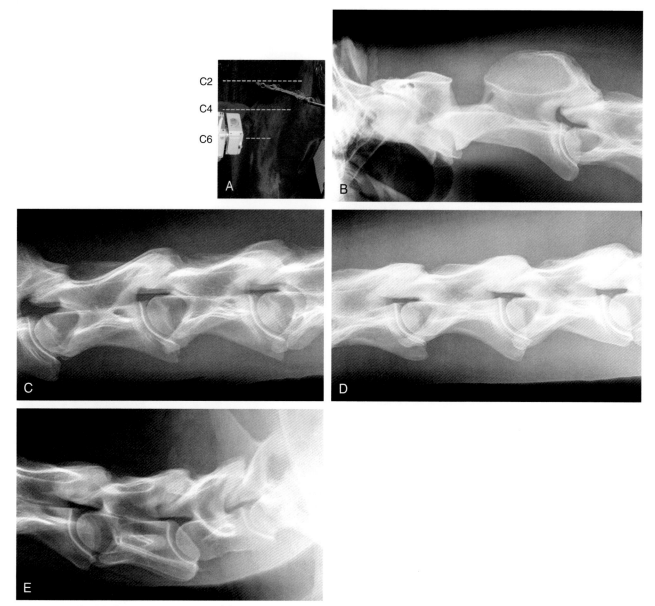

FIGURE 26-55 A, Positioning of the cervical vertebrae. Note the three areas of centering, C2, C4, and C6. Radiographs of the lateral cervical spine series: **B,** C1 and C2; **C,** C3 and C4; **D,** C4 and C5; **E,** C6 and C7.

alternate limb through ropes, may be required. The use of a lift table enables the limbs to be secured in a motionless fashion and increases positioning options since the patient can be lifted and tilted off the ground. The lifting of the alternate limb may increase the safety of maneuvering around distal extremities.

Sedation or rapid general anesthesia may be used with the bovine patient. The combined use of restraint devices and sedation can significantly increase the safety of personnel, equipment, and the patient for bovine radiographs. Care must be taken to consider the stage of gestation, if applicable, and the potential for recovery trauma.

Before a digit radiograph is taken in the bovine patient, the interdigital space and both claws should be cleansed thoroughly, and both claws should be lightly trimmed. If this

step is not taken, false images or shadows may mask abnormalities present in the claws. The digits can be viewed radiographically using four angles or projections.[7]

Equipment requirements and positioning techniques for bovine radiography are the same as those for equine radiography. Handling restrictions may hinder the options and available positions. See Table 26-4 for the common views. Center on the area of interest. For a joint, include up to one-third of the bones proximal and distal; for a bone, include the joints proximal and distal. Pelvis, skull, spine, thorax, and abdomen radiographs are completed much like those in horses.

In the case of a small calf, radiographs may be performed in the clinic with use of positioning and techniques similar to those used for a large dog. A mobile x-ray

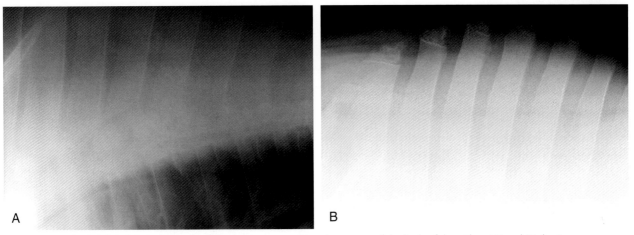

A

B

FIGURE 26-56 Radiographs of the thoracic spine. Note the images of the body of the withers (**A**) and (**B**) the tips.

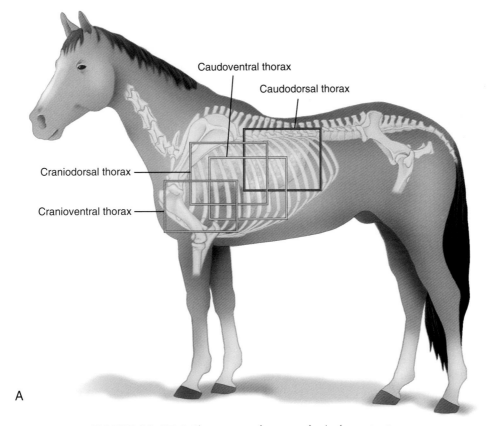

Caudoventral thorax

Caudodorsal thorax

Craniodorsal thorax

Cranioventral thorax

A

FIGURE 26-57 A, Thorax areas of centering for the four main views.

machine can be used to take thoracic or abdominal radiographs in a small calf (Figure 26-59).

Ovine/Caprine/Porcine

Small ruminant patients (sheep/goats) and swine can be radiographed much like small animals. Because they can be easily transported, small ruminant patients are often radiographed within the clinic setting. Because of their minimal handling experience, however, care must be taken to prevent injury due to patient response to fear (i.e., thrashing of limbs). If the patient is horned, special precautions to prevent injury to staff must be taken. Sedation is recommended to produce quality radiographs in an efficient manner.

Care must be taken with the fleece of the ovine patient. The fleece is dense and may contain dirt and debris (i.e., twigs, clumps of mud/stones). Before imaging, carefully

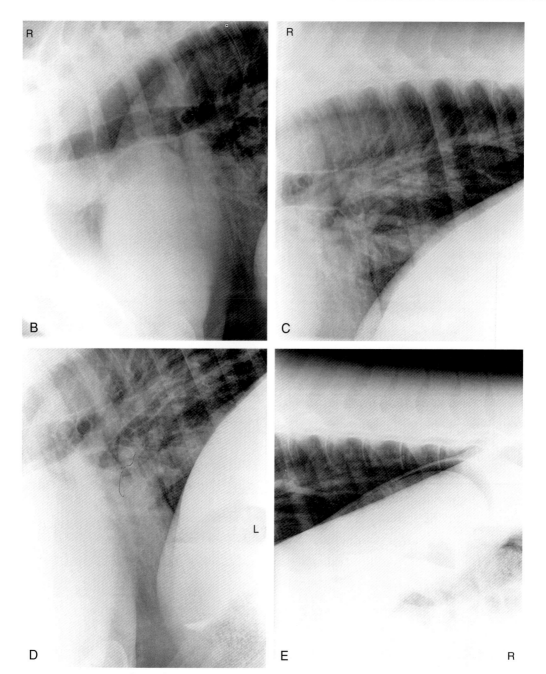

FIGURE 26-57, cont'd Lateral radiographs of the cranioventral thorax (**B**), craniodorsal thorax (**C**), caudoventral thorax (**D**), and caudodorsal thorax (**E**).

inspect for and remove debris that may produce artifacts within the image.

Alternate Modality Images

It is beyond the scope of this text to discuss alternate modalities (Figure 26-60) in this edition. Additional imaging, such as nuclear scintigraphy, infrared thermal imaging, and MRI, show more features for diagnosis but are considerably more expensive than imaging with the use of x-radiation.

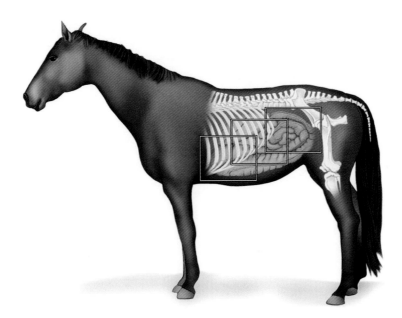

FIGURE 26-58 Abdomen.

TABLE 26-4	Suggested Views for the Bovine Limb Examination	
EXAMINATION	**STRUCTURES EVALUATED/ COMMENTS**	**VIEWS***
Digit/foot P3 (distal phalanx)	Standard: Lateral, DP	Lateromedial
		Dorsal 45-degree proximal–palmarodistal (D45Pr-PaDi)
	Optional, lateral-interdigit	Lateromedial (mediolateral) with interdigital film
	Lateral and medial oblique	Dorsoproximal 45-degree lateral–palmarodistomedial oblique (DPr45L-PaDiMO)/(DPr45M-PDiLO)
Digit/foot P2 and P3	Standard: Lateral, DP	Lateromedial
	Optional: Medial and lateral oblique	Dorsal 45-degree proximal–palmarodistal (D45Pr-PaDi)
		Dorsoproximal 45-degree lateral–palmarodistomedial oblique (DPr45L-PaDiMO) (medial oblique)
		Dorsoproximal 45-degree medial–palmarodistolateral oblique (DPr45M-PaDiLO) (lateral oblique)
Fetlock	Standard Views: Metacarpophalangeal/ metatarsophalangeal articulation: DP, lateral, medial, and lateral oblique	Dorsopalmar DP: Dorsoproximal-palmarodistal (DPr-PaDi)
		Lateromedial extended (LM)
		Dorsoproximal 30-degree lateral–palmarodistomedial oblique (DPr30L-PaDiMO) (medial oblique)
		Dorsoproximal 30-degree medial–palmarodistolateral oblique (DPr30M-PaDiLO) (lateral oblique)
Carpus	Standard views: DP, lateral	DP: Dorsoproximal-palmarodistal (dorsopalmar) (DPr-PaDi)
		Lateromedial extended (LM)
	Optional views: lateral flexed, medial, and lateral oblique	Lateromedial flexed (LM)
		Dorsolateral-palmaromedial oblique (DL-PMO) (medial oblique)
		Dorsomedial-palmarolateral oblique (DM-PLO) (lateral oblique)
Elbow joint	Standard	Caudocranial standing (CrCd)
		Lateromedial standing (LM)
	Optional views	Craniocaudal standing (CrCd)
		Obliques (O)
Shoulder	Standard view	Obliques standing (O)
	Optional	Mediolateral recumbent (ML)
Stifle	Standard	Caudocranial (CdCr)
		Lateromedial
	Optional	Lateromedial (LM) patella
		Craniolateral-caudomedial oblique (CrLCdMO)

**Palmar(o)* is used with the understanding that *plantar(o)* can be substituted when referring to the hind limb.

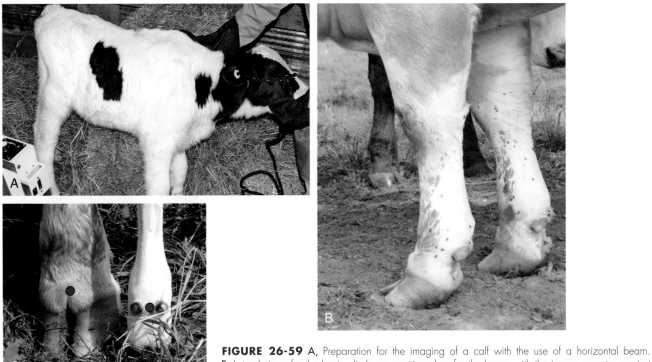

DP   PD

FIGURE 26-59 A, Preparation for the imaging of a calf with the use of a horizontal beam. B, Lateral views for the bovine limb are positioned as for the horse, with the image receptor against the medial aspect, parallel to the area of interest and perpendicular to the ground. The central ray is 90 degrees to the midsagittal plane, parallel to the ground, and perpendicular to the cassette. C, DP: Dorsopalmar (forelimb)/dorsoplantar (hind limb) front to back and PD: palmarodorsal (forelimb)/plantarodorsal (hind limb) back to front.

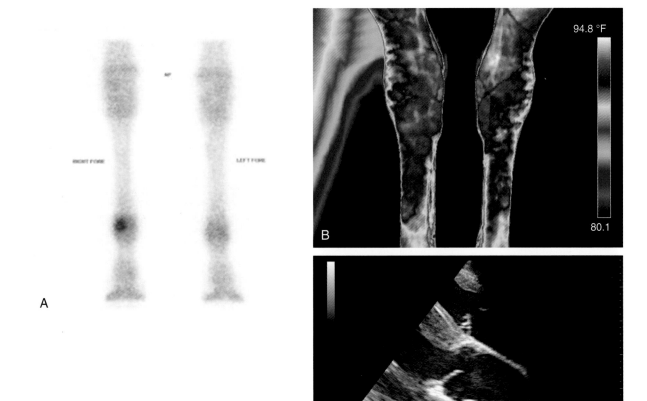

FIGURE 26-60 A, Nuclear scintigraphy of the carpus of a horse. The dark areas indicate "hot spots" or inflammation. B, Infrared thermal image of another horse. The *red areas* indicate "hot spots" or inflammation. C, Ultrasound image of the equine heart.

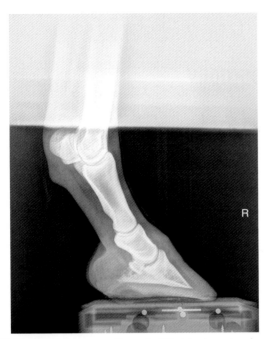

FIGURE 26-61 Mystery radiograph. What body part and position is this? Where is the plate placed?

---

1. Patience, planning, proper preparation, and knowledge of anatomy and directional terms are all required for diagnostic large animal radiographs.
2. Most of the positions in large animals are standing which necessitates the use of the horizontal beam.
3. Radiation, patient, and human safety need to be kept in mind at all times.
4. Because of the unique anatomy of the equine limb, a minimal of four positions is required: dorsopalmar/dorsoplantar, lateromedial, and two oblique views, one on either side of the midsagittal plane taken between the DP and lateromedial positions.
5. If joints are to be examined, further positions may include a flexed lateral, skyline or flexor view.
6. The same principles of radiography apply to all species. Thus the angle of the beam is always perpendicular to the area of interest, but in the equine patient the angle of the beam to the ground for dorsopalmar/dorsoplantar and oblique radiographs may vary according to the foot trimming and anatomy. For lateromedial views, the beam is always parallel to the ground.
7. Standard radiographs for cloven-footed large animals are generally the dorsopalmar/dorsoplantar and lateromedial views with occasional oblique projections for joints.

References

1. Bassert JM, McCurnin DM: *McCurnin's Clinical textbook for veterinary technicians*, ed 7, St. Louis, 2010, Saunders.
2. Weaver M, Barakzai S: *Handbook of equine radiography*, London, 2010, Saunders Elsevier.
3. Morgan JP: *Techniques of Veterinary Radiography*. Ames, Iowa, 1993, Iowa State University Press.
4. Butler JA, Coles CM, Dyson SJ, et al: *Clinical radiology of the horse*, Osney Mead, Oxford, 1993, Blackwell Science Ltd.
5. Han C, Hurd C: *Practical diagnostic imaging for the veterinary technician*, St. Louis, 2005, Elsevier Mosby.
6. Thrall DE: *Textbook of veterinary diagnostic radiology*, ed 5, St. Louis, 2007, Saunders.
7. The Merck veterinary manual. http://www.merckvetmanual.com/mvm/index.jsp?cfile=htm/bc/90504.htm.

Bibliography

American College of Veterinary Radiology (ACVR): *Radiology 2—equine*, 2009, ACVR.

Anderson KL: *Equine Proximal Limb Normal Radiographic Anatomy*, College of Veterinary Medicine, University of Minnesota. http://www.cvm.umn.edu/vetrad/prod/groups/cvm/@pub/@cvm/@vetrad/documents/asset/cvm_asset_360311.pdf

Aspinall V, Cappello M: *Introduction to veterinary anatomy*, London, 2009, Butterman-Heineman.

Bassert JM, McCurnin DM: *McCurnin's Clinical textbook for veterinary technicians*, ed 7, St. Louis, 2010, Saunders.

Colville T, Bassert J: *Clinical anatomy and physiology for veterinary technicians*, St. Louis, 2008, Elsevier.

Done SH, Goody PC, Stickland NC, Evans SA: *Color atlas of veterinary anatomy, the dog and cat*, London, 2009, Mosby.

Douglas SW: *Principles of veterinary radiography*, London, 1980, Bailliere Tindall.

Dyce KM, Sack WO, Wensing CJG: *Textbook of veterinary anatomy*, ed 4, St. Louis, 2010, Saunders.

Lavin L: *Radiography in veterinary technology*, ed 3, St. Louis, 2007, Saunders.

O'Brien T: *O'Brien's Radiology for the Ambulatory Equine Practitioner*, Jackson, 2005, Tewton NewMedia.

Radiology of the equine limbs. (n.d.). http://www.quia.com/files/quia/users/medicinehawk/2407-Vet/Radiology-2.pdf

Redding WR: *Radiographic Examination of the Equine Foot*. College of Veterinary Medicine, North Carolina State University, Raleigh, NC. http://www.equipodiatry.com/Radio.htm

Reid CF, Bathurst NW: *Large animal radiography nomenclature*. 1995, University of Pennsylvania School of Veterinary Medicine. http://cal.vet.upenn.edu/projects/larad/names/name.htm

Romich J: *An illustrated guide to veterinary medical terminology*, Clifton, NY, 2009, Delmar Cengage Learning.

Smallwood JE, Shively MJ, Rendano VT, Habel RE: A standardized nomenclature for radiographic projections used in veterinary medicine, *Vet Radiol* 26:2-9, 1985.

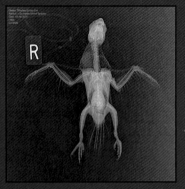

KEY TERMS

Orthogonal
Positional terminology

TECHNICAL NOTE

To preserve space, the radiographs presented in this chapter do not show collimation. For safety, always collimate so that the beam is limited to within the image receptor edges. You should see a clear border of collimation on every radiograph. In some jurisdictions, use of collimation is the law.

Avian and Exotic Radiography

Be as a bird perched on a frail branch that she feels bending beneath her, still she sings away all the same, knowing she has wings.

—Victor Hugo, French writer, 1802–1885

OUTLINE

LEARNING OBJECTIVES

Upon completion of this chapter the reader should be able to:

1. Produce diagnostic high-quality radiographs of birds, small mammals, and reptiles with special emphasis on:
   - Understanding of common anatomical species-specific terms.
   - Radiographic concerns related to the anatomy of the species.
   - Common reasons for imaging.
   - Machine and positioning considerations.
   - Patient preparation and concerns.
   - Normal views and protocol for the various species and positions.
   - Familiarity of the normal species imaging with special emphasis on measuring, centering, inclusion, positioning, and how to tell whether the image will be parallel to the image receptor and if both will be perpendicular to the central ray.
   - Identify normal avian and exotic species anatomy found on a radiograph.

Medical imaging is an important diagnostic tool in avian and exotic animal medicine (Table 27-1). The anatomy of the respiratory tract limits auscultation, and it is also difficult to palpate much of the viscera. Radiographs are often required by the veterinarian for avian patients that show obscure clinical signs. The bird's system of air sacs provides enhanced contrast in areas that are not well visualized in mammals.

Very small variations in x-ray output are more noticeable in the avian patient than in cats and dogs because of their smaller size; thus, a high-frequency unit with uniform output is required. The machine should be capable of producing at least 300 milliamperes (mA), have an exposure time of 1/60 sec (0.17 sec) or faster, and a kilovolt peak (kVp) range of 40 to 60 kVp that should be adjustable in 2-kVp increments. Short exposure times are essential to minimize the motion artifacts associated with a rapid respiratory rate and muscle tremors that are common in birds as well as in some small mammals.

Because of lower bone density than in reptiles or mammals, less exposure is needed for flight birds of the same thickness. Wing radiographs are often overpenetrated, making this area appear excessively dark with low contrast. Unlike with dogs and cats, the determination of the exposure is not usually based on measurement, because most exposure charts are based on species and size. If there is not a specific avian or small mammal chart, the cat abdomen chart for that thickness is useful. Then start with decreasing the milliampere-seconds (mAs) by at least 50%. Alternatively the feline extremity chart can be used. If a measurement is taken for any of the species, it should be at the thickest body part of the area to be examined.

The general principles of canine and feline radiography apply to avian, as well as rodent and rabbit imaging. Two orthogonal views should also be taken.

A longer scale of contrast associated with lower kVp in the 40 to 60 kVp range is preferred. Non-screen film (larger dental film, size 4) is useful, and high-detail film screen systems produce images with better detail than digital systems. Use of mammography cassettes with a single screen and with single emulsion film is especially diagnostic. As a guide, about four times the mAs will be required over a regular 400 speed system.

Digital radiography systems usually use higher kVp techniques than the film/screen systems, possibly leading to lower contrast, but incremental changes of 2 kVp will help with adjustments of proper contrast. However, a greater image contrast range, resulting in improved image quality, is more possible in digital radiography than with film imaging. Special algorithms for digital units are required that are often provided by the manufacturers.[1]

Further detail can also be achieved with smaller focal spots. Grids are not typically used because most patients are less than 11 cm wide. For avian patients wider than 11 cm, the air within the air sacs of birds does not generate noteworthy scatter radiation.

The tube stand should have source-image distance (SID) adjustments that can compensate for changing the mAs to decrease the exposure time. Remember from Part Two that mAs is inversely proportional to the square of the distance from the x-ray source (focal spot), so that as you decrease the distance from the source, you can also decrease the mAs. However, remember also that as the SID decreases, the magnification increases which affects penumbra. The minimum

TABLE 27-1	Recommended Views of Exotic Species for Complete Body Study	
SPECIES	**RECOMMENDED VIEW**	**OPTIONAL**
Avian	VD: coelom (whole body) Lateral: coelom (whole body) with wing superimposition	Modified lateral: whole body; wings not superimposed Wing: CdCr and mediolateral Lateral and VD Foot: lateral and CrCd Contrast study for GI tract Urography for urinary tract
Small mammals	DV: whole body (smaller mammals) Lateral: whole body	VD: whole body or site of interest Extremities: lateral and ventral recumbency Contrast study for GI
Larger pocket pets—rabbits, ferrets, guinea pigs	VD: site of interest Lateral: site of interest Skull: DV and lateral Extremities: both views	Contrast study for GI Further skull views
Lizards	Whole body: DV with vertical beam Whole body: lateral with horizontal beam	Extremities: vertical beam Contrast study for GI
Turtles or tortoises	DV with vertical beam Lateral: horizontal (preferred). Rostrocaudal: horizontal beam (preferred)	Contrast study for GI
Snakes	DV: whole body for GI, cranial 2/3 for respiratory Whole body for GI: lateral view, with horizontal beam	Contrast study for GI

Cd, caudal; Cr, cranial; DV, dorsoventral; GI, gastrointestinal; VD, ventrodorsal.

SID used should be 30 inches (76 cm) unless a magnification study is required.

Dental units can be used, provided that the patient is small (typically less than 20 g for birds), the area localized, and the patient anesthetized to minimize respiratory movements. Portable units used for large animals typically do not produce sufficient mA values at the required short exposure times without drastically reducing the SID.

Ultrasound, computerized tomography (CT), and magnetic resonance imaging (MRI) are more diagnostic modalities but are relatively expensive and not always readily available.

Avian

Patient Preparation

A bird is best fasted so that the crop (for those species that possess one) feels empty on palpation. The time to achieve this will vary greatly with species and can range from 1 hour to multiple hours. The radiographic appearances of the internal organs are affected by digestive tract contents, possibly leading to misdiagnosis.[1] Avoid gavaging prior to radiography; especially in debilitated birds. The crop and proventriculus emptying times may be prolonged in dehydrated birds. Stress associated with the procedure, increases the likelihood of regurgitation and airway aspiration.

Recall that in canine and feline patients, thorax radiographs should be taken at peak inspiration. In the avian patient, however, the air is continuously moving into the pulmonary parenchyma, and the air sacs and the lungs are nonexpansile; thus, the effect of the respiratory cycle on the radiographic appearance is less noticeable. However, in some cases, distention of the abdominal air sacs may enhance the contrast of the abdominal viscera, especially those with abundant coelomic fat. Positive-pressure ventilation can be applied to an intubated, anesthetized bird for air sac inflation, and the radiographic exposure timed accordingly to correspond with increased air in the sacs. Regardless, respiratory movements should be minimized, if possible, by trying to coordinate the exposure time during a pause in the respiratory cycle.

Anesthesia and Positioning Devices

Anesthetizing a healthy bird with inhalation gas anesthesia is generally less stressful for the patient than taking radiographs unanesthetized. Accurate positioning with near-perfect alignment is essential for correct interpretation of avian images. In addition, the radiographs are generally of higher quality and fewer images need to be taken because

there is less chance of motion artifacts. The birds are easily positioned, there is less potential for iatrogenic fractures, and the air sacs can be inflated in the intubated patient. Anesthesia and stress may further compromise debilitated patients.

Precautions should be taken. Many of these considerations apply not only to birds but also to any species undergoing radiography.

The following suggestions apply particularly to the handling of wild birds that are fully conscious[2]:
- Have everything organized prior to the procedure to minimize the time required for restraint or anesthesia.
- Wear protective clothing, gloves, and headgear as appropriate with the species:
  - Wear protective eye wear and long protective gloves over the lower arms for raptor restraint. Never leave talons unrestrained. Once the feet have been radiographed, wrap the talons closed for added handler safety.
  - When working with raptors, never leave talons unrestrained. Once the feet have been radiographed, it is advisable to wrap the talons closed for added handler safety.
  - A full face shield is suggested for water birds with long beaks. Never leave dangerous beaks such as those of herons unrestrained.
- Work in a dimly lit room, and minimize unnecessary noise and movement.
- Ensure that the area is contained, avoiding escape routes and areas in which the patient can hide or injure itself. Have capture devices, such as nets, on hand in case of escape.
- Cover the bird's head and torso with a towel.
- If taping the bird down, ensure that the tape will not rip out feathers (See Figure 27-1). Stress can be fatal, especially for debilitated birds so reduce stress and minimize handling time.
- If anesthetizing, have everything prepared previously, working quickly and accurately, to minimize the anesthetic time.
- An anesthetized bird should be monitored very closely and regularly, and kept warm.
- For small ill birds, such as canaries or budgies, the veterinarian will not likely recommend anesthesia; excessive handling will cause further stress. Consider using a horizontal beam while the bird is either perching or placed in a small box or plasticware (e.g., Tupperware) container, where it can be wedged in the corner with pieces of foam. The images are not ideal but they may be diagnostic enough to indicate the problem.
- Make sure that the radiographs and the number of views are satisfactory prior to recovering the patient.
- Minimize manual restraint.

Small birds weighing less than 100 g can be positioned directly on the image receptor with masking tape,

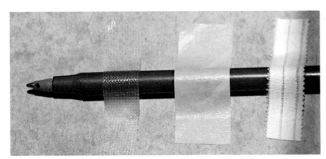

FIGURE 27-1 Three types of tape used for avian and exotic restraint. *Left,* Transparent medical tape is best as it does not pull the feathers off birds. *Center,* Paper masking tape or autoclave tape also minimizes hair and feather loss. *Right,* Adhesive tape could pull off feathers and hair. Floral tape is also effective.

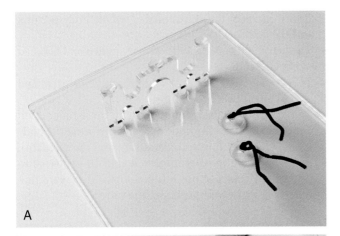

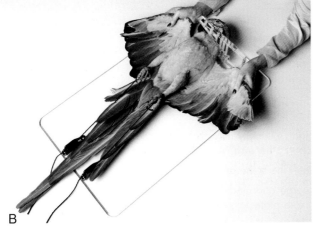

FIGURE 27-2 Two types of avian restrainers. **A,** VSP Avian Neck Restraint & VSP Avian Restraint Board (Veterinary Specialty Products, Shawnee, KS). Different-sized collars or suction cups are available. **B,** Starting to get the bird in position with use of the Miami Vice positioner.

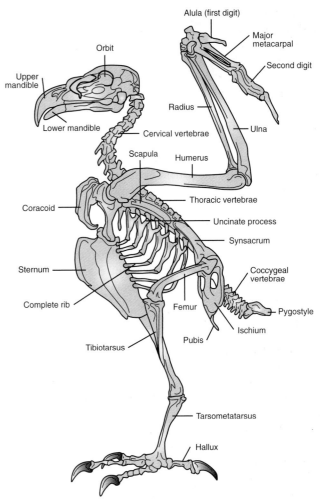

FIGURE 27-3 Skeleton of a hawk.

transparent medical tape, or a floral Millipore tape. This paper tape is less likely to damage the skin and feathers (Figure 27-1). Using bird positioning devices or restraint boards simplifies the positioning and reduces the time for correct positioning.

Use of a plexiglass or other acrylic restraint device (Figure 27-2) often requires an increase of 2-4 kVp, especially if the lower range of kVp is used. Extensions such as intravenous

(IV) tubing, rope, or gauze can be used in lieu of tape to attach the limbs to the positioner or to the table. Alternatively, sandbags can be gently placed over the extensions. Cardboard shoeboxes or plasticware containers can restrain ill birds that cannot tolerate anesthesia (Figure 27-16A). Be careful with patient stress and possible injury that may result from struggling.

As with mammals, two projections, made at a 90-degree angle (orthogonal projections), are recommended unless the patient is compromised. Standard views include lateral and ventrodorsal studies of the coelom. Because of the curvature of the skeletal structures of the wing, both orthogonal projections of the wings, taken while the patient is in either ventrodorsal (VD) or lateral recumbency, will turn up as lateral views. If a pectoral extremity is required, the standard is the mediolateral and caudocranial of the wing.

In between imaging and during recovery, ensure that the bird is placed in a normal sternal position to aid breathing efforts. A towel "donut" (twisted towel to support the bird) can help with this. Do not place the bird on a perch until the patient is fully recovered. Because recovery can be rapid, ensure that hands are on the larger patient especially, to prevent a fall.

Radiographic Views

Lateral View of the Avian Coelom

Positioning

Place the patient in right lateral recumbency. Use a radiolucent or cardboard sheet on the cassette to tape the patient to this sheet to facilitate moving the patient if another exposure is required. Gently extend the bird, and with precut strips of tape, carefully tape the patient on the radiolucent plexiglass or cardboard sheet in the following order if the patient is not chemically restrained:

Head: Tape is gently placed across the neck at the base of the skull. If the tape is too tight, tracheal collapse may result.

Wings: Extend the wings dorsally in full extension; tape the dependent wing first and then superimpose the upper wing. Avoid excessive pressure to the upper wing to prevent rotation.

Pelvic limbs: Extend and superimpose the pelvic limbs slightly caudally, secure the tape or gauze to the distal tarsometatarsal bones, and extend the limbs. Tape the dependent limb first.

Tail: Taping of the tail is optional but should be close to the base. Include the correct positional marker, and place it on the cranial aspect of the film.

If the bird positioner (commercial or homemade guillotine device [bird board]) is being used:
- Place the neck in the cervical restraint portion; then gently move the body caudally to reduce the curvature of the neck.
- Immobilize the rest of the body as just described, using tape, gauze, or tubing to secure the limbs to the cleats.

Comments and Tips

- If the patient is anesthetized, the order of taping or positioning is not important.
- Be gentle; luxation of the shoulder can result if the position is forced. Consider increasing the plane of anesthesia, but keep in mind there may be an anatomical inability to position the limb properly.
- Superimposition of the extremities helps minimize rotation. If pelvic limb or wing images are required, the limbs are not superimposed; instead they are positioned as described later for the modified whole-body/pectoral limb lateral view.
- The pelvic limbs need to be securely pulled and fastened to straighten the femur.
- The sternum and vertebral column can be palpated and should be on the same plane.
- The tail can be taped, and more tape can be placed on either the humeral portions of the wings or on the body if needed. Be careful to avoid pressure over the chest area.
- If the lungs are to be examined, it may be beneficial to deliberately underexpose a lateral view. Make sure that the wings are drawn away from the torso.

> **TECHNICIAN NOTES**   When working with raptors, make sure to tape the talons or use Vetwrap to keep them restrained once the feet have been imaged.

MEASURE: If a variable chart is available or a modified cat abdominal/extremity chart is being used: At the thickest part of chest (over the keel if it is a larger bird). Use the species and size chart otherwise.

CENTRAL RAY: At the level of the xiphoid (caudal tip of keel), between the spine and keel.

BORDERS: For small birds, the whole body should be included. For large and medium birds, include the coelom, proximal extremities, and caudal cervical regions, or the area of interest. Multiple plates are needed for larger birds, especially long-necked patients such as swans.

Lateral View of the Avian Coelom—*cont'd*

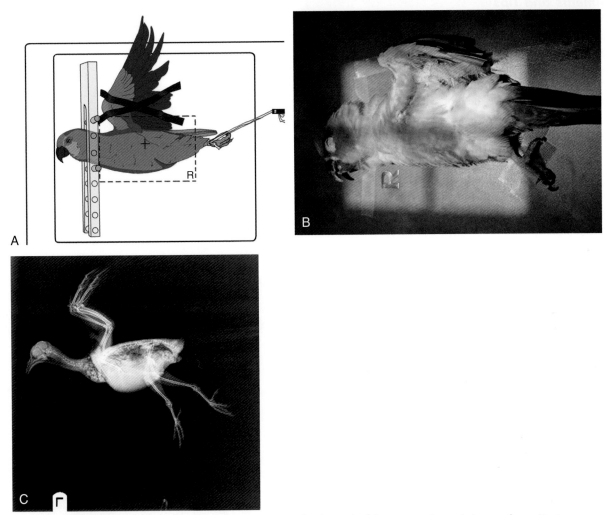

FIGURE 27-4 **A,** Positioning technique for a right lateral radiograph of the avian coelom with the use of a positioning device.[5] **B,** Positioning for a lateral whole-body radiograph of a Sun Conure with the use of tape. If the extremities are superimposed, there will be less rotation of the bird's body. **C,** Radiograph of the lateral view of an adult bird with the wings superimposed. Superimposition of the pelvic limbs also assists in minimal rotation.

Modified Whole-Body/Pectoral Limb Lateral View

Comments and Tips

- If the pectoral or pelvic limbs of small birds need to be radiographed, the limbs and wings can be separated in the lateral view to minimize the number of images needed. Position in lateral recumbency as described previously, with the following exceptions:
    - Do not superimpose the limbs; instead separate both the wings and the legs.
    - The extremities on the dependent side should be pulled and taped cranially, with padding placed between the perspective limbs to avoid rotation of the body.
    - Secure the contralateral limbs caudally (leg) and dorsally (the wing) to minimize superimposition.
- In this view, the contralateral wing is in a mediolateral view but there will be increased object-film distance (OFD); thus the patient is best placed in a VD position for the mediolateral pectoral limb.
- There is more rotation of the body when the limbs are not superimposed.

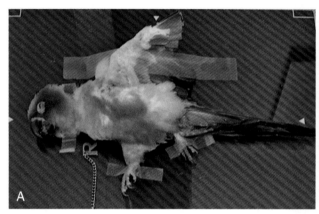
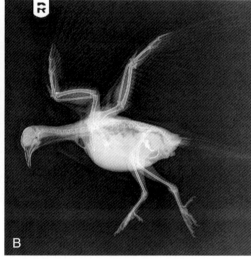

FIGURE 27-5 A, Modified positioning technique for a right lateral radiograph of the avian, if separation of the extremities is required. B, Radiograph of the modified lateral view of an adult bird with the wings separated.

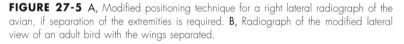
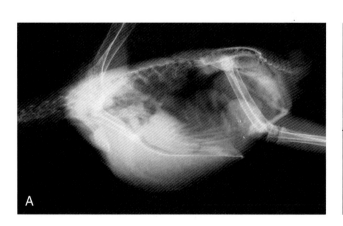
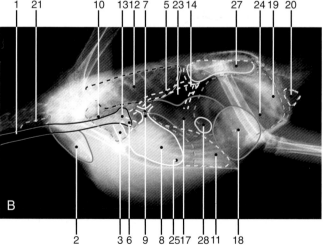

FIGURE 27-6 Radiographic anatomy of the lateral view of the adult Lovebird. Projection: Laterolateral (right lateral recumbency). 1, Trachea; 2, crop; 3, brachiocephalic artery and aorta; 4, brachiocephalic artery; 5, aorta; 6, pulmonary artery; 7, pulmonary vein; 8, heart; 9, left atrium; 10 esophagus; 11, liver; 12, lung; 13, syrinx; 14, gonad; 15, ovary; 16, testes; 17, proventriculus; 18, ventriculus; 19, intestines; 20, cloaca; 21, cervical air sac; 22, clavicular air sac; 23, thoracic air sac; 24, abdominal air sac; 25, apex of heart; 26, interface between caudal thoracic and abdominal air sacs; 2,7 kidneys; 28, spleen.

Ventrodorsal View of the Avian Coelom

Positioning

Place the patient in dorsal recumbency. Have precut paper tape ready. If the positioning board is used, the fabric gauze or IV tubing found on the board can be attached to the cleats or suction cups in lieu of tape (See Figure 27-7).

Gently extend and carefully secure the patient in the following order if the bird is not chemically restrained:

Head: If using a bird positioning board, gently place the head in the cervical restrainer portion in a true rostrocaudal position. Otherwise place tape at the mandibular articulation at the base of the skull.

Wings: Open the wings at a 90-degree angle to the body with two pieces of tape crossed at the carpal region of each wing. *Never* tape over the chest: because of the delicate air sacs, respiration is impacted.

Pelvic limbs: Apply tape or tubing separately around each tarsometatarsus and pull caudally and symmetrically.

Tail: Tape close to the base of the tail if needed.

Comments and Tips

- Place an indicator marker on the appropriate side.
- If the patient is anesthetized, the order of taping or positioning is not important.
- To position the leg caudally without moving the bird's body, gently place a finger at the tip of the sternum for resistance, making sure not to press dorsally on the sternum while doing so; otherwise the bird could suffocate.

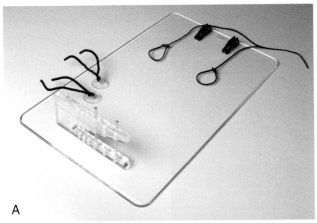

A

> ### TECHNICIAN NOTES
> - To ensure that a VD coelom or whole-body view is symmetrical:
>   - The keel (sternum) is directly over the spine.
>   - The scapula, acetabulum, and femur are parallel, equidistant, and symmetrical.
>   - The wings are open at 90 degrees to the body.

MEASURE: If a variable chart is available or if a modified cat abdominal/extremity chart is used: At the thickest part of chest (over the keel if it is a larger bird). Use the species and size chart otherwise.

CENTRAL RAY: Over the midline at the caudal tip of sternum.

BORDERS: Include the whole body for a small bird. For a large or medium sized bird, include the coelom, proximal extremities, and caudal cervical regions, or the area of interest. Multiple plates are needed for larger birds, especially long-necked patients such as swans.

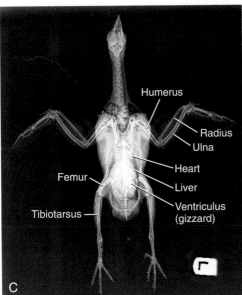

Humerus

Radius
Ulna

Heart

Femur

Liver

Ventriculus
(gizzard)

Tibiotarsus

C

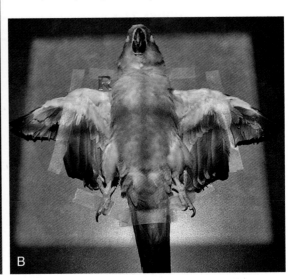

B

FIGURE 27-7 A, VSP Miami Vise Avian Restraint. Another type of positioner is the Auspex Avian Positioner (Jorgensen Laboratories, Inc., Loveland, CO; *not shown*), which has two short slots and four longer slots machined through the board with several pieces of strategically placed hook-and-loop hook-type fasteners permanently attached to the bottom of the board. B, Positioning for the ventrodorsal view of a Sun Conure with the use of tape. C, Radiographic anatomy of the ventrodorsal view of an adult Lovebird.

Mediolateral View of a Wing in Isolation

Positioning

For a true mediolateral view of the wing with decreased object-film distance (OFD), place the bird in dorsal recumbency. Position the body as in the VD view of the coelom.

- Position the body to the side of the cassette to allow the affected wing and area of interest to be centered. Tape at the mandibular articulation at the base of the skull. Open the wings at a 90-degree angle to the body with two pieces of tape crossed at the carpal region of each wing. Separate and tape the pectoral limbs at the tarsometatarsal bones.

Tape the tail close to the base. Additional tape can be applied to the proximal and distal portions of the affected wing if needed (See Figure 27-8).

Comments and Tips

- The positioning of the affected wing is more crucial, but keep the patient's injuries in mind.
- A decrease of 2 to 4 kVp from the coelomic view prevents overexposure.

CENTRAL RAY: Mid-wing or the area of interest.

BORDERS: Include the entire wing, including the scapulohumeral joint. For large birds, the wings may have to be positioned diagonally across the image receptor to maximize the x-ray field.

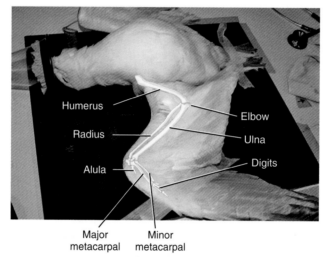

FIGURE 27-8 Positioning for a mediolateral view of avian wing in isolation.

Caudocranial View of the Wing

The caudocranial (CdCr) view of the wing is taken to see a true orthogonal view because both the lateral and VD coelom positions show the wings in a lateral projection. This view is also referred to as a "leading edge or hanging drop view,"[2] because the cranial edge of the wing is placed just above the cassette. The patient should be sedated or anesthetized. Unfortunately, to obtain a true caudocranial view the patient needs to be held (See Figure 27-9).

Positioning

Carefully position the patient upside down with the head directed to the floor. Have the long axis of the body parallel to the vertically directed x-ray beam. Extend the wing fully with its cranial edge in contact with the image receptor.[3]

Comments and Tips

- To prevent variable OFD, it is important to keep the wing as close and as parallel to the image receptor as possible.
- Distortion may occur toward the edges of the radiograph of birds with large wings because of beam divergence.
- For direct digital units, the CdCr view may be difficult because the x-ray sensor may not move to the edge of the table.
- The craniocaudal (CrCd) view is not as practical and would have an increased OFD because of the length of the flight feathers.

CENTRAL RAY: On the area of interest.

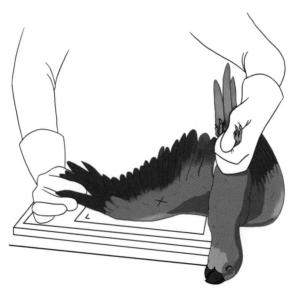

FIGURE 27-9 Positioning for a caudocranial view of the avian wing. The patient does need to be sedated and is held to ensure the proper orientation.

Lateral View of the Avian Head

Positioning

Place the patient in right lateral recumbency with the head either positioned through the cervical restrainer of the acrylic positioning board or taped to a sheet or image receptor. Collimate, and keep the head on the plate, carefully supporting the rest of the body with a towel or other positioner, depending on patient size. Secure the head by separately applying tape to the mandible and maxilla. A species and size exposure chart will likely be used otherwise measure at the thickest part (See Figure 27-10).

CENTRAL RAY: Ventral to the eye.

BORDERS: Include the entire head extending to the cervical region.

Ventrodorsal View of the Head

Positioning

Place the patient in dorsal recumbency as for the VD view of the coelom. Ensure the head is in a true rostrocaudal position. Apply radiolucent tape to the ventral aspect of the rhinotheca to bring the maxilla closer to the cassette (See Figure 27-11).

CENTRAL RAY: Midline between the eyes.

BORDERS: Include the entire head.

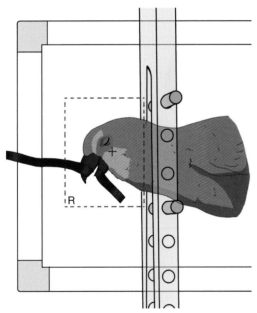

FIGURE 27-10 Positioning for a lateral view of the avian head.

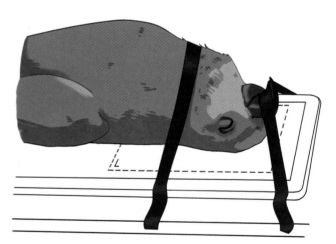

FIGURE 27-11 Ventrodorsal positioning for a radiograph of the avian head.

Mediolateral of the Foot

Depending on the size of the patient, the image of the foot can be combined with a full body view as described for the modified whole body/limb view. Larger patients may require a separate film, or a coelom view may not be required (See Figure 27-12).

Positioning

Place the patient in right lateral recumbency via an acrylic positioning board or taped to a sheet or the image receptor. If the positioning board is utilized, use tape, not the cleats, to secure the feet directly to the board. Separate the digits of the affected limb to minimize superimposition by applying radiolucent tape on each toe. The tape allows for more precise positioning than gauze. Tie and secure the unaffected limb caudally. Extend the dependent limb cranially to prevent superimposition.

Comments and Tips

* A decrease of 2 to 4 kVp from the coelomic view prevents overexposure.

CENTRAL RAY: On the condyles of the tarsometatarsal bone.

BORDERS: Include all of the phalanges.

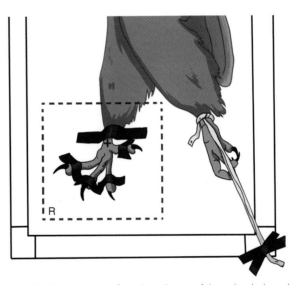

FIGURE 27-12 Positioning for a lateral view of the pelvic limb and foot.

Craniocaudal View of the Avian Pelvic Limb

Positioning

Place the patient in dorsal recumbency. Position as for the VD view of the coelom, securing the head and pectoral limbs. Separate and use tape or gauze or tubing at the tarsometatarsal bones of the pelvic limbs and caudally extend them. Separate the toes with tape or cotton to prevent superimposition, being careful of any injury.

Comments and Tips

* Place an R or L marker on the appropriate limb, and center accordingly.
* If needed tape the tail close to the base and additional tape can be applied to the proximal portions of the affected limb.

CENTRAL RAY: On the affected limb(s).

BORDERS: Include just beyond the affected area.

Contrast Study of the Gastrointestinal Tract

Birds generally have a rapid digestive tract transit time, although it varies greatly among species. This feature, plus the anatomy, makes a single protocol for a contrast study possible, unlike for most mammals. Oral contrast media can be administered to study the digestive tract from the esophagus to the large intestine, and occasionally the cloaca. However, for true cloacal studies, contrast medium should be administered retrograde directly into the cloaca.

Preparation

Ideally the crop and the proventriculus should be empty, provided that the bird can tolerate fasting. The fasting period depends on the size, metabolic requirements, and health of the bird. Food in the ingluvies (crop) decreases the volume of contrast media that can be safely administered. Food in the gastrointestinal (GI) tract prevents full contact of the contrast medium with the digestive tract mucosa and may delay passage of the contrast medium.

Birds weighing more than 300 g should not be fed pelleted foods within 4 hours of the contrast study. When food is mixed with the contrast medium, the patterns shown on radiographs are unpredictable.

Anesthesia and Positioning Devices

If health of the bird permits, anesthesia is suggested. Tracheal intubation is ideal to prevent aspiration. Anesthetic masks are used for many small birds. Some birds may vomit upon recovery from anesthesia because of hypersensitivity to the gas anesthetic, but anesthetized birds do tend to regurgitate less than non-anesthetized birds.[1]

If regurgitation does occur, remove the medium immediately from the oropharynx with cotton-tipped applicators to prevent the contrast medium from passing through the choanal slit into the nasal cavity. Monitor the oral cavity carefully for any regurgitated contrast medium. In all situations, the cranial portion of the body should be raised.

Barium sulfate 30% weight to volume (w/v) is recommended at a general calculation of 20 to 50 mL/kg; however, it is better to estimate the volume of food that can be safely administered via crop gavage, and to give the contrast medium at only 50% to 75% of this amount.[1]

Warm the medium to room temperature by immersing the syringe in warm water. Make sure to mix the warmed liquid well and to test the temperature prior to administration to prevent crop burn, which can precipitate severe metabolic and fluid imbalances as well as decrease the mucosal detail.

Administer the contrast media via a rigid or soft gavage tube passed into the crop, being careful to verify that the tube is correctly palpated and placed. An increase of 2 to 4 kVp over that used in the survey study is suggested, because of the greater opacity of the contrast medium (Figure 27-13).

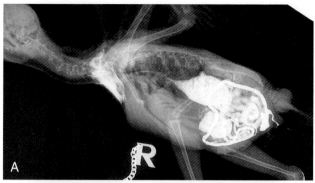

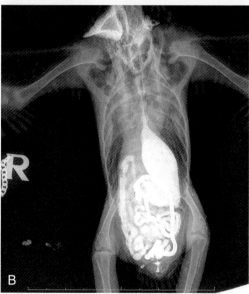

FIGURE 27-13 Gastrointestinal barium study with contrast medium administered about 3 hours previously. **A,** Right lateral; **B,** ventrodorsal. Barium is in the crop, proventriculus, ventriculus, intestines, and cloaca.

Considerations

BORDERS: Include the caudal cervical area and the entire coelom.

Technique

Produce survey ventrodorsal and right lateral radiographs just prior to the contrast study to indicate the current status of the digestive tract. If the esophagus, crop, and proventriculus are of interest, lateral and ventrodorsal radiographs should be taken immediately. There are significant species variations in transit time, so depending on the type of bird, further lateral and ventrodorsal radiographs can be taken at 15 minutes and 30 minutes.

Further 30-minute radiographs can be taken as needed, and if continued anesthesia allows. The procedure is technically finished when the contrast medium has entered the colon. Digestive transit time is generally more rapid than in mammals.

Positioning Concerns

Position as for the lateral and ventrodorsal coelom. To prevent retrograde flow of contrast medium, either raise the cranial portion of the body or apply a bandage to the cervical esophagus.

To raise the cranial body, slide either a radiolucent positioning device under the cranial aspect of the body or under the acrylic positioning device.

A bandage can partially occlude the cervical esophagus to minimize retrograde flow of contrast medium. Take care that any bandage material around the neck does not occlude the trachea. Diligently monitor the anesthesia level and the cavity for any regurgitation.

Double-Contrast Study

A double-contrast study gives superior mucosal detail and usually has a shorter transit time. Anesthesia is frequently required because the gas infused into the crop would be immediately expelled in most awake birds. Less contrast medium is used, lessening the potential for contrast medium to be aspirated into the respiratory tract than with positive-contrast studies. If air is regurgitated, further air can be administered to distend the crop.[1]

Cloacagram

Hollow organs are best viewed if properly distended; thus retrograde administration of barium into the vent is required to fully visualize the cloaca, rather than relying on the antegrade GI dispension.

Procedure

Prior to administration of the barium, gently flush the cloaca with isotonic saline. Positive- and double-contrast cloacagrams can be performed. The common dosage of barium sulfate is 0.025 to 0.05 mL per g body weight.

If a double-contrast study is to be completed, perform the positive-contrast study first, and then remove all of the barium pooled in the cloaca prior to introducing the negative-contrast medium (room air or carbon dioxide). The cloacal mucosal surface is better visualized in this way. Research indicates that carbon dioxide creates less potential for intravascular air emboli to occur. Also, it should be kept in mind that technically, fecal matter can be refluxed into the ureters when retrograde vent procedures are performed.[1]

CENTRAL RAY: Cranial to the cloaca (vent).

BORDERS: Include the cranial third of the coelom.

Positioning

As described for VD and lateral views of the coelom.

Urography

Urography can also be completed through the use of an intravenous contrast medium to evaluate the urinary tract, especially if an abnormal mass is palpated, the droppings volume and consistency have changed, or there is paresis. If anesthesia or sedation cannot be used or if the bird will be stressed out, the procedure should not be completed. The water-soluble iodinated solution (non-ionic preferred) is injected and VD radiographs are rapidly imaged at 10, 60, and 120 seconds after administration. A further VD radiograph can be taken at 5 to 7 minutes to show the contrast agent at the cloaca or rectum.

Radiographic Anatomy

Radiographic anatomy of the avian skeleton is very straightforward but radiographic anatomy and interpretation of the internal structures is more complicated. Radiographically, the viscera are tightly packed together, making it difficult to identify anatomy. There is a minimal amount of perivascular fat and what is present is similar in radiographic density to other soft tissues, making differentiation difficult.

Also, there is no true division of thoracic and abdominal structures because the bird does not have a diaphragm. The advantage for birds and reptiles in not having a diaphragm, is the ability to expand abdominal contents into the respiratory system without any major compromise. Anatomically the coelom is not divided in birds, but for discussion purposes, it is often separated into the thoracic and abdominal regions.

Many features of birds are different from those of mammals and are important in birds. Because many people are not familiar with the anatomy of the avian, more information on anatomy is provided in this chapter. There are lots of differences but also some similarities between birds and mammals.

The skeletal system is different in birds. The anatomy of most birds has been modified for flight either through fusion of bones, reduction in the number of bones, hollowing of bones filled with air spaces, or less bone density through a network of internal bony braces. There are also changes in density that occur with reproduction because of the deposition of medullary bony tissue prior to egg laying.

Appendicular Skeleton

The appendicular skeleton consists of the shoulder bones, wings, pelvic bones, and legs.

Pectoral Girdle and Wing

The shoulder or pectoral girdle consists of three pairs of bones—the clavicle, coracoids, and scapula (Figure 27-14):

- The right and left clavicles are fused to form the furcula (wishbone).
- The strong coracoid extends from the shoulder joint to the cranial end of the sternum.
- The scapula is a flat rod that lies lateral and parallel to the vertebral column extending to the pelvis.

Where the coracoids and scapula are joined on each side, a depression called the glenoid cavity or triosseal canal exists. The wing forms a highly flexible joint in this cavity.

The humerus extends from the shoulder to the elbow joint. The length varies depending on the species. It is longer in birds that soar and glide but short in birds that need to

Coracoid   Clavicle   Scapula

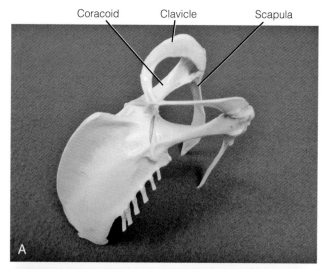

Fused clavicles - furcula

Humerus

Coracoid

Scapula

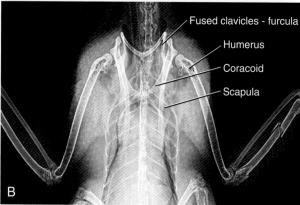

FIGURE 27-14 A, Anatomy of the pectoral girdle of a rough-legged hawk. B, Radiograph showing the pectoral girdle of a red-tailed hawk.

flap during flight. The distal end of the humerus joins at the elbow to a separate radius and ulna (forearm). The distal wing consists of a fused carpus, metacarpal bones, and digits, which all support and control the larger flight feathers.

- The elbow of the bird, called the cubital joint, can be compared to the elbow of the mammal, although there are marked differences. The avian olecranon is short and broad, not tall and narrow.
- The ulna is slightly arched, is longer and generally twice as thick in comparison with the nearly straight radius of mammals. In most birds, the radius and ulna are about 15% larger than the humerus. The radius and ulna are about two-thirds larger than the metacarpus.
- Because of fusion, there are only two carpal bones in the proximal row, the radial and ulnar carpal bones. The distal row has fused with the metacarpus.
- The metacarpal bones consist of the major metacarpus and minor metacarpus, which extend from the carpus.
- There are three avian digits, which along with the metacarpal bones support the primary flight feathers. The stubby first digit, or alular, also originates from the proximal metacarpal tubercle near the carpus and carries the feathers responsible for steering. It is a small rudder-like structure. The second and third digits, respectively,

articulate at the distal portions of the major and minor metacarpus.
- An additional phalanx, sometimes referred to as the fourth digit, is the most terminal skeletal element in the wing.
- Immature wings have blunted bone ends, not obvious joints.

Pelvic Girdle and Legs and Feet

Each side of the pelvic girdle is made up of three bones that join where the leg attaches to the body.

- The broad ilium is fused to the synsacrum; and the thin and long ischium and pubis are fused to the anterior ilium. The ischium and pubis direct caudally and are parallel to the vertebrae. The distal portions are not fused. The hind limb consists of the following:
- Femur, which generally resembles the mammalian bone. At the distal portion of the femur there is a lesser and greater trochanter.
- Patella, which is also similar to the patella in mammals.
- Tibia, which fuses with the tarsus and is called the tibiotarsus. The tibiotarsus is much longer than the femur with which it articulates.
- The smaller-in-diameter fibula also articulates with the femur and almost acts like a splint as it tapers to a sharp point about three quarters of the way down the tibiotarsus. This part of the thigh is known as the drumstick.
- The tibiotarsus and fibula end at the hock, a single elongated fused bone called the metatarsus.
- The distal tarsus merges with the metatarsus to join the tarsometatarsus, which in turn extends to the ground and generally ends in four digits, although some species may have two or three toes. Typically there are three toes pointing forward and one toe pointing backward as an adaptation for perching in many species, but there are exceptions, such as the parrot and budgerigar, both of which have two toes pointing forward and two toes pointing backward.
- Hallux, which is one of the digits and generally points backwards. It is considered the equivalent of the human big toe.
- Phalanx or claw at the end of each digit.

Axial Skeleton

> **TECHNICIAN NOTES**   The axial skeleton follows the same concept as in mammals, in which the bones that make up the general framework are the skull, vertebral column, and sternum.

The Skull

As with other anatomical adaptations, the skull is made for lightness. The bones are thinner and there are no teeth.

- The mandible and maxilla extend into a beak of varying size, depending on the species.
- There are large orbits or eye sockets that are protected by bony plates called the sclerotic ring. Radiographically the eyes may appear nearly as large as the adjacent brain.

- Facial sinuses may be significant in some birds, such as parrots.
- Radiographically these sinuses appear radiodense, and smaller individual structures may be hard to identify.

Vertebral Column

Birds also have the five general groups of vertebrae found in mammals—cervical, thoracic, lumbar, sacral, and coccygeal or caudal. What does differ is the number of vertebrae. There are fewer in the thorax, lumbar, and sacral regions and more in the neck and caudal region in the bird. The numbers and formulae do vary with the species.

- Small birds may only have 8 cervical vertebrae but swans may have 25.
- The atlas or C1 has a ball-and-socket type of structure (condyle) attachment to the head so that there is greater range of motion. Except for the dens, which attaches to the atlas, the axis is similar to the remaining cervical vertebrae, which are uniformly cylindrical with prominent articular processes and rudimentary caudally directed cervical ribs.[4]
- There may be from three to seven thoracic vertebrae. In many species, the first three thoracic vertebrae are fused into a single bone, or notarium, to provide a rigid beam.[4] There is a single free mobile vertebra and then the last one or two thoracic vertebrae fuse with the lumbar, sacral, and first caudal vertebrae to form the synsacrum.
- The synsacrum extends laterally and caudally to fuse with the long hip bones to form support of the legs.
- There are an average of 5 to 6 free caudal vertebrae for movement of the tail and then further fusion of the caudal vertebrae, called the pygostyle (supports the tail feathers), for an average of about 12 caudal vertebrae.
- The combination of the notarium, synsacrum, and pygostyle makes it difficult to see the vertebral column. The sacrum is disproportionately large, and there is minimal tissue density. Trauma can be hard to note, especially at the caudal spine.[2]

Sternum and Ribs

- The unsegmented sternum in most species is large and concave to protect the chest and to serve as the origin for the flight feathers. Strong fliers have a large bony ridge or keel often referred to as the carina.
- The first few ribs from the last cervical vertebrae generally float. They are relatively short or complete. Five or six pairs of complete ribs connect the sternum with the thoracic vertebrae. The sternal portion corresponds to the cartilaginous part of the mammalian rib. The osseous vertebral portion generally possesses a caudodorsally directed (uncinate) process that overlaps the next rib.

The Torso

Birds do not possess a diaphragm but do have a thin sheet of connective tissue called the horizontal septum that separates the lung from the remaining viscera (Figure 27-15). The single cavity is termed a coelom or the coelomic cavity and contains the air sacs and abdominal organs.

TECHNICIAN NOTES As with radiography in mammals, a minimal of two views perpendicular to each other are required.

Because of the superimposition of the organs, two perpendicular views, and perhaps an oblique view, may be needed to hopefully visualize at least the larger organs, such as the heart and liver, and the natural contrast of the gizzard and bowel (See Figure 27-15).

Terminal Tracheal, Syrinx, and Mainstem Bronchi

- In the lateral view, the terminal portion of the trachea, syrinx, and mainstem bronchi are found dorsal to the heart. On the VD projection, they are superimposed on the heart.
- Visibility of the respiratory structures on a radiograph does depend on the size and species.

Lung and Air Sacs

- The smaller, dorsally located lungs are hard to see on a radiograph, especially in a VD view, because of superimposition of the peripheral portion of the heart over the muscles, making the lungs appear dense and even opaque. They appear honeycomb-like.
- In the lateral projection there is less superimposition, but the wings need to be pulled away from the torso.
- Depending on the species there are generally nine air sacs in birds. The thin-walled sacs are enlargements of the bronchial system that extend beyond the lung and are closely connected with the thorax and abdominal viscera (see Figure 27-15B).
- The air sacs can easily be seen on the radiograph because of the radiolucency, and provide negative contrast for the abdominal and thoracic organs.

Heart

- Superimposition of other organs, such as the liver at the caudal portion of the heart, makes it difficult to visualize the heart well in birds.
- The heart and liver fill the cranioventral portion of the body cavity and often blend into a single shadow on the radiograph.
- One indicator to determine disease, is the variation in the central visceral silhouette of the superimposed heart and liver, as noted on a VD view. This feature is not totally reliable, however, because the outline varies among species. The symmetry of the silhouette is also affected by improper positioning, and surrounding viscera such as the stomach.
- If the exposure is increased over the coelom values on the VD view, the aorta and the two main branches of the left and right brachiocephalic trunks can be visualized. The right and left vertebral and common carotid arteries could possibly be identified as they branch from the brachiocephalic arches,[2] especially if they appear head on.

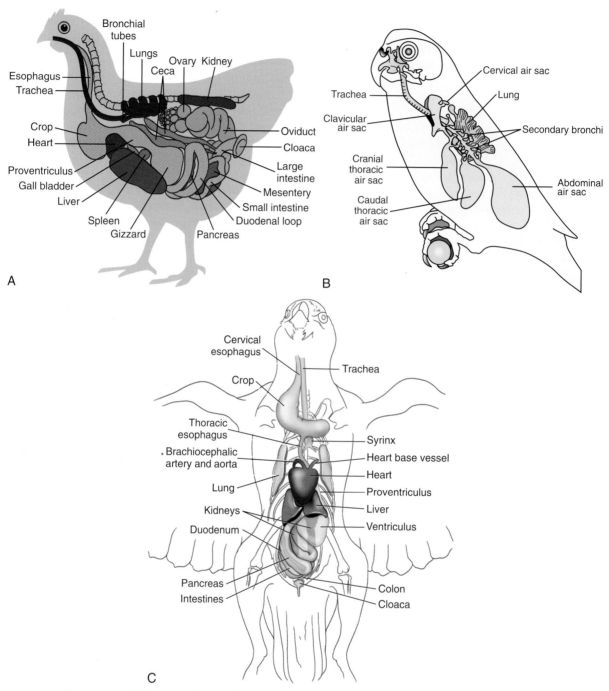

FIGURE 27-15 A, Anatomical drawing of the viscera of an adult chicken in lateral view. **B,** Diagram of the lateral view of the avian respiratory system. **C,** Anatomical drawing (ventrodorsal view) of the viscera of an adult bird.

Liver

The liver is the lower portion of the single shadow of the central visceral silhouette (heart and liver) that, when imaged in a VD view, vaguely resembles an hourglass.

Spleen and Pancreas

- The spleen is quite small, variable in shape though generally round, and located near the stomach just caudal and slightly dorsal to the liver shadow. It is better seen on the lateral view.

- A healthy pancreas is not radiographically detected and may also be difficult to note ultrasonographically.

Digestive Tract

- The lateral view of the torso better shows the caudal esophagus, ventriculus, and bowel mass, although they are not always visible.
- The digestive system is well seen, with the rather long esophagus leading to the ingluvies (crop) at the thoracic inlet of those species that possess a crop.

- The stomach of the bird is divided by a constriction into a predominantly glandular proventriculus, which is small and spindle-shaped, and a muscular ventriculus or gizzard, which is round or oblong and usually identified by the radiodense grit it contains.
- The proventriculus ventrally contacts the lobe of the left liver. The larger gizzard is more caudal and also touches the left liver lobe as well as contacting the sternum and the lower section of the left lateral wall.
- The crop and ventriculus are easier viewed if a recent meal (especially bones) has been ingested. There will be more breakdown of the meal when the stomach is reached. High-density material such as bone or grit may be noted in the bowel. Lead will be noted but most pesticides ingested by wild birds will not.[2]
- The intestines are in the caudal part of the coelom contacting the gizzard and reproductive organs. The intestines are composed of the tubular duodenum, jejunum, ileum, ceca, and rectum, which are difficult to separate on a survey radiograph. Herbivorous birds have two ceca that form from the ileocolic junction and traverse with the ileum in a retrograde direction. They are vestigial in the canary and pigeon and absent in the budgerigar.

Kidneys

- The elongated avian kidneys are found tight on either side of the caudal abdomen and lie almost to the caudal limit of the synsacrum, embedded in a depression on its ventral surface. The adrenal glands and gonads are also crowded in with the kidneys and hard to separate on a radiograph.
- Abdominal air sacs lie against the ventral surfaces of the kidneys and extend diverticula that penetrate through the dorsal renal surfaces.

Reproductive Organs

- The generally dominant left ovary lies slightly cranial to the left kidney. The oviduct occupies the left dorsal part of the body cavity, extends from the ovary to the cloaca, and is more evident during the reproductive[4] season.
- Once shell formation has occurred in the uterus, the egg is radiographically evident. Some calcification may occur in the caudal portion of the oviduct.
- The paired bean-shaped testes are adjacent to each cranial pole of the kidney just caudal to the adrenal gland. These are best noted on the lateral view and are often mistaken for kidneys on the radiograph. The testicles are more visible radiographically during breeding season.

Small Mammals

With the smaller rodents, such as rats, mice, hamsters, gerbils, or small rabbits and guinea pigs, the two orthogonal views generally are the DV and lateral. With the DV view, the animals are not as stressed, and the patient's small size does not really contribute to abnormal distortion or magnification. Also, interpretation seems to be easier on the DV rather than the VD view for these species. A horizontal beam can be used to obtain a lateral while the patient is in the DV position if manipulation of the tube head is possible. For the horizontal beam, the patient and the image receptor may both have to be raised by being placed on a wooden block with the image receptor placed vertically behind the animal and the beam perpendicular to both. Larger small mammals, such as rabbits and ferrets, are best positioned like cats, in lateral and VD recumbency.

Anesthesia and Positioning Concerns

Many of the small mammals can be brought into the room for the anesthesia induction and recovery. They are generally not fasted and are either placed in a properly ventilated "cat anesthesia box" and then connected to an anesthesia mask, or are directly masked. These patients can be taped to either the image receptor or a plastic positioner, are radiographed, and then allowed to recover. The full process can be completed in 10 minutes. Other chemical restraint can also be utilized. Make sure to keep the patients warm, because they can quickly become hypothermic owing to their small size.

Plasticware containers, cardboard shoe boxes, paper tape, gauze, and IV tubing are all simple positioning devices that are extremely useful in conjunction with anesthesia for radiography of small mammals (Figure 27-16). As with the avian patient, it is important to be as quick and efficient as possible to minimize stress to the animal. Masking tape or transparent medical tape is less likely to remove the animal's fur and is also less likely to be radiodense at lower kVp settings.

> **TECHNICIAN NOTES** The radiographic use of smaller mammals are generally the lateral and DV, while the radiographic views of larger small mammals are the VD and lateral.

If a small guinea pig or rodent cannot be sedated or anesthetized, it can be radiographed while naturally crouched in the DV position in a small cardboard box, plasticware container, or disposable plastic container used for packaging foods and found in delicatessens. If a properly sized container cannot be found to contain the animal, foam blocks can be used to make a corral. The lateral image can also be obtained with this position by using the horizontal x-ray beam. Clean, loose-fitting stockinet, pinched at both ends to prevent escape, is also effective to restrain the limbs and torso. If needed, a wooden spatula or a tongue depressor can be used to keep the patient in place.

Any lumps or subcutaneous masses should be identified by some sort of lead marker on the overlying skin especially in the reptilian species.

The dorsal half of a hedgehog's body is covered by a thick coat of long protective spines. When threatened, hedgehogs roll into a tight ball. If not anesthetized, they are often positioned in a small container with a horizontal beam used for the lateral view.

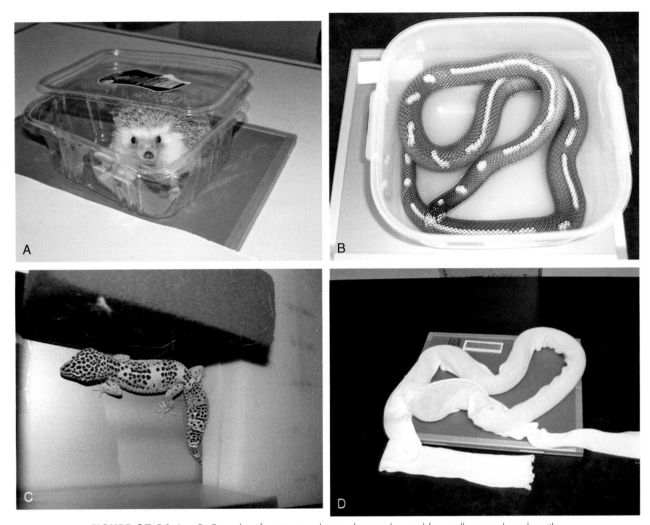

FIGURE 27-16 A to D, Examples of positioning devices that can be used for small mammals and reptiles.

Ultrasonography

Ultrasonography is a useful diagnostic tool for pocket pets. Guinea pigs, rabbits, and small rodents are difficult to examine with ultrasound because of their small size and reluctance to keep still. They are often best restrained in an upright position in the lap of or against the body of a restraining assistant. The restrainer will support the upper limbs and head with one hand and the rear limbs with the other. If further support for a larger patient is needed for ultrasonography, the lower limbs can be grasped by another person.

Small Pocket Pets

The main reason for admitting rats and other pet rodents for treatment is trauma, often due to being stepped on, crushed, or attacked by other pets mostly cats. Trauma to the chest or diaphragm is often involved. Abdominal distention and tumors are also reasons for medical imaging. Malignant tumors in the form of cranial mediastinal masses are not uncommon, with some tumors being the size of the heart.

Radiographic Views

Dorsoventral View of the Small Rodent

Positioning

Place in ventral recumbency. If the patient is anesthetized, place it on the table on a sheet of plastic or cardboard if preferred. Secure the head and neck with precut tape. Gently move the limbs away from the body to prevent their superimposition over the abdomen and thorax. Tape over the shoulders behind the level of the elbow to stretch the forelimbs. Tape over the pelvis (Figure 27-17).

Comments and Tips

To ensure that the DV or whole-body view is symmetrical:

- The vertebrae are directly over the sternebrae in a vertical plane.
- The acetabula are symmetrical.
- The animal is as straight as possible from head to tail.

If the patient is too ill to be anesthetized, it can be placed in an appropriate-size plasticware or plastic container, or cardboard box in its natural ambulatory position:

- Gently corral to a section of the container to limit its movement by using cotton or foam wedges. The disadvantage of the natural DV positioning is that there is superimposition of the front and hind limbs over the cranioventral viscera and caudal abdomen.

For the natural DV position:

- Place the container with the corralled patient on the image receptor.
- Use a vertical beam.

Depending on the type of container, 2 to 4 kVp may need to be added to the original setting.

- The image will not be as diagnostic as the regular DV due to superimposition.

MEASURE AND CENTRAL RAY: Over the thoracolumbar (TL) junction.

BORDERS: Include the whole body or the area of interest.

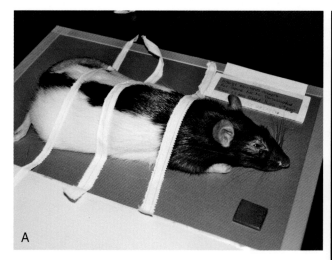
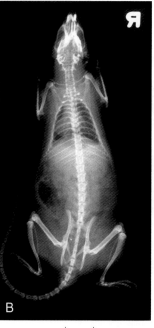

FIGURE 27-17 A, Positioning for the dorsoventral view of the rat. The patient was anesthetized via gas anesthetic chamber and quickly positioned and radiographed. Ideally the forelimbs should be extended more. **B,** Dorsoventral radiograph of the rat in **A.** The artifacts are the adhesive tape which is more evident at lower exposure factors.

Lateral View of a Small Rodent

Positioning

Place in lateral recumbency with the affected side down. Secure the head and neck with precut tape. Pull the pectoral limbs cranially and the pelvic limbs caudally, superimposing each set. Tape or use IV tubing or gauze to secure the patient to the image receptor or sheet. Tape over the tail if there is any chance of tail movement. Have the sternebrae and vertebrae on the same plane by placing a small sponge under the sternum and some cotton between the limbs (Figure 27-18).

Comments and Tips

- Superimposition of the limbs leads to less rotation of the torso and the hind limbs are more out of the field of view than if the dependent limb is pulled cranial.
- If radiographs of the limbs are required and extra radiographs are not practical, the limbs can be separated. The dependent limb should be pulled slightly cranially in each case.

To ensure that the lateral view is symmetrical:
- The head is slightly extended.
- The respective acetabula and ribs are superimposed.
- The sternum and vertebral column are on the same horizontal plane.

If the patient is too ill to be anesthetized, it can be placed in an appropriate-size plasticware or plastic container, or cardboard box in its natural ambulatory position:
- Gently corral to a section of the container to limit its movement by using cotton or foam wedges. The

disadvantage of the natural DV positioning is that there is superimposition of the front and hind limbs over the cranioventral viscera and caudal abdomen.

For the natural DV position:
- Place the container with the corralled patient on the image receptor.
- Use a vertical beam.

For the lateral view with a horizontal beam (Figure 27-19):
- Keep the corralled patient in the natural DV position in the container.
- Move the tube head to the horizontal position. Depending on how low the tube head will move, the container may have to be placed on a block or positioning device.
- Place the image receptor vertically against the side of the container away from the beam. Keep the cassette as close and parallel to the container as possible, to minimize OFD and distortion.
- The cassette may have to be taped or held in position by a device.
- The horizontally placed beam will be perpendicular to both the image receptor and the patient.
- Due to superimposition of the limbs, this view will not be as diagnostic as the regular lateral.

> **TECHNICIAN NOTES**　Remember to place an appropriate left or right marker for each radiograph.

CENTRAL RAY: TL junction.

BORDERS: Include the whole body or the area of interest.

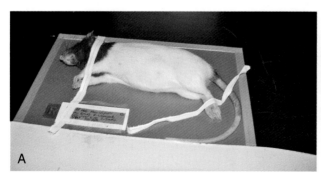
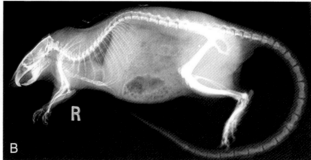

FIGURE 27-18 **A,** Positioning for the lateral view of the full body of a rat. **B,** A lateral radiograph of the rat in **A.**

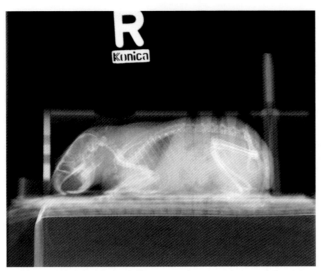

FIGURE 27-19 Use of a horizontal beam for the lateral view of a hamster in ventral recumbency. The patient is in a disposable container that was placed on a plastic-covered foam pad.

Normal Rat Radiographic Anatomy

Most radiographic examinations require chest or abdominal radiographs. Cardiopulmonary examinations are particularly difficult to interpret. Proper positioning is essential, especially for viewing the cranial cardiac border in a lateral view, on which improper positioning makes determining the size of the heart more difficult. Postural atelectasis due to gaseous anesthesia also makes optimal visualization of the dependant lung difficult because it collapses. The heart then shifts to the partially collapsed portion of the lung. This is called a cardiac shift. The displacement of the heart from the center causes rotation of the heart on its vertical axis. These processes contribute to changing of the cardiac silhouette, which may cause misdiagnosis.[2]

The cranial mediastinum width can be four times greater than that of a cat. Further interpretive challenges include those that occur in the VD or DV views. The right side of the heart also appears larger and more conical in a VD/DV view appearing close to the right chest, which is even more evident if the rat is not symmetrically positioned.

Distention of the gastrointestinal tract, especially the stomach and cecum, forces the diaphragm forward, making the diaphragm often appear nearly vertical. This causes the heart to appear larger because the lung is less visible. This relationship is often referred to as the cardiac-thoracic ratio. The intestinal tract, especially the well-developed cecum, often obscures other peritoneal cavity anatomy, especially when the tract is full of food or feces (Figure 27-20). The placement of the kidneys is similar to that in dogs and cats. Males have numerous accessory sex glands that are generally found in the caudoventral abdomen. To best differentiate the gastrointestinal tract from surrounding viscera, consider contrast media.

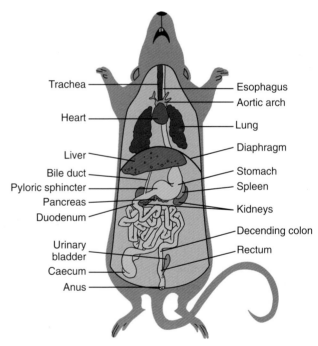

FIGURE 27-20 Anatomy of the rat.

> *TECHNICIAN NOTES* Tape, especially porous or paper masking tape, is very useful in positioning pocket pets, giving the patient the illusion that it is being controlled.

Other Small Pocket Pet Anatomy

The internal radiographic anatomy of smaller pocket pets is difficult to differentiate on a radiograph because of their smaller size. The skull of the hamster is relatively shorter, wider, and rounder than that of the rat and guinea pig. The narrow, tapered trunk of the hamster is similar to that of a rat. The overall body shape of the gerbil is longer and thinner than that of the hamster. Members of the order *Rodentia* (rat, mice, hamster, and gerbil) do not have any canine or premolar teeth. There is a diastema or space between the incisors and molar teeth (See Figure 27-24).

Larger Pocket Pets: Rabbits, Ferrets, Guinea Pigs

Rabbit

Common reasons for radiographing rabbits are generally fractures or dislocations of the extremities, pelvic fractures, chest trauma, and bruises, scrapes, and minor lacerations of the face. Dental disease is of concern, and radiographs are often required. Though there are exceptions, most middle ear infections in rabbits appear radiographically normal. Gastric dilation often the result of transient atony, is not uncommon to view on a radiograph, and it is not necessarily a mechanical obstruction. Massive fluid distension of the stomach can make peritoneal fluid diagnosis difficult.

Rabbits are generally docile and can be easily handled. To minimize radiation exposure for the radiographer, however, a healthy patient is best anesthetized and positioned according to principles similar to those used for rodents and cats. Rabbits are generally not routinely fasted prior to anesthesia, because they do not regurgitate or vomit. In addition, fasting in the rabbit is not likely to reduce gastrointestinal volume significantly, and can contribute to ileus.

Ferret

Ferrets are often brought in with complaints of trauma, gastrointestinal obstruction, cancer, or heart disease.[2] As with other small animals, they often get underfoot and experience limb fractures. Thoracic crush injuries, in which widespread lung bruising is capable of causing severe dyspnea, are often more serious. Because of their curiosity and ability to hide in narrow places, ferrets often swallow small objects, many of which can cause obstruction. They do suffer from various congenital and acquired heart diseases, cardiomyopathy being the most common.

Dental radiographs may be needed in ferrets. Occlusal dental film is preferred, but oblique extraoral projections can be made. Follow the same procedure as suggested for the dental radiography of cats (see Chapter 24). At least four views should be taken.

Ferrets are relatively easy to handle because they are friendly and inquisitive but, as with rabbits, healthy ferrets are best anesthetized or sedated. They can be squirmy and will not remain still in a container similar to that used for smaller pocket pets. If anesthetized, a ferret should be fasted for 3-4 hours beforehand. Check for hidden food in the cage of a ferret that is to be fasted.

Guinea Pig

Guinea pigs often are admitted for injuries, usually caused by a dog or cat or by accidental injuries such as being stepped on, being caught in a door, or being crushed. Suspected bloat and urinary tract calculi are other common reasons for diagnostic imaging.

Guinea pigs are not aggressive but do stress easily and try to escape when scared. They are best sedated or anesthetized for radiography. Generally they are not fasted.

Radiographic Position

Positioning for radiography is fairly consistent for the slightly larger pocket pet patients. What does vary is where the patient is measured and centered and what the peripheral borders are, depending on the site of interest. Table 27-2 indicates the differences. See the particular views for how to position.

TABLE 27-2	Where to Measure, Center and What to Include When Radiographing Slightly Larger Small Mammals or Rodents			
SPECIES	**VIEW**	**WHERE TO MEASURE**	**WHERE TO CENTER**	**WHAT TO INCLUDE**
Guinea pig, chinchilla, and small rabbits	Ventrodorsal (VD) of full body	At the last rib (thickest part of the body)	Thoracolumbar (TL) junction	Minimum of shoulder joint to caudal to ilium, including the limbs
	Lateral of full body	Last rib (thickest part of the body)	TL junction for a full-body view	Depends on size (similar to small cat)
Ferrets and larger rabbits	VD of abdomen	Last rib (thickest part of the body)	Caudal to last rib	Cranial from xiphoid process to caudal to pubis
	Lateral of abdomen	Last rib (thickest part of the body)	Caudal to last rib	Cranial from xiphoid process to caudal to pubis
	VD of thorax	Last rib (thickest part of the body)	At xiphoid of sternum	Shoulder joint to slightly caudal to last rib
	Lateral of thorax	Last rib (thickest part of the body)	Caudal sternum	Shoulder joint to slightly caudal to last rib

Ventrodorsal View of Whole Body/Abdomen/Thorax of a Larger Pocket Pet

Place the patient in dorsal recumbency assuming a chemically restrained patient, and gently extend the pectoral limbs cranially. Slightly rotate the pelvic limbs medially and pull them caudally keeping the limbs equidistant. Tape the legs to a plastic sheet, image receptor, or table, and keep them symmetrical.

Alternatively, place gauze or tubing around the hocks and elbows and extend it to either a cleat at each end of the table or a positioning device. A sandbag can be placed over the gauze stretching the limbs, or on the hind limbs for the larger patients. Keep the head straight and secure it with tape if needed (Figures 27-21 and 27-22).

> **TECHNICIAN NOTES** To ensure that the ventrodorsal/ dorsoventral view is symmetrical:
> - The vertebrae are over the sternebrae on the same vertical plane.
> - The spinous processes are aligned in the center of the vertebral bodies.
> - The acetabula are symmetrical and the femurs parallel, if possible.
> - The animal is as straight as possible from the head to its tail, avoiding any rotation.

Comments and Tips

- An acrylic or foam positioning device similar to that used for cats can also be utilized.
- The exposure factors may have to be increased by 2 to 4 kVp if a positioning device is used.
- The extended VD can be painful if there is any injury. This pain can be slightly alleviated by not fully extending the legs and by placing the patient on a medium-density foam pad.
- Keep the patient warm, and monitor if anesthetized.
- The same positioning applies for the DV, except that the patient is in sternal recumbency.
- If limb studies are required either the VD or DV position can be used. In the VD position, slightly rotate the patient to the opposite side to minimize soft tissue superimposition. Extend the limbs and secure with tape or tubing, so that the affected forelimb is extended cranially and the hind limb caudally.

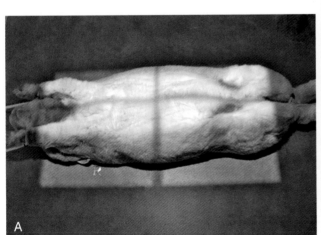
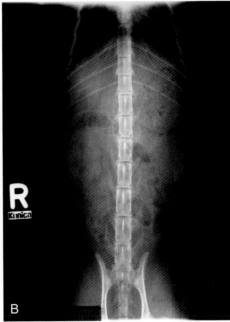

FIGURE 27-21 A, Positioning for a full-body ventrodorsal (VD) view of a rabbit. The same positioning applies for abdomen, thorax, VD skull, pelvis, and proximal limbs. **B,** Radiograph of the VD view of the abdomen of a rabbit.

Continued

Ventrodorsal View of Whole Body/Abdomen/Thorax of a Larger Pocket Pet—*cont'd*

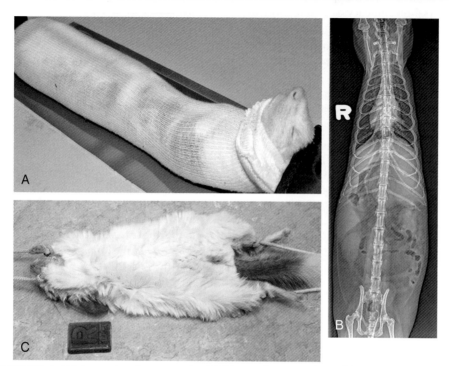

FIGURE 27-22 A, Utilizing stockinet for a ventrodorsal (VD) view of an unanesthetized ferret. Sandbags can be placed at either end. **B,** VD radiograph of the ferret. **C,** Positioning for a VD view of a chinchilla. Place the central ray over the area of interest and collimate appropriately.

Lateral View of the Whole Body/Abdomen/Thorax of a Larger Pocket Pet

Place the patient in lateral recumbency. A right lateral view is often preferred but be consistent. Position the head laterally and secure with tape if needed. Place a small foam wedge under the sternum to keep the sternum and vertebrae on the same horizontal plane.

Fully extend and tape the dependent limbs—the pelvic limbs caudally and pectoral limbs cranially. Superimpose the contralateral pelvic and pectoral limbs and tape separately. Use padding between the legs if needed (Figure 27-23). Use a vertical beam (Figures 27-23).

Comments and Tips

* If limb radiographs are required and two extra views are not practical, separate the limbs. The dependent limb will be pulled slightly cranial in each case.
* Applying and securing tape around the contralateral limb, and rotating the body slightly, minimizes superimposition.
  A lateral view can also be obtained with a horizontal beam (see Figure 27-23D) as described in small pocket pets.
* Keep the corralled patient in the natural DV position in the container.

* Place the image receptor vertically against the opposite side close and parallel to the container to minimize OFD and distortion. The horizontal central ray is perpendicular to the image receptor and patient.
* There may be superimposition of the limbs on the area of interest.

> **TECHNICIAN NOTES**
> To ensure that the lateral view is symmetrical:
> * Sternebrae and vertebrae are on the same plane.
> * The ribs are superimposed and straight.
> * Intervertebral foramina are the same size.
> * The acetabula are superimposed.
> * Ventral processes are superimposed.

> **TECHNICIAN NOTES** Be sure to fully extend the front limbs cranially on the lateral projection, especially for a rabbit, so that you have optimum radiographic detail of the cranial thorax. Hind limbs not properly extended, interfere with the caudal abdomen vsicera.

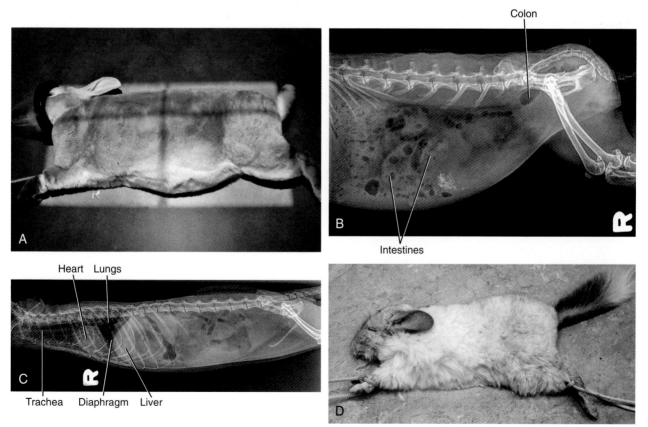

FIGURE 27-23 A, Positioning for the lateral full-body view of the rabbit. The same positioning applies for abdomen, thorax, skull, pelvis, and limbs (if separated). **B,** Radiograph of the lateral view of a rabbit. **C,** Right lateral view of the thorax and abdomen of a male ferret. **D,** Positioning for a lateral view of a chinchilla. Place the central ray over the area of interest, and collimate appropriately.

Lateral View of the Skull

Positioning

Place the patient in lateral recumbency with affected side down. Position the head so that the mandible is parallel to the long edge of the image receptor. Use a foam pad or cotton under the nose and neck to superimpose the rami and to prevent rotation of the skull and tape in place to align the skull parallel to the table. Keep the ears dorsal and caudal so they are out of the field of view. Place the label dorsal to the nose (Figure 27-24).

Comments and Tips

- How to tell whether the image will be symmetrical: Draw an imaginary line between the medial canthi and make sure this line is perpendicular to the table. In the image the left and right halves of the skull of a normal animal should be superimposed.

MEASURE: The thickest part of the skull.

CENTRAL RAY: Mid-skull just rostral and ventral to the eye.

BORDERS: Include from the tip of the nose to C2 (the base of the skull).

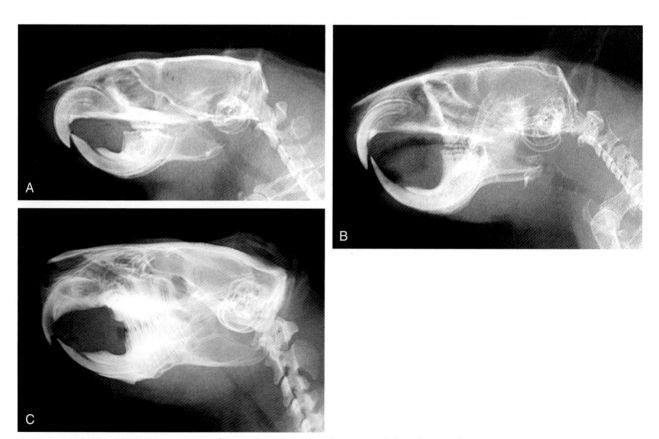

FIGURE 27-24 Comparisons of some of the skulls of pocket pets. Right lateral views of a rat (**A**), hamster (**B**), guinea pig (**C**),

Lateral View of the Skull—*cont'd*

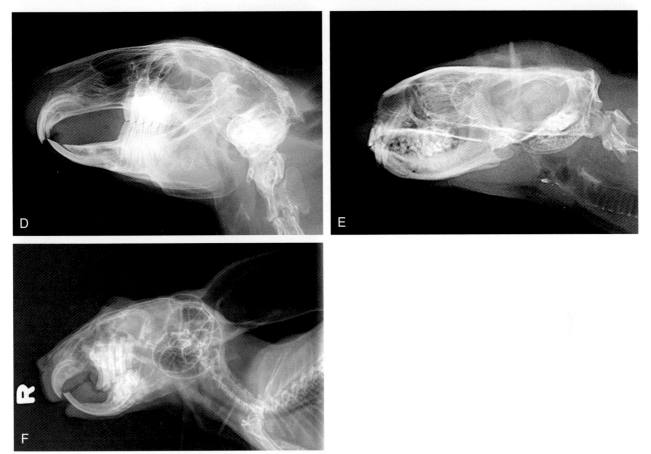

FIGURE 27-24, cont'd rabbit (D), and ferret (E). **F,** Lateral view of the skull of a chinchilla.

Dorsoventral or Ventrodorsal View of the Skull

Positioning

Place the patient directly on the table in ventral recumbency for a DV view and dorsal recumbency for a VD view. Sandbags or foam pads can be placed on either side to prevent rotation, ensuring that they are not in the field of view (Figure 27-25).

For the DV view: Position the head flat on the cassette and tape across the nasal septum and the cranium to keep the sagittal plane of the head perpendicular to the image receptor.

For the VD view: Position a foam pad or cotton under the neck so that the hard palate is parallel with the image receptor. Put tape caudal to the ears. Tape across the mandible to keep the head aligned with the table.

Comments and Tips

- Place the label lateral to the nose.
- Make sure the ears are positioned laterally, equidistant from the head.
- How to tell whether the image will be symmetrical:
- Draw an imaginary line between the medial canthi, and make sure this line is parallel to the table.
- If there is symmetry on the final image of a normal animal:
  - The left and right half of the skull should be a mirror image of each other.

MEASURE: The thickest part of the skull.

CENTRAL RAY: Midline between the eyes.

BORDERS: Include the tip of the nose to C2 (base of the skull).

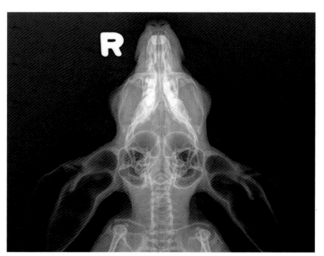

FIGURE 27-25 Ventrodorsal view of the skull of a chinchilla.

Lateral Oblique (Oblique Dorsoventral) Views of the Skull for Tympanic Bullae, Dental Arcade, and Temporomandibular Joint

Positioning

Place the patient in left or right lateral recumbency. Place sponges under the skull, creating a 30-degree angle[6] to the cassette, with the nose touching the cassette. This position will also produce a radiograph of the lower dental arcade. Ensure that the ears are out of the field of view. Place a label dorsal to the nose.

If the patient is lying on its right side, this position is technically referred to as the LeD30-RtVO or right oblique DV view. (See Chapter 23 for a review of oblique terminology).

Comments and Tips

- If the upper dental arcade is of interest, place foam pads under the nose, creating a 30 to 45 degree angle to the table, with the back of the skull touching the image receptor and the nose in the air. Secure with tape if needed (Figure 27-26). If the patient is lying on its right side, this position is technically referred to as the LeV30-RtDO or right oblique VD view.
- A complete radiographic study of the skull should include extraoral lateral, oblique, dorsoventral (or ventrodorsal); and rostrocaudal head views as well as intraoral views (Table 27-3).[5] See Chapters 23 and 24 for further information on radiographing the canine or feline skull, which can be applied to smaller mammals as well (Figure 27-26).
- Magnification of rodent and rabbit skulls may be required. This can be obtained by using a small focal spot and increased OFD/decreased SID. The patient can be positioned on a radiolucent foam sponge on top of the image receptor. If the OFD is 12 inches and the SID is 20 inches, the magnification is about 2.0.[6]

MEASURE: The thickest part of the skull.

CENTRAL RAY: Mid-skull just rostral and ventral to the eye.

BORDERS: Include the tip of the nose to C2 (the base of the skull).

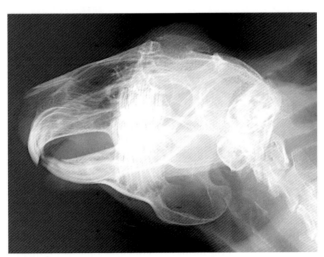

FIGURE 27-26 Oblique (30 degree) ventrodorsal view of the skull of an adult rabbit.

TABLE 27-3	Dentition of Some Common Rodents and the Rabbit*				
	PERMANENT	PERMANENT INCISORS	PERMANENT CANINES	PERMANENT PREMOLARS	PERMANENT MOLARS
Hamsters, gerbils, rodents	16	2/2	0/0	0/0	6/6
Guinea Pigs	20	2/2	0/0	2/2	6/6
Rabbits	28	4/2	0/0	6/4	6/6

*Number before slash indicates total maxillary teeth; number after indicates total mandibular teeth.

Anatomy of the Guinea Pig

Laterally, the skull of the guinea pig looks like a surgical towel clamp (see Figure 27-25C).[2] It is flattened dorsally with a small cranium that blends in. The elongated face that terminates in a rostral hook is met with the curve of the mandibular incisors and a large interdental gap.

The thorax, being about one-sixth of the total length of the torso, is disproportionately small in comparison with the abdomen. The poor contrast between the heart and lung makes the thoracic viscera difficult to view. Also, the limbs often superimpose over the thorax, and the thoracic portion of the trachea in the cranial mediastinum is often invisible. The diaphragm is best seen on a lateral view (Figure 27-27). For these reasons, which can also apply to other rodents, accurate thoracic diagnosis can be difficult.[2]

The large gas-filled viscera—the stomach and cecum—visually dominate and make up the majority of the abdomen. The liver is easy to identify mainly because it lies between the air-filled lungs and the stomach in the lateral view, and cranially and caudally in the DV position. Depending on the amount of surrounding gas, the kidneys and urinary bladder may or may not be identifiable.

Unless guinea pigs and other rodents are chemically restrained, the limbs may be difficult to extend because they are small and physically difficult to isolate. The limbs can be taped to the image receptor if the animal is unconscious. If manual restraint is required, a tongue depressor can be used to gently pull the limbs away from the body and held. Because guinea pigs are easily stressed, make sure that everything is prepared prior to bringing the patient into the radiography room.

Normal Chinchilla Anatomy[2]

The most common reason for radiographing a chinchilla is generally injury from being stepped on by the owner.

Chinchillas are often compared to guinea pigs, but there are differences. They are distinguished by the large tympanic bullae, which are four to five times larger than those of any of the other comparably sized rodents (see Figures 27-24F and 27-25). Their hind legs are also more muscular than and twice as long as their forelimbs, a difference that may necessitate increasing the exposure for proper imaging of the hind limbs.

The heart in the chinchilla, particularly the cranial border, is generally more radiographically visible than in mice, rats, or hamsters. As with the small rodents, the heart appears comparatively larger than the lungs, giving the false illusion of cardiac enlargement.

As with the guinea pig, a full stomach or cecum dominates the chinchilla's digestive tract. A wrinkled or haustrated appearance of the colon is normal.[2]

Normal Anatomy of the Rabbit

The large diastema (interdental space) accentuates the long curved upper incisors and the shoveled lower incisors (see Figure 27-24D). The premolars and molars have a lengthy, complex root system. Malocclusion is common in rabbits.

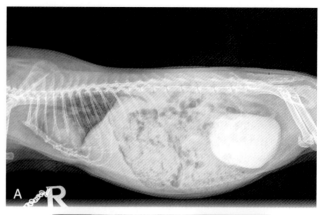

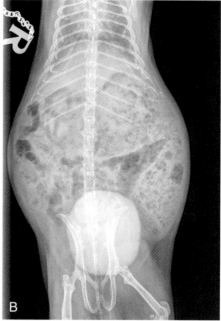

FIGURE 27-27 **A,** Lateral view of a guinea pig showing urinary sediment. **B,** Ventrodorsal view of the same guinea pig.

Dental abscesses and resultant osteomyelitis are also of concern. The nasal cavity is expansive with prominent conchae, and the cranial portion of the mandible is smaller than the caudal portion of the mandible. This makes the lateral rabbit skull look like an asymmetrical egg (Figure 27-28).[2]

The long and distinctive ears of a rabbit could superimpose anatomy to be imaged if not correctly positioned.

The hips of an immature rabbit appear differently from those of immature dogs and cats. Normal anatomical variations can sometimes be confused for femoral head fractures. The immature rabbit's femoral head appears to be in two sections because of unique epiphyseal anatomy. Hips in mature rabbits are generally set deep in their sockets. Excessive rotation can give false bowing of the femurs known as positional curvature.

In an immature thorax, the thymus and its fat is sometimes mistaken for a tumor such as a thymoma. This normal

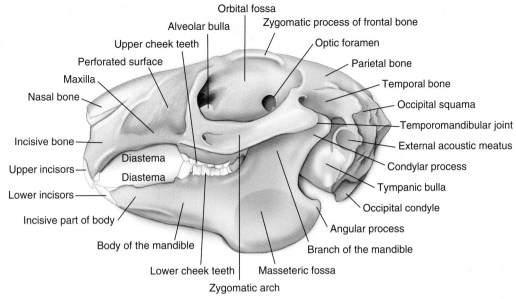

Orbital fossa
Zygomatic process of frontal bone
Alveolar bulla
Optic foramen
Upper cheek teeth
Perforated surface
Parietal bone
Maxilla
Temporal bone
Nasal bone
Occipital squama
Temporomandibular joint
Incisive bone
External acoustic meatus
Diastema
Condylar process
Upper incisors
Diastema
Tympanic bulla
Lower incisors
Occipital condyle
Incisive part of body
Angular process
Body of the mandible
Branch of the mandible
Lower cheek teeth
Masseteric fossa
Zygomatic arch

FIGURE 27-28 The anatomy of the skull of the rabbit.

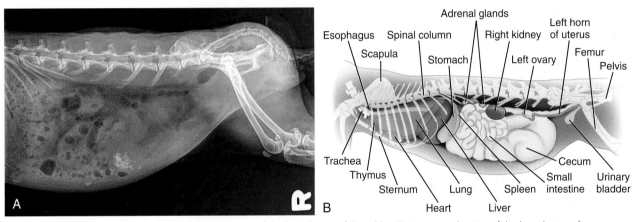

Adrenal glands
Left horn of uterus
Esophagus Spinal column Right kidney
Scapula Femur
Stomach Left ovary
Pelvis

Trachea
Cecum
Thymus
Small
Urinary
Sternum Lung Spleen intestine bladder
Heart Liver

A B

FIGURE 27-29 A, Radiographic anatomy of the lateral view of the rabbit. B, Anatomic drawing of the lateral view of the rabbit.

Continued

anatomy also contributes to the wide cranial mediastinum in an immature rabbit (Figure 27-29).

In the mature thorax, the cranial and precardiac parts of the mediastinum have a localized fat deposition with a thoracic narrowing, further giving the perception of a cranial mediastinal mass. Perithoracic fat also adds to the low contrast that is often evident on the radiographs. No cranial mediastinum is really seen because the heart is positioned cranially, close to the thoracic inlet. The cardiac borders are often relatively indistinct, especially if a large amount of fat is present. Large caudal lung fields are not evident, and the scapulas are superimposed on the dorsal thorax. Distinct bronchial markings are not evident, nor do the lungs inflate greatly. If the feline thoracic chart is used, kVp may have to be raised slightly.

As with other small mammals, the stomach and its contents of food, fluid, and gas and the cecum do influence the radiographic appearance. The intraabdominal fat and, to a lesser extent, the amount of extraabdominal fat also affect the image.

Normal Anatomy of the Ferret

Ferrets are generally radiographed similar to cats. Anatomically the torso is elongated and tapered at each end for both species. The skull of the ferret, however, is longer, with a more dorsally flattened cranium (Figures 27-22B, 27-23C and 27-24D).

Reptiles

Radiographic imaging is frequently required in pursuing reptile diagnostics. Knowledge of reptiles' unique anatomical characteristics is essential for providing a technically

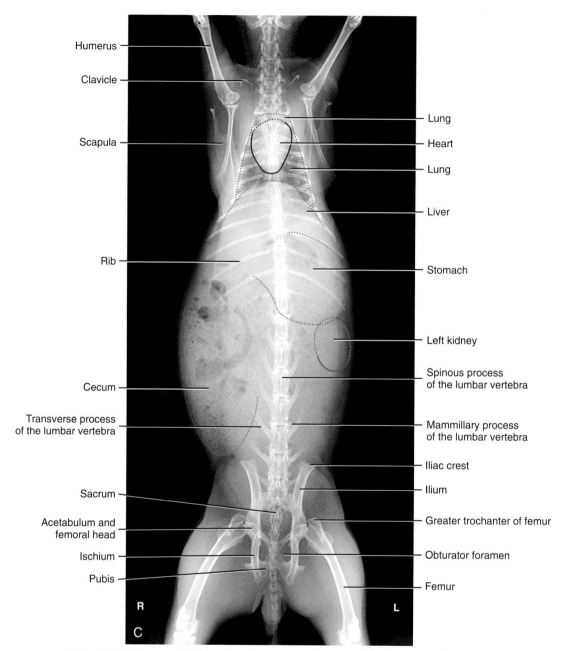

Humerus

Clavicle

Scapula

Rib

Cecum

Transverse process
of the lumbar vertebra

Sacrum

Acetabulum and
femoral head

Ischium

Pubis

Lung

Heart

Lung

Liver

Stomach

Left kidney

Spinous process
of the lumbar vertebra

Mammillary process
of the lumbar vertebra

Iliac crest

Ilium

Greater trochanter of femur

Obturator foramen

Femur

R   L

C

FIGURE 27-29, cont'd C, Radiographic anatomy of the ventrodorsal (VD) view of the rabbit.

proficient image. Traumatic injuries, gravidity evaluation, impactions, lung evaluation for pneumonia, and urinary calculi are common reasons that a radiograph may need to be acquired in a reptile.

Chelonians (tortoise and turtles) present a unique challenge in radiography, in that their ribs and sternum are fused to form the carapace and plastron. As such, coelomic detail is difficult to view.

Positioning of snakes to obtain two views is often problematic and frequently requires aids such as tubes to enable a lateral view to be taken.

Ultrasound and endoscopy are also diagnostic tools in reptilian medicine. Endoscopy is particularly useful.

Coelioscopy, or internal examination of the coelomic cavity, provides direct view of the liver, lungs, kidneys, heart, spleen, bladder, gastrointestinal tract, pancreas, and gonads, although it requires an incision. In lizards, the incision for coelioscopy is generally made in the lateral body wall just caudal to the last rib. In chelonians, the incision is at the center of the pre-femoral fossa, and in snakes, at the junction of the ventral and lateral scales at the expected site of interest. Endoscopy can also be used in reptiles to visualize the trachea and bronchi for evaluation of respiratory disease, to retrieve foreign bodies from the gastrointestinal tract, and to obtain tissue specimens of diseased organs.[7]

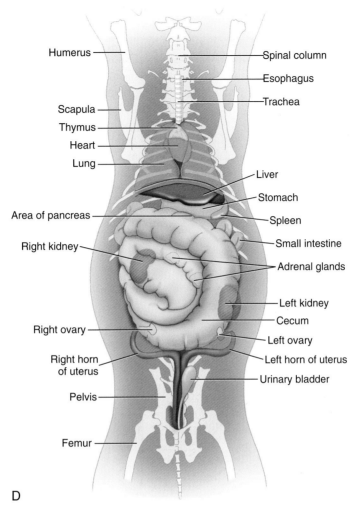

Humerus — Spinal column

Esophagus

Trachea

Scapula —

Thymus —

Heart —

Lung —

— Liver

— Stomach

Area of pancreas — — Spleen

Right kidney — — Small intestine

— Adrenal glands

— Left kidney

— Cecum

Right ovary — — Left ovary

Right horn of uterus — Left horn of uterus

— Urinary bladder

Pelvis —

Femur —

D

FIGURE 27-29, cont'd D, Anatomical drawing of the viscera of the thorax and abdomen of an adult female rabbit in VD view.

Turtle and Tortoise

Positioning Concerns

Turtles are generally easy to restrain for radiography because many species are lethargic. One challenge can be keeping the limbs in extension. Taping the carapace caudally to the plate can help with this, as turtles often pull against the force of the tape and in doing so extend their limbs (see Figure 27-30A). Raising the body up higher than the legs can reach can also be used for a dorsoventral radiograph. A small radiolucent object can be placed under the central plastron. If possible, lowering the temperature helps decrease the activity without changing the metabolic rate.

A short-acting anesthetic agent such as alfaxalone can also facilitate proper positioning. With turtles, it is important to obtain a rostrocaudal (craniocaudal) view in addition to dorsoventral and lateral views. The rostrocaudal view enables unobstructed vision of both lungs. The horizontal beam should be considered for the rostrocaudal as well as lateral views, if the machine allows.

A grid is not likely needed except for the larger species. Nonscreen dental film or a digital dental unit can be used for smaller patients, and a high-detail system should be used for the larger patients. A positive-contrast study can be completed if the GI tract is of concern. If GI contrast studies are completed, the time scale for passage of the medium is longer than in mammals.

Radiographic Positions

Dorsoventral View

Positioning
Position the patient on its plastron and use tape if required at the caudal aspect (Figure 27-30).

Comments and Tips
- A small radiolucent device can be used under the plastron to raise the body so that the limbs are not touching the plate. Tape over the shell caudally to keep the patient from wandering.

- The turtle can be turned on its back and then flipped upright just before taking the image. This may disorient the patient so as to cause momentary extension of the appendages and head.
- An appropriate-size container or a foam wedge barricade can also be used to keep the turtle in a limited area.
- As long as the central ray is in the center of the shell, most chelonian images show symmetry.

MEASURE: The thickest part of the body.

CENTRAL RAY: The center of the shell.

BORDERS: Include the whole body.

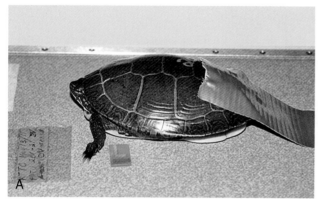
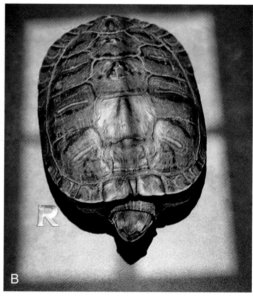

FIGURE 27-30 A, Strategic use of tape keeps the turtle in position and also encourages it to extract its limbs as it tries to walk away. B, Dorsoventral view of a painted turtle.

Dorsoventral View—cont'd

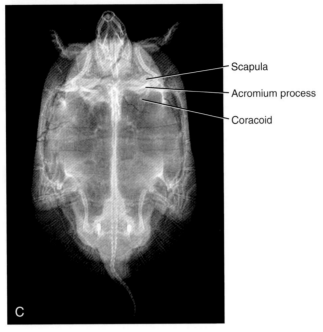

Scapula

Acromium process

Coracoid

C

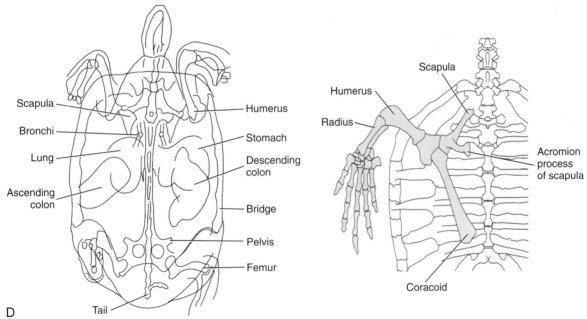

Scapula

Humerus

Bronchi

Stomach

Lung

Descending colon

Ascending colon

Bridge

Pelvis

Femur

Tail

D

Scapula

Humerus

Radius

Acromion process of scapula

Coracoid

FIGURE 27-30, cont'd C, Dorsoventral radiograph of a painted turtle. D, Radiographic anatomy of the snapping turtle.

Lateral View

Positioning for a Lateral View with a Horizontal Beam

Use of the lateral decubitus view (dorsoventral position with a horizontal beam) is preferred for the lateral view of a turtle or tortoise.

Place the turtle or tortoise in ventral recumbency on top of a foam pad or acrylic positioning device or on a small radiolucent object so the legs are exposed. Tape over the shell caudally to prevent the patient from wandering. Place the image receptor perpendicular to the table directly behind the turtle's lateral side opposite to the beam. Position the beam parallel to the table so that the central ray is midway between the plastron and carapace, in full view of the image receptor. The beam should bisect the plastron and carapace for the image to be symmetrical (Figure 27-31).

Positioning for a Lateral view with a Vertical Beam

Place the turtle in ventral recumbency on its plastron, and securely tape the patient to a foam pad or acrylic positioning device or secure between two devices. Then turn the pad so that the lateral side of the turtle is positioned on the image receptor: The turtle is lying laterally on its "side." The beam passes vertically between the carapace and plastron. The beam should bisect the plastron and carapace for the image to be symmetrical.

> **TECHNICIAN NOTES**   As with other positions, the lateral decubitus view is labeled according to the side against the image receptor. In a right lateral, the right side is against the plate. Technically this is called a left to right lateral decubitus view (dorsoventral position) with a horizontal beam.

MEASURE: The thickest part of the shell.

CENTRAL RAY: The center of the body between the carapace and plastron.

BORDERS: Include the whole body.

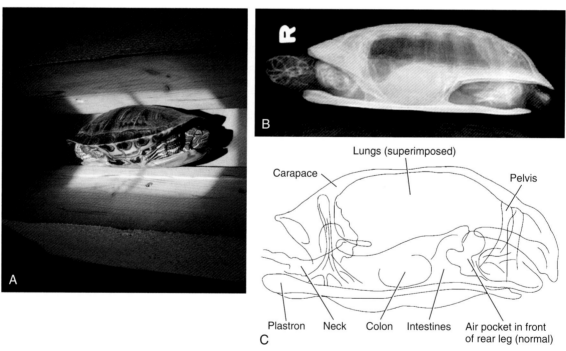

FIGURE 27-31 A, Positioning for a lateral view of a painted turtle with the use of a horizontal beam. **B,** Radiograph of a lateral view with the use of the horizontal beam of the painted turtle, using a wooden block on which to position the turtle. **C,** Lateral radiographic anatomy of a painted turtle.

Rostrocaudal View

Positioning for a Rostrocaudal View with a Horizontal Beam

Place the turtle in ventral recumbency and tape it to a foam pad or block, putting both on the table. Have the image receptor caudal to and as close to the patient as possible. Direct the beam horizontally from a cranial direction through to the tail (see Figure 27-32).

Positioning for Rostrocaudal View with a Vertical Beam

Place the turtle in ventral recumbency and tape the turtle to a foam pad or block. Place and position the turtle and block so that the caudal portion of the body is resting on the cassette and table and the nose is pointing up to the beam. Direct the beam vertically from the head through the tail.

MEASURE: The thickest area of the body.

CENTRAL RAY: Through the middle of the head.

BORDERS: Include the whole body.

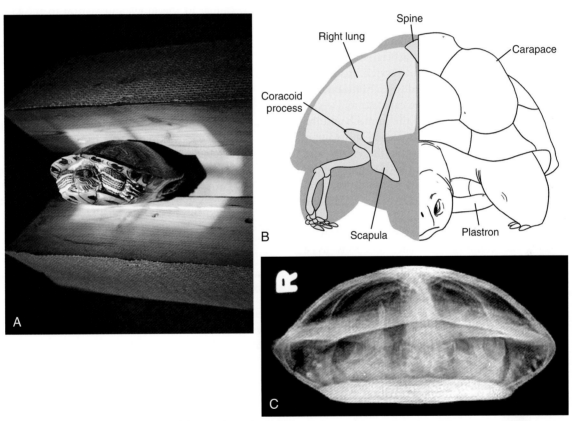

FIGURE 27-32 A, A rostrocaudal view of a turtle. **B,** Radiographic anatomy and overlay of the rostrocaudal view of the painted turtle. **C,** Rostrocaudal radiograph of a painted turtle.

Normal Anatomy of Chelonians

The skeletal anatomy of chelonians as do other animals consist, of an appendicular and axial skeleton. The axial skeleton is composed of the skull, ribs, carapace, vertebrae, and derivative of the ribs, and the appendicular includes the forelimbs, hind limbs, and supporting structures. The plastron is a combination of both the ventral ribs and the pectoral girdle. Because of all the bone, soft tissue DV radiographs are difficult to diagnose. Scales and scute nomenclature assists species and medical identification.

The terminology of the limbs in turtles and tortoises is quite similar to that in mammals. The differences are the size, shape, fusion, and process attachments. The vertebral number is such that turtles have 7 mobile cervical vertebrae, with the 8th cervical vertebrae being fused to the carapace, 10 thoracic vertebrae, 2 sacral vertebrae, and 12 or more caudal vertebrae. Chelonians do not have teeth but do have keratinized beaks.

The respiratory system consists of a glottis, trachea, a bronchus to each lung, and right and left lungs. Unlike other reptiles, chelonians do have complete cartilaginous tracheal rings. Tracheal bifurcation occurs in the cervical area.

The multichambered lungs (referred to as multicameral) are found dorsally and attached to the carapace and vertebrae. Ligaments attach the left lung to the stomach and the right lung to the right side of the liver. Caudally the lungs are attached to the peritoneum to overlie the kidney and adrenal glands. The lungs are adjacent to the gonads. The medial border of each lung is attached to the dorsolateral surfaces of the vertebral column. There is no diaphragm (Figure 27-33).

As with most reptiles the three-chambered heart, with two atria and one common ventricle, functions as a four-chambered heart because of the regions within the single ventricle that prevent mixing of oxygenated and deoxygenated blood. The chelonian heart is located in the pericardium on the midline. The heart is bordered ventrally by the acromion and coracoid, dorsally by the lungs, and laterally by the lobes of the liver. On a craniocaudal radiograph, the heart and greater vessels are difficult to determine.

In some species the esophagus is quite long, traversing almost half of the body before it finally enters the stomach, which is located on the left cranioventral side of the coelomic cavity.

The small intestine is relatively short. The two-lobed liver is large, saddle-shaped, and located ventrally under the lungs. The cecum is not well developed. The kidneys are dorsally located. The urinary bladder is dorsal to the rectum, lateral to the ilia and sacrum, and ventral to the proximal caudal vertebrae.

The gonads of both sexes are located dorsally in the body cavity, caudal to the lungs and ventral to the kidney and peritoneal wall. The cranial poles of the ovary and testes are found caudal to the lungs and extend caudomedial to the cloaca. However, they are not visualized very well radiographically.

TECHNICIAN NOTES   In female turtles, the caudal vertebrae are short and decrease in size distally, whereas in males, the lateral and dorsal processes are stout. As a general rule the vent of a female is found at or within the carapace perimeter. The male generally has a long tail, and the vent (cloacal opening) is generally more caudal than in the female or nearer the tip of the tail. Males may have strong curved claws on the second digit, and during mating season the mid-ventral plastron becomes soft. Male painted turtles have very long front toenails.

Lizard

Positioning of lizards (order *Squamata*) for radiography utilizes the conventional DV and lateral views. They are the most straightforward of the reptiles to image, and many of the concepts employed for small mammal radiography can be utilized.

Many species can be radiographed awake, although anesthesia aids in obtaining diagnostic radiographs. Lowering the environmental temperature may make lizards more lethargic. Strategically placed tape can be employed to stabilize the patient on the plate. Placing a blindfold of some sort over the eyes of the lizard may minimize movement. This can be achieved by placing eye lubricant in the eyes and wrapping the head with Vetwrap.[8] Applying pressure over the both eyeballs through closed lids can also be effective. The response to this pressure is the vasovagal reflex, which can induce a drop in heart rate and blood pressure and a catatonic state.

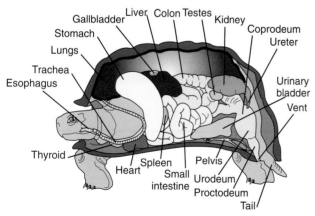

FIGURE 27-33 Cross section of the internal anatomy of a chelonian.

Radiographic Positions

Dorsoventral View

Positioning

Place the lizard in sternal recumbency with limbs lateral to the body. Put masking tape over the neck, caudal to the pectoral limbs and over the pelvis, if needed. Use a vertical beam (Figure 27-34).

Comments and Tips

- The limbs are naturally positioned lateral to the body, so superimposition with viscera does not usually occur.

- Watch the stress level of lizards.
- If only the extremities are of interest, tape as already described and extend the limb of interest with masking tape, gauze, or rope.

TECHNICIAN NOTES How to tell whether the image is symmetrical:
- The spine is superimposed over the sternum.
- The patient is straight from head to tail.

MEASURE: The thickest point of the body.

CENTRAL RAY: Over the midline of the body about the level of the TL junction, unless the tail is of interest.

BORDERS: Include the whole body.

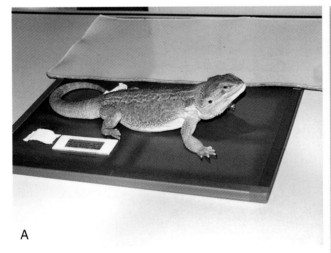
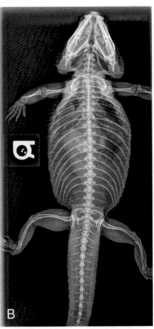

FIGURE 27-34 A, Dorsoventral positioning for the lizard species of a bearded dragon. If the head is raised, there will be more magnification and less sharpness of that area. Tape should be used to keep the head and neck more parallel to the cassette. **B,** Dorsoventral radiograph of the bearded dragon.

Lateral View

To image the lateral view, the lateral decubitus (dorsoventral position with horizontal beam) is less stressful for the patient.

Positioning

Place the patient in ventral recumbency on a raised sponge block or plastic sheet. Tape the neck, shoulders, and pelvis if needed. Position the beam so it is horizontal with the table and perpendicular to the image receptor, which is placed as close as possible to the side of the lizard that is being radiographed. Mark the side closer to the cassette (see Figure 27-35).

Comments and Tips

- Keep the body of the patient close to the cassette and the spine straight and parallel to minimize OFD and distortion.
- The tails of larger lizards can be taped.
- How to tell whether the image will be symmetrical: The patient should have equal weight on its feet and the spine should be as parallel to the casette and perpendicular to the central ray as possible.

MEASURE: The thickest point of the body

CENTRAL RAY: Over the midline of the body.

BORDERS: Include the whole body.

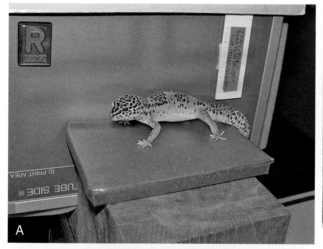

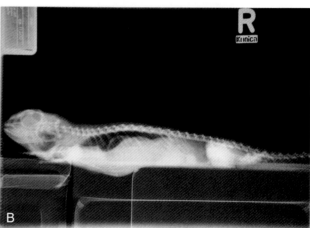

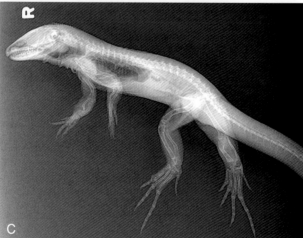

FIGURE 27-35 A, Horizontal beam for the right lateral view of a gecko. B, Lateral view of a bearded dragon on positioning devices with use of a horizontal beam and the patient in ventral recumbency. C, Radiograph of a lizard in regular lateral position with the use of a vertical beam.

Normal Anatomy of the Lizard

Because lizards do not have mesenteric fat storage, there is minimal contrast between the tissues. The viscera are not well differentiated. The lack of a diaphragm and bones that are less radiopaque than mammals also make interpretation more difficult (Figure 27-36).

As with most reptiles, the pectoral girdle consists of a scapula and coracoid bone that attaches to the body with muscles. The limb consists of the same bones as in mammals and articulates with the pectoral girdle. The pelvic limb consists of the femur, tibia, tarsal bones, metatarsal bones, and phalanges and is joined to the pelvis, which articulates with the sacral vertebrae. Lizards have five digits on each foot.

In normal iguanas the kidneys are found in the intrapelvic canal.[8] The liver is fairly large and usually consists of at least two lobes. Most lizards have oblong smooth-surfaced kidneys located in the caudal coelom. Depending on the diet, the colon can be more complex, and the cecum may or may not be present. Ceca are found in herbivores such as the green iguana and are absent or rudimentary in carnivorous

species. Some lizards have a urinary bladder connected to the urodeum of the cloaca by a short broad urethra.

Ultrasound[7] is more diagnostic and can be used to evaluate various systems, such as the reproductive, as well as the heart and other viscera. The heart, as in most reptiles, is three-chambered. In most lizards it is situated in the pectoral girdle. Place the transducer in the axillary region and rotate it to evaluate all three chambers. The viscera in the caudal coelom can be examined, and ultrasound can be used to help collect fine-needle biopsy specimens or aspirates. Ovulation can be determined by placing the transducer over the ovary on the lateral body wall just caudal to the last rib and noting the follicle measurement. Both ovaries should be examined. Depending on the species, this comparison may help determine when the male and female should be placed together.

Snake

Snake species (order *Squamata*) are extremely variable in size, and thus restraint devices in many sizes are required for them. Small snakes can be coiled on the cassette or in a box such as a plastic container. Disposable containers used for salads found in deli sections are ideal (once they are washed) as the material is radiolucent and the containers can be disposed of after use. The snake could also be stretched and taped to a long plastic sheet or supported in a tubed stockinet (see Figure 27-16D). If the stockinet is used, the position will be fairly well maintained provided that the patient is not able to rotate its head inside the tube. Keeping the body elongated and not coiled is especially important for the lateral view with horizontal beam. Placing metallic pellets may assist with "dividing" the body for easier identification.

Manual restraint may be needed for some of the larger species in order to position the body correctly. It is important in snakes to have the body in a straight line, and thus multiple exposures may be required to allow the entire body to be imaged. Knowledge of the location of the various organs is essential for proper positioning. Lateral recumbency is needed to visualize the organs properly. A horizontal beam for the lateral radiograph is recommended for accurate imaging of this view in reptiles. The dorsoventral view is more useful for imaging the spine and ribs.

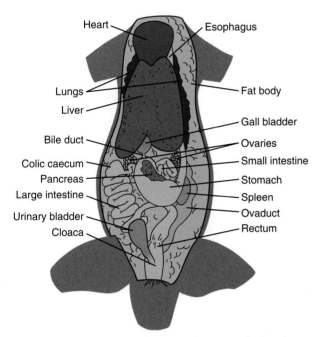

FIGURE 27-36 Simplified internal anatomy of a lizard.

Radiographic Positions

Dorsoventral View

Positioning

* Keep the patient in sternal recumbency in a natural position: inside a plastic box, in a tube or stockinet, or taped down. Use a vertical beam (Figure 27-37).
* How to tell whether the image will be symmetrical: There should not be overlapping of the vertebrae and the ribs should appear equidistant on each side of the vertebrae.

Comments and Tips

Multiple handlers may be required for safe radiography of a large snake.

CENTRAL RAY: Over the area of interest.

BORDERS: Include the area of interest (anterior, middle, caudal end).

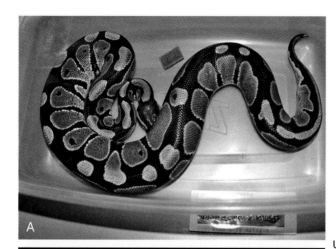

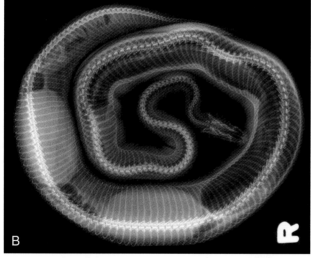

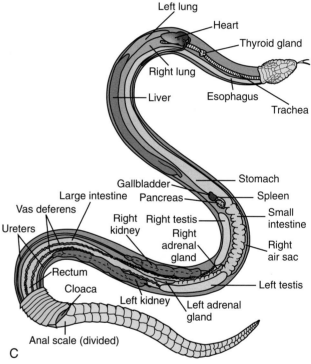

FIGURE 27-37 A, Positioning for a dorsoventral view of a boa constrictor. The same positioning can be used for the lateral with the use of a horizontal beam, but there will be some overlap of the cranial half in this particular case. B, Radiograph of a dorsoventral view of an egg-bound ball python. C, Ventral view of a male snake showing internal anatomy.

Lateral View

Lateral decubitus (dorsoventral position with horizontal beam).

Positioning

- Place the patient in a DV position as described above, and use a horizontal beam, putting the image receptor vertically on the side of interest.

- How to tell whether the image will be symmetrical: The snake is stretched out, with no coiling of the body. The vertebrae appears on the dorsal aspect.

CENTRAL RAY: Over the area of interest.

BORDERS: Include the area of interest (anterior, middle, caudal end).

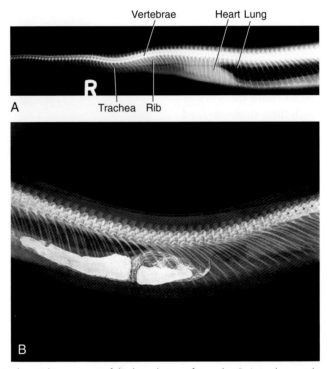

FIGURE 27-38 **A,** Radiographic anatomy of the lateral view of a snake. **B,** Lateral view taken during a contrast study of a snake.

Normal Snake Anatomy

Imagine the snake as a long tube.[9] The major organs of the cranial quarter of the snake are the head, esophagus, trachea, and heart. Snakes have six rows of teeth, two rows on the mandible, two on the maxilla, and two on the palantine/pterygoid bones. The esophagus, as with most reptiles, is thin and distensible. The tracheal rings are incomplete. The heart is three-chambered and is usually at the junction of the first and second thirds of the body length. It is fairly mobile within the coelomic cavity (see Figure 27-37C).

The next quarter consists of the cranial portion of the lungs, the liver, and the stomach. The lung is considered quite primitive and is a simple, saclike structure (unicameral lung). The cranial portion of the lung is the site of gas exchange, and the caudal portion found in the third quarter, is comparable to the avian air sac. Like other reptiles, snakes do not have a true diaphragm. The stomach is distensible but difficult to differentiate from the esophagus and duodenum. The liver is large, elongated, and single-lobed. The intestinal tract is relatively straight.

The third quarter of the snake extends from the cranial aspect of the gallbladder, spleen, and pancreas (or spleno-pancreas depending on the species) to either the testes or ovaries. The small intestine is between these structures, and the right lung is adjacent to them. In some species, such as boas and pythons, the left lung is reduced in size. The gallbladder is found caudal to the liver near the spleen and pancreas. The pancreas is near the pylorus of the stomach by the gallbladder and spleen.

The caudal quarter contains the junction between the small and large intestines, the cecum (if present), the kidneys (with the right being more cranial), and finally the cloaca. The kidneys are lobulated, resembling stacks of melted coins.[10] Snakes do not have a urinary bladder. The urine is stored in the cloaca. Most of the anatomy is visible on a radiograph.

Amphibians

Radiography Comments and Tips

- Amphibians such as toads and frogs (order *Anura*), salamanders and newts (order *Caudata*) can be imaged much like other species.
- Depending on the size of the species, Petri dishes or containers can be used.
- The most commonly used view is the DV. If required, lateral views are completed with the patient in a DV position with the use of a horizontal beam (Figure 27-39).
- Anurans are able to prolapse the stomach after eating undesirable food, after some methods of anesthesia, and when they are dying.

Anatomy

The amphibian intestinal tract is not as distinct as that of mammals. The esophagus is short and wide in anurans (frogs and toads). The liver and gallbladder are close together,

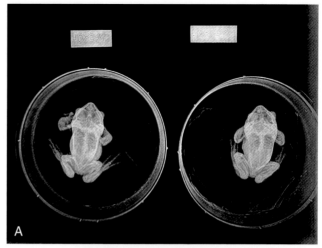

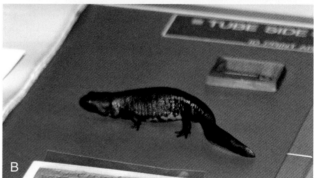

FIGURE 27-39 A, Dorsoventral views of South American Tree Frogs being restrained in Petri dishes. **B,** Dorsoventral view of a red spotted newt (caudata species of amphibian).

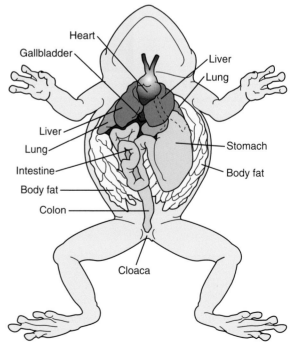

FIGURE 27-40 Ventral view of the frog showing internal anatomy.

and the pancreas is usually found between the stomach and proximal segments of the intestine (Figure 27-40).

The kidneys of amphibians are usually lobulated and found in the caudodorsal coelom. Amphibians have urinary bladders and cloacal anatomy similar to that of reptiles. The lungs are generally simple saclike structures with very little partitioning. Most amphibians have teeth. Anurans have an ossified pectoral girdle and an elongated pelvic girdle. Typically there are four toes on the front feet of anurans and salamanders and five on the hind feet.

Fish

Fish medicine is a fast growing area in veterinary medicine, with ever-increasing knowledge in the area of diagnostics. As such, radiography is becoming more commonly performed. Common reasons for radiography include trauma, swim bladder issues, and neoplasia.

When handling fish, keep in mind that the skin and scales provide a protective barrier and are quite sensitive to handling. Scales grow continuously throughout the life of the fish and are not regenerated if lost. They must continuously be kept moist and not exposed to air for more than a few seconds. If a temporary aquarium or bucket with some of the aquarium water is used, it will be difficult to keep the fish stationary and there will likely be movement artifacts. The exposure factors will also have to be altered.

Generally fish require anesthesia with an agent such as tricaine methanesulfonate (MS-222) in the water to enable proper positioning. Using a moist baggy with the MS-222 for the procedure will keep the patient comfortable and minimize movement. It is vital that the patient be returned to its environment as quickly as possible.

Radiographic Positions

Dorsoventral and Lateral Views

Positioning
Place the fish in a bag with water from its aquarium (Figure 27-41). Complete the procedure quickly. For both views, use a vertical beam. The lateral view is more practical but if the DV is required, support the bag so the fish is upright.

CENTRAL RAY: The middle of the body.
BORDERS: Include the whole body.

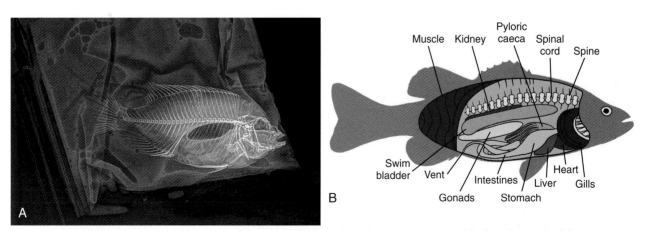

FIGURE 27-41 A, Lateral view of a fish radiographed in a bag of water. **B,** Anatomy of the lateral view of a fish.

Normal Radiographic Anatomy of the Fish[11,12]

Depending on the species, there are various types and pairs of fins, including the usually paired pectoral and pelvic fins, and unpaired cranial, caudal dorsal, anal, and caudal fins. The anal urogenital openings are cranial to the anal fin.

The skeleton of bony fish is composed of bone and cartilage and is not as radiopaque as that of mammals. The axial skeleton consists of the skull, vertebral column, and unpaired fins, and the appendicular skeleton is composed of the pelvic and pectoral girdles and their appendages or fins.

Fish breathe through the gills, which are found caudal to the head and located under the operculum. There are no lungs but there is a gas bladder, or swim bladder, which is located immediately dorsal to the peritoneal cavity. This long saclike organ normally contains a mixture of gases that contributes to the ability of a fish to control its buoyancy. Some fish have primitive lungs.

The coelom can be vaguely separated into the smaller pericardial portion and the peritoneal cavity. The small two-chambered heart—a thin-walled atrium and single thick-walled ventricle—is in the pericardial cavity ventral and caudal to the gills. Along with the heart there are two other chamber-like structures, the saclike sinus venosus and a muscular tube called the bulbous arteriosus. Blood enters the atrium from the sinus venosus and leaves the ventricle via the bulbous arteriosus.

The large liver is found at the cranial end of the peritoneal cavity and partially superimposes on a portion of the stomach and other organs. Three short sacs called pyloric caeca attach the stomach to the cranial end of the small intestine, which then leads to the large intestine. The length of the small intestine varies depending on the diet with the small intestine of the herbivores being the longest.

The spleen is located along the caudal surface of the stomach. A pair of elongated slender kidneys, which end in the urinary bladder, course adjacent to the spine and dorsal to the swim bladder. Both organs traverse practically the full length of the coelom. Wastes pass from the kidneys through the wolffian ducts and into the urinary bladder. From the bladder, wastes pass to the outside through the urinary pore in males and through the common urogenital pore in females. The paired testes in the male are located caudal to the stomach and ventral to the air bladder. The single large ovary of the female is in the same location.

> **KEY POINTS**
>
> 1. Generally, avian radiography requires chemical restraint for diagnostic results. The time for fasting of birds prior to anesthesia is variable and species specific.
> 2. Ensure handler safety when radiographing birds by always restraining their particular weapons, which vary by species.
> 3. For proper diagnosis, the positions must be exactly perpendicular, especially with the avian ventrodorsal view, to avoid misinterpretation of the radiograph.
> 4. Rodents and rabbits also generally require chemical restraint for adequate radiographs, but they are not usually fasted prior to sedation or anesthesia.
> 5. Dental concerns are extremely common in rodents and rabbits, and so excellent skull radiographs are essential.
> 6. Good coelomic detail is difficult to visualize during radiography of turtles. A rostrocaudal view is essential to obtain an unobstructed view of the lungs.
> 7. Lateral radiographs of snakes are necessary to adequately visualize internal structures. Consider use of a horizontal beam.
> 8. Almost any species can be radiographed if the behavior and important radiographic principles are kept in mind.

Acknowledgements

Special thanks to Sue Carstairs, DVM, of Seneca College, Toronto Wildlife Centre and Kawartha Turtle Trauma Centre for her assistance with the chapter.

References

1. Silverman ST: *Radiology of birds, an atlas of normal anatomy and positioning*, St. Louis, 2010, Elsevier.
2. Farrow C: *Diagnostic imaging-birds, exotic pets and wildlife*, St. Louis, 2009, Elsevier.
3. Morgan JP: *Techniques of veterinary radiography*, Ames, Iowa, 1993, Iowa State University Press.
4. Dyce KM, Sack WO, Wensing CJG: *Textbook of veterinary anatomy*, ed 4, St. Louis, 2010, Saunders.

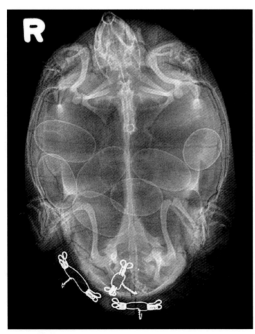

FIGURE 27-42 Mystery radiograph: How many eggs does this turtle have? What are the artifacts?

5. Gracis MD: Clinical technique: Normal dental radiography of rabbits, guinea pigs, and chinchillas, *J Exotic Pet Med* 17:78-86, 2008.

6. Silverman S, Tell L: *Radiology of rodents, rabbits and ferrets: an atlas of normal anatomy and positioning*, St. Louis, 2005, Saunders

7. Innis CD: *Reptile medicine.* Cummings School of Veterinary Medicine at Tufts University, 2008. http://ocw.tufts.edu/Content/60/lecturenotes/828884.

8. Mitchell M: Diagnostic imaging of lizards. In: *NAVC Conference: Small Animal and Exotics.* Orlando, FL, 2007, North American Veterinary Conference, pp 1590-1591.

9. Mitchell, MA, Tully, TN: *Manual of Exotic Pet Practice*, St. Louis, 2009, Saunders.

10. Colville T, Bassert J: *Clinical anatomy and physiology for veterinary technicians*, St. Louis, 2008, Elsevier.

11. Peterson K: Biology 453, Comparative Vertebrate Anatomy course notes, Autumn 2012, University of Washington, Seattle. http://courses.washington.edu/chordate/453labs/453lab1-fall2012.pdf Retrieved Nov/2012.

12. Mayer J: Clinical anatomy and physiology of fish. CVC in Kansas City proceedings. Aug 1, 2012. http://veterinarycalendar.dvm360.com/avhc/Veterinary+Exotics/Clinical-anatomy-and-physiology-of-fish-Proceeding/ArticleStandard/Article/detail/738519

Bibliography

Valente AL: Cervical and coelomic radiologic features of the loggerhead sea turtle, Caretta caretta, *Can J Vet Res* 70:285-290, 2006.

Aspinall V, Cappello M: *Introduction to veterinary anatomy*, London, 2009, Butterman Heineman.

Avian respiration. (n.d.). Retrieved 10/20/2011. http://people.eku.edu/ritchisong/birdrespiration.html.

Ballard B, Cheek R: *Exotic Animal medicine for the veterinary technician*, Ames, IA, 2003, Iowa State University Press.

Done, SH, Goody PC, Stickland NC, Evans SA: *Color atlas of veterinary anatomy, the dog and cat*, London, 2009, Mosby.

Han C, Hurd C: *Practical diagnostic imaging for the veterinary technician*, ed 3, St. Louis, 2005, Mosby.

Hernandez-Divers S: Reptile radiology: techniques, tips and pathology. In: *NAVC Conference: Small Animal and Exotics*, Orlando, FL, 2006, North American Veterinary Conference, pp 1626-1630.

Hernandez-Divers S: Snake radiology: the essentials. In: *NAVC Conference: Small Animal and Exotics*, Orlando, FL, 2008, North American Veterinary Conference, pp 1772-1774.

Kaufman GD: Avian radiology, Published 2008. http://ocw.tufts.edu/Content/60/lecturenotes/832723.

Lavin L: *Radiography in veterinary technology*, ed 3, St. Louis, 2007, Saunders.

Mitchell M: Diagnostic imaging of lizards. In: *NAVC Conference: Small Animal and Exotics*, Orlando, FL, 2007, North American Veterinary Conference, pp 1590-1591.

Mitchell, MA, Tully, TN: *Manual of Exotic Pet Practice*, St. Louis, 2009, Saunders.

Morgan JP: *Techniques of veterinary radiography*, Ames, IA, 1993, Iowa State University Press.

Romich J: *An illustrated guide to veterinary medical terminology*, Clifton, NY, 2009, Delmar Cengage Learning.

Setter M: Radiology of reptiles and amphibians. In: *NAVC Conference: Small Animal and Exotics*, Orlando, FL, 2003, North American Veterinary Conference, pp 1231.

Setter M: Ultrasound in reptiles and amphibians. In: *NAVC Conference: Small Animal and Exotics*, Orlando, FL, 2003, North American Veterinary Conference, pp 1232-1233.

Sirois M: *Principles and practice of veterinary technology*, ed 3, St. Louis, 2011, Mosby.

Sirois M, Anthony E, Mauragis D: *Handbook of radiographic positioning for veterinary technicians*, Clifton Park, NY, 2010, Delmar Cengage Learning.

Smallwood JE, Shively MJ, Rendano VT, Habel RE: A standardized nomenclature for radiographic projections used in veterinary medicine, *Vet Rad* 26:2-9, 1985.

Thrall DE: *Textbook of veterinary diagnostic radiology*, ed 5, St. Louis, 2007, Saunders.

Tighe M, Brown M: Mosby's comprehensive review for veterinary technicians, ed 3, St. Louis, 2008, Mosby.

15% rule Changing the kilovoltage peak by 15% has a similar effect on radiographic density as doubling the milliampere-seconds (mAs) or reducing the mAs by 50%.

Absorbing layer A light-absorbing dye used in the screen to absorb light directed toward it by the phosphor layer.

Absorption As the energy of the primary x-ray beam is deposited within the atoms comprising the tissue, some x-ray photons are completely absorbed. Complete absorption of the incoming x-ray photon occurs when it has enough energy to remove (eject) an inner-shell electron.

Acidifier Stops the development process and creates an acid pH environment for the fixing agent.

Acromion process The outer end of the scapula, extending over the shoulder joint and forming the highest point of the shoulder, to which the collarbone is attached. *Process* is a prominence or projection, as from a bone.

Actual focal spot size The size of the area on the anode target that is exposed to electrons from the tube current.

Added filtration The filtration that is added to the port of the x-ray tube. Aluminum is the material primarily used for this purpose because it absorbs the low-energy photons while allowing the useful higher-energy photons to exit.

Air gap technique Method for limiting the scatter reaching the image receptor. Scatter radiation exiting the patient will miss the image receptor if there is increased distance between the patient and image receptor (increased OID).

Air sacs The nine air sacs or bags found in birds provide a unidirectional flow of air to the lungs, making more oxygen available to flow into the lungs.

Algorithm Mathematical formulae used to specify image reconstruction.

Alveolar bone The compact bone composing the alveolus (tooth socket). It is supported by trabecular bone and the fibers of the periodontal ligament insert into it (from the Latin *alveoli/o*, "small sac").

Alveolar pattern Change in opacity resulting from abnormal cells or fluid within the terminal air spaces of the lung.

Anatomic programming/anatomically programmed radiography (APR) A radiographic system that allows the radiographer to select a particular button on the control panel that represents an anatomic area; a preprogrammed set of exposure factors is displayed and selected for use based on patient measurement.

Anconeal The projection of the ulna that occupies the olecranon fossa of the humerus when the elbow is extended and which develops as a separate ossification center in some dogs (from the Greek *ankon*, "elbow").

Angiocardiography Radiography of the heart and great vessels after the introduction of an opaque contrast medium into a blood vessel or a cardiac chamber (from the Greek *angeion*, "vessel," + *kardia*, "heart," and *graphein*, "to record").

Angiography Radiographic examination of the vascular system after the intravenous injection of positive-contrast medium.

Anode A positively charged electrode within the x-ray tube. It consists of a target and, in rotating anode tubes, a stator and rotor.

Anode heel effect Because of the angle of the anode target, the x-ray beam has greater intensity (number of x-rays) on the cathode side of the tube, with the intensity diminishing toward the anode side.

Antebrachium The radius and ulna, that part of the arm or forelimb between the brachium (humerus) and the carpus (from the Latin *ante* "fore," and *brachium*, "arm").

Antegrade urethrogram Radiographic examination of the urethra in which positive-contrast medium is injected vascularly and voided from the urinary bladder (from the Latin *ante*, "before," and *gredi*, "to go").

Anticlinal vertebrae A point in the caudal thoracic vertebral column at which vertebral anatomic features change. In quadrupeds, the spinous process extends vertically (from the Greek *cline*, "that upon which one lies").

Antilog The number corresponding to a given log of exposure. Used to determine the factorial change in intensity of exposure.

Aperture diaphragm The simplest type of beam-restricting device, constructed of a flat piece of lead that has a hole in it.

Apical In dental radiography, the direction toward the root of a tooth (from Latin *apex*, "tip, extreme end").

Appendicular The part of the skeleton that contains the bones of the limbs that functionally are involved with locomotion. Compare with the axial skeleton, which contains the bones of the skull, vertebrae, ribs, and sternum (from the noun *appendage*, "a part that is joined to something large").

Arch The dentition together with the alveolar ridge regardless of the number of teeth present (from the Latin *arc/o*, "bow or arch").

Arthrography Radiographic examination of the articular cartilage, joint space, and joint capsule after the sterile injection of contrast medium.

Artifact Any accidental or unintentional image on a radiograph.

Attenuation Reduction in the energy of the primary x-ray beam as it passes through a filter or anatomic tissue.

Automatic collimator Device attached below the x-ray tube that automatically limits the size and shape of the primary beam to a preset size and shape.

Automatic exposure control (AEC) A system used to consistently control radiographic density by terminating the length of exposure according to the amount of radiation reaching the image receptor.

Automatic processor A device that encompasses chemical tanks, a roller transport system, and a dryer system for the processing of radiographic film.

Average gradient   The slope of the straight-line region of a sensitometric curve.

Backup time   The maximum length of time the x-ray exposure will continue when an automatic exposure control system is used.

Barium sulfate   Positive-contrast medium that is often used as a suspension in a radiographic contrast study to evaluate the gastrointestinal tract.

Base   The bottom layer of the intensifying screen, found farthest from the film. The material that comprises the foundation of the x-ray film and upon which the emulsion is coated.

Base plus fog (B + F)   The minimum amount of optical density on the processed radiographic film.

Beam restriction/collimation   Used interchangeably, these words refer to a decrease in the size of the projected radiation field.

Beam-restricting device   Device that changes the shape and size of the primary beam; located just below the x-ray tube housing.

Binary number system   Combination of zeros and ones to process and store computer information.

Bisecting angle   A dental radiographic technique in which the central x-ray beam is positioned perpendicular to the line that bisects the angle formed by the long axis of the tooth and the film.

Bit   The computer's basic unit of information, either 0 or 1.

Bit depth   The number of bits that determines the precision with which the exit radiation is recorded and thus controls the exact pixel brightness that can be specified.

Blur   Unsharpness resulting from patient motion. It is the most detrimental factor to maximizing recorded detail.

Body habitus   The general form or build of the body, including size. There are four types: sthenic, hyposthenic, hypersthenic, and asthenic.

Brachycephalic   Having a short and wide head, such that the length of the cranium is shorter than the width (from the Greek *brachy*, "short," and *cephal*, "head").

Bremsstrahlung interactions   Occur during the production of x-rays when a projectile electron completely avoids the orbital electrons of the tungsten atom and travels very close to its nucleus. The very strong electrostatic force of the nucleus causes the electron to suddenly "slow down." As the electron loses energy, it suddenly changes its direction and the energy loss then reappears as an x-ray photon.

Brightness gain   The product of both flux gain and minification gain, which results in a brighter image on the output phosphor.

Bronchial pattern   Abnormal lung opacity caused by thickened bronchi or abnormal cells and/or fluid immediately adjacent to the bronchi.

Buccal   The outer surfaces of the premolars, molars, and the lateral aspects of the canine teeth that face toward the cheek (from the Latin *bucca*, "cheek").

Bucky   In veterinary medicine the Potter Bucky diaphragm has been removed and the unit is equipped with a sliding drawer to hold the x-ray cassette.

Byte   A combination of 8 bits.

Calipers   Devices that measure anatomical part thickness.

Carapace   A hard bony or chitinous outer covering, such as the fused dorsal plates of a turtle; a protective, shell-like covering. It consists of an external layer of horny material divided into plates called scutes and an underlying layer of interlocking bones (from the Latin *capa*, "cape").

Carina   A structure with a projecting central ridge, often in reference to the keel of a bird. The carina of the trachea is the ridge at the lower end of the trachea that separates the openings of the two primary bronchi [from the Latin *carina*, "nut-shell", (keel)].

Carnassial tooth   A large, shearing cheek tooth; the upper fourth premolar and lower first molar in dogs and cats. Also referred to as a sectorial tooth.

Cathartic   A purgative; an agent for purging the bowels, especially a laxative (from the Greek *katharsis* "to purge, cleanse, purify").

Cathode   A negatively charged electrode within the x-ray tube. It comprises a filament and a focusing cup.

Caudal   A location toward the tip of the tail. Also refers to the parts of the limb above (proximal to) the carpal and tarsal joints that face toward the tail (from the Latin *cauda*, "tail").

Caudocranial (CdCr)   Passing of the x-ray beam from the caudal surface to the cranial surface of a structure. Technically used for radiographing extremities that are proximal to the carpus or tarsus. Common (though incorrect) terminology for this view is posterior-anterior (PA).

Caudomedial-craniolateral oblique (CdM-CrL)   The beam enters from the back of the limb at the medial side and exits at the front of the limb on the lateral side, where the cassette is placed. The alternate view is the caudolateral-craniomedial oblique (CdL-CrM). *Oblique* means that the central ray will be angled.

Cementoenamel junction (CEJ)   An anatomical border identified on a tooth. It is the location where the enamel, which covers the anatomical crown of a tooth, and the cementum, which covers the anatomical root of a tooth, meet.

Characteristic interactions   Produced when a projectile electron interacts with an electron from the inner (K) shell of the tungsten atom. When the K-shell electron is ejected from its orbit, an outer-shell electron drops into the open position and thereby creates an energy difference. The energy difference is emitted as an x-ray photon.

Charge-coupled device (CCD)   Detector used in direct digital radiography that records flashes of light produced by the exit x-rays interacting with a screen that scintillates.

Choanal slit   The sagittal slit in the hard palate of the normal bird.

Cholecystography   Radiographic examination of the bile ducts and gallbladder following administration of an oral or intravenous positive-contrast agent.

Cloaca   The common cavity or vestibule into which the intestinal, urinary, and generative canals open in birds, reptiles, amphibians, many fishes, and certain mammals (from the Latin *cloaca* "sewer, drain," from cluere "to cleanse," "sewer or drain," or the Greek *klyzein*, "to wash away").

Coelom   The body cavity of the developing embryo situated between the layers of lateral mesoderm; in mammals, the coelom gives rise to the pericardial, pleural, and peritoneal cavities. In birds, because there is no diaphragm, the pleural and peritoneal cavities are one (from the Greek *koilos*, "hollow").

Coherent scattering   An interaction with low-energy x-rays, below the diagnostic range. The incoming photon interacts with the atom, causing it to become excited. The x-ray does not lose energy but changes direction.

Collimator A device located immediately below the tube window that has two or three sets of lead shutters. The variable entrance shutters limit the x-ray beam to the size of the image receptor.

Comparative anatomy Similar exposure techniques can be used for similar anatomic parts to achieve diagnostic radiographs.

Compensating filter A special filter added to the primary beam to alter its intensity. Such filters are used to image anatomic areas that are non-uniform, helping create a radiographic image with a uniform density.

Compton effect The loss of energy of the incoming photon when it ejects an outer-shell electron from the atom. The remaining lower-energy x-ray photon changes direction and may leave the anatomical part.

Compton electron/secondary electron The ejected electron resulting from the Compton effect interaction.

Concave Curving in or hollowed inward (from the Latin *concavus* "hollow").

Conchae A nasal concha (or turbinate) is a long, narrow, spongy and curled bone shelf shaped like an elongated seashell that protrudes into the breathing passage of the nose (from the Greek *konkhe*, "shell").

Cone An aperture diaphragm that has an extended flange. The flange can also be made to telescope, thereby increasing its total length.

Coned-down view Image of a specific body part focussed on a particular area of anatomy that is smaller than the original view.

Congenital hip dysplasia (CHD) A degenerative, developmental condition leading to painful hip osteoarthritis, stiffness, and diminished quality of life.

Congruity In reference to pelvic anatomy, how neatly the rounded femoral head fits into the curve of the acetabulum or socket. In its abstract form, the term means similarity between objects (from Latin *congruere*, "to come together or agree").

Congruity Alignment Occurs when the x-ray beam is superimposed exactly on the collimator light beam.

Contralateral Relating to the other side of the body (from Latin *contra*, "against").

Contrast medium (agent) A substance that can be instilled into the body by injection or ingestion to create higher subject contrast.

Contrast resolution The ability of the imaging system to distinguish between small objects with similar subject contrast.

Convergent line An imaginary line if points were connected along the length of the grid.

Convergent point An imaginary point if imaginary lines were drawn from each of the lead lines in a linear focused grid.

Convex Curving out or bulging outwards (from Latin convexus "vaulted, arched").

Coracoid A well-developed beak-shaped cartilage bone that is part of the pectoral girdle of birds and many lower vertebrates; it articulates with the scapula and sternum (from Greek for "crow"). In mammals, it is a bony process on the scapula with no articulation with the sternum.

Coronal surface The surface toward the crown of a tooth (from Greek and Latin *coron/o*, "crown").

Coronoid process A wide, flaring projection of the proximal end of the ulna. The proximal surface of the process forms the lower part of the trochlear notch (from Greek *korono* "something hooked, like a crow's beak").

Costochondral Pertaining to a rib and its cartilage (from Latin *costa*, "rib," and Greek *chondros*, "cartilage").

Cranial (Cr) The parts of the neck, trunk, and tail positioned *toward the head* from any given point. In limbs, *cranial* refers to the parts above (proximal to) the carpal and tarsal joints that face toward the head (from Latin *cranio*, "head").

Craniocaudal (CrCd) Passing of the x-ray beam from the cranial surface to the caudal surface of a structure. Technically, the craniocaudal projection is used for radiographing extremities that are proximal to the carpus or tarsus. Common (though incorrect) terminology for this view is anterior-posterior (AP).

Crena The large notch in the solar border of the equine sole (from the Latin *crena*, "to split").

Crossed/cross-hatched grid A grid in which lead lines are positioned vertically as well as horizontally.

Crossover Light that has been produced by an intensifying screen that exposes one emulsion and then "crosses over" the base layer of the film to expose the other emulsion.

Crossover roller An assembly within the automatic film processor that moves the film from one tank to another and into the dryer assembly.

Crura of the diaphragm (singular: crus) Tendinous structures that extend from the diaphragm to attach to the vertebral column and form a tether for muscular contraction (from Latin *crus*, "leg").

Cupula The ventral dome of the diaphragm (from Latin *cupula*, diminutive of *cupa* for "small, inverted cup or dome-shaped cap over a structure").

Cusp In dental radiography, a pointed or rounded area on or near the masticating surface of a tooth (from Latin cuspis "point, spear, head").

Cylinder An aperture diaphragm that has an extended flange attached to it. The flange can also be made to telescope, thereby increasing its total length.

Cystography Radiographic contrast study evaluating the urinary bladder (from Greek *cyst/o*, "urinary bladder").

Densitometer A device used to measure optical densities on radiography film.

Density maintenance formula Also known as *mAs/distance compensation formula*; a mathematical calculation for adjusting the mAs (milliamperes-seconds) if it is necessary to change the source-image distance (SID).

Detectors Radiation exposure measuring devices.

Developing agents Chemicals used in the developer to reduce exposed silver halide to metallic silver and to add electrons to exposed silver halide.

Diastema (plural diastemata) A space between two teeth found in many species of mammals, most commonly between the incisors and molars (from the Greek *dia*, "through or apart," and *stomat/o-*, "mouth").

Differential absorption A process whereby some of the x-ray beam is absorbed in the tissue and some passes through the anatomical part.

Diffusion The process by which the x-ray film is developed, fixed, and washed. The chemicals are diluted in water and saturate the emulsion of the film.

Digital imaging Recording radiographic images as numerical data.

Dimer   A compound formed by the union of two radicals or two molecules of a simpler compound. A polymer formed from two molecules of a monomer.

Direct-exposure film   Single-emulsion, nonscreen film that is significantly thicker than screen film and requires more exposure time.

Distal   Situated farthest from the center, median line, or point of attachment or origin. In dental radiography, the direction toward the last tooth in each quadrant of a dental arch; farthest from the median line (from Latin *dist/o*, "far").

Distolateral oblique   Direction of the x-ray beam at an oblique angle from the distal aspect (rear of the animal). Used in reference to dental radiography.

Distortion   Results from the radiographic misrepresentation of either the size or shape of the anatomic part.

D$_{max}$ The point on the sensitometric curve at which maximum density has been produced.

D$_{min}$ The point on the sensitometric curve at which minimum amount of optical density is measured.

Dolichocephalic   Having a long, narrow head such that the cranial length is greater than the cranial width (from Greek *dolich/o-*, "long," and *cephal-*, "head").

Dorsal (D)   Toward the back; thus, dorsal describes the upper aspect of the head, neck, trunk, and tail. In limbs, *dorsal* refers to those areas of the legs distally from the carpus and tarsus joints that face cranially or towards the head (from Latin *dors/o*, "back").

Dorsal plane   Divides the body into back and ventral (belly parts).

Dorsolateral-palmaromedial oblique (DLPMO)   A term commonly used in equine radiography. *Oblique* means that the central ray will be angled between the dorsopalmar and lateral side of the limb. In a dorsolateral-palmaromedial oblique projection, the central ray enters the equine limb dorsally toward the lateral side. The beam exits on the palmar portion of the limb toward the medial side. The film is placed against the palmaromedial aspect. *Plantar* can be substituted for *palmar*.

Dorsomedial-palmarolateral oblique (DMPLO)   A term commonly used in equine radiography. *Oblique* means that the central ray will be angled between the dorsopalmar and lateral side of the limb. In a dorsomedial-palmarolateral oblique projection, the central ray enters the equine limb dorsally toward the medial side. The beam exits on the palmar portion of the limb toward the lateral side. The film is placed against the palmarolateral aspect. *Plantar* can be substituted for *palmar*.

Dorsopalmar (DPa)   Radiographs that are taken distal to and including the carpus of the front limb. The x-ray beam passes from the dorsal surface (the cranially facing surface) to the palmar surface of the forelimb. Common (though incorrect) terminology is anterior-posterior (AP).

Dorsoplantar (DPl)   Radiographs that are taken distal to and including the tarsus of the hind limb. The x-ray beam passes from the dorsal (toward the head) surface of the hind limb to the plantar surface. Common (though incorrect) terminology is anterior-posterior (AP).

Dorsoproximal-palmarodistal (DPr-PaDi)   The correct term for describing the dorsopalmar projection for views of and distal to the carpus. The beam enters the front or dorsal portion of the limb and exits at the back or palmar side. *Plantar* can be substituted for *palmar*. The terminology then applies to views of and distal to the tarsus.

Dose creep   A term used in digital radiography to describe incremental increases in exposure in an attempt to reduce the amount of "noise" affecting the image quality. This will increase patient dose.

Dosimeter   A radiation dose measuring device.

Double contrast   A radiographic contrast technique that uses a combination of positive- and negative-contrast media to better evaluate organs.

Double-contrast cystogram   A radiographic study of the urinary bladder that involves distending the bladder with a gas and then adding a small amount of iodinated positive-contrast medium.

Double-emulsion film   Radiographic film that has an emulsion coating on both sides of the base.

Dynamic studies   Motion studies such as flexion and extension of the cervical and lumbosacral vertebrae (from Greek *dynamis*, "power, might, strength").

Dynamic range   Range of values that can be displayed by an imaging system; shades of gray.

Dyschezia   Difficult or painful defecation (from Greek *dys*, "bad or difficult," and *chezein*, "stool").

Dysplasia of the hip   Abnormal or faulty development of the acetabulum and the spherical end or caput of the femoral head. It is a polygenic trait affected by environmental factors in the production of the final phenotype that in its more severe form can cause crippling lameness and painful arthritis (from Greek *dys* "disordered or abnormal," and *plassein*, "to form").

Effective focal spot size   The focal spot size as measured directly under the anode target.

Electromagnetic radiation   Oscillating electric and magnetic fields that travel in a vacuum with the velocity of light. Includes x-rays, gamma rays.

Electrostatic focusing lenses   Lenses that focus the electrons through the image intensifier toward the anode.

Elongation   Effect in which images of objects appear longer than the original object.

Elongation of the teeth   A dental radiographic image error that results when the x-ray beam is perpendicular to the tooth instead of to the bisecting angle. The teeth appear longer than they actually are.

Emulsion   The radiation-sensitive and light-sensitive layers of film and intensifying screens spread evenly across a polyester or Mylar base.

Enamel bulge   Normal expansion of the crown at the gingival margin, designed to deflect food particles away from the gingival sulcus.

Entrance roller assembly   Rollers at the entrance to a film processor.

Epicondyle   A rounded projection at the end of a bone, located on or above a condyle and usually serving as a place of attachment for ligaments and tendons (from Greek *kondulos*, "knuckle of a joint," and *epi*, "upon or superimposition").

Esophageal hiatus   A hole in the diaphragm through which the esophagus passes. It is located in the right crus of the diaphragm.

Esophagography   Radiographic examination of the esophageal function and morphology following the administration of contrast medium.

Excretory urography   Radiographic examination of the kidneys and ureters following an injection of an intravenous positive-contrast medium. Originally referred to as intravenous urogram (IVU) or intravenous pyelogram (IVP).

Exit radiation   The attenuated x-ray beam that leaves the patient; it is composed of both transmitted and scattered radiation also known as remnant radiation.

Exposure latitude   The range of exposures that produce optical densities within the straight-line region of the sensitometric curve.

Exposure technique charts   Preestablished guidelines used by the radiographer to select standardized manual or automatic exposure control exposure factors for each type of radiographic examination.

Extraabdominal tissue   The tissues outside the abdomen that should also be evaluated when one is examining abdominal views; they include the pelvis and pelvic limbs, lumbar and caudal thoracic vertebrae, ribs, diaphragm, caudal thorax, abdominal musculature and wall, and the soft tissues dorsal to the thoracic and lumbar spine.

Extraoral   Outside the mouth (from Latin *extra,* "outside or beyond," and *oris,* "mouth").

Extrapolation   A process to mathematically estimate exposure techniques.

Facial   In dental radiography, the side of a tooth that is adjacent to (or the direction toward) the inside of the cheek or lips. This term is an umbrella term for both *buccal* and *labial* (from the Latin *faci,* "face or form").

Falciform ligament   A ligament that attaches the liver to the anterior body wall and is "falciform" (Latin for "sickle-shaped"); its base being directed downward and backward and its apex upward and backward.

Feed tray   In a film processor, a flat metal surface with an edge on either side that permits the film to enter the processor easily and aligned correctly.

FIFO   An acronym for "first in/first out." This film storage system requires that film received first be the film that is moved first into the working film supply.

Filament   A coiled tungsten wire that is the source of electrons during x-ray production.

Filament current   Electric current induced across the filament in the cathode when the rotor, or prep button, is pushed. This current is relatively low, approximately 3 to 5 amps, and operates at about 10 V.

Filling defect   Anything that occupies space within the lumen of an organ, thus preventing normal filling from occurring, such as a blood clot. Filling defects of the bladder, for example, are not radiolucent on a survey radiograph but do appear radiolucent when filled with positive-contrast medium.

Film contrast   The result of the inherent properties manufactured into the type of film and how it is radiographed (direct exposure or with intensifying screens), along with the processing conditions.

Film-screen contact   The amount of direct contact between the film and intensifying screens.

Film speed   The degree to which the film emulsion is sensitive to x-rays. Indicates the amount of optical density produced for a given amount of radiation exposure.

Fistula   An abnormal tubelike passage within body tissue; usually the result of an injury or congenital abnormality (from Latin *fistula,* "pipe, ulcer").

Fistulography   A positive or negative radiographic contrast study used to determine the depth and origin of a fistulous tract.

Fixed kVp/variable mAs technique chart   A type of exposure technique chart in which the optimal kVp value for each part is indicated, and the milliamperes-seconds (mAs) value is varied as a function of part thickness.

Fixing agent   Chemical used in the film fixer to clear undeveloped silver halide from the film.

Flat panel direct capture detector   An image receptor used in direct digital radiography that absorbs radiation and converts the energy into electrical signals.

Flexor view   Usually in reference to an oblique projection taken at the posterior aspect of the equine foot for the navicular and fetlock.

Flocculation   Clumping.

Flood replenishment   The addition of fresh chemicals that occurs at timed intervals, independent of the size or number of films processed.

Fluorescence   The ability of phosphors to emit visible light only while exposed to x-rays.

Fluoroscopy   Real time imaging of the movement of internal structures with a continuous beam of x-rays.

Flux gain   Increase in light intensities at the output phosphor as a result of acceleration of the electrons in the image intensifier.

Focal distance   The distance between the grid and the anode focal spot. Also known as the grid radius.

Focal film distance (FFD)   The distance between the anode and the image receptor; also referred to as SID or source-image distance.

Focal range   The recommended range of source-image distances that can be used with a focused grid.

Focal spot   The physical area of the target that is bombarded by electrons during x-ray production.

Focused grid   A grid in which the lead strips are angled to approximately match the angle of divergence of the primary beam.

Focusing cup   A device in the x-ray tube positioned to focus the stream of electrons. It has a negative charge, which maintains the direction of the electron cloud.

Fog   Unwanted density on the radiographic image caused by extraneous heat, light, or chemical fumes.

Foreshortening   Reduction in projected image size related to the angle of inclination of the object.

Foreshortening of the teeth   A radiographic image error resulting from the x-ray beam's being perpendicular to the film instead of to the bisecting angle. On a foreshortened dental film, the teeth appear shorter than they actually are.

Foundation layer   Polyester (Mylar) that gives the film physical stability.

Frequency   The number of waves passing a given point per given unit of time. Frequency is represented by a lowercase f or by the Greek letter *nu* (n), and values are given in units of Hertz (Hz). X-rays used in radiography range in frequency from about 3×10^{19} to 3×10^{18} Hz.

Frenulum   A band of tissue that attaches the lip in the region of the mandibular canine tooth to the mandible (from the Latin *fren/o*, "bridle, or device that limits movement").

Functional study   Contrast radiographic studies that evaluate the activity, purpose, or reason; relating to the way something works or operates (from Latin *funct/o*, "to perform").

Furcation   Anatomical area of a multi-rooted tooth where the roots diverge.

Furcula   A forked bone found in birds, it is formed by the fusion of the two clavicles that is part of the pectoral girdle; wishbone (from Latin word for "little fork").

Gamma   The slope calculated within the straight-line region of the sensitometric curve from points surrounding the optical density of 1.0.

Gastric rugae   The folds that provide the stomach with increased surface area. When food enters the stomach, these rugal folds become stretched, allowing the stomach to expand without increased pressure (from Latin, *ruga* "a wrinkle in the face").

Gastrography   Radiographic examination of the size, shape, position, and morphology of the stomach following administration of contrast medium (from Greek *gaster* "belly, paunch").

Geometric properties   The sharpness of structural lines recorded in the radiographic film image.

Geometric unsharpness   A result of the relationship between the size of the focal spot, the source-image distance, and the object-image distance that causes lack of recorded detail in the image.

Glenoid   The articular depression of the scapula entering into the formation of the shoulder joint (from Greek *glene*, "joint socket").

Gnathotheca   The horny sheath of the lower beak or mandibular rhamphotheca.

Gradient point   A slope calculated at any point along the sensitometric curve.

Granuloma   A tumor composed of granulation tissue produced in response to chronic infection, inflammation, a foreign body, or unknown causes (from Latin *granulum*, "granular-grain or seed," and *oma*, "lump, tumor or mass").

Grid   A device that has very thin lead strips with radiolucent interspaces located between the table top and the image receptor. It is used to absorb scattered radiation.

Grid cap   A film cassette holder that contains a permanently mounted grid and allows the image receptor to slide in behind it. Usually used in portable radiography.

Grid cassette   An image receptor that has a grid permanently mounted to its front surface.

Grid conversion factor (GCF)   A factor that can be used to determine the adjustment in milliampere-seconds (mAs) needed when one is changing from using a grid to not using a grid (or vice versa) or changing to a grid with a different grid ratio.

Grid cutoff   A decrease in the number of transmitted photons that reach the image receptor because of misalignment of the grid.

Grid factor (Bucky factor)   Used to determine the adjustment in mAs needed when one is changing from using a grid to not using a grid (or vice versa) or changing to a grid with a different grid ratio.

Grid focus   The orientation of the lead lines to one another. Two types of grid focus exist: parallel (non-focused) and focused.

Grid frequency   The number of lead lines per unit length, in inches, or millimeters.

Grid pattern   The linear arrangement of the lead lines of a grid. Two types of grid pattern exist: linear, crossed or crosshatched.

Grid ratio   The ratio of the height of a grid's lead strips to the distance between them.

Guide plates   In a film processor, slightly curved metal plates that properly guide the leading edge of the moving film through the roller assembly.

Half-value layer (HVL)   The amount of filtration that reduces the intensity of the x-ray beam to half its original value.

Hallux   The first or most medial digit. In tetrapods, this is referred to as the big toe (from Latin *allex*, "great toe").

Haustra (singular: haustrum)   Small pouches of the colon, caused by sacculation, which give the colon its segmented appearance (from Latin *haustor*, "drawer").

Heat unit (HU)   The amount of heat produced at the anode from any given x-ray exposure.

High-contrast radiograph   A radiograph with few densities but great differences between them; also described as a short-scale contrast radiograph.

Hilum (plural: hila)   The root of the lungs at the level of the fourth and fifth dorsal vertebrae. The hilum on the medial side of each lung is where the main bronchus, pulmonary arteries, bronchial arteries, and nerves enter the lung and where the pulmonary veins, bronchial veins, and lymphatic vessels leave it (from Latin- for "a trifle").

Histogram   Graphic display of the distribution of pixel values in the image receptor. A pattern of contrast on the image receptor.

Image intensification   A method of amplifying the brightness of the fluoroscopic image to reduce patient dose.

Image receptor   A device that receives the remnant radiation and produces the image.

Image receptor contrast   A result of the inherent properties manufactured into the type of image receptor and how it is radiographed (direct exposure or with intensifying screens), along with the processing conditions.

Imaging plate (IP)   The flexible plate inside the computed radiography cassette where the photon intensities are absorbed by the photostimulable phosphor.

Immersion heater   In a film processor, a heating coil that is immersed in the bottom of the developer and fixer tank. It is thermostatically controlled to heat the solution to the correct temperature and maintain that temperature as long as the processor is turned on.

Incisal   In dental radiography, either the direction toward the biting edge of anterior teeth or to something relating to this edge, as in "incisal guidance" or "incisal edge." This is comparable to *occlusal*, which is related to the analogous location on posterior teeth (from Latin *incis/o*, "cutting into").

Ingluvies   Also known as the crop in a bird's digestive system, an outpouching of the esophagus, located near the throat, that is used to store food when the stomach is full. Not present in all birds, and the size and shape does vary.

Inherent filtration   The filtration that is permanently in the path of the x-ray beam. Three components contribute to inherent filtration: (1) the glass envelope of the tube, (2) the oil that surrounds the tube, and (3) the mirror inside the collimator (beam restrictor located just below the x-ray tube).

Input phosphor Light-emitting material in the image intensifier that converts exit radiation into visible light.

Instantaneous load tube rating chart A reference used to determine whether a particular exposure will be safe to make and to determine what limits on kV, mA, and exposure time must be made to make a safe exposure.

Intensification factor (IF) A formula that represents the degree to which exposure factors are reduced when intensifying screens are used.

Intensifying screen A device found in radiographic cassettes that consists of an emulsion spread on a polyester base containing phosphors that convert x-ray energy into light, which then exposes the radiographic film.

Intensity of radiation exposure The measurement of the quantity of radiation.

Interspace material Radiolucent strips between the lead lines of a grid, usually aluminum.

Interstitial pattern Change in opacity of the interstitium. The pattern can be either structured (nodular or masses) or unstructured.

Interstitium The non–air-containing elements of the lungs, including the alveolar septum, interlobular septum, and microscopic blood vessels. It does not include the macroscopic blood vessels.

Intraoral The inside of the mouth (from Latin *intra*, "inside, within," and *oris*, "mouth").

Inverse square law States that: The intensity of the x-ray beam is inversely proportional to the square of the distance from the source.

Ionization The ability to remove (eject) electrons; a property of x-rays.

Ionization/ion chamber A hollow cell that contains air and a wire detector attached to a dosimeter. Typically used to measure radiation dose.

Ipsilateral Relating to the same side of the body.

Kyphosis The curvature of the thoracic vertebrae. Dogs and cats have a natural kyphosis in the mid to caudal thoracic vertebrae (from Greek, *kyphos*, "bent").

Labial In dental radiography, surfaces of the canine and incisor teeth that face the lip (from Latin *labi/o*, "lip").

Lamina dura The dental radiographic term used for the cribriform plate and dense alveolar bone surrounding the root. The lamina dura appears as a dense white line adjacent to the periodontal ligament space.

Latent image The invisible image that exists on the exposed film before it has been chemically processed.

Latent image centers Several sensitivity specks with many silver ions attracted to them.

Lateral (L) Side. The x-ray beam either enters through the left or right side of the body and emerges on the opposite side, where the cassette is positioned. In strict American College of Veterinary Radiology (ACVR) nomenclature, if a patient is lying on its left side, this view would be referred to as a "right-to-left lateral." However, convention refers to a this as a "left lateral." A "left lateral" limb in small animal radiography means that the patient is lying on its left side with the left limb against the image receptor. The x-ray beam penetrates from medial to lateral (technically called a mediolateral) (from Latin *later/o*, "side").

Lateromedial (LaM) Projection in which the x-ray beam enters a limb through the lateral side and exits on the medial side. In equine radiography, most lateral radiographs of the limbs are taken in a lateromedial projection.

Leakage radiation Any x-rays, other than the primary beam, that escape the tube housing.

Line focus principle The relationship between the actual and effective focal spots in the x-ray tube. If the face of the anode is angled, the actual focal spot can remain relatively large, whereas the effective focal spot is reduced in size.

Linear grid A grid with lead lines that run in only one direction and are not focussed.

Lingual In dental radiography, the side of a tooth adjacent to (or the direction toward) the tongue (from Latin *lingu/o*, "tongue").

Log relative exposure Measurement of the intensity of radiation exposure in increments of a constant change.

Logarithmic scale Relating to Logarithmic Relative Exposure; the change in optical density over various exposure intervals plotted on a graph.

Long-scale contrast radiograph A radiograph with a large number of densities but little density difference between them, and described as a low-contrast radiograph.

Lookup table A reference that allows one to alter the digital image to change its display.

Lordosis The state of the spine in which it is bent inward as opposed to outward (from Greek *lordos* "bent inwards").

Low-contrast radiograph A radiograph with a large number of densities but little differences among them, and described as a long-scale contrast radiograph.

Lower gastrointestinal (LGI) study Radiographic examination of the rectum, colon, and cecum following the administration of contrast medium. Commonly referred to as a barium enema study.

Luminescence The emission of light from the screen when it is stimulated by radiation.

Luxation The displacement or misalignment of a joint. A *subluxation* is a partial dislocation (from Latin *luxatio*, "out of place, crooked").

Lymphography Radiographic examination of the lymphatic vessels and lymph nodes following the administration of contrast medium.

Magnification factor (MF) A factor that indicates how much size distortion or magnification is demonstrated on a radiograph. Magnification factor equals source-image distance divided by source-object distance.

Malocclusion Poor fitting of the upper and lower teeth when the animal closes its mouth (from Latin *mal*, "bad, poor," and *occluso*, "to close up").

Manifest image The visible image on film after processing.

mAs conversion formula for screens A formula used to determine how to compensate or adjust milliampere-seconds (mAs) when changing intensifying screen system speeds.

Matrix The combination of rows and columns (array) of pixels.

Maximum contrast The greatest difference in optical densities achieved within the straight-line region of the sensitometric curve.

Medial (M) The direction toward the animal's midline. For limb radiographs, the beam enters from the medial side and exits the lateral side. Technically this is a mediolateral (ML) projection, but generally it is referred to as a lateral especially in small animals (L) (from Latin *medi/o*, "middle").

Mediastinum The potential space between the right and left pleural sacs that divides the thorax into right and left sides. It is formed by the parietal pleura of the right and left hemithoraces and contains the trachea, esophagus, heart, aorta and its major branches, thoracic duct, lymph nodes, and nerves.

Mental foramina Radiolucent openings in the bone located on the lateral surface of the mandible in the region of the first three mandibular premolars.

Mesial In dental radiography, the direction toward the anterior midline in a dental arch, as opposed to *distal*, which refers to the direction toward the last tooth in each quadrant. Each tooth can be described as having a mesial surface and, for posterior teeth, a mesiobuccal (MB) and a mesiolingual (ML) corner or cusp (from Greek *mesi*, "middle, midline").

Mesiobuccal (MB) Pertaining to or formed by the mesial and buccal surfaces of a tooth.

Mesiolateral oblique Directing the x-ray beam at an oblique angle from the mesial aspect (front of the animal). Usually used in reference to dental radiography.

Mesiolingual (ML) Pertaining to or formed by the mesial (towards the anterior midline) and lingual surfaces of a tooth.

Mesocephalic Describes the majority of dogs with medium or average head shape in which the width and length of the head are in balance, normal occlusion and function of a scissor or shear bite with the maxillary incisors rostral to the mandibular incisor teeth (from Greek *mesi*- "middle," and *cephal*, "head"). Sometimes also referred to as *mesaticephalic*.

Midsagittal plane A vertical plane through the midline of the body; divides the body into right and left halves. Also called the median plane (from Latin *sagitta*, "arrow").

Minification gain An increase in light intensities as a result of the reduction in size of the output phosphor image in comparison to the input phosphor image.

Minimum response time The shortest exposure time that the automatic exposure control system can produce.

Morphological studies Contrast studies looking at the form and structure, including size and shape (from Greek *morpho*, "shape or form").

Myelography Radiographic examination of the subarachnoid space surrounding the spinal cord following the administration of contrast medium (from Greek *myel/o*, "spinal cord or bone marrow," "white substance").

Negative-contrast agents Gases that are more radiolucent to x-rays than soft tissues and thus appear black on a radiograph. Air, carbon dioxide, and nitrous oxide are such agents.

Nephrogram A phase of an excretory urogram characterized by the diffuse opacification of the functional renal parenchyma, which shows the vascular supply and kidney perfusion. This phase is immediately noted in a normal contrast study of the kidneys (from Greek *nephr/o*, "kidney").

Numerical exposure indicator An instrument that indicates the level of x-ray exposure received by the computerized radiography (CR) imaging plate.

Oblique (O) Positioning in which the primary beam enters the body at an angle other than 90 degrees to the anatomical area of interest. It is used primarily in dental and large patient limb radiographs (from Latin *obliquus*, "slanting, sidelong, indirect").

Occlusion The contact between the upper and lower teeth when the mouth is closed. Dogs and cats have sectorial occlusion (from Latin *occlus/o*, "close up").

Object-film distance (OFD) The distance from the image detector to the part of the body being radiographed.

Optical density (OD) A measurement of the amount of light transmitted through the film.

Optimal density Radiographic densities that lie within the straight-line region of the sensitometric curve.

Optimal kVp The kilovoltage power (kV) value that is high enough to ensure penetration of the part but not too high to diminish radiographic contrast.

Oropharynx The oral part of the pharynx, which reaches from the soft palate to the level of the hyoid bone. It is one of the three anatomic divisions of the pharynx, lying posterior to the mouth and is continuous above with the nasopharynx and below with the laryngopharynx (from Latin *oris*, "mouth," and Greek, *pharynx*, "throat").

Orthogonal views Two projections made at a 90-degree angle (right angle), which are recommended for two-dimensional imaging of three-dimensional objects (from Greek *ortho*, "straight," and *gonia*, "angle").

Osmolality The concentration of an osmotic solution, usually in terms of osmoles. The osmolality of blood is the osmotic pressure of blood and is usually expressed in terms of osmoles. Osmolality measures the amount of solute concentration per unit of total volume of a particular solution (from Greek, *osmos*, "impulsion or pushing").

Output phosphor Light-emitting material in the image intensifier that converts accelerated electrons into visible light.

Palatal surface The side of a tooth adjacent to (or the direction toward) the palate. This term is strictly used in the maxilla (from Latin *palat/o*, "roof of mouth").

Palmar (Pa) The caudal surface of the forelimb from and including the carpal joint distally (from Latin *palmar*, "hollow of hand").

Palmarodorsal (PaD) Describes radiographs that are taken of and distal to the carpus of the front limb. The x-ray beam passes from the palmar (towards the tail) surface of the forelimb to the dorsal (toward the head) surface. Common (though incorrect) terminology is posterior-anterior (PA).

Palmaroproximal–palmarodistal (PaPr-PaDi) oblique view Usually in reference to equine. Also referred to as skyline or flexor view. The central ray is on the palmar aspect of the limb and is angled down to the fetlock or navicular. The image receptor is under the foot.

Parallel grid A nonfocused grid that has lead lines running parallel to one another.

Parallel technique In dental radiography, placement of the film parallel to the long axis of the tooth with the central x-ray beam positioned perpendicular to the film.

Parasympatholytic agents Drugs that reduce the activity of the parasympathetic nervous system, and also referred to as anticholinergics.

Parenchyma The essential parts of the organ that are concerned with its function (from Greek *parenkhyma* "something poured in beside)." It was believed that the insides of the organs formed from blood strained through the capillaries and congealed.

Penetrometer A device constructed of uniform absorbers of increasing thicknesses also called a stepped wedge.

Periapical The area surrounding the apex of the tooth.

Peritoneum The serous membrane that forms the lining of the abdominal cavity or the coelom. It consists of the outer layer (parietal peritoneum), which is attached to the abdominal wall, and the inner layer (visceral peritoneum), which is adhered to the internal organs that are located inside the intraperitoneal cavity. The potential space between these two layers is the peritoneal cavity, which usually contains a very small amount of fluid.

Pes The scientific term for foot (or footlike part) of an animal (from Latin *pes,* "foot").

Phosphor A chemical compound that emits visible light when struck by radiation.

Phosphor layer Active layer of the intensifying screen that contains the phosphor material that absorbs the transmitted x-rays and converts them to visible light.

Phosphorescence Emission of visible light during and after stimulation.

Photocathode Device that converts the visible light in the image intensifier into electrons.

Photoelectric effect Complete absorption of the incoming x-ray photon when it has enough energy to remove (eject) an inner-shell electron. The ionized atom has a vacancy, or electron hole, in its inner shell and a secondary photon is created when the vacancy is filled by an outer-shell electron.

Photoelectron The ejected electron resulting from total absorption of the photon during the photoelectric effect interaction.

Photographic properties Visibility of the recorded image; determined by the extent to which the structural components of the anatomical area of interest can be seen.

Photomultiplier (PM) tube An electronic device that converts visible light energy into electrical energy.

Phototimer A device used in first-generation automatic exposure control systems that includes a fluorescent (light-producing) screen and a photomultiplier tube.

Photon A small, discrete bundle of energy.

Picture archiving and communications system (PACS) A computer system designed for digital imaging that can capture, store, display, and distribute digital images.

Pixel The smallest component (picture element) of the matrix.

Plantar (Pl) The caudal surface of the hind limb from the tarsal joint distally (from Latin *plantar,* "sole of the foot").

Plantarodorsal (PlD) Radiographs that are taken distal to and including the tarsus of the hind limb. The x-ray beam passes from the plantar (towards the tail) surface of the hindlimb to the dorsal (toward the head) surface. Common (though incorrect) terminology is posterior-anterior (PA).

Plastron The nearly flat bottom part of the shell structure of a turtle or tortoise that is similar in composition to the carapace and protects the abdomen of chelonians (from French *plastron,* "breastplate").

Pneumocystogram Radiographic examination of the urinary bladder following the administration of a radiolucent or negative-contrast medium (from Greek *pneum/o,* "air").

Pneumoperitoneography Radiographic examination of the peritoneal cavity following the administration of negative-contrast medium or gas (from Greek *pneum/o,* "air").

Position indicating device (PID) The cone portion of the x-ray tube head.

Positive beam-limiting device A device that automatically limits the size and shape of the primary beam to the size and shape of the image receptor.

Positive-contrast agents Substances containing elements of high atomic number that are more radiopaque to x-rays than they are to tissue or bone so they appear white on a radiograph.

Positive-contrast cystogram Distention of the bladder with iodinated positive-contrast medium for a radiographic study.

Postprocessing Manipulation of the digital image after the original result has been reviewed.

Processing cycle The amount of time it takes to process a single sheet of x-ray film.

Processor capacity The number of films that can be processed per hour.

Protective layer The outermost layer of the screen, found closest to the film and made of plastic to protect the fragile phosphor material beneath it. Modern screens incorporate this layer into the emulsion.

Proventriculus The elongated, spindle-shaped, glandular stomach of birds, which may store and/or commence digestion of food before it progresses to the gizzard, or muscular stomach (from Latin *pro,* "before" and *venter,* "belly").

Proximal (Pr) Nearer to the middle or the point of origin of a structure (from Latin *proxim/o,* "next").

Proximal surface Surface of a tooth that normally lies adjacent to another tooth. It is an umbrella term that includes both mesial and distal (from Latin *proxim/o,* "near").

Pyelogram A phase of an excretory urogram showing the opacification of the renal collection system—the renal pelvis, pelvic recesses, and ureters.

Quantum A small, discrete bundle of energy.

Quantum mottle The statistical fluctuation in the quantity of x-ray photons that contribute to image formation per square millimeter that results in a radiographic image that is grainy, or noisy, in appearance.

Radicular groove A channel evident on the lower first molar tooth and the upper forth premolar tooth in dogs. Visible as a double periodontal ligament space on radiographs but is a normal anatomical feature caused by indentations in the roots structure with a corresponding alveolar ridge.

Radiographic contrast The degree of difference between adjacent densities.

Radiographic density The amount of overall blackness produced on the image after processing.

Radiolucent A substance that allows x-rays to penetrate with less absorption than soft tissues and will thus appear black on a radiograph. Air, carbon dioxide, and nitrous oxide are such agents (from Latin *radiare,* "to emit rays," and *lucere,* "to shine").

Radiopaque A substance such as barium that contains elements of high atomic number that will absorb more x-rays than tissue or bone so it appears white on a radiograph (from Latin *radiare,* "to emit rays," and *opacus,* "to obscure").

Rare earth element Phosphor materials ranging in atomic number from 57 to 71 on the periodic table. These elements are used in the manufacture of intensifying screens.

Reciprocity law Principle states that the optical density on a radiograph is proportional only to the total energy imparted to the radiographic film.

Recirculation system A system of pumps within the automatic processor designed to stabilize temperature, pH of the chemicals, dilution of the chemicals, and filter the solutions. Each separate tank contains one pump.

Recorded detail The distinctness or sharpness of the structural lines that make up the recorded film image. Usually expressed as line pairs per millimeter.

Recumbent Lying down. Most radiographs of the dog and cat are made in this position. In small animals, it is the assumed position unless otherwise noted (from Latin *recumbentem*, "back" + "to lie down").

Reducing agents Chemicals used in the radiographic developer to reduce exposed silver halide to metallic silver and to add electrons to exposed silver halide.

Reflecting layer Either a magnesium oxide or titanium dioxide material used in the screen to reflect all of the light toward the film.

Relative speed The ability of the screen to produce visible light, and therefore density. Relative speed results from comparing screen-film systems on the basis of the amount of light (and density) produced for a given exposure.

Remnant radiation The attenuated x-ray beam that leaves the patient; is composed of both transmitted and scattered radiation.

Replenishment The replacement of fresh developer and fixer solutions after the loss of chemicals during processing.

Resolution The ability of the imaging system to resolve or distinguish between two adjacent structures; can be expressed in the unit line pairs per millimeter (Lp/mm).

Retrograde contrast studies Infusion of either a positive- or negative-contrast agent, in reverse to how the discharge normally flows (from Latin *retr/o*, "behind or backwards," and *gredi*, "to go").

Retrograde urography Radiographic examination of the urinary tract following injection of contrast medium directly into the urethra or bladder.

Retroperitoneum The space between the peritoneum and the dorsal abdominal wall that contains the kidneys, the adrenal glands, the aorta caudal vena cava, lymph nodes and vessels, and portions of the nervous system.

Rhinotheca The horny sheath of the upper beak, also known as the maxillary rhamphotheca.

Rodentia An order of mammals also known as rodents, characterized by two continuously growing incisors in the upper and lower jaws that must be kept short by gnawing (Latin *rodere*, "to gnaw").

Rostral Toward the tip of the nose (from Latin rostrum "beak").

Rostrocaudal oblique In dental terminology, the direction of the beam coming from the nose to the throat at an angle to the 90-degree lateral (from Latin *rostri*, "beak," and *caud/o*, "toward the tail").

Rotor Rotates the anode in an x-ray tube. Rotating part of an electromagnetic induction motor contained within the glass envelope of the x-ray tube.

Sagittal plane The plane that divides the body into unequal right and left parts (from Latin *sagitta*, "arrow").

Scapulohumeral articulation The shoulder joint.

Scattering When some incoming photons are not absorbed, but instead lose energy during interactions with atoms making up the tissue, change direction, and are scattered within the anatomic part. They may have enough energy to leave the patient's anatomy and affect the image receptor.

Screen film X-ray film that is manufactured to be used with either one or two intensifying screens placed in an x-ray cassette.

Screen speed The capability of a screen phosphor to produce visible light. A faster screen produces more light than a slower screen for the same radiation exposure.

Sectorial occlusion The upper fourth premolar overlaps the lower first molar in a scissor type of occlusion, so that the food is processed on the sides of the teeth in a chopping fashion (from Latin *sect/o*, "cutting").

Sensitometer A device used to expose x-ray film to light. When the film is processed it will demonstrate consistent stepped densities.

Sensitometric curve A graphic display of the relationship between the intensity of radiation exposure to film and the resultant optical densities.

Sensitometric strip A stepped-wedge density image produced after exposing the film in a sensitometer and then processing the film.

Sensitometry The study of the relationship between the intensity of radiation exposure to the film and the amount of blackness produced after processing (density).

Sharpness of recorded detail The distinctness of structural lines recorded in the radiographic image.

Short-scale contrast radiograph A radiograph with few densities but great differences among them and described as a high-contrast radiograph.

Shoulder region An area on the sensitometric curve where changes in exposure intensity no longer affect the optical density.

Sialography A radiographic contrast study evaluating the salivary glands and ducts (from Greek *sialon*, "duct" + *graphein*, "to record").

Source-image distance (SID) The distance between the source of the radiation (anode) and the image receptor.

Silver halide The material in the film's emulsion that is sensitive to radiation and light.

Silver recovery The removal of silver from used fixer solution.

Single-emulsion screen film Radiographic film having only one emulsion layer that is used with a single intensifying screen.

Size distortion/magnification An increase in the object's image size compared with its true, or actual, size.

Skyline view Tangential radiographic view of any structure; taken to provide more information than the standard projections. Usually used to examine the trochlear groove of the stifle in dogs and carpal slab fractures in horses.

SLOB rule In dental radiography, an acronym meaning "same lingual, opposite buccal," in reference to the position of the tube head and the determination of the root. This term is used in the radiography of three-rooted teeth to determine the identity of the roots.

Slope A mathematical calculation of the tilt or slope of a line on a graph.

Source-object distance (SOD) The distance from the x-ray source (focal spot) to the object being radiographed.

Space charge The electrons liberated from the filament during thermionic emission that form a cloud around the filament.

Space charge effect Phenomenon of the space charge to limit subsequent electrons to be emitted by the filament because of electrostatic repulsion.

Spatial resolution The smallest detail that can be detected in an image. Normally expressed as line pairs consisting of one white line and one black line.

Spectral emission The color of light produced by a particular intensifying screen.

Spectral matching Correctly matching the color sensitivity of the film to the color emission of the intensifying screen.

Spectral sensitivity The color of light to which a particular film is most sensitive.

Speed Sensitivity of radiographic film to radiation exposure.

Speed exposure point The point on a sensitometric curve that corresponds to the intensity of exposure needed to produce a density of 1.0 plus B + F (speed point).

Speed point The point on a sensitometric curve that corresponds to the optical density of 1.0 plus B + F.

Standby control On an automatic processor the electric circuit that shuts off power to the roller assemblies when the processor is not being used.

Stator An electric motor that turns the rotor at very high speed during x-ray production.

Stepped wedge Also called a penetrometer. Filter that varies in height used during testing of radiographic film screen systems to compare contrast and densities. Typically consists of aluminium and contains 10 to 21 steps.

Stepped-wedge densities A graded series of uniform densities of film that increase from light to dark. (Densities of a film alphabetized).

Straight-line region The area on a sensitometric curve where the diagnostic or most useful range of densities is produced.

Subject contrast A result of the absorption characteristics of the anatomic tissue radiographed and the level of kilovoltage used.

Sulcus (plural: sulci) The central grove of the frog that extends up between the bulbs (from Latin meaning "furrow, rut").

Superadditivity Chemicals which have a greater effect when combined than they would individually.

Supercoat A durable protective layer on film that is intended to prevent damage to the sensitive emulsion layer underneath it. Modern films incorporate this layer into the emulsion.

Supratrochlear foramen A small hole located above the trochlea of the humerus. It is covered by a layer of connective tissue (from Latin, *supra*, "above", + Greek *trochos*, "wheel" + Latin *forare*, "bore, to pierce").

Swim bladder An internal gas-filled organ that contributes to the ability of a fish to control its buoyancy to stay at the current water depth. The bladder also is a stabilizing agent and a resonating chamber to produce or receive sound.

Syrinx The vocal organ of birds, formed by the terminal part of the trachea and the first part of the primary bronchi.

Tangential In a direction perpendicular to the line of sight. Anything in the direction that is at a 90-degree angle to the radius of a circle is tangential. It is the plane that "just touches" the surface at that point (from Latin *tangere*, "to touch").

Target A metal that abruptly decelerates and stops electrons at the anode, thereby allowing the production of x-rays.

Tenesmus Generally, painful or ineffective defecation, but can also mean painful, ineffective urination (from Greek *teinesmos*, "to stretch").

Thermionic emission Emission of electrons from a heated surface.

Toe region The area of low density on a sensitometric curve.

Total filtration The sum of the added filtration and the inherent filtration.

Transmission The passage of the x-ray beam through an anatomic part with no interaction with atomic structures.

Transport rollers The roller assembly in an automatic film processor that moves the film through the chemical tanks and dryer assembly.

Transverse plane The plane that divides the body into cranial and caudal parts. This is also called the horizontal plane or cross-sectional plane and can describe a perpendicular cross section to the long axis of the limb (from Latin *transversus*, "turned or directed across").

Triiodinated compound A common component of iodinated positive-contrast media that contains three atoms of iodine per molecule.

Tube current The flow of electrons from cathode to anode; measured in units called milliamperes (mA).

Turnaround roller Rollers at the bottom of the roller assembly in a film processor that reverse the direction of the film in the the transport assembly.

Ungular or collateral cartilage Foot cartilage (from Latin nail or claw- *unguis*).

Upper gastrointestinal (UGI) study Radiography of the stomach and small intestines following injestion of contrast medium, usually barium sulfate.

Urethrography Radiography of the urethra following administration of a contrast agent.

Vaginocystourethrography Radiographic examination of the vagina, bladder, and urethra following retrograde administration of a radiopaque medium.

Vaginography Radiographic examination of the vagina after the injection of radiopaque contrast media.

Variable kVp/fixed mAs technique chart A type of exposure technique chart that changes the kilovoltage (kV) as the part thickness changes. The mAs remains constant.

Vent A term often used for the cloaca of birds, reptiles, amphibians, many fishes, and certain mammals. The vent is actually the anal region, whereas the cloaca is the actual vestibule (from Latin vent, "hole, opening, outlet").

Ventral (V) Lower or toward the lower aspect of the body (from Latin *venter*, "belly").

Ventriculus The muscular-walled, avian stomach used for grinding up food, also known as the gizzard. It is well developed in herbivorous species such as geese and swans, and less so in carnivorous species such as hawks and owls (from Latin *ventricul/o,* "small cavity or chamber").

Visibility of recorded detail Photographic properties of the recorded image; determined by the extent to which the structural components of the anatomic area of interest can be seen.

Voltage ripple Description of voltage waveforms in terms of how much the voltage varies during x-ray production.

Wafer grid A stationary, nonmoving grid placed on top of the image receptor.

Wavelength The distance between two successive crests or troughs. Wavelength is represented by the Greek letter *lambda* (λ), and values are given in units called angstroms (Å). X-rays used in radiography range in wavelength from about 0.1 to 1.0 Å.

Wedge filter The most common type of compensating filter. The thicker part of the wedge filter is lined up with the thinner portion of the anatomical part.

Window level Location on the digital image number scale at which the levels of gray are assigned. It regulates the optical density of the displayed image and identifies the type of tissue to be imaged.

Window width Specific number of gray levels or digital image numbers assigned to an image. It determines the grayscale rendition of the imaged tissue and therefore the image contrast.

X-ray emission spectrum The x-ray beam is polyenergetic (consists of a wide range of energies) of a wide range of energies. X-ray energy is measured in kiloelectron-volts (keV) (1000 electron volts).

X-ray quality Penetrability of the x-ray beam.

X-ray quantity Output intensity of an x-ray imaging system.

X-ray tube rating charts Charts that guide the technician in the use of x-ray tubes.

Page numbers followed by "f" indicate figures, "ef" with numbers indicate online figures, "t" indicate tables, and "b" indicate boxes.